THE JOHNS HOPKINS WHITE PAPERS

2005

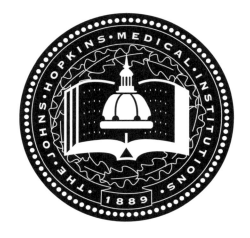

Heart Attack Prevention

Hypertension and Stroke

Lung Disorders

Memory

Nutrition and Weight Control

Prostate Disorders

Vision

VOLUME 2

Prepared by the Editors of
The Johns Hopkins White Papers
Published by Medletter Associates, Inc.

JOHNS HOPKINS MEDICINE
BALTIMORE, MARYLAND

THE JOHNS HOPKINS MEDICAL LETTER
HEALTH AFTER 50

THE JOHNS HOPKINS WHITE PAPERS *are published in association with* THE JOHNS HOPKINS MEDICAL LETTER: HEALTH AFTER 50. *This monthly eight-page newsletter provides practical, timely information for anyone concerned with taking control of his or her own health care. The newsletter is written in clear, nontechnical, easy-to-understand language and comes from the century-old tradition of Johns Hopkins excellence. For information on how to subscribe to this newsletter, please write to Health After 50, P.O. Box 420179, Palm Coast, FL 32142.*

Get subscription information—along with the latest perspectives from our experts—at our Web site:

www.hopkinsafter50.com

Please visit
www.hopkinswhitepapers.com

for articles, updates, special reports, information on our other products, including the Heart, Memory, and Prostate quarterly bulletins, and more.

Published in the United States in 2005 by Medletter Associates, Inc., 325 Redding Road, Redding CT 06896

Copyright 2005 Medletter Associates, Inc.

ISBN: 1933087153 Johns Hopkins White Papers, Volume Two

Printed in the United States

Note

This book is not intended as an alternative to personal medical advice. The reader should consult a physician in all matters relating to health and particularly in respect of any symptoms that may require diagnosis or medical attention. While the advice and information are believed to be accurate and true at the time of going to press, neither the authors nor the publisher can accept any legal responsibility or liability for any errors or omissions that may have occurred.

HEART ATTACK PREVENTION

Roger S. Blumenthal, M.D.

and

Simeon Margolis, M.D., Ph.D.

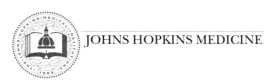

JOHNS HOPKINS MEDICINE

Dear Readers:

Heart attacks continue to be the nation's number one killer—and if you've never had a heart attack but are at elevated risk for one, this White Paper could help save your life. By focusing on the most important research findings of the past year, it gives you the tools—from the latest medication recommendations to advice on changing your lifestyle—to reduce your risk of a heart attack. You'll also learn why blood cholesterol testing doesn't tell the whole story about heart attack risk, and what other screening tests are on the horizon.

Here are some of this year's highlights:

- Why **calling 911** is still the best approach for people with chest pain. (page 5)
- Calculating your **risk of having a heart attack** in the next 10 years. (page 10)
- The surprising link between **osteoporosis** and heart disease risk. (page 17)
- **Apo B**: A better predictor of heart attacks than LDL cholesterol? (page 19)
- The **smoking ban** that produced a dramatic effect on heart attack rates. (page 25)
- How useful are **coronary calcium scans** for detecting heart disease? (page 26)
- **Trans fats**: Learn how to banish these fats from your diet. (page 31)
- **Cholesterol-busting foods** to add to your diet now. (page 43)

I hope that, as a result of this new information, you can work with your doctor to develop your own program for heart attack prevention.

Sincerely,

Roger S. Blumenthal, M.D.

Roger S. Blumenthal, M.D.
Director, Ciccarone Preventive Cardiology Center
Associate Professor of Medicine
Johns Hopkins University School Of Medicine

P.S. Don't forget to visit HopkinsWhitePapers.com for the latest news on heart disease and other information that will complement your Johns Hopkins White Paper.

THE AUTHORS

Roger S. Blumenthal, M.D., F.A.C.C., F.A.H.A., F.C.C.P., received his M.D. from Cornell University Medical College and did his internal medicine and cardiology fellowship training at Johns Hopkins, where he then joined the medical school faculty. He is currently an associate professor of medicine in the Division of Cardiology at Johns Hopkins Hospital and the director of the Johns Hopkins Ciccarone Preventive Cardiology Center.

Dr. Blumenthal's clinical and research interests include noninvasive detection of coronary atherosclerosis and the development of new strategies for the optimal management of cardiovascular disease risk factors. He has written numerous articles and editorials dealing with coronary heart disease and the prevention and management of atherosclerosis. He is also on the editorial board of several professional journals, including *Preventive Cardiology, Cardiology Review,* and *Today in Cardiology.*

Dr. Blumenthal is a fellow of the American College of Cardiology, the American College of Chest Physicians, and the American Heart Association's Epidemiology and Prevention Council. He is a member of the National Lipid Education Council (NLEC) and is on the steering committee of the Emerging Science of Lipid Management (ESLM) Council and the Coalition for the Advancement of Cardiovascular Health (COACH). He is also an official national spokesperson for the American Heart Association (AHA).

■ ■ ■

Simeon Margolis, M.D., Ph.D., received his M.D. and Ph.D. from the Johns Hopkins University School of Medicine and performed his internship and residency at Johns Hopkins Hospital. He is currently a professor of medicine and biological chemistry at the Johns Hopkins University School of Medicine and medical editor of *The Johns Hopkins Medical Letter: Health After 50.* He has served on various committees for the Department of Health, Education, and Welfare, including the National Diabetes Advisory Board and the Arteriosclerosis Specialized Centers of Research Review Committees. In addition, he has acted as a member of the Endocrinology and Metabolism Panel of the U.S. Food and Drug Administration.

A former weekly columnist for *The Baltimore Sun,* Dr. Margolis lectures regularly to medical students, physicians, and the general public on a wide variety of topics, such as the prevention of coronary heart disease, the control of cholesterol levels, the treatment of diabetes, and the use of alternative medicine.

CONTENTS

Who Gets Heart Attacks? . . . . p. 1

The Importance of Primary Prevention . . . . p. 2

What Is A Heart Attack? . . . . p. 4

Causes of Heart Attack . . . . p. 5

Risk Factors for Heart Attack . . . . p. 8

Risk Factors That Cannot Be Changed, Risk Factors That Can Be Changed

Screening Tests for Coronary Heart Disease . . . . p. 20

Lipid Profile, C-reactive Protein (CRP), PLAC Test, Electrocardiogram (ECG or EKG),
Exercise Stress Test, Further Evaluation (Nuclear Imaging, Echocardiography,
Electron-Beam Computed Tomography and Multidetector Computed Tomography)

Lifestyle Measures To Prevent Heart Attack . . . . p. 25

Cigarette Smoking, Dietary Fat and Cholesterol, Dietary Fiber, Soy Products,
Antioxidants, Sodium and Potassium, Physical Activity, Weight Control, Alcohol,
Stress Reduction

Medications To Prevent Heart Attack . . . . p. 36

Lipid-Lowering Medications, Medications To Lower Blood Pressure,
Aspirin Therapy for Primary Prevention, Hormone Replacement Therapy and CHD

Chart: Lipid-Lowering Drugs 2005 . . . . p. 38

Chart: The ABCs of Heart Attack Prevention . . . . p. 46

Glossary . . . . p. 49

Health Information Organizations and Support Groups . . . . p. 51

Leading Hospitals for Cardiology and Heart Surgery . . . . p. 52

Selected Medical Journal Article . . . . p. 53

HEART ATTACK PREVENTION

Diseases of the heart take many forms, but the most common—and life threatening—is a heart attack, technically called a myocardial infarction (meaning death of heart muscle). Each year, approximately 565,000 Americans have a heart attack for the first time and another 300,000 have a recurrent attack. About one fifth of these heart attacks are fatal.

Fortunately, the death rate from heart attacks has been declining steadily for many years, owing to a combination of better medical care and increased efforts to identify and control risk factors associated with heart attacks. But heart attacks remain the leading cause of death in Americans—and the death rate rises as people get older.

WHO GETS HEART ATTACKS?

More than half the people who have heart attacks—and four out of five who die of a heart attack—are over age 65. More men than women have heart attacks each year, and men suffer from heart attacks at a much earlier age than women. For example, a 40-year-old woman has only about one fourth the chance of dying of heart disease than a man of the same age. After menopause, however, a woman's risk of a heart attack begins to climb substantially, and by age 75 heart attacks are the chief killer of women. In fact, women are six times more likely to die of a heart attack than of breast cancer.

Most heart attacks result from coronary heart disease (CHD), a condition characterized by a progressive narrowing of the coronary arteries. Over the past four decades, scientists and physicians have identified many risk factors for CHD. A risk factor is an indication of probability—having a risk factor increases the likelihood of developing CHD but doesn't make a heart attack inevitable; conversely, the absence of any or all risk factors does not guarantee that someone won't have a heart attack. A recent study found that 90% of people who have a heart attack have at least one major risk factor—hypertension (high blood pressure), elevated cholesterol levels, diabetes, or smoking. But a substantial number with one or more of these risk factors never develop CHD.

Obviously some risk factors—such as getting older or being male—can't be changed. But a number of risk factors can be

NEW RESEARCH

More Than 10% of U.S. Adults At High Risk for a CHD Event

About 3% of adults in the United States are at high risk for having a CHD event in the next 10 years, and nearly 16% face an intermediate risk, according to a report from the National Health and Nutrition Examination Survey (NHANES III).

This estimate does not include people who already have cardiovascular disease or diabetes. When these individuals are taken into account, about 12% of U.S. adults are considered to have a high 10-year risk.

The researchers estimated risk among 13,769 people age 20 to 79 based on their age, cholesterol levels, smoking status, and blood pressure. They defined high-risk individuals as those with a more than 20% chance of having a CHD event in the next decade, intermediate as a 10% to 20% risk, and low as less than a 10% risk.

The percentage of people at high risk increased with age and was higher among men than among women, but did not vary substantially with race or ethnicity.

According to an accompanying editorial, the figures likely underestimate the percentage of people at high and intermediate risk because they don't take into account important risk factors such as abdominal obesity and family history of early CHD.

JOURNAL OF THE AMERICAN
COLLEGE OF CARDIOLOGY
Volume 43, pages 1791 and 1797
May 19, 2004

modified, and studies have shown that people can dramatically lower their likelihood of having a heart attack by avoiding, controlling, or eliminating certain risk factors. In addition, research is focusing not only on well-established risk factors, such as hypertension and high levels of blood cholesterol, but also on newly discovered risk factors, such as C-reactive protein and specific forms of cholesterol-carrying particles.

THE IMPORTANCE OF PRIMARY PREVENTION

This White Paper emphasizes the primary prevention of heart attacks—that is, prevention for people who have not been diagnosed with CHD or had a heart attack, but rather have one or more risk factors that can be modified to lower their risk. Tens of millions of Americans fall into this category.

The government's National Cholesterol Education Program (NCEP) has estimated that at least 36 million people—about two thirds of them age 45 or older—have blood cholesterol levels high enough to merit treatment with cholesterol-lowering drugs. Yet only 12 to 15 million of them are currently taking such medication, and many (probably most) are taking too small a dose. This pronouncement was echoed in the landmark Heart Protection Study, published in *The Lancet* in 2002, which concluded that cholesterol-lowering drugs called statins can produce substantial benefits in a much wider range of high-risk people than had been previously thought—including people over age 70, women, and anyone with vascular disease or diabetes, regardless of whether they have high cholesterol levels.

Similarly, of the 50 million Americans estimated to have hypertension, about 33 million do not have the condition under control. Millions of Americans are overweight, sedentary, or both. All of these individuals are at risk for a heart attack, yet they are not taking potentially lifesaving preventive measures known to reduce the risk of CHD.

The following pages discuss in detail all of the risk factors associated with CHD and heart attacks and the recommended strategies for prevention. (These strategies are also recommended as part of the treatment and management of known CHD and its complications, usually in combination with additional medical therapies.) Screening tests for CHD are also described, because such tests, along with a medical history and physical exam, can help reveal problems that increase the risk of a heart attack. Using this information to determine the degree of CHD risk, doctor and patient can work

Changes in the Coronary Arteries That Lead to a Heart Attack

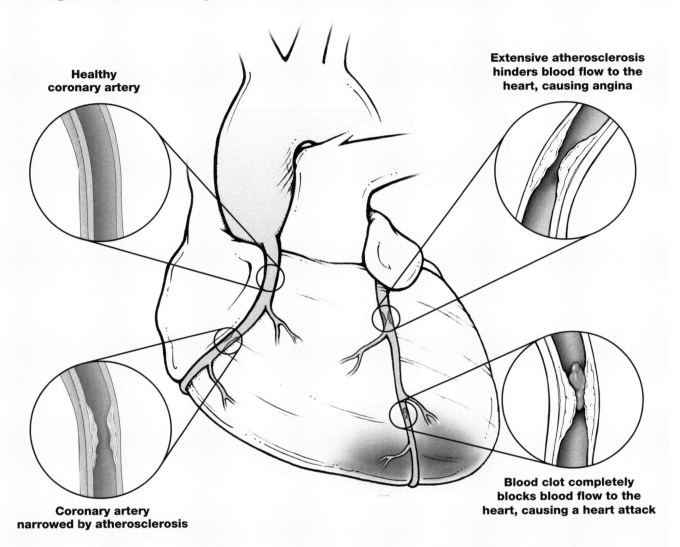

Healthy coronary artery

Extensive atherosclerosis hinders blood flow to the heart, causing angina

Coronary artery narrowed by atherosclerosis

Blood clot completely blocks blood flow to the heart, causing a heart attack

The heart is a hollow muscular organ with a straightforward purpose: to pump blood containing oxygen and nutrients to tissues throughout the body. To function properly, the heart requires a continuous supply of oxygenated blood provided by the coronary arteries, which are located on the surface of the heart and branch off into a system of smaller vessels and capillaries that extend into the heart muscle itself.

As we grow older, healthy coronary arteries may become narrowed by atherosclerosis, the underlying cause of coronary heart disease (CHD). Atherosclerosis is an ongoing process that begins in childhood and takes years to develop. The process involves the formation of deposits called plaques within the walls of arteries.

The plaques are composed of cholesterol-laden foam cells, smooth muscle cells, fibrous proteins, and calcium. As the plaques build up, the arterial walls thicken and narrow.

Symptoms of CHD, including angina, result when an advanced plaque narrows a coronary artery so much that it hinders blood flow to the heart. Blood clots can form on the exterior of a plaque—particularly if the plaque ruptures. Complete blockage of a coronary artery by a clot can cause a heart attack. A clot can also cause a heart attack when a portion of the clot breaks loose from its place of origin and lodges in a narrower section of the coronary artery or in a smaller vessel supplying blood to the heart.

2005 ♨ HopkinsWhitePapers.com

together to develop a customized program for heart attack prevention. This White Paper can serve as the first step in that direction.

WHAT IS A HEART ATTACK?

The heart is a muscular pump that is responsible for supplying blood rich with oxygen and nutrients to all the body's tissues and organs—including the heart muscle itself. With every heartbeat, oxygenated blood is pumped through the aorta—the body's largest artery—to smaller arteries throughout the body. These arteries, in turn, branch into even smaller vessels, called arterioles, and eventually into the microscopic capillaries that deliver oxygen and nutrients to every cell.

The heart receives its own oxygenated blood supply via the coronary arteries, which emerge from the base of the aorta. The two primary coronary arteries—the left main coronary artery and the right coronary artery—lie on the surface of the heart and branch off into a series of smaller blood vessels, the smallest of which extend deep into the heart muscle. In a healthy heart, the flow of blood through the coronary arteries can increase to meet the demand for more oxygen (as it does during exercise). But in people with CHD, the coronary arteries have narrowed and blood flow to the heart cannot increase enough to satisfy such extra needs.

A heart attack typically occurs when an artery becomes completely—or almost completely blocked—cutting off the blood supply to part of the myocardium, the muscular layer of the heart wall that is responsible for the heart's pumping action. The result of this blockage—which is often signaled by a crushing pain or pressure in the middle of the chest—is tissue death (infarction) in portions of the myocardium.

Many people who suffer a heart attack have a history of angina (episodes of chest pain associated with CHD) and may experience more frequent or severe anginal pain in the days preceding the attack. Others may have ill-defined warning symptoms such as shortness of breath, dizziness, or nausea. In many cases, however, a heart attack strikes suddenly and without warning. Once the heart muscle is deprived of oxygen, irreparable damage can develop within a few hours or even minutes. Therefore, it is essential to get immediate medical help when symptoms suggest a heart attack (for a list of possible symptoms, see the feature on page 7). Half of the deaths from heart attacks occur within the first hour, before the victim gets to a hospital, where the chances of survival are greatly improved.

see the feature on page 7

CAUSES OF HEART ATTACK

The blockage that ultimately triggers a heart attack is most often a blood clot that forms at a site where a coronary artery has developed atherosclerosis, the underlying cause of CHD. Atherosclerosis tends to occur as people grow older, but it is an ongoing process that begins in childhood and takes years to develop. The process involves the formation of deposits called plaques within the walls of arteries. The plaques are composed of cholesterol-laden foam cells, smooth muscle cells, fibrous proteins, and calcium. As the plaques build up, the arterial walls thicken and narrow.

Symptoms of CHD, including angina, result when an advanced plaque narrows a coronary artery so much that it hinders blood flow to the heart. Plaque deposits also roughen arterial walls and make it easier for a blood clot to form along their surface. Complete blockage of a coronary artery by a clot can cause a heart attack. A portion of a clot can also break loose from its place of origin and cause a heart attack by lodging in a narrower section of the artery or in a smaller artery supplying blood to the heart.

A number of factors play key roles in the stages leading up to a heart attack:

Cholesterol. Cholesterol is a white, waxy lipid (fat) that is present in the tissues of humans and other animals and, thus, in all foods from animal sources. Cholesterol is essential for many bodily functions: It is a building block for hormones and for vitamin D; it is a component of the outer membranes of cells; and it is a part of the insulation sheath around nerve fibers that enables nerves to communicate.

Despite its importance to life, cholesterol isn't an essential nutrient, meaning that the diet does not need to contain cholesterol to meet the body's requirements. The liver manufactures all the cholesterol the body needs. Particles called lipoproteins, formed in the liver, transport cholesterol and other fats through the bloodstream. The three lipoproteins are named according to their density: very–low-density lipoprotein (VLDL), low-density lipoprotein (LDL), and high-density lipoprotein (HDL). Most cholesterol is transported by LDL.

The liver secretes VLDL, which is converted to LDL in the bloodstream. The cholesterol on LDL is used to form membranes in cells throughout the body, and it also serves as the starting molecule for the formation of several hormones, such as estrogen, androgen, and cortisol. Deposits of LDL cholesterol in the arterial

NEW RESEARCH

EMS Bring Faster Care for Chest Pain Than Private Transportation

People with chest pain often take private transportation to the hospital in the belief that this approach will be faster than calling 911 and waiting for an Emergency Medical Services (EMS) ambulance. But quicker care comes through EMS, a new study shows.

The study involved 5,581 patients in 20 U.S. cities who had gone to a hospital emergency department with chest pain.

The results confirmed the common view that private transportation often gets a person to the emergency room faster than an ambulance. But the time difference is small and may not be clinically significant: Private transportation took 35 minutes compared with 39 minutes for EMS.

Because EMS personnel can initiate diagnosis and treatment on the scene, patients who called on EMS received initial care within six minutes, much less than those relying on private transportation, who had to wait until they reached the hospital. Also, patients who used EMS got from the emergency room door to thrombolytic therapy faster (32 minutes) than those who used private transportation (49 minutes).

The study underscores the wisdom of relying on EMS for chest pain. Trying to outrace the ambulance can in fact delay treatment.

AMERICAN HEART JOURNAL
Volume 147, page 35
January 2004

walls initiate the formation of plaques.

HDL also carries cholesterol in the blood; however, HDL has the beneficial capacity to pick up cholesterol from cells and atherosclerotic plaques and bring it back to the liver for reprocessing or excretion. Therefore, HDL cholesterol is often referred to as "good" cholesterol, because it clears cholesterol from the arteries, while LDL cholesterol has been called "bad" because it deposits cholesterol in the arteries.

Because elevated cholesterol levels contribute to the development of atherosclerosis, reducing cholesterol levels can help prevent CHD and heart attacks.

Triglycerides. Triglycerides are another type of lipid, which the body uses for energy. Like cholesterol, triglycerides are obtained from food and produced in the liver, and they are transported in the blood by lipoproteins, mostly VLDL.

High triglyceride levels are a risk factor for CHD, partly because elevations in triglycerides are commonly associated with low HDL cholesterol levels. However, research over the last decade indicates that elevated triglyceride levels are also an independent risk factor for CHD, although how they increase the risk isn't quite clear. One possible explanation is that elevations in blood triglycerides alter the size, density, and composition of LDL—changes that may promote atherosclerosis.

Inflammation and C-reactive protein. About half of all heart attacks occur in people with normal or even low cholesterol levels. In fact, despite dramatic advances in the understanding and control of known risk factors for CHD—which include smoking, obesity, a high-fat diet, lack of exercise, diabetes, and high blood pressure as well as high cholesterol and triglyceride levels—some people who develop CHD show no evidence of these predictors. This suggests that other factors are likely involved in causing heart attacks.

Evidence now indicates that chronic inflammation within artery walls is associated with the development of atherosclerosis and an increased risk of CHD and heart attack. C-reactive protein (CRP), a protein produced by the liver, is a blood marker for low levels of chronic inflammation. A high CRP level indicates excessive inflammation within the walls of arteries, where it appears to cause plaque instability. Unstable plaques are more likely to rupture and initiate the formation of blood clots that can trigger a heart attack.

Blood clot formation (coronary thrombosis). Formation of a blood clot (thrombus) is initiated after an atherosclerotic plaque ruptures, which triggers a cascade of events at the site of the injury

How To Recognize a Heart Attack

Chest pain and shortness of breath aren't the only possible symptoms.

Most people associate a heart attack with crushing chest pain. But not all people having a heart attack experience chest pain, and a 2003 study found that nearly half of women who had a heart attack had no chest discomfort at all. Instead, a large number of women had unusual fatigue (71%), sleep disturbances (48%), and/or shortness of breath (42%) for more than a month before their heart attack.

In fact, heart attacks can have a variety of symptoms, particularly in women. It is essential to familiarize yourself with all possible heart attack symptoms—both typical and atypical—and to be aware that women tend to have more vague symptoms that may delay a trip to the hospital and therefore delay prompt diagnosis and treatment.

When a heart attack occurs, it's an emergency situation that requires immediate medical attention. If you experience any of the symptoms below for more than 10 minutes, call an ambulance (dial 911 in most areas of the United States). Many Emergency Medical Services (EMS) vehicles carry emergency cardiac equipment, so treatment can begin on the way to the hospital.

If it's clear that an ambulance will not be available within 20 to 30 minutes, another person should drive the victim to the nearest emergency room. Under no circumstances should the victim drive to the hospital.

Unless there is a contraindication, the person with symptoms should immediately chew on an aspirin—which may start to dissolve the blood clot causing the arterial blockage until stronger drugs can be administered. Emergency personnel will need to know that an aspirin has been taken.

It's normal for people to deny the possibility of something as serious as a heart attack. If someone you are with experiences symptoms, don't take no for an answer. Insist on prompt action.

Typical Symptoms	Atypical Symptoms
Uncomfortable pressure, fullness, squeezing, or pain in the center of the chest	Mild or no chest pain
Pain spreading to the shoulders, jaw, neck, arms (especially the left arm), back, or upper abdomen	Breathlessness, dizziness, or light-headedness
Chest discomfort accompanied by light-headedness, sweating, nausea, shortness of breath, or fainting	Nausea or heartburn

within the artery. Once a plaque ruptures, clot-producing blood cells called platelets attach to the inner lining of the artery, known as the endothelium. This encourages the adherence of more platelets to the endothelial wall and leads to the formation of a clump of platelets called a platelet aggregate. The platelet aggregate activates procoagulating proteins, which promote the formation of a blood clot. If the clot blocks the flow of blood within a coronary artery, a heart attack will occur.

Coronary artery spasm. In some cases, a heart attack results from severe contraction or spasm of a coronary artery, which narrows the affected artery and decreases or halts blood flow to the heart muscle. A spasm can occur in blood vessels that appear normal as well as in vessels that show signs of atherosclerosis. The cause of spasms is often unknown.

RISK FACTORS FOR HEART ATTACK

The presence of certain risk factors increases the likelihood of developing CHD and thus a heart attack. The more risk factors a person has, the greater his or her chance of developing CHD. Of course, people who already have had a heart attack or have diabetes or evidence of atherosclerosis at other sites (such as an aortic aneurysm, history of a stroke or transient ischemic attack, or peripheral arterial disease) are at greatest risk for a heart attack. People with evidence of significant atherosclerosis in other arteries invariably have atherosclerosis in the coronary arteries as well.

Risk factors for CHD can be divided into two categories: those that cannot be changed and those that can.

Risk Factors That Cannot Be Changed

Even though nothing can be done to alter the following risk factors, their presence should alert people to consider taking preventive steps.

Age. CHD incidence increases with age, especially in men age 45 and older and women age 55 and older. Women who experience menopause before age 40 are also at increased risk.

Gender. Before age 50, CHD is far more common in men than in women. After menopause, however, when decreasing levels of estrogen lead to an increase in LDL cholesterol and a drop in HDL cholesterol, women's risk of CHD increases. After age 65, CHD occurs in one in four women. In fact, CHD is the major cause of death in women after menopause—every year, just as many women as men die of a CHD event (such as a heart attack). The risk of CHD in younger women who undergo premature menopause (before age 40) owing to surgical removal of the ovaries or spontaneous ovarian failure is similar to that of postmenopausal women.

Heredity. People are at increased risk for CHD if they have a male first-degree relative (a father or brother) who experienced a CHD event before age 55 or a female first-degree relative (a mother or sister) who had a CHD event before age 65. (For recent studies on heredity and CHD risk, see the sidebar at right and on page 9.)

Diabetes. People with diabetes are two to four times more likely to develop CHD than people without diabetes. The increase in the

NEW RESEARCH

Parents' Early CHD an Important Risk Factor for Some People

New research confirms that many adults with a parent who suffered a heart attack or stroke at a relatively young age are themselves at risk.

The research, based on 2,302 mostly middle-aged men and women from the Framingham Heart Study, shows that premature cardiovascular disease in at least one parent—before age 55 for a father or age 65 for a mother—doubles a son's risk of suffering a CHD, stroke, or peripheral arterial disease event over the next eight years, and boosts a daughter's risk by 70%.

However, overall risk factor status was a key ingredient: Parents' cardiovascular disease did not substantially raise the risk in adults who lacked other risk factors or in those with a large number of risk factors. Instead, people with a moderate number of risk factors were most affected by a parent's history; the greatest impact was seen in those with "borderline" cholesterol and blood pressure levels.

This middle group, the authors note, often present the toughest treatment decisions—such as whether lifestyle changes or drugs are needed to prevent cardiovascular disease. They conclude that the study findings underscore the importance of considering parental history in such patients.

JOURNAL OF THE AMERICAN MEDICAL ASSOCIATION
Volume 291, page 2204
May 12, 2004

incidence of CHD is especially great in women with diabetes. One reason for the increased risk is that elevated triglycerides, low HDL cholesterol, high blood pressure, and obesity, all of which are risk factors for CHD, are more common in people with diabetes. In addition, diabetes itself imparts other, as-yet-unidentified mechanisms for increasing the risk of CHD. For example, young women with diabetes lose the protection that other premenopausal women have against CHD; in fact, these women have the same frequency of CHD as do men of the same age without diabetes.

Moreover, people with pre-diabetes (blood glucose levels higher than normal but not quite in the diabetes range) are at increased risk for CHD. Pre-diabetes is diagnosed when blood glucose levels are between 100 and 125 mg/dL on a fasting blood glucose test or between 140 and 199 mg/dL on an oral glucose tolerance test.

Careful control of blood glucose levels with diet and drug therapy may reduce the increased risk of CHD associated with diabetes, but it does not completely eliminate the risk. Therefore, it is particularly important for people with diabetes or pre-diabetes to control other risk factors for CHD.

Cerebrovascular disease. CHD is the most likely cause of death in people with cerebrovascular disease (blockage of an artery that supplies blood to the brain). People with evidence of blockage in these arteries invariably have CHD as well.

Peripheral arterial disease. CHD is also the most likely cause of death in people with peripheral arterial disease (narrowing of the arteries that supply blood to the extremities, especially the legs). Just as with cerebrovascular disease, people with narrowed peripheral arteries also have CHD. Reduced blood pressure measured at the ankles or painful cramping in the legs upon exertion are signs of peripheral arterial disease.

Blood-clotting factors (fibrinogen, factor VII, platelets, PAI-1, and PLA-2). Efforts to find a consistent clotting abnormality in people prone to heart attacks have not been successful. However, a number of studies have found an association between increased heart attack risk and an elevation in blood levels of fibrinogen or factor VII (two clotting proteins), or an over-responsiveness of platelets to certain stimuli. Elevated levels of plasminogen activator inhibitor type 1 (PAI-1), a substance that inhibits the breakdown of blood clots, are also associated with increased cardiovascular risk, including heart attack risk.

A variation in platelet antigen-2 (PLA-2), one of the proteins involved in platelet binding of fibrinogen, was the first inherited

NEW RESEARCH

Premature CHD in Sibling Raises Risk of Atherosclerosis

A new study from Johns Hopkins finds that the risk of coronary artery calcification—a sign of atherosclerosis—is particularly high if the person has a sibling history of premature CHD.

The study involved 8,549 people, average age 52, with no symptoms of CHD. Of those, 27% had a family history of premature CHD—a heart attack, bypass surgery, or angioplasty before age 55. The researchers used electron-beam computed tomography to detect calcium deposits in the coronary arteries.

Calcium deposits were more frequent in people with a family history of premature CHD than in those without such a history. The prevalence of calcium deposits was 30% higher if the family history was in a parent, but was more than twice as high if the family history occurred in a sibling. Compared with people without a family history of premature CHD, the risk of advanced calcified plaques was four times greater in people with a sibling history and two times greater in people with a parental history.

It is unclear why sibling history may play a greater role in atherosclerosis than parental history. One possible explanation is that siblings are more likely than parents and children to share environmental CHD risk factors, such as smoking, obesity, and a high-fat diet, since they grow up in the same household.

CIRCULATION
Volume 110, page 2150
October 12, 2004

Your Risk of a Heart Attack in the Next 10 Years

Using a system called Framingham risk scoring, you can estimate your risk of experiencing a coronary heart disease (CHD) event—a heart attack, unstable angina, the need for angioplasty or bypass surgery, or CHD-related death—over the next 10 years.

To use the scoring system, first review how many of the following traditional CHD risk factors you have:

- cigarette smoking;
- high blood pressure (140/90 mm Hg or higher) or use of blood pressure-lowering medication;
- high-density lipoprotein (HDL) cholesterol level less than 40 mg/dL;
- family history of early heart disease (heart disease in father or brother before age 55; heart disease in mother or sister before age 65); and
- being age 45 or older if you're a man or age 55 or older if you're a woman.

Standard recommendations state that if you have two or more of these risk factors, you can use the scoring system printed below. The Johns Hopkins Ciccarone Preventive Cardiology Center takes a more aggressive approach, however, and recommends that you use the scoring system if you have even one of these risk factors. Those without any traditional CHD risk factors are considered at low risk and need not use the Framingham risk scoring system.

To estimate your 10-year risk of a CHD event, just add up the points you receive for each of the five factors in section I. Then use the sum to find your 10-year risk by gender in section II. The number in the right-hand column in section II indicates the likelihood that you will experience a CHD event in the next 10 years.

To get the most accurate estimate, your total cholesterol and HDL cholesterol levels should be the average of two or more readings. A person is considered a smoker if he or she has smoked at all in the previous month. Blood pressure also should be the average of at least two readings. In each blood pressure category, extra points are added for taking blood pressure-lowering medication because high blood pressure—even when reduced by medication—is still associated with some additional risk.

According to guidelines published by the National Cholesterol Education Program (NCEP), people are candidates for cholesterol-lowering drug therapy if they are:

- at high risk (have cardiovascular disease, diabetes, or a greater than 20% risk of a CHD event in the next 10 years) and have a low-density lipoprotein (LDL) cholesterol level of 100 mg/dL or more. (Drug therapy may also be considered when LDL cholesterol is less than 100 mg/dL.);
- at moderately high risk (two or more risk factors or a 10% to 20% risk of a CHD event in the next 10 years) and have a LDL cholesterol level of 130 mg/dL or higher. (Drug therapy may also be considered when LDL cholesterol is between 100 and 129 mg/dL.);
- at moderate risk (two or more risk factors and less than a 10% risk of a CHD event in the next 10 years) and have a LDL cholesterol level of 160 mg/dL or higher; or
- at low risk (one or no risk factors) and have a LDL cholesterol level of 190 mg/dL or higher. (Drug therapy may also be considered when LDL cholesterol is between 160 and 189 mg/dL.)

Section I: Determine the points you should receive for each of the following five risk factors associated with CHD.

1.

Age	Men	Women
20–34	-9	-7
35–39	-4	-3
40–44	0	0
45–49	3	3
50–54	6	6
55–59	8	8
60–64	10	10
65–69	11	12
70–74	12	14
75–79	13	16

2.

Total Cholesterol (mg/dL)	Age 20–39 Men	Women	Age 40–49 Men	Women	Age 50–59 Men	Women	Age 60–69 Men	Women	Age 70–79 Men	Women
<160	0	0	0	0	0	0	0	0	0	0
160–199	4	4	3	3	2	2	1	1	0	1
200–239	7	8	5	6	3	4	1	2	0	1
240–279	9	11	6	8	4	5	2	3	1	2
≥280	11	13	8	10	5	7	3	4	1	2

3.

Smoking Status	Age 20–39 Men	Women	Age 40–49 Men	Women	Age 50–59 Men	Women	Age 60–69 Men	Women	Age 70–79 Men	Women
Nonsmoker	0	0	0	0	0	0	0	0	0	0
Smoker	8	9	5	7	3	4	1	2	1	1

Section I. (continued)

4.

HDL Cholesterol (mg/dL)	Men	Women
≥60	-1	-1
50-59	0	0
40-49	1	1
<40	2	2

5.

Systolic Blood Pressure (mm Hg)*	If Untreated		If Treated	
	Men	Women	Men	Women
<120	0	0	0	0
120-129	0	1	1	3
130-139	1	2	2	4
140-159	1	3	2	5
≥160	2	4	3	6

Section II: Add up points from section I. Then use the appropriate table below to determine your 10-year risk of a CHD event.

Men

Point Total	10-Year Risk (%)
<0	<1
0	1
1	1
2	1
3	1
4	1
5	2
6	2
7	3
8	4
9	5
10	6
11	8
12	10
13	12
14	16
15	20
16	25
≥17	≥30

Women

Point Total	10-Year Risk (%)
<9	<1
9	1
10	1
11	1
12	1
13	2
14	2
15	3
16	4
17	5
18	6
19	8
20	11
21	14
22	17
23	22
24	27
≥25	≥30

* The upper number in a blood pressure reading.

Source: Adapted from *Journal of the American Medical Association*, May 16, 2001, p. 2497.

A more precise way to calculate CHD risk is with the "10-Year Heart Attack Risk Calculator," available on-line under "Health Assessment Tools" at www.nhlbi.nih.gov/health/index.htm.

platelet factor to be identified as a risk factor for heart disease. A study conducted by a team of Johns Hopkins researchers found that heart attacks at an early age occurred more often in people who had the PLA-2 variant than in those who did not. (The PLA-2 variant is also known as the Grinkov risk factor, after the famous Olympic skater Sergei Grinkov, who died in 1995 at age 28 of a massive heart attack and was found to have the PLA-2 variant.)

Chronic kidney disease. Adults with chronic kidney disease have a markedly increased risk of CHD and death from a heart attack; in fact, people with chronic kidney disease are more likely to die of CHD than of kidney disease itself.

One of the reasons for this association is that people with chronic kidney disease have a higher prevalence of risk factors for CHD, including hypertension, elevated lipid levels, diabetes, physical inactivity, and older age. Chronic kidney disease increases the synthesis and decreases clearance of lipoproteins, and so people with the disease have elevated levels of VLDL and LDL. They also have increased blood levels of an amino acid called homocysteine that promotes atherosclerosis. In addition, these individuals have greater procoagulant activity, which results in platelets that are more apt to clump and form clots. At the same time, chronic kidney disease also seems to play a role independent of these risk factors, though the exact mechanisms have yet to be clearly established.

Even people with early kidney disease—marked by the presence of small quantities of the protein albumin in the urine (microalbuminuria)—are at increased risk for developing CHD and its complications. Microalbuminuria raises CHD risk even in the absence of other CHD risk factors.

Because chronic kidney disease is associated with such a high risk of CHD and its complications, clinical practice guidelines issued by the National Kidney Foundation recommend that all such patients be screened for other risk factors for CHD, and be considered in the highest risk group for CHD, irrespective of other risk factors. The guidelines also stress the importance of aggressively controlling modifiable risk factors for CHD in people with chronic kidney disease.

Risk Factors That Can Be Changed

It is important to control or eliminate as many of the following risk factors for CHD as possible.

Cigarette smoking. Smoking cigarettes is a dangerous risk factor for CHD as well as for lung cancer and many other disorders, especially in younger people. (Cigar and pipe smoking also seem to increase the risk of CHD, but not to the same degree as cigarette smoking, probably because cigar and pipe smokers are less likely to inhale the smoke.) Substances in smoke not only reduce the amount of oxygen in the blood, but also promote the buildup of plaques in coronary arteries.

A smoker's risk of a heart attack is more than twice that of a nonsmoker's, and smokers are more likely to die of a heart attack than nonsmokers. Fortunately, much can be gained by stopping smoking. Even after many years of smoking, the risk of a heart attack or other CHD event returns to that of a nonsmoker within about five years of quitting smoking. (However, the elevated risk of developing lung cancer persists.)

Hypertension. Hypertension is defined as a systolic blood pressure of 140 mm Hg or higher or a diastolic blood pressure of 90 mm Hg or higher. Systolic blood pressure, the upper number in a blood pressure reading, is the pressure in the arteries while the heart is pumping blood to the body; diastolic blood pressure, the lower number, is the arterial pressure while the heart relaxes between beats.

High blood pressure causes the left ventricle of the heart to enlarge and require more blood. At the same time, hypertension increases the rate of atherosclerosis, thus limiting the heart's blood supply. Lowering blood pressure with medication in people who have hypertension decreases the likelihood of a heart attack, reduces the incidence of heart failure and stroke, and slows the progression of kidney disease.

People with a condition called prehypertension—defined as a systolic blood pressure of 120 to 139 mm Hg or a diastolic blood pressure of 80 to 89 mm Hg—are more likely to develop high blood pressure and have a greater risk of heart attack than those with lower blood pressures. These individuals should attempt to lower their blood pressure to less than 120/80 mm Hg through such lifestyle measures as diet, exercise, and smoking cessation.

Studies now demonstrate that elevated systolic blood pressure alone (called isolated systolic hypertension) is also risky—and, in fact, elevated systolic pressure, rather than elevated diastolic pressure, is the most important risk determinant. Treating isolated systolic hypertension (which is the most common form of high blood pressure in the elderly) can have a major impact on preventing a heart attack: In one study, lowering blood pressure with medication in people with isolated systolic hypertension decreased the frequency of fatal and nonfatal heart attacks by 27%.

NEW RESEARCH

Depression Increases Women's Risk of Cardiovascular Disease

Postmenopausal women with a history of depression are at increased risk for cardiovascular disease and death, according to a large study. The results support previous findings of a significant link between depressive symptoms—even when they fall short of full-blown clinical depression—and cardiovascular disease.

Researchers investigated the relationship between depression and cardiovascular disease over more than four years among nearly 94,000 women who participated in the Women's Health Initiative Observational Study. Cardiovascular disease includes both CHD and stroke.

According to the results, women with depression were significantly more likely to have risk factors for cardiovascular disease and were 60% more likely to have a history of cardiovascular disease than those who did not have depressive symptoms. In addition, women with depression were 50% more likely to die of cardiovascular disease and 32% more likely to die of any cause.

The authors conclude that depression is an important risk factor for cardiovascular disease. More research is needed, however, to determine if treatment with antidepressants would help lower the risks.

ARCHIVES OF INTERNAL MEDICINE
Volume 164, page 289
February 9, 2004

Abnormal levels of cholesterol, triglycerides, and lipoproteins. Knowledge of the effects of abnormalities in lipids and lipoprotein blood levels has grown rapidly. In response to this knowledge, the NCEP recently updated its guidelines for the detection, evaluation, and treatment of abnormal levels of blood lipids and lipoproteins. The guidelines and specific risks of the different lipid and lipoprotein abnormalities are as follows:

Increased total and LDL cholesterol levels boost the risk of CHD by increasing the amount of cholesterol deposited within the walls of the arteries. The NCEP guidelines recommend that total cholesterol levels be kept below 200 mg/dL to reduce the risk of CHD. The target for LDL cholesterol depends on how many of the following risk factors are present:

- cigarette smoking;
- high blood pressure (140/90 mm Hg or higher) or use of blood pressure-lowering medication;
- HDL cholesterol level below 40 mg/dL;
- family history of a premature CHD event (under 55 years old in men, under 65 in women) in a first-degree relative; and
- older age (45 years or older in men, 55 or older in women).

For people with none or one of these risk factors, LDL cholesterol levels should be less than 160 mg/dL. In individuals who do not have known cardiovascular disease or diabetes but have two or more of these risk factors, LDL cholesterol levels should be kept below 130 mg/dL. In all people with known cardiovascular disease or diabetes, LDL cholesterol levels should be lowered to less than 100 mg/dL, with an optional goal of less than 70 mg/dL. This new, optional goal was added to the guidelines in 2004 because several studies have shown that more aggressive lipid lowering in people who have recently had a heart attack or episode of unstable angina reduces their risk of future CHD events and death.

A low HDL cholesterol level (less than 40 mg/dL) is considered a risk factor for CHD. In fact, a total blood cholesterol level of 200 mg/dL or lower—the level considered desirable—may still be associated with an increased risk of CHD if HDL cholesterol levels are below 40 mg/dL, particularly in women. A high level of HDL cholesterol (60 mg/dL or higher), however, is considered protective against CHD and cancels out the effects of one other CHD risk factor (such as increased age) when determining one's total number of risk factors.

Triglyceride levels between 150 mg/dL and 199 mg/dL are considered borderline, and levels between 200 mg/dL and 500 mg/dL

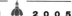

Evaluating Your Blood Lipid Levels

Cholesterol and triglycerides are fatty substances called lipids. Both are essential for proper body functioning, but elevated blood levels of these lipids increase the risk of coronary heart disease (CHD) and heart attacks.

According to current guidelines from the National Cholesterol Education Program (NCEP), everyone who is 20 years of age or older should have a blood test called a lipid profile (sometimes called a lipoprotein profile) at least once every five years. This test, which measures blood levels of total cholesterol, low-density lipoprotein (LDL) cholesterol, high-density lipoprotein (HDL) cholesterol, and triglycerides, should be performed at your doctor's office. You will probably be asked to fast for at least 12 hours before the test, since what you eat can affect levels of blood triglycerides.

If fasting isn't possible, then only the values for total cholesterol and HDL cholesterol are obtained. If you are considered at low risk for CHD

	Desirable	Borderline	Increased Risk
Total cholesterol	<200 mg/dL	200–239 mg/dL	≥240 mg/dL
LDL cholesterol	100–129 mg/dL*	130–159 mg/dL	≥160 mg/dL
HDL cholesterol	≥60 mg/dL	40–59 mg/dL	<40 mg/dL
Triglycerides	<150 mg/dL	150–199 mg/dL	≥200 mg/dL

*LDL <100 mg/dL is optimal. For people with diabetes, peripheral arterial disease, history of stroke or aortic aneurysm, or known CHD, and for some people with two or more CHD risk factors, a target of LDL <70 mg/dL should be considered.

and the test results confirm this assumption, no further testing may be required. Otherwise, your doctor may ask you to return for a fasting lipid profile.

Your doctor will use the test results—along with the presence of other risk factors for CHD (such as age, family history of premature heart disease, cigarette smoking, blood pressure, and diabetes)—to estimate your CHD risk. If your total cholesterol, LDL cholesterol, or triglyceride levels are elevated (or if your HDL

level is too low), your doctor will determine the most effective risk reduction measures for you to take. These could involve changes in your diet, increasing physical activity, quitting smoking, moderating alcohol intake, taking medication, or a combination of these measures.

The table above shows the risk classifications of blood lipid and lipoprotein levels for people without CHD. Because everyone's situation is different, be sure to talk to your doctor about interpreting your test results.

are high. (Levels greater than 500 mg/dL are very high.) About 35% of men and 24% of women are thought to have triglyceride levels above 150 mg/dL. However, it has been difficult to determine whether high triglyceride levels directly raise the risk of CHD, since elevated triglycerides are frequently accompanied by low HDL cholesterol levels. But the latest research indicates that high triglyceride levels are a risk factor even when HDL cholesterol levels are normal.

The CHD risk of elevated triglycerides is especially great when combined with low levels of HDL cholesterol and small, dense LDL particles (see page 16). This pattern is common in people who are obese or have diabetes or pre-diabetes. Elevated triglycerides also impart high risk when associated with a high ratio of LDL to HDL cholesterol or when due to one of two inherited conditions—familial combined hyperlipidemia or dysbetalipoproteinemia. Both of these disorders cause high blood cholesterol and/or high blood triglyceride levels.

Elevated levels of triglycerides may interfere with the normal widening of coronary arteries that occurs, for example, during physical exertion, or may increase the risk of blood clots. Lowering triglycerides with weight loss, control of diabetes (if present), and lipid-lowering medications (when necessary) may raise HDL cholesterol levels and reduce the risk of CHD.

Size and density of LDL particles can also affect CHD risk. LDL particles vary in size and density to produce two patterns: A and B. People with pattern A have mostly large LDL particles, while people with pattern B have a predominance of small, dense particles. Pattern B patients have a higher risk of CHD than pattern A patients. The majority of people with triglyceride levels above 150 mg/dL have pattern B. Men are more likely than women to have pattern B, which may be genetic or develop as a result of elevated triglycerides or diabetes.

The reason for the increased risk of CHD with pattern B is that smaller LDL particles enter the arterial wall more easily and are more prone to oxidation than larger LDL particles. However, the presence of mostly small LDL particles is often linked to higher triglyceride and lower HDL cholesterol levels, as well as to a greater number of LDL particles, and this combination may have a more important effect on CHD risk than particle size alone.

High levels of lipoprotein(a), also known as Lp(a), are another risk factor for CHD. The structure of Lp(a) is similar to LDL, except that it contains another protein called apo(a), which resembles the blood protein plasminogen. Plasminogen is converted into the enzyme plasmin, which plays a role in eliminating arterial blockage by breaking down fibrin, a major component of blood clots.

Two explanations have been proposed for why Lp(a) increases the risk of CHD. First, because of the similarity of apo(a) to plasminogen, Lp(a) might interfere with the conversion of plasminogen to plasmin, thus promoting the persistence of blood clots by reducing the beneficial action of plasmin. Second, like LDL, Lp(a) can deposit in arterial walls and contribute to plaque formation.

Unfortunately, Lp(a) levels are difficult to lower. Mild reductions have been achieved with high doses of niacin in some patients and with estrogen replacement in postmenopausal women (although hormone replacement therapy is no longer recommended for the prevention of CHD and heart attack, as explained on pages 47–48).

Obesity. Being overweight or obese increases the risk of CHD. Federal guidelines issued jointly by the National Heart, Lung, and Blood Institute and the National Institute of Diabetes and Digestive and Kidney Diseases use body mass index (BMI) to determine which people are considered overweight or obese. BMI is calculated by multiplying weight in pounds by 704 and dividing the result by the square of height in inches. Overweight is defined as a BMI of 25 to 29.9, and obesity as a BMI of 30 and over. Therefore, someone who is 5 feet 10 inches tall is overweight at 174 lbs. and obese at 209 lbs.; someone 5 feet 4 inches tall is overweight at 145 lbs. and obese at 174 lbs.

Data from a National Health and Nutrition Examination Survey showed a direct relationship between BMI and both blood pressure and LDL cholesterol levels. As BMI rises, blood pressure and LDL cholesterol levels increase. Moreover, increasing BMI is associated with a decrease in HDL cholesterol levels. Such changes in blood pressure and lipid levels are associated with an increased risk of CHD and heart attack.

Waist circumference is another method of judging CHD risk. The adverse effects of obesity depend not only on the amount of excess body fat but also on how it is distributed. Abdominal obesity is particularly dangerous because it causes insulin resistance (the reduced ability of the body to respond to insulin, a hormone that regulates blood glucose levels). Insulin resistance leads to elevated blood levels of insulin, which are associated with high triglyceride and low HDL cholesterol levels, hypertension, and increased CHD risk.

A waist circumference of greater than 40 inches in men or 35 inches in women indicates abdominal obesity and a heightened CHD risk. To measure waist circumference, wrap a tape measure around the waist at the level of the top of the hip bones; the tape should feel snug without compressing the skin. Measure after exhaling normally.

Metabolic syndrome. A person is considered to have metabolic syndrome if he or she has at least three of the following five findings:

- abdominal obesity (a waist circumference greater than 40 inches in men or greater than 35 inches in women);
- triglyceride level of 150 mg/dL or greater;
- HDL cholesterol level of less than 40 mg/dL in men or less than 50 mg/dL in women;
- blood pressure of 130/80 mm Hg or higher, or taking a blood pressure-lowering medication; and
- fasting blood glucose level of 100 mg/dL or greater.

Metabolic syndrome affects about 25% of American adults and nearly 50% of those over age 50. The condition increases the risk of CHD as well as diabetes and stroke.

Virtually all individuals with metabolic syndrome have insulin

Thin Hand Bones Linked To Women's CHD Risk

Although staying lean is one road to a healthy heart, thin hand bones due to osteoporosis may be a sign of trouble ahead for women, according to a study.

Researchers found that middle-aged and older women whose hand x-rays revealed low bone mass 30 years earlier were more likely than other women to develop CHD. The reason for the link is not fully clear, but the authors say the findings echo existing evidence that atherosclerosis and osteoporosis may have common underlying causes.

What's more, they note, the research suggests that preserving women's bone mass may reduce their risk of CHD. However, long-term studies using more modern techniques than x-rays to measure bone mass are needed to test this possibility.

The study involved 1,236 women and 823 men age 47 to 80 who had hand x-rays taken between 1967 and 1970. Women with the thinnest bones were 27% more likely than those with the thickest bones to develop CHD over the next three decades. No such relationship was seen in men, which may reflect gender differences in how bone mineralization, cardiovascular disease, or both take shape, the researchers note.

AMERICAN JOURNAL OF EPIDEMIOLOGY
Volume 159, page 589
March 15, 2004

resistance—a decreased ability of the body's tissues to respond to insulin, a hormone that enables cells to take up glucose from the blood for use as a source of energy. Treatment of metabolic syndrome involves lifestyle measures such as weight loss, exercise, a fiber-rich diet, and smoking cessation. Medications to improve lipid levels, lower blood pressure, and control blood glucose levels may also be needed.

Physical inactivity. Research shows that regular physical activity and physical fitness help prevent a first heart attack, and the American Heart Association cites physical inactivity as an important risk factor for CHD. As a result, the American Heart Association recommends at least 30 minutes of moderate-intensity physical activity such as brisk walking on most—preferably all—days of the week. This level of activity not only reduces CHD risk but also helps to control weight, lower blood pressure, and produce a more favorable lipid profile.

Homocysteine. Elevated levels of the amino acid homocysteine are associated with an increased risk of CHD. It is not known how homocysteine adversely affects the arteries, but high levels may promote atherosclerosis by damaging the endothelium and stimulating the growth of smooth muscle cells in the arteries.

Homocysteine levels can be lowered with folic acid supplements, but to date, there is no proof that this therapy will reduce the risk of CHD or heart attacks. People concerned about homocysteine can safely take 400 to 2,500 micrograms (mcg) of folic acid daily, either as a single tablet or in a multivitamin. Folic acid should be taken along with 1 mg of vitamin B_{12} since folic acid can mask the typical blood changes of pernicious anemia that are caused by a deficiency of vitamin B_{12}. Taking 50 mg a day of vitamin B_6 is often recommended as well to help lower homocysteine levels.

C-reactive protein (CRP). The liver produces CRP when inflammation occurs anywhere in the body—for example, within the walls of arteries. People with even small elevations of CRP appear to be at increased risk for CHD and its complications regardless of their age, gender, general health, or the presence of other CHD risk factors. In fact, elevated CRP levels (above 3 mg/L) are found in up to 50% of heart attack patients. The combination of elevated cholesterol and a high CRP level increases the risk of a heart attack severalfold.

CRP levels can be lowered with physical activity, weight loss, aspirin, and statin drugs. But it is not known whether reducing

A Better Marker for Heart Attack Risk?

Apo B may be a more accurate predictor of heart attacks than LDL cholesterol, but experts aren't ready to use it in place of testing for LDL.

A high level of low-density lipoprotein (LDL, or "bad") cholesterol is an important risk factor for a heart attack. Yet about half of the people who develop coronary heart disease (CHD) have normal or even low LDL levels. Some research suggests that a component of LDL—called apolipoprotein B, or apo B—may be more accurate at predicting CHD.

Room for Improvement
The problem with using LDL cholesterol levels to determine heart attack risk is that the test measures only the amount of cholesterol in the LDL particles, not the number or size of these particles. Apo B measurements, on the other hand, provide information on the number of LDL particles.

Apo B is a protein found on the surface of LDL particles. Because each LDL particle contains only one molecule of apo B, the total amount of apo B in the blood is equivalent to the number of LDL particles. The size of these particles can sometimes be inferred from the total amount of apo B and the LDL cholesterol level. For example, people

with a higher apo B value than LDL cholesterol value tend to have smaller, denser LDL particles. Studies have shown that small, dense LDL particles are more strongly associated with heart attack risk than large, "fluffy" LDL particles.

Preliminary But Compelling Evidence
Research published in 2003 in *The Lancet* reviewed five studies of LDL and apo B in nearly 200,000 people. The researchers concluded that high levels of apo B were more strongly linked with future heart attack risk than LDL cholesterol levels.

A second 2003 report published in *Circulation* studied more than 1,500 adults. The participants were categorized based on their LDL and apo B levels. Those with normal LDL and high apo B levels were more likely to have other heart attack risk factors—such as low high-density lipoprotein (HDL) cholesterol and high triglyceride levels, abdominal obesity, and high fasting insulin levels—than those with high LDL and normal apo B levels. The researchers pointed out that if apo B levels were used to

determine who needs cholesterol-lowering medication, 25% of the participants with normal LDL levels would meet the criteria.

The Bottom Line
Apo B is measured with a simple blood test. Proponents of apo B argue that the test is accurate, inexpensive, and does not require fasting, as LDL cholesterol testing usually does. However, the American Heart Association has determined that the evidence to date is not strong enough to recommend that apo B testing become standard procedure.

Even apo B researchers recognize that LDL is an important predictor of heart attack risk and suggest that apo B is most helpful for predicting risk in people with normal or low LDL levels but high triglyceride levels. Overall, if one's LDL cholesterol value is high, an apo B measurement is not necessary. Another important consideration is that LDL levels can be used to guide therapeutic interventions to decrease heart attack and stroke risk, but no data have shown that apo B levels can be used in the same way.

levels of CRP decreases the risk of CHD.

Stress. Over the past 30 years, studies by many investigators have shown a relationship between mental stress and various aspects of CHD. Physiological responses to stress include the release of adrenaline (epinephrine) and other hormones that speed heart rate, raise blood pressure, and may cause constriction or spasm of a coronary artery. If a coronary artery is already narrowed by atherosclerosis, spasm can lead to episodes of angina or, if an artery is almost completely blocked, a heart attack. Nonetheless, stress is not generally accepted as a causal risk factor for CHD, partly because it is so difficult to quantify the amount of stress in an individual's life.

SCREENING TESTS FOR CORONARY HEART DISEASE

For most healthy people free from CHD-related symptoms, a lipid profile, along with a comprehensive physical examination and medical history, remains the standard of good preventive cardiac care. But the presence of more than one or two risk factors can be cause for concern, and additional tests may be advisable, as discussed below.

Lipid Profile
All adults age 20 and older should have a lipid profile at least once every five years. This simple blood test, which measures levels of total cholesterol, LDL cholesterol, HDL cholesterol, and triglycerides, is performed after an overnight fast. The tests results—along with the presence of other CHD risk factors—are used to estimate CHD risk.

C-reactive Protein (CRP)
To address accumulating evidence showing an association between inflammation and CHD, the American Heart Association and Centers for Disease Control and Prevention recently issued a joint statement about CRP testing. According to their guidelines, testing for CRP is only beneficial for people who have an intermediate risk of CHD—that is, a 10% to 20% risk of a heart attack in the next 10 years. In these individuals, a CRP test can help guide decisions about evaluation and treatment. The test involves drawing blood from a vein in the arm.

PLAC Test
The platelet-activating factor acetylhydrolase (PLAC) test is a new laboratory blood test, approved by the U.S. Food and Drug Administration (FDA) in 2003. The test measures a "novel" independent risk factor for CHD—an enzyme in the blood called lipoprotein-associated phospholipase A2, or Lp-PLA2. Studies have shown that elevated levels of this enzyme are associated with an increased risk of CHD, even in individuals who do not have elevated levels of LDL cholesterol. (Some studies have shown that the test is not as strong a predictor of risk in women as in men, however.) The PLAC test is not a stand-alone test but should be used in conjunction with established tests in helping a physician determine a patient's risk profile and the appropriate preventive therapy.

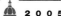

Electrocardiogram (ECG or EKG)

An electrocardiogram (ECG) is the most common test ordered to evaluate people with suspected CHD. According to recommendations released by the U.S. Preventive Services Task Force in 2004, however, ECG testing is not recommended for people at low risk for CHD who have no symptoms of the disease.

In an ECG, small metal sensors (electrodes) are applied to the skin to detect and record electrical signals from the heart. An ECG is especially valuable in detecting abnormal heart rhythms and a recent or ongoing heart attack. It also indicates areas of previously damaged heart muscle (as from a prior heart attack). Additional relevant information obtained with an ECG includes thickening (hypertrophy) of the wall of the left ventricle and defects in conduction of electrical impulses from the atria to the ventricles.

A normal resting ECG does not eliminate the possibility of myocardial ischemia (inadequate blood flow to the heart), which may occur and cause chest pain only during increased physical activity. Silent ischemia (impaired blood flow to the heart without causing symptoms) can be detected using a Holter monitor (also called an ambulatory ECG), which continuously records the heart's electrical activity over a 24-hour period. Holter monitoring is useful in evaluating people with unexplained light-headedness, fainting, or heart palpitations and in determining the effectiveness of drug therapy for abnormal heart rhythms.

Exercise Stress Test

An exercise stress test involves administering an ECG while an individual walks on a treadmill or pedals a stationary bicycle as the intensity of the workout is gradually increased. During exercise, the heart's workload increases and the coronary arteries widen to allow more blood to reach the heart. Because narrowed coronary arteries do not dilate as much as healthy ones, heart muscle fed by narrowed arteries receives less blood than heart muscle supplied by healthy arteries. Heart muscle that receives too little blood may produce changes that can be detected with an ECG.

In people who are at high risk for CHD or have chest pain that might be angina, an exercise stress test can detect the presence of blocked arteries better than a resting ECG. Recent studies from Johns Hopkins and other institutions have found that the length of time on the treadmill or bicycle (exercise capacity) and the amount that the heart rate declines in the first two minutes after exercise (heart rate recovery) predict future risk of cardiovascular

NEW RESEARCH

Findings Question Value of C-Reactive Protein Testing

In recent years, mounting evidence has indicated that individuals with high blood levels of C-reactive protein (CRP), a measure of inflammation in the body, are at increased risk for heart attacks. But a new study carried out in people from Iceland suggests that the test's value may have been overstated.

The researchers measured levels of C-reactive protein in 2,459 people who went on to suffer a nonfatal heart attack or die of CHD, as well as in nearly 4,000 people who did not develop CHD.

Patients with the highest CRP levels were 45% more likely to have a heart attack during 19 years of follow-up than those with the lowest CRP values—a smaller risk of CRP than that reported in previous research. In addition, CRP was just as good as traditional risk factors, such as high cholesterol levels and cigarette smoking, in predicting CHD risk.

The author of an accompanying editorial writes that further research is needed to clarify the relationship between CRP and heart attack risk.

THE NEW ENGLAND
JOURNAL OF MEDICINE
Volume 350, pages 1387 and 1450
April 1, 2004

What To Expect From an Exercise Stress Test

This diagnostic tool can help determine how well your heart is functioning.

In people who have chest pain or are at risk for coronary heart disease (CHD), an exercise stress test can be used to detect the presence of CHD. The test uses an electrocardiogram (ECG) to record the electrical impulses from the heart during exercise.

If the results of the exercise stress test are inconclusive, your doctor may recommend a nuclear medicine stress test, which involves the use of a radioactive substance to evaluate blood flow to the heart during exercise. Another option is a treadmill stress echocardiogram, in which an ultrasound test is done before and immediately following exercise.

Exercise Stress Test

During exercise, the heart's workload increases and the coronary arteries widen to allow more blood to reach the heart. Narrowed coronary arteries do not dilate as much as healthy ones. As a result, heart muscle fed by narrowed arteries receives less blood than heart muscle supplied by healthy arteries. Heart muscle that receives too little blood may produce symptoms, such as chest pain or shortness of breath, as well as changes that can be detected with an ECG.

During the test. Electrodes will be placed on your chest, shoulders, and hips to record the electrical activity of your heart. A baseline reading of your heart rate and blood pressure will be taken before you start exercising.

The stress test is usually performed on a treadmill, although a stationary bicycle may be used. You will be asked to begin walking on the treadmill or pedaling the bicycle. Gradually, the speed and incline of the treadmill or the resistance of the bicycle are increased until you reach your target heart rate (at least 85% of your maximal heart rate).

If you are unable to exercise, you may be given a drug called dobutamine instead. Dobutamine simulates the effects of exercise by increasing the heart's workload.

During the test, the doctor will monitor your ECG, blood pressure, heart rate, and breathing for any changes. You also may be asked to breathe into a tube for a few minutes while exercising to measure how much oxygen your body is using.

Depending on your fitness level, the exercise may last up to 15 minutes. The exercise may be terminated before you reach your target heart rate if you become fatigued or experience symptoms such as chest pain, shortness of breath, dizziness, or an irregular heartbeat. Changes in your ECG or blood pressure also may prompt the doctor to stop the test.

After the test. You will be asked to rest until your blood pressure and heart rate return to normal. After the electrodes are removed, you may return home or to work. The entire test takes approximately 30 minutes.

Risks. The test is no more dangerous than engaging in moderately vigorous exercise. The risks include falling off the treadmill or experiencing a heart attack and its complications. The risk of a fatal heart attack during a stress test is very small—about 1 in 10,000. Medical personnel are on hand should chest pain occur. Side effects from dobutamine are temporary and can include headache, dizziness, chest discomfort, nausea, and vomiting.

The results. Although an exercise stress test can be helpful in diagnosing CHD, the results do not always lead to an accurate diagnosis. The test may occasionally be normal when the person does have coronary artery obstruction (false negative), or the test may be abnormal even though the person's coronary arteries are not

events. For more information on exercise stress testing, see the feature above.

Further Evaluation

If a resting or exercise ECG test shows equivocal results or more information is needed to confirm a diagnosis, either nuclear imaging or echocardiography can often provide the necessary information. Coronary calcium scans using electron-beam computed tomography (EBCT) or multidetector computed tomography (MDCT) may also prove helpful in determining if someone has significant CHD when standard tests don't provide sufficient information about a

narrowed (false positive). False positives occur most often when the test is performed in young women and other individuals at low risk for CHD.

Nuclear Medicine Stress Test

In a nuclear medicine stress test (also called nuclear imaging), a radioactive substance—usually thallium but sometimes Cardiolite—is injected into the bloodstream and travels to the heart. Heart muscle supplied by blocked coronary arteries receives less of the radioactive substance than heart muscle fed by healthy arteries.

During the test. In most ways, the nuclear medicine stress test is identical to the standard exercise stress test. ECG electrodes are put in place, and you begin walking on a treadmill or pedaling a stationary bicycle. If you are unable to exercise, a drug called dobutamine may be used to simulate the effects of exercise on the heart.

Once your target heart rate is reached, a small amount of thallium or Cardiolite is injected into a vein in your arm. The radioactive substance is distributed within the heart muscle in proportion to the blood flow (that is, areas of the heart that receive more blood also receive more thallium or Cardiolite). You then lie on an examination table, and a special camera is used to take pictures of your heart. The pictures reveal the distribution of the

---

How To Prepare

The preparations for both the exercise and the nuclear medicine stress tests are the same:

- Do not eat or drink anything but water for a few hours before the test.
- Avoid smoking cigarettes and drinking caffeine or alcohol for at least four hours before the test.
- You will be exercising during the test, and the doctor needs to have access to your chest, arms, and legs to place the ECG electrodes. So wear loose-fitting clothing and comfortable shoes.
- Do not use any lotions, oils, or powders on your chest; they could interfere with the ECG electrodes.
- If you have diabetes, talk to your doctor in advance about how to adjust your food intake and the dosage of your insulin or oral diabetes medication prior to the test.
- Talk to your doctor about whether or not you should adjust any other medications before the stress test.

---

radioactive substance in your heart.

In some cases, a second set of pictures is taken on the same or next day when the heart is at rest to determine which areas of the heart are still not getting enough blood. Such areas may contain scar tissue from a previous heart attack.

After the test. As with a standard exercise stress test, you will need to rest until your heart rate and blood pressure have returned to normal. Then you can return home or to work. Over the next few hours, drink extra fluids to help your body get rid of the radioactive material.

Risks. The risks of the nuclear medicine stress test are the same as those for a standard exercise stress test. The dose of radiation is similar to that from a series of chest x-rays and is not considered dangerous.

The results. Your doctor can give you preliminary results immediately, but a full report may take a day. The nuclear medicine stress test can be more accurate than a standard exercise stress test. It detects coronary artery obstruction in 20% of patients with narrowed coronary arteries who have normal results on a standard stress test.

---

patient's risk status.

Both nuclear imaging and echocardiography are usually performed first while the patient is at rest and then during exercise. As with a regular exercise stress test, there is a very small risk of a heart attack or cardiac arrest during the exercise portion of the test. If exercise is too difficult or impossible for the patient, a drug such as dobutamine, which mimics the effects of exercise, can be used instead. This so-called pharmacological testing is recommended for those who do not or cannot exercise to their full capacity during exercise stress testing (for example, because of age, frailty, arthritis, or other health problems) and is often the most accurate approach for women.

Nuclear imaging. This test indicates how well blood flows to the heart muscle (myocardial perfusion). It involves injecting a mildly radioactive substance into a vein and then using a special type of camera that can locate the radioactive substance in the heart. The camera works in conjunction with computers to produce images.

Besides revealing likely sites of blockages in the arteries and the general presence of heart damage, nuclear imaging can show the extent and location of damage and help predict the likelihood of future heart attacks. Nuclear imaging is generally accurate and equally effective in men and women. Specifically, it detects CHD in about 20% of people whose resting and exercise ECG are normal despite narrowing of their coronary arteries. Although the amount of radioactivity is greater than that from an x-ray, it is not considered a cause for concern.

Echocardiography. In this test, ultrasound waves are used to create images of the heart at rest and during activity. Echocardiography reveals the size and shape of the heart's chambers, the activity of the chambers and valves, and how much blood is ejected with each contraction (ejection fraction). It can also detect blood clots within the heart and, sometimes, evidence of scarring. In addition, echocardiography is helpful for diagnosing heart valve disorders, left ventricular hypertrophy (enlargement of the heart muscle), cardiomyopathy (disease of the heart muscle), chronic bronchitis or emphysema, and congenital disorders. The test is considered highly accurate because of its low rate of false-positives.

Coronary calcium scans. New imaging technologies—electron-beam computed tomography (EBCT) and multidetector computed tomography (MDCT)—are now available to measure calcium in the coronary arteries. Calcium is usually a major component of arterial plaque and is not present in healthy arteries. Therefore, if coronary calcification is present, it indicates atherosclerosis.

EBCT and MDCT are easy to perform: The patient simply lies face up on a table for five to eight minutes during a circular x-ray scan. Calcium in the coronary arteries appears as whitish spots or streaks on the x-rays. A technician then uses a computer program to derive a calcium score; higher scores are associated with a greater degree of atherosclerosis.

To date, the link between coronary calcium and future heart attacks appears strongest in people who have at least one traditional CHD risk factor. Consequently, the U.S. Preventive Services Task Force recently recommended against the routine use of coronary calcium scans in people at low risk for CHD. For more information on the use of EBCT and MDCT for predicting heart attack risk, see the feature on pages 26–27.

LIFESTYLE MEASURES TO PREVENT HEART ATTACK

Lifestyle measures can have a greater impact on the prevention of CHD and heart attack than on practically any other disorder. For example, lifestyle changes can reduce elevated blood pressure and cholesterol levels. Even when such changes are not completely effective by themselves, and medication is required to lower cholesterol or blood pressure to acceptable levels, lifestyle measures may allow a patient to take smaller amounts of medication (which in turn can reduce the risk of side effects). In addition, the combination of lifestyle changes and medication is often more effective than either alone. The most effective preventive lifestyle measures are quitting smoking, eating a diet low in saturated fats, and engaging in regular physical activity. (The same lifestyle measures for preventing CHD are also effective in preventing future coronary events in people with established CHD.)

Cigarette Smoking

Smoking is a difficult habit to break because of the powerful physical and psychological addiction to nicotine. Giving up cigarettes requires a tremendous amount of determination, and only about 5% to 10% of people successfully quit on their own, without any kind of aid or reinforcement. Fortunately, there are several options that can dramatically increase a smoker's chances of quitting. These options include nicotine replacement therapy, drug therapy, and counseling. Combining all three increases the likelihood of quitting to about 35%.

Nicotine replacement therapy minimizes the symptoms of nicotine withdrawal and helps control cravings. Many forms of nicotine replacement therapy are available—gums, skin patches, nasal sprays, inhalers, and lozenges. Some are sold over the counter; others must be prescribed by a doctor. A prescription drug called bupropion (Zyban) also helps reduce cravings and withdrawal symptoms. It works by disrupting the pleasurable feelings that cigarette smoking typically produces in the brain. Counseling—either in a group or one-on-one with a therapist—can be helpful as well. People learn coping skills, relapse prevention, and stress management as well as receive social support and encouragement.

NEW FINDING

Smoking Ban Produces Rapid Heart Benefits

When the city of Helena, Montana, passed a law banning smoking in the workplace and all public places, it took only six months before opponents won a court order to suspend the law. But while the ban was in effect, hospital admissions for heart attacks dropped by a whopping 40%, according to researchers.

The investigators compared the number of hospital admissions for heart attacks during the smoking ban with the number of admissions during the same six-month periods in years before and after the ban.

They found that before and after the ban, an average of 40 patients were admitted to hospital for heart attacks during those six months, while only 24 were admitted while the ban was in effect. A similar decrease in hospital admissions was not observed in communities outside of Helena that did not enact a ban.

The author of an accompanying editorial notes that the findings underscore the dangers of secondhand smoke, and that people who have or are at high risk for CHD should avoid all indoor environments where smoking is permitted.

BMJ
Volume 328, pages 977 and 980
April 24, 2004

How Useful Are Coronary Calcium Scans?

This simple test can identify atherosclerosis but may not accurately predict heart attack risk.

Most healthy people who are concerned about their risk of a heart attack are familiar with their cholesterol and blood pressure measurements. Now many are asking: Should they also know their calcium scores?

Calcium in the coronary arteries indicates atherosclerosis—the buildup of plaques that can lead to heart attacks. New imaging technologies called electron-beam computed tomography (EBCT) and multidetector computed tomography (MDCT) are now available to measure coronary calcium. This development has led to hospitals and testing clinics advertising EBCT and MDCT scans that may provide a quick, easy, accurate way to assess the presence and severity of coronary atherosclerosis and the risk of a heart attack.

Yet earlier this year, the government's Preventive Services Task Force recommended that EBCT not be used to screen healthy people unless they have known coronary heart disease (CHD) risk factors or symptoms—and that even then, the usefulness of the test is unclear.

What Are EBCT and MDCT?

EBCT and MDCT, also known as ultra-fast CT, are painless, five- to eight-minute tests. The patient lies face up on an examination table under a CT scanner. An electron beam generates x-rays (four times as strong as a simple chest x-ray) that pass through the patient's body. Calcium in artery walls appears as whitish spots or streaks on the x-rays.

Technicians identify the calcium deposits in the images, then use a computer program to derive a coronary artery calcium score that reflects the total calcium "load" in the coronary arteries. Scores of 0 to 10 reflect arteries largely free from coronary plaque (minimal coronary calcification). Scores of 11 to 400 indicate mild to moderate plaque buildup; scores above 400 indicate extensive plaque.

What the Score Reveals ...

Many studies have shown that people with higher calcium scores are at greater risk for heart attacks and strokes and that those with very low scores are at relatively low risk over the next five years. What has been controversial is whether calcium screening with EBCT or MDCT adds useful information beyond that provided by standard risk factors (cholesterol, blood pressure, triglycerides, obesity, smoking, diabetes, age, and family medical history).

A September 2003 study in *Radiology* showed that calcium screening adds considerable predictive value. Researchers tested more than 10,000 people between the ages of 30 and 85 who were at above-average risk for CHD but had no symptoms. Increased calcium scores were associated with substantially worse survival five years later.

A January 2004 study in the *Journal of the American Medical Association (JAMA)* revealed similar findings: In testing 1,461 asymptomatic adults with at least one CHD risk factor, a calcium score above 300 was associated with a large increase in the risk of heart attacks (or other CHD-related deaths) compared with risk predicted by the Framingham Risk Score, which uses age, blood pressure, cholesterol levels, and smoking.

... And What It Doesn't

While there is widespread agreement among cardiologists that EBCT and MDCT can correctly identify the presence and extent of atherosclerosis, there is less agreement over what to do with the information and how accurately the results can predict the risk of a heart attack. Increasingly,

Dietary Fat and Cholesterol

The average American diet contains about 35% to 40% of calories from fat. Not all of this fat is bad—in fact, some types of fat, such as mono- and polyunsaturated fat, have a beneficial effect on blood lipids and may lower the risk of developing CHD or dying of it. But the prevalent type of fat in the American diet is saturated fat, the major dietary factor that raises blood cholesterol levels. In fact, saturated fat has a bigger impact on blood cholesterol levels than dietary cholesterol itself. Saturated fat includes most animal and dairy fats and some oils, such as palm and coconut oils.

experts have recognized that a heart attack most commonly occurs when a soft, unstable plaque in the artery wall breaks open and causes the formation of an artery-plugging blood clot. But EBCT and MDCT, as well as other types of imaging studies, can't reliably distinguish between stable and unstable plaques. In the *JAMA* study, for example, low calcium scores did not totally preclude heart attack risk. However, it is clear that the more calcified plaque that is present, the more numerous are the softer, noncalcified plaques.

In addition, because EBCT and MDCT are relatively new, researchers are still refining the implications of different calcium scores. Generally, an individual's score is compared with the average score for someone the same age and gender. But more clinical data are needed to establish standardized risk thresholds and treatment guidelines for specific scores.

What To Do Now

Because no study has examined the outcome of using calcium scores as a guide in determining treatment for asymptomatic individuals, the U.S. Preventive Services Task Force has recommended against routine EBCT and MDCT screening for the general population—arguing that screening may occasionally cause unnecessary further invasive testing and treatment in patients with positive calcium scores.

The American College of Cardiology and the American Heart Association also argue that more data are needed to clearly determine who will benefit from EBCT or MDCT screening and whether the tests are significantly better as screening tools than standard, less expensive, readily available tests with decades of research behind them.

Many experts feel that ECBT and MDCT should not be stand-alone tests—they should be done with your doctor's supervision and interpretation. And even in a comprehensive clinical setting, scanning doesn't necessarily provide useful additional information for everyone. For example, most (though not all) patients at low risk according to Framingham scores will also have low calcium scores (unless they have a family history of premature CHD), while high-risk patients should be treated aggressively no matter what a calcium scan would show. In the *JAMA* study cited above, knowing the calcium scores did not substantially change the predicted risk for patients considered at low risk or high risk according to their Framingham scores.

But for the many adults at intermediate risk—with a Framingham score showing a 10% to 20% risk of a CHD event in the next 10 years—screening can be valuable. Such patients potentially could be candidates for aggressive preventive therapy with aspirin and blood pressure- and cholesterol-lowering medication (if they have a very high calcium score for their age).

Knowledge of calcium scores might also motivate intermediate-risk patients to comply with healthier lifestyle habits and medical therapy, though research into the roles EBCT and MDCT might play in patient compliance has only just begun. Others who could potentially benefit from EBCT and MDCT are people at low risk according to Framingham scores but with other well-established risk factors not utilized by Framingham, such as metabolic syndrome, obesity, or a family history of premature CHD.

Developing a consensus on guidelines concerning the role of EBCT and MDCT in primary heart attack prevention will require a number of carefully conducted trials. The clearest picture yet should emerge from the Multi-Ethnic Study of Atherosclerosis (MESA), an ongoing National Institutes of Health study of various imaging technologies that will include the most rigorously conducted assessment to date of EBCT in 6,700 asymptomatic people with different ethnic and racial backgrounds. Johns Hopkins is one of seven participating research centers, and results from this study are expected in 2008.

The simplest dietary measure to lower the risk of CHD and heart attack is limiting saturated fat intake. The 2001 NCEP guidelines recommend reducing total fat to between 25% and 35% of total calories, with the majority of fat calories coming from mono- or polyunsaturated fat. Also advised is limiting the intake of saturated fat to less than 10% of total calories in order to reduce blood cholesterol levels—specifically LDL cholesterol.

The guidelines recommend these dietary measures even when cholesterol levels are normal, since a modified fat intake can help maintain optimal cholesterol levels. A reduction in saturated fat may also help to maintain an ideal weight, because a gram of fat contains more than twice as many calories (9 calories) as a gram of carbohydrates or protein (4 calories). (Fat and protein are more filling than carbohydrates, however.)

The NCEP guidelines also recommend limiting dietary cholesterol to less than 300 mg per day. But if LDL cholesterol levels remain high, saturated fat should be further restricted to less than 7% of calories and cholesterol to less than 200 mg per day.

While modifying fat intake is desirable, it is important not to get too carried away with restricting fat in the diet. According to the American Heart Association, short-term studies reveal that lowering fat intake to 15% or less of total calories does not reduce LDL cholesterol levels much further than a standard low-fat diet. In addition, very–low-fat diets decrease HDL cholesterol (see the sidebar at right) and increase triglyceride levels, whereas the moderate-fat diet recommended by the NCEP guidelines can help reduce triglycerides and raise HDL cholesterol, particularly in people with metabolic syndrome.

Mono- and polyunsaturated fats. When fat is consumed, monounsaturated fats should be chosen whenever possible so that they contribute up to 20% of total calories. Olive and canola oils, almonds, and avocados contain large amounts of monounsaturated fat. When they are substituted for saturated fat in the diet, monounsaturated fats can lower LDL cholesterol levels, reduce the likelihood of LDL oxidation, and stabilize or even raise HDL cholesterol levels. Polyunsaturated fats—found in safflower, sunflower, and corn oils—also lower LDL cholesterol levels.

Omega-3 fatty acids, another type of polyunsaturated fat, seem to have cardioprotective benefits beyond LDL cholesterol lowering. There are three types of omega-3 fatty acids: eicosapentaenoic acid (EPA), docosahexaenoic acid (DHA), and alpha-linolenic acid (ALA). EPA and DHA, found only in fish (particularly fatty fish), can reduce the tendency for blood to clot, decrease the risk of arrhythmias (abnormal heart rhythms), and lower triglyceride levels; the benefits of ALA are unclear. The American Heart Association recommends consuming at least two servings of fish per week to benefit from the cardioprotective effects of omega-3 fatty acids.

Trans fats. Just as with saturated fats, people should minimize their intake of trans fats—fats that are found in foods made with hydrogenated or partially hydrogenated oils. Some examples are margarine and commercial baked goods. Trans fats (also known as

NEW RESEARCH

Very–Low-Fat Diets Lower HDL Cholesterol Levels

Very–low-fat diets tend to be poor in certain nutrients and can reduce levels of HDL ("good") cholesterol, a new study shows.

Cutting fat intake is often recommended as a way to reduce the risk of CHD, lose weight, and avoid obesity-related health problems, but fat-containing foods are rich in energy, essential fatty acids, and certain vitamins.

The researchers randomly assigned 11 healthy, sedentary individuals to a diet with either 19% or 50% of calories from fat for three weeks. After a one-week "washout" on a 30%-fat diet, they were switched to the other diet.

No detrimental effects of the 50%-fat diet were found on blood pressure, lipoprotein levels, and other cardiovascular risk factors. On the other hand, levels of HDL cholesterol were significantly lower among those on the 19%-fat diet.

Very–low-fat diets do little to improve CHD risk factors and are difficult to follow over the long term. The study authors recommend that people eat a mix of beneficial fats and lose weight by increasing physical activity.

JOURNAL OF THE AMERICAN COLLEGE OF NUTRITION
Volume 23, page 131
April 2004

trans fatty acids) are formed during the addition of hydrogen atoms to unsaturated oils to make them more saturated and therefore solid at room temperature and more shelf-stable. Trans fats may be even more harmful to health than saturated fats because these fats raise the ratio of LDL to HDL cholesterol levels more than saturated fats. The Institute of Medicine, a branch of the National Academy of Sciences, recommends that trans fat consumption be as low as possible. To learn more about trans fats and how to avoid them, see the feature on page 31.

Dietary Fiber

Experts recommend that adults consume at least 25 to 30 g of dietary fiber each day. Fiber is an indigestible component of many foods, primarily grains, legumes, fruits, and vegetables. Fiber comes in two forms: soluble, the type in oatmeal that gets sticky when wet; and insoluble, the sponge-like version in bran and in fruit and vegetable skins that absorbs water and helps to prevent constipation. Both types of fiber are important, but soluble fiber is especially effective in lowering blood cholesterol levels. Foods containing soluble fiber—such as oats, oat bran, barley, legumes, dried plums (prunes), apples, carrots, and grapefruits—should be included in the diet each day.

It is best to get your fiber from foods, because they contain a variety of nutrients, rather than from supplements. Some people find it difficult to get enough fiber from foods, however. As an alternative, regular use of products that contain soluble fiber from psyllium seeds—such as Metamucil—can lower cholesterol levels by 5% to 10%.

Just how soluble fiber reduces cholesterol levels is unclear. Researchers theorize that it works in much the same way as a class of lipid-lowering drugs called bile acid sequestrants. Normally, bile acids are reabsorbed from the intestine and returned to the liver for reprocessing. Bile acid sequestrants bind bile acids in the intestine and remove them in the stool. As a result, the liver converts more cholesterol to bile acids and removes more LDL from the blood by developing more LDL receptors on its surface.

Soy Products

Soy products may also lower blood cholesterol levels. An analysis of 38 studies in which soy protein replaced animal protein in people's diets found that eating an average of 47 g (about 10 oz.) of soy protein per day lowered levels of total cholesterol by about 9%, LDL

NEW RESEARCH

Dietary Fiber Protects Against CHD

After combining the results of 10 prospective studies, researchers conclude that dietary fiber intake from cereals and fruits decreases the risk of CHD in both men and women.

A total of 336,244 people participated in the studies, which measured the amount of fiber in the participants' diets and analyzed links between fiber intake and CHD events and deaths.

For each 10 g of fiber consumed per day, the risk of CHD events dropped 14%, and the risk of dying from CHD dropped 27%. Fiber from cereal reduced the risk of CHD events by 10% and the risk of CHD death by 30% for each 10 g per day, while the same amount of fruit fiber reduced the risk of CHD by 16% and the risk of death of CHD by 30%. Vegetable fiber did not affect CHD risk.

The authors note that recommendations to consume a diet rich in high-fiber food, particularly whole grains and fruits, are based on "a wealth of consistent scientific evidence" showing that these foods provide significant health benefits.

ARCHIVES OF INTERNAL MEDICINE
Volume 164, page 370
February 23, 2004

cholesterol by 13%, and triglycerides by 11%. The substitution of unsaturated for saturated fat (38% of the calories in soybeans come from fat, mostly unsaturated) may account for some of this benefit, but soy also contains phytochemicals (plant chemicals)—isoflavones, in particular—that may contribute to the cholesterol-lowering effect. Isoflavones are estrogen-like compounds present in soy foods such as tofu and soy milk; estrogen lowers LDL cholesterol and boosts HDL cholesterol levels.

Antioxidants

Numerous studies have shown that people who eat a diet rich in fruits and vegetables are at reduced risk for developing CHD. Some researchers attribute this benefit to antioxidants. These substances, which are plentiful in fruits and vegetables, help the body neutralize free radicals—by-products of normal metabolism that oxidize LDL and make it more likely to deposit in the arteries.

In studies that measured dietary intakes or blood levels of antioxidants, high levels of vitamin E, beta-carotene, and other carotenoids were associated with a reduced risk of CHD. It was hoped that supplementation with these nutrients would slow the development of atherosclerosis by preventing LDL oxidation. However, clinical trials have not shown this to be the case. In fact, a recent analysis of previous research found that, compared with a placebo, vitamin E supplementation did not reduce the risk of death from CHD, and beta-carotene supplementation increased the risk of lung cancer. (No studies have been conducted on the cardiovascular effects of supplemental vitamin C, another antioxidant.)

The U.S. Preventive Services Task Force concluded in 2003 that there is insufficient evidence for or against the use of vitamins A, C, or E for the prevention of cardiovascular disease. In addition, the Task Force recommended that people not take beta-carotene supplements to reduce their cardiovascular risk, since the supplements are unlikely to provide important benefits and may increase the risk of lung cancer. Therefore, people should eat a diet rich in fruits and vegetables rather than using antioxidant supplements to reduce their risk of CHD.

Sodium and Potassium

Limiting dietary sodium and increasing the intake of potassium-rich foods can help control high blood pressure and, in turn, lower the risk of CHD.

The typical daily intake of sodium in the United States is 3,000 to

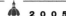

Bringing Trans Fats Into the Open

These heart-harmful fats won't stay hidden for long, thanks to new food labeling required by the FDA.

Trans fatty acids—also known as trans fats—are formed when food manufacturers add hydrogen atoms to unsaturated vegetable oils (a process called hydrogenation) to make them more saturated and therefore more solid and shelf-stable. These synthetic trans fats are found in nearly all commercially prepared foods. In addition to margarines, trans fats are often found in frozen dinners, dry mixes, snack foods (including chips, crackers, and baked goods), and fried fast food. Trans fats also occur naturally, primarily in dairy products, beef, and pork. About a quarter of the trans fats in the diet are from natural sources; the remainder are synthetic.

Why Are Trans Fats So Bad?

Trans fats not only raise low-density lipoprotein (LDL) cholesterol, but they also lower high-density lipoprotein (HDL) cholesterol levels. A 2004 study in the *Journal of Nutrition* found that recent heart attack victims had significantly more trans fats in their fat tissue than did healthy people. In addition, people who reported the highest intake of trans fats were more than twice as likely to have a heart attack as people who reported the lowest.

The research on trans fats and heart disease is so convincing that one expert from the U.S. Food and Drug Administration (FDA) estimated that removing all trans fats from margarine and just 3% of trans fats from baked items would prevent more than 17,000 heart attacks and more than 5,000 deaths related to coronary heart disease (CHD) a year. In fact, Denmark recently banned hydrogenated fats from all foods sold in that country.

Reading Labels

Prepared foods currently list the types of oils they contain and whether any oils have been hydrogenated, but there is no requirement to list the amount of trans fats. The FDA recently altered this policy, however.

In the biggest change to food labeling since 1993, all food manufacturers will be required to list the amount of trans fats per serving by

Nutrition Facts

Serving Size 1 cup (228g)
Servings Per Container 2

Amount Per Serving			
Calories 260		Calories from Fat 120	
		% Daily Value*	
Total Fat 13g			20%
Saturated Fat 5g			25%
Trans Fat 2g			
Cholesterol 30mg			10%
Sodium 660mg			28%
Total Carbohydrates 31g			10%
Dietary Fiber 0g			0%
Sugars 5g			
Protein 5g			

Vitamin A 4%	•	Vitamin C 2%	
Calcium 15%	•	Iron 4%	

* Percent Daily Values are based on a 2,000 calorie diet. Your Daily Values may be higher or lower depending on your calorie needs.

	Calories	2,000	2,500
Total Fat	Less than	65g	80g
Sat Fat	Less than	20g	25g
Cholesterol	Less than	300mg	300mg
Sodium	Less Than	2,400mg	2,400mg
Total Carbohydrates		300g	375g
Dietary Fiber		25g	30g
Calories per gram:			
Fat 9	Carbohydrate 4		Protein 4

January 1, 2006. Some manufacturers are already including this listing, while others have removed trans fats from their manufacturing processes.

The amount of trans fats in a food product will be listed below the amount of saturated fats (see the sample nutrition label above). A "% Daily Value" is not indicated for trans fats because they are not recommended at all. A recent report from the Institute of Medicine concluded that there is no safe level of trans fat intake, so it's important to limit your consumption of trans fats as much as possible.

The new labeling will make it easier to choose products that have no trans fats—or have very few. But foods with less than 0.5 g of trans fats can round down to 0. Therefore, if a single serving of cookies contains 0.4 g of trans fats, and you eat a whole box (the equivalent of 10 servings), you will have consumed not 0 g of trans fats, but a total of 4 g.

Even foods that contain no trans fats still have calories, which all add up and can lead to weight gain, so it's important to eat in moderation. Remember that all fat is equally high in calories, and saturated fat is also detrimental to your health. Keep daily saturated and trans fat intake to 20 g or less. People with CHD, diabetes, or elevated LDL cholesterol levels should aim even lower, getting less than 15.5 g of saturated and trans fats a day.

Don't Wait for the Labeling Changes

Although the amount of trans fats is not yet included on most nutrition labels, you can limit them in your diet by:

- Avoiding stick margarine. Instead, use tub or liquid products like olive oil, which contain fewer hydrogenated oils.
- Checking ingredient lists for fully or partially hydrogenated vegetable oils and for shortening—all of these foods contain trans fats. The higher they are on the ingredient list, the more plentiful they are in the food.

5,000 mg, although the body needs only about 200 mg of sodium a day. Cutting back to less than 2,000 mg of sodium daily by following a "no-added-salt diet" lowers systolic and diastolic blood pressure by 3 to 5 mm Hg, on average. Sodium restriction is particularly effective in reducing blood pressure in older individuals with hypertension.

The U.S. government currently recommends that people consume no more than 2,400 mg of sodium per day. But the Institute of Medicine released new guidelines in 2004 stating that daily sodium intake should be even lower: 1,500 mg for adults under age 50; 1,300 mg for people age 50 to 70; and 1,200 mg for those over 70 years old.

Salt added to foods during cooking or at the table is an obvious source of sodium in the diet. However, sodium occurs naturally in many foods and is used extensively in food processing. Cold cuts, canned vegetables, canned soups, cheeses, and snack foods can all be concentrated sources of sodium. Check nutrition labels for the amount of sodium in foods and, when buying packaged or processed foods, choose the low- or no-salt versions whenever possible.

A number of studies show that a low potassium intake can raise blood pressure, while increased potassium intake can lower blood pressure. People with high blood pressure should increase their intake of fresh fruits and vegetables, which are high in potassium and have the added benefit of being low in sodium and rich in dietary fiber and antioxidants. Citrus fruits and bananas are particularly good sources of potassium.

According to 2004 guidelines from the Institute of Medicine, people should consume at least 4.7 g of potassium per day. Except when prescribed by a doctor, potassium supplements are not recommended for blood pressure control and may even be dangerous for some people with high blood pressure and kidney disease.

Physical Activity

Regular exercise has many advantages. It helps to control body weight, can raise HDL cholesterol, improves the work capacity of the heart, reduces blood pressure and blood glucose, and relieves stress.

Many people feel that they must engage in strenuous physical activity for exercise to provide any benefit. But even brisk walking can be a healthy form of exercise if performed regularly. One study of postmenopausal women found that an amount of physical activity equivalent to walking 30 to 45 minutes, three times a week, reduced the risk of a heart attack by 50%.

In 1995, the Centers for Disease Control and Prevention and the American College of Sports Medicine developed a set of exercise recommendations. In reviewing all of the available evidence on physical activity and health, an expert panel convened by these two organizations concluded that adults should get 30 minutes or more of physical activity on most, preferably all, days of the week. The activity should be performed at moderate intensity—the equivalent of walking at a pace of three to four miles per hour.

Differing from many previous recommendations, the panel concluded that the 30 minutes of activity need not take place at one time. Short bursts of activity for 8 to 10 minutes, three times a day, are enough to reduce the risk of CHD, as long as they are performed at moderate intensity. Such activities include walking up stairs, walking short distances instead of driving, and doing calisthenics or pedaling a stationary bicycle while watching television. Gardening, housework, raking leaves, dancing, and playing with children can also count as part of the 30-minute total—if they are performed at a level of intensity that corresponds to brisk walking. According to the panel, those who perform lower-intensity activities should do them more often, for longer periods of time, or both. The Institute of Medicine recently recommended getting even more exercise—an hour a day—but this goal may not be realistic for most adults.

Men over age 40 and women over age 50 who plan to begin a vigorous exercise program should consult their doctor first, particularly if they have previously led a sedentary lifestyle. Those who have CHD or are at high risk for developing it should also see a doctor before beginning any new physical activities, even moderate ones. Though rare, heart attacks may be triggered by unusually high amounts of exertion in individuals with a previously sedentary lifestyle. Thus, physical activity should be incorporated gradually into one's lifestyle, and its intensity increased slowly and steadily.

Weight Control

A low-fat diet combined with regular exercise will help people maintain an appropriate weight or lose weight, if necessary. Weight loss is the most effective way to lower elevated triglyceride levels. It also helps to raise HDL cholesterol levels: In one study, a 5-lb. weight gain lowered HDL levels by 4% in men and 2% in women; losing weight counteracted this effect.

Weight loss is one of the first steps in the treatment of type 2 diabetes, and a weight loss of as little as 5 to 10 lbs. may lower blood

NEW RESEARCH

Physical Fitness Helps Counter Risks of Metabolic Syndrome

Being physically fit may lessen the consequences of having a cluster of risk factors known as metabolic syndrome, a large study suggests.

In a study that followed more than 19,000 men for up to 17 years, physical fitness cut the risk of death in those with metabolic syndrome. People with this syndrome have at least three of the following factors—abdominal obesity, high blood pressure, abnormal blood glucose levels, high triglyceride levels, and low HDL cholesterol levels—and are at increased risk for type 2 diabetes, CHD, and stroke.

Men in the study who had metabolic syndrome were 89% more likely to die of cardiovascular disease than were healthy men. But when the researchers factored in physical fitness—as measured by treadmill tests at the study's start—they found that fit men with metabolic syndrome had death risks similar to those without metabolic syndrome.

Overall, fitness appeared to lower a man's death risk regardless of his body weight, supporting the notion that fitness brings health benefits even when a person remains overweight, the researchers note. It's not clear exactly how fitness may counter the effects of metabolic syndrome, but the authors conclude that exercise may be a "valuable tool" in treating metabolic syndrome and preventing its complications.

ARCHIVES OF INTERNAL MEDICINE
Volume 164, page 1092
May 24, 2004

A Drink a Day To Keep Heart Attacks at Bay?

Alcoholic beverages appear to lower the chances of having a heart attack, even for people at high risk—unless you drink too much.

"Whether wine is a nourishment, medicine, or poison is a matter of dosage," the German physician Paracelsus wrote in the 16th century. Some 500 years later, his words still ring true, especially when it comes to alcohol and preventing heart attacks. Study after study has shown that people who drink moderately—about a drink or two per day—have a significantly lower risk of having a heart attack than people who drink infrequently or not at all. But you can't save these drinks up for the weekend: Binge drinking is associated with numerous health risks, including liver disease and accidents.

Recent Evidence

A number of recent studies have attempted to tease out some of the details of how moderate alcohol intake helps prevent heart attacks—including the pattern in which people drink and what they drink.

A recent report from the March 2004 issue of *Addiction* compared 427 men who had suffered a recent nonfatal heart attack with 905 similar men who had never had a heart attack. Men who drank daily in the previous two years were 59% less likely to have a heart attack than lifelong abstainers. People who drank somewhat less frequently—even those who drank less than once a week—also had a decreased risk of heart attacks. But men who consumed alcohol only on weekends (and who were often binge drinkers) elevated their risk of a heart attack compared with daily or less-than-once-weekly drinkers. Although this study also found that alcohol was only beneficial when consumed with meals, other studies have not demonstrated such a link.

Some experts have suggested that the reduced rate of heart attacks associated with alcohol consumption is offset by increases in death from other causes. But according to another article in the same issue of *Addiction*, middle-aged men who drank about two drinks a day were still 50% less likely to die of any cause over 10 years compared with those who drank once per week or less. Women who drank about one to six drinks per week (spread out across the week) were 28% less likely to die of any cause than those who drank less frequently.

Some, but not all, research has indicated that red wine is modestly better for the heart than other alcoholic beverages. This line of thinking began when investigators discovered that the French have a lower rate of heart attacks than Americans despite the fact that both countries consume similar amounts of animal fat—a phenomenon known as the "French paradox." Some experts have suggested that red wine, which is favored by the French, is the factor that lowers their heart-attack risk, but many subsequent studies, including a 2003 report in *The New England Journal of Medicine*, have found that any type of alcoholic beverage—beer, wine, or spirits—has the same potential to reduce the risk of a heart attack.

How Alcohol Lowers Risk

Alcohol may lower the chance of a heart attack through many mechanisms. Most important is its effects on high-density lipoprotein (HDL, or

pressure enough to make blood pressure-lowering medication unnecessary. Blood pressure drops even more with a combination of weight loss and medication than with medication alone.

Improving insulin sensitivity, by combining weight loss with increased physical activity, is critical in managing metabolic syndrome. Even modest weight loss—in the range of 5% to 10% of body weight—can help restore insulin sensitivity and greatly lower the chances that the syndrome will progress to type 2 diabetes. If a lifestyle approach does not reduce risk factors sufficiently, cholesterol-lowering drugs may be added to improve lipid levels. A blood pressure-lowering drug may also be needed to treat high blood pressure. There is also evidence that the insulin-sensitizing drug metformin (Glucophage), ordinarily used to treat type 2 diabetes,

"good") cholesterol. Moderate drinking increases HDL by about 12%. Alcohol also may protect against heart attacks by inhibiting constriction of the coronary arteries, limiting clot formation, and decreasing levels of homocysteine—an amino acid linked to increased heart-attack risk. Some evidence has also linked moderate intake of alcohol to a lower rate of obesity.

Researchers are unlikely to ever conduct a clinical trial in which people would be randomly assigned either to drink alcohol or to abstain. In the absence of such trials, however, there is no way to be entirely certain whether the effects of alcohol are due to the drink itself or to other factors that may be common in moderate drinkers.

Should You Imbibe?

Although much evidence points toward the heart benefits of alcohol, experts do not recommend that people who abstain start drinking to improve their heart health. Instead, the American Heart Association recommends the traditional methods for preventing heart disease, including consuming a healthy diet, exercising, and controlling blood cholesterol, weight, and blood

---

The Negative Effects of Alcohol

Of course, alcohol abuse can be detrimental to your health. Excessive alcohol intake has been linked to alcohol cardiomyopathy (a weakening of the heart muscle), hemorrhagic (bleeding) stroke, cirrhosis of the liver, pancreatitis (inflammation of the pancreas), certain cancers, trauma (such as in car accidents), suicide, and homicide. Heavy alcohol intake can also cause or exacerbate high blood pressure. The American Heart Association recommends that people with the following conditions not drink alcohol:

- A personal or strong family history of alcoholism;

- Uncontrolled high blood pressure (however, moderate alcohol intake appears helpful in men with controlled hypertension);

- High blood triglyceride levels;

- Pancreatitis;

- Liver disease;

- Porphyria (a genetic disorder of metabolism);

- Heart failure;

- Pregnancy; and

- Use of medications that can have adverse interactions with alcohol.

---

pressure. But for people who do drink moderately, a drink or two per day for men and no more than a drink a day for women can be one of the many ways to maintain heart health. (More than one drink a day for women may increase the risk of breast cancer; because women tend to weigh less, heavier drinking is also more likely to lead to cirrhosis of the liver in women than in men.) One drink is generally defined as 12 oz. of beer, 5 oz. of wine, or 1.5 oz. of spirits.

---

may be helpful in preventing the progression of metabolic syndrome to type 2 diabetes.

Alcohol

Consuming one or two alcoholic drinks a day is associated with a reduced heart attack risk. Researchers are not sure why, but alcohol increases HDL cholesterol levels, inhibits the constriction of coronary arteries, and limits blood clot formation. But because of the health risks of alcohol—heavy drinking can damage the heart and liver and cause accidents and hemorrhagic (bleeding) strokes—the American Heart Association does not recommend drinking alcohol for heart attack prevention. In fact, controlling other risk factors for CHD has a greater impact on CHD risk than moderate alcohol consumption. For more information on alcohol and your heart, see the feature on pages 34–35.

Stress Reduction

A variety of approaches can help one cope with stress. Regular aerobic exercise—even a daily walk—can ease stress. A network of supportive family or friends can also help reduce stress. Relaxation techniques such as yoga, tai chi, and transcendental meditation, as well as more formal programs in which a therapist teaches relaxation exercises, can be useful as well. Some people may benefit from behavior modification techniques—for example, biofeedback, anxiety management, and stress management.

MEDICATIONS TO PREVENT HEART ATTACK

Lifestyle measures are typically considered the first step and the cornerstone for preventing heart attacks—and they may be all that are needed. But if they fail to adequately control blood lipid levels and high blood pressure (usually within three to nine months), medication is often recommended in addition to lifestyle changes.

Lipid-Lowering Medications

The benefits of reducing total and LDL cholesterol levels with medication have been clearly demonstrated by a number of well-designed studies. Recently, results from the Heart Protection Study, which examined the effects of long-term therapy with simvastatin in more than 20,500 people, found that statin therapy reduced the incidence of heart attacks and strokes by about one third. Statins were effective not only in people with existing heart disease, but also in people at high risk for heart attack, including those with diabetes, peripheral arterial disease, or a history of stroke. Moreover, people with pretreatment LDL cholesterol levels within the normal range—or even less than 100 mg/dL—benefited from statin therapy.

Despite these benefits, studies have shown that as many as half of the people prescribed lipid-lowering medications stop taking them after one year, even though these drugs should be continued indefinitely. And people who adhere to taking the medications are often on too low a dose to achieve adequate reduction of LDL cholesterol levels.

The following five classes of lipid-lowering drugs are available: HMG-CoA reductase inhibitors, better known as statins; bile acid sequestrants; nicotinic acid, or niacin; fibrates; and cholesterol absorption inhibitors. (See below and the chart on pages 38–39.)

Statins (HMG-CoA reductase inhibitors). About 90% of the cholesterol-lowering drugs taken by Americans are statins. The drugs in this class are associated with few side effects and are the most effective drugs for lowering total and LDL cholesterol levels and for reducing the risk of heart attack. Statins also help lower the risk of stroke and, in people with CHD, the need for bypass surgery and angioplasty.

The statins include atorvastatin (Lipitor), fluvastatin (Lescol), lovastatin (Mevacor), pravastatin (Pravachol), simvastatin (Zocor), and the most recent addition, rosuvastatin (Crestor), which was approved in 2003. Lovastatin, the only statin available as a generic, is also available in combination with extended-release niacin and is sold under the brand name Advicor. In addition, the FDA recently approved a pill called Caduet, which combines atorvastatin and the blood pressure-lowering drug amlodipine, for the treatment of elevated cholesterol levels in people who also have hypertension. And more recently the FDA approved Vytorin, a pill containing both simvastatin and the cholesterol absorption inhibitor ezetimibe.

Statins produce about a 25% to 55% reduction in levels of LDL cholesterol, a 5% to 15% increase in HDL cholesterol levels, and a 10% to 25% reduction in triglyceride levels. The relative efficacy of the statins for lowering LDL cholesterol and triglyceride levels is as follows: rosuvastatin has the most potent effect, followed by atorvastatin, simvastatin, pravastatin, lovastatin, and fluvastatin. The ability to lower LDL cholesterol levels is usually the most important factor to consider when choosing a statin, but other considerations include a patient's level of CHD risk, differences in side effects, drug interactions, cost, results of clinical trials, and the time of day a dose should be taken.

In addition to their positive effects on blood lipid levels, the statins also appear to improve the function of the endothelium in the arteries. Specifically, they help arteries regain at least some of their normal ability to widen and permit increased blood flow during exercise. Statins also reduce the risk of plaque rupture by decreasing the cholesterol content and amount of inflammation in the arterial wall.

Side effects are uncommon, occurring in only 1% to 2% of people. The most common side effect is muscle aches. Others include bloating or upset stomach and increases in liver enzymes, usually when a patient is also taking other medications. In rare cases, most

NEW RESEARCH

Intensive Lipid-Lowering Improves Cholesterol Levels

In a head-to-head comparison of two statin drugs, researchers determined that an intensive regimen resulted in significantly lower LDL cholesterol levels and less progression of atherosclerosis than a more moderate regimen.

In the study, 329 patients with elevated LDL cholesterol levels were randomly assigned to take 40 mg daily of pravastatin (Pravachol; the moderate regimen), and 328 were assigned to take 80 mg daily of atorvastatin (Lipitor; the intensive regimen).

After 18 months, patients who took atorvastatin had lower LDL cholesterol levels compared with patients who received pravastatin (79 mg/dL vs. 110 mg/dL). In addition, the amount of plaque buildup in the coronary arteries (as measured by intravascular ultrasound) was unchanged in the atorvastatin group, while it increased nearly 3% in the pravastatin group.

These findings provide evidence that intensive treatment using the maximum approved dosage of a statin slows progression of atherosclerosis in the coronary arteries. However, an accompanying editorial states that until longer studies comparing statins are completed, physicians should not immediately begin prescribing higher doses of these drugs in people who've not had a recent heart attack or episode of unstable angina.

JOURNAL OF THE AMERICAN MEDICAL ASSOCIATION
Volume 291, pages 1071 and 1132
March 3, 2004

Lipid-Lowering Drugs 2005

Drug Type	Generic Name	Brand Name	Average Daily Dosage*	Average Retail Price†
Statins (HMG-CoA reductase inhibitors)	atorvastatin	Lipitor	10 to 80 mg	10 mg: $68
	fluvastatin	Lescol	20 to 80 mg	40 mg: $58
	fluvastatin, extended-release	Lescol XL	80 mg	80 mg: $74
	lovastatin‡	Mevacor	20 to 80 mg	20 mg: $70 ($30)
	pravastatin	Pravachol	10 to 40 mg	40 mg: $126
	rosuvastatin	Crestor	5 to 40 mg	10 mg: $71
	simvastatin§	Zocor	10 to 80 mg	20 mg: $122
Bile acid sequestrants	cholestyramine	Questran	8 to 24 g	4 g‖: $80 ($40)
		Questran Light	8 to 24 g	4 g‖: $66 ($45)
	colestipol	Colestid	10 to 30 g	5 g‖: $60
		Colestid Flavored	10 to 30 g	5 g‖: $66
		Colestid pills	10 to 30 g	1 g: $20
	colesevelam	WelChol	3.75 to 4.375 g	0.625 g: $27
Nicotinic acid	niacin	Niacor	3 to 6 g	500 mg: $7 ($5)
	niacin, extended-release‡	Niaspan	375 to 2,000 mg	500 mg: $43
Fibrates	fenofibrate	Lofibra	67 to 200 mg	67 mg: $26
		Tricor	54 to 160 mg	54 mg: $35
	gemfibrozil	Lopid	1,200 mg	600 mg: $47 ($9)
Cholesterol absorption inhibitor	ezetimibe§	Zetia	10 mg	10 mg: $75

* These dosages represent an average range for the treatment of elevated lipid levels. The precise effective dosage varies from patient to patient and depends on many factors. Do not make any changes in your medication without consulting your doctor.

† Average price for 30 tablets or capsules (unless otherwise indicated) of the dosage strength listed. Actual price may vary. If a generic version is available, the cost is listed in parentheses. Sources: drugstore.com, eckerd.com, and walgreens.com.

‡ A combination of lovastatin and extended-release niacin (brand name Advicor) is available.

§ A combination of simvastatin and ezetimibe (brand name Vytorin) is available.

‖ Amount of the active ingredient.

How They Work	Advantages	Disadvantages
HMG-CoA reductase is required for the liver to produce cholesterol. Statins block the action of this enzyme. As a result, the liver makes less cholesterol and more LDL receptors, which remove LDL from the blood.	The most effective drugs to lower total and LDL cholesterol. Can lower LDL cholesterol by 25% to 55% and triglycerides by 10% to 25%. Can increase HDL cholesterol by 5% to 15%. Side effects are uncommon. Better tolerated than bile acid sequestrants or nicotinic acid. Reduce the risk of heart attacks, strokes, and death.	Gastrointestinal symptoms or reversible liver injury occurs in 1% to 2% of people. Muscle soreness also can occur, more often when statins are used in combination with nicotinic acid, fibrates, erythromycin, antifungal agents, or cyclosporine. When severe, muscle inflammation can cause kidney damage.
Bile acids, made from cholesterol by the liver, are released from the gallbladder into the intestine after meals. Normally, bile acids are reabsorbed from the intestine and returned to the liver for reprocessing. Bile acid sequestrants bind bile acids in the intestine and remove them via the stool. As a result, the liver converts more cholesterol to bile acids and removes more LDL from the blood.	Long-term safety and effectiveness have been established. Can be combined with any other lipid-lowering drug. Used for people with elevated LDL cholesterol levels but normal triglyceride levels. On average, bile acid sequestrants reduce LDL cholesterol by 15% to 25%. Used alone, these drugs reduce the risk of heart attacks. Bile acid sequestrants also slow the progression of plaques and may even cause plaque regression when combined with other cholesterol-lowering drugs.	Constipation is common, especially at higher doses. This side effect may be temporary and can be relieved with a high-fiber diet or stool-softening pills. May cause heartburn or a feeling of fullness. Triglyceride levels may rise. Rarely, bile acid sequestrants can interfere with the absorption of folic acid. Proper timing of drug dosage is important to avoid interference with the absorption of other drugs.
Nicotinic acid decreases the production of VLDL by the liver. VLDL is the major carrier of triglycerides in the blood.	Safe and effective, niacin is used to treat high LDL cholesterol levels, high triglyceride levels, and/or low HDL cholesterol levels. The most effective drug to raise HDL levels (about 20% on average), it also reduces LDL cholesterol on average by 10% to 20% and triglycerides by 20% to 30%. Used alone, it decreases heart attacks and heart attack deaths. When combined with bile acid sequestrants, it slows progression and contributes to regression of plaques in the coronary arteries.	Skin flushing and itching may occur about half an hour after taking the drug. These side effects often decrease with time and can be greatly reduced by starting on a low dose and gradually increasing the dose, taking an extended-release formulation, taking the drug with meals, or taking an aspirin half an hour before taking the drug. Should not be used by people with peptic ulcers or a history of ulcers or by people with liver disease or gout. Should be used with caution in people with diabetes or pre-diabetes. In rare cases, sustained-release formulations can cause liver injury.
These drugs stimulate the activity of lipoprotein lipase. This enzyme breaks down triglycerides and thus lowers VLDL and triglyceride levels.	Fibrates are safe for long-term use. They are the most effective drugs to lower triglycerides, producing reductions of 30% to 50%. They also raise HDL cholesterol by about 10%. Fenofibrate may be more effective than gemfibrozil in lowering total and LDL cholesterol. Gemfibrozil reduces the risk of heart attacks.	Total and LDL cholesterol may increase. Feelings of fullness, diarrhea, gas, muscle aches, and reversible liver injury may occur. Long-term use can lead to gallstones. When taken with a statin, fibrates (especially gemfibrozil) increase the risk of severe muscle inflammation and kidney damage.
Ezetimibe inhibits the intestinal absorption of cholesterol from the diet and from bile acids.	Safe and effective, ezetimibe lowers total cholesterol by 13%, LDL cholesterol by 15%, and triglycerides by 8%. When used in combination with a statin, total cholesterol is reduced by 17%, LDL cholesterol by 25%, and triglycerides by 14%. May be useful in people who experience intolerable side effects with statins or cannot reach desirable lipid levels with a statin alone.	People with liver disease or elevated liver enzymes should not take ezetimibe in combination with a statin. Side effects are uncommon; they include back pain, joint pain, diarrhea, and sinus inflammation.

often when a statin is taken along with certain other medications, the kidneys can become damaged by the release of the protein myoglobin from severely inflamed muscles (rhabdomyolysis). Anyone taking a statin who experiences unusual or unexplained muscle aches should call a doctor.

Bile acid sequestrants. The bile acid sequestrants, cholestyramine (Questran) and colestipol (Colestid), have proven long-term safety and effectiveness. A newer sequestrant called colesevelam (WelChol) became available in 2000. Sequestrants effectively lower LDL cholesterol levels, especially when taken in combination with statins or niacin. A number of studies have shown that such combinations slow the progression—or even cause modest regression—of plaques. Bile acid sequestrants can modestly raise triglyceride levels, however.

Common side effects include constipation, heartburn, bloating, belching, and abdominal discomfort. Intestinal obstruction is a rare adverse effect; stop taking the drug and contact a doctor if you experience severe abdominal pain. Rarely, bile acid sequestrants can also interfere with the absorption of folic acid. Taking the sequestrants at the proper times is important to avoid interfering with the absorption of other drugs.

Niacin. Large doses of this B vitamin are the most effective therapy to raise HDL cholesterol levels. Niacin can also lower triglyceride and LDL cholesterol levels but frequently causes adverse effects, especially when dosages higher than 2 grams a day are taken.

Skin flushing and itching are common but not dangerous. More serious side effects include liver toxicity, peptic ulcers (ulcers in the stomach or upper intestine), gout, and an increase in blood glucose levels. Doctors cannot predict who will experience these side effects. Niacin should not be taken by those with a current or past peptic ulcer, liver disease, or gout. It should be used with caution in people with diabetes or pre-diabetes; generally, these individuals are advised to take no more than 1 gram a day.

Extended-release niacin (Niaspan) causes less flushing than immediate-release niacin (Niacor) and has the added advantage of once-daily dosing at bedtime, rather than three times a day with meals. Older, sustained-release niacin preparations increase the risk of liver toxicity and should only be taken under a doctor's supervision. Extended-release niacin is also available in combination with lovastatin (brand name Advicor). Although niacin is available over the counter, all preparations should be used under a doctor's supervision.

Fibrates. The fibrates, fenofibrate (Lofibra, Tricor) and gemfibrozil (Lopid), are the treatment of choice for those with markedly increased blood triglyceride levels. But any reduction in triglycerides with fibrates may be accompanied by a slight rise in LDL cholesterol. When this problem occurs, the addition of a statin can improve LDL cholesterol levels but may cause muscle inflammation in about 1% of people. (The problem is more common with gemfibrozil than with fenofibrate.) Muscle inflammation is reversible, but both drugs must be promptly discontinued, since persistent, severe muscle inflammation can cause kidney failure. Call your doctor right away if you experience unusual or unexplained muscle aches. Uncommon side effects of fibrates include diarrhea, nausea, gas, skin rash, infection, and flu-like symptoms.

Cholesterol absorption inhibitors. An inhibitor of cholesterol absorption is the newest type of lipid-lowering medication. As the name implies, these drugs work by blocking the intestinal absorption of cholesterol from the diet and bile acids. Ezetimibe (Zetia) is the first and only drug to be approved in this class. The drug lowers LDL cholesterol levels by about 15%, and when used in combination with a statin, LDL levels may be reduced by up to 55%. Side effects are infrequent and include back pain, joint pain, diarrhea, and sinus inflammation.

Stanols and sterols. In 1999, the FDA approved cholesterol-lowering food additives called stanols and sterols, which help lower cholesterol levels by blocking the absorption of cholesterol in the small intestine. So far these substances have been added to margarines (Benecol, Take Control, and SmartBalance OmegaPlus) and orange juice (Minute Maid Premium Heart Wise). The margarines can reduce LDL cholesterol levels by 7% to 14% when used daily for a year or longer in combination with a low-saturated fat, low-cholesterol diet and regular exercise. In a recent study, sterol-fortified orange juice reduced LDL cholesterol by 12% when participants drank two 8 oz. glasses each day with meals for eight weeks. Don't forget that stanol- and sterol-fortified foods contain calories and can cause weight gain when consumed in large quantities or in addition to the usual diet.

Medications To Lower High Blood Pressure

Five classes of drugs, used individually or in combination, are most frequently prescribed for the treatment of high blood pressure: diuretics, beta-blockers, ACE inhibitors, angiotensin II receptor blockers, and calcium channel blockers.

NEW RESEARCH

Experimental Drug Found To Boost HDL Cholesterol

An experimental drug may raise heart-healthy HDL cholesterol in people with low levels, according to a small study.

Researchers found that in 19 people with HDL levels below 40 mg/dL the drug torcetrapib increased HDL cholesterol, with or without the help of a statin drug. After four weeks, HDL levels rose 46% in patients who took torcetrapib alone once a day, while those who also took the cholesterol drug atorvastatin (Lipitor) had a 61% gain. In a subgroup who did not take atorvastatin and was given torcetrapib for another four weeks, this time twice a day, HDL cholesterol increased by 106%.

Torcetrapib reduces the activity of a blood protein called CETP that helps transfer cholesterol from HDL to LDL. While the new findings suggest such drugs can boost HDL cholesterol, further clinical trials are needed to determine whether they actually help prevent heart attacks and strokes.

Statins cut the risk of heart attacks, but they work mainly by lowering the "bad," LDL, cholesterol. According to an accompanying editorial, the development of HDL-raising drugs represents an "exciting" new treatment strategy.

The study received partial funding from Pfizer, Inc., the manufacturer of torcetrapib and atorvastatin.

THE NEW ENGLAND JOURNAL OF MEDICINE
Volume 350, pages 1491 and 1505
April 8, 2004

Diuretics. By increasing the amount of sodium excreted in the urine, diuretics promote water loss and decrease blood volume. Diuretics can also widen small blood vessels, which increases blood flow. Thiazides are the most commonly used diuretics. They are inexpensive and only need to be taken once a day.

Possible side effects include weakness; fatigue; erectile dysfunction; higher levels of blood glucose, uric acid, and triglycerides; lower HDL cholesterol levels; and excessive loss of potassium in the urine. Potassium depletion can be prevented by combining a thiazide with a potassium-sparing diuretic such as triamterene (Dyrenium), by taking potassium supplements, or by adding an ACE inhibitor or an angiotensin II receptor blocker.

Low-dose thiazide diuretics are often the first medication tried in people with high blood pressure. In addition to their blood pressure-lowering effect, these drugs may reduce the risk of heart attack, heart failure, and stroke. In a recent study, called the Antihypertensive and Lipid-Lowering Treatment to Prevent Heart Attack Trial (ALLHAT), people taking a thiazide diuretic were less likely to develop or be hospitalized for heart failure than people taking a calcium channel blocker. The study also showed that a thiazide diuretic was slightly more effective than an ACE inhibitor for reducing the risk of heart failure, being hospitalized or treated for angina, needing to undergo angioplasty or bypass surgery, and having a stroke.

Beta-blockers. These drugs, which impede the actions of adrenaline, lower blood pressure by slowing heart rate and decreasing cardiac output (the amount of blood pumped by the heart). Beta-blockers can also alleviate the symptoms of angina, help treat heart failure, and reduce the risk of death and future heart attacks in people who have had a heart attack. Possible adverse effects of beta-blockers include fatigue, depression, erectile dysfunction, a mild rise in blood glucose and triglyceride levels, a slight fall in HDL cholesterol levels, and wheezing in people with asthma. In people taking medication for diabetes, beta-blockers may mask the warning symptoms of hypoglycemia (low blood glucose) by interfering with the actions of adrenaline.

ACE inhibitors. ACE stands for angiotensin-converting enzyme. One way ACE inhibitors decrease blood pressure is by inhibiting the formation of angiotensin II, a substance that constricts blood vessels and stimulates the adrenal glands to release the hormone aldosterone, which promotes sodium retention. ACE inhibitors generally cause fewer adverse effects than diuretics or beta-blockers; a dry

Cholesterol-Busting Foods

Some foods can lower cholesterol levels effectively and will fit easily into your diet.

When people need to reduce their cholesterol, they often think about eliminating some foods from their diet. But research increasingly shows that adding certain foods can also lower cholesterol levels significantly. In fact, a 2003 study in *Metabolism* found that people with high cholesterol who ate a diet not only low in saturated fat but high in plant sterols, soluble fibers, soy protein, and almonds effectively lowered their low-density lipoprotein (LDL or "bad") cholesterol levels by 35%. (Although this diet would be very difficult to follow for long periods, the study illustrated the feasibility of lowering LDL cholesterol through diet.)

To avoid consuming excess calories, it's important to substitute the cholesterol-busting foods described below for other foods (preferably those high in saturated fat and cholesterol) rather than simply add them to the diet.

Plant Sterols and Stanols

Plant sterols and stanols, plant compounds that are structurally similar to cholesterol, partially block the absorption of cholesterol from the small intestine. They lower levels of LDL cholesterol without adversely affecting high-density lipoprotein (HDL or "good") cholesterol levels.

The American Heart Association states that people whose elevated cholesterol levels are not controlled by increased physical activity, weight loss, and dietary changes (decreasing saturated fat and cholesterol intake) might consider adding about 2 g of plant sterols or stanols daily to their diet. This dietary change can lower LDL cholesterol levels by about 10% and, over a lifetime, may decrease the risk of a heart attack by up to 20%. However, consuming more than 2 g per day of plant sterols or stanols will not lower cholesterol any more effectively and may lead to excess caloric intake.

What foods contain sterols and stanols? The margarines Benecol, Take Control, and SmartBalance OmegaPlus are fortified with either sterols or stanols. And a new orange juice, Heart Wise by Minute Maid, has added sterols.

In a March 2004 study from *Arteriosclerosis, Thrombosis, and Vascular Biology,* daily consumption of 16 oz. of orange juice fortified with plant sterols (for a total of 2 g of sterols daily) decreased total cholesterol levels by 7% and LDL cholesterol levels by 12% over eight weeks.

Other types of food fortified with stanols or sterols, like salad dressings, cereals, breads, and yogurt, may become available. (Please note that these fortified products tend to be more expensive than the nonfortified versions.)

Soluble Fiber

The American Heart Association also recommends that people who are unsuccessful in lowering their cholesterol through lifestyle changes boost their intake of soluble fiber to 10 to 25 g each day. Good sources of soluble fiber include legumes such as peas and beans; cereal grains such as oats and barley, and vegetables and fruits such as carrots, apples, and dried plums (prunes).

A 2002 study from the *Journal of the American Dietetic Association* found that eating four servings of high fiber foods per day for seven weeks and receiving guidance about other lifestyle changes to lower cholesterol decreased total cholesterol levels by almost 6% and LDL cholesterol levels by over 7%. Fiber may help lower cholesterol by interfering with the reabsorption of bile acids from the intestine, so the liver converts more cholesterol to bile acids.

Soy Protein

Populations such as the Japanese and Chinese, which regularly eat soy products, have a lower rate of heart disease than people who follow a Western diet. One reason for this association appears to be soy's effect on cholesterol levels: Replacing food high in saturated fat and cholesterol with those high in soy protein helps reduce LDL cholesterol levels. In fact, eating four 6.25-g servings of soy protein a day—equivalent to four cups of soy milk daily—will bring LDL cholesterol levels down by 5% to 7%. It is not clear whether the protein or other components of soy products are responsible for lowering cholesterol levels. In fact, cholesterol may decrease with soy intake because people who eat soy tend to consume fewer meat products, which can contribute to high cholesterol levels.

Nuts

Although nuts are high in fat, the fats are predominantly monounsaturated and polyunsaturated, which are known to decrease LDL cholesterol levels. Although a number of types of nuts have been shown to help lower LDL cholesterol levels—including walnuts, peanuts, pecans, macadamias, and pistachios—the best evidence exists for almonds. In one report, from a 2002 issue of *Circulation,* people with high cholesterol levels who added 37 g of almonds (about a handful) per day to their diet lowered their LDL cholesterol levels by 4%; 74 g of almonds daily lowered LDL cholesterol levels by 9%. People should be sure to choose dry roasted or natural nuts and not ones that contain added oil and salt.

cough is the most frequent side effect. Uncommon side effects are an increase in blood potassium levels and impaired kidney function.

ACE inhibitors are also effective in preventing CHD events. In 2000, the Health Outcomes Prevention Evaluation (HOPE) study showed that the ACE inhibitor ramipril (Altace) significantly reduced the incidence of CHD events and strokes over a five-year period in people with vascular disease or diabetes plus one of the following CHD risk factors: high blood pressure, elevated total cholesterol levels, cigarette smoking, low HDL cholesterol levels, or microalbuminuria (protein in the urine). ACE inhibitors may also reduce the risk of diabetes, kidney disease, and stroke.

Angiotensin II receptor blockers. These drugs work by interfering with the action of angiotensin II. They may also halt the growth of smooth muscle cells in blood vessel walls. Rare side effects include headache and digestive upset, although these problems also occurred at about the same frequency in people who received a placebo in one study. Individuals who develop a cough while taking an ACE inhibitor can be prescribed an angiotensin II receptor blocker instead. Angiotensin II receptor blockers and ACE inhibitors should not be used by women who are pregnant or planning a pregnancy.

Researchers have found that angiotensin II receptor blockers can also protect the heart. One recent study found that an angiotensin II receptor blocker was helpful in the treatment of heart failure. In addition, these drugs can help prevent kidney disease in people with diabetes, and there is some evidence they may help prevent diabetes. They may also help prevent stroke in people with hypertension and thickening of the heart muscle.

Calcium channel blockers. These drugs lower blood pressure by dilating arteries and, possibly, by decreasing cardiac output. Like beta-blockers, calcium channel blockers help alleviate the symptoms of angina. They are also sometimes used to reduce the risk of stroke and kidney disease.

Long-acting calcium channel blockers are safer and more effective than short-acting calcium channel blockers. In addition, because long-acting calcium channel blockers need to be taken only once a day, people are less likely to miss doses. Flushing and swelling of the legs are occasional side effects.

Aspirin Therapy for Primary Prevention

Aspirin is an antiplatelet agent: It can reduce the stickiness of blood platelets and prevent them from clumping together to initiate clot

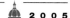

formation. Because of this antiplatelet effect, low-dose aspirin therapy has long been recommended for secondary prevention—to help reduce the risk of additional heart attacks and ischemic strokes in people who have already experienced one of these life-threatening events.

Recently, the U.S. Preventive Services Task Force declared that millions more Americans can benefit by taking aspirin to help reduce the risk of a first heart attack. Their guidelines, published in 2002, strongly recommend that healthy people take aspirin, but only if they have a significant risk of a heart attack within the next 10 years. This limitation was placed on aspirin use because it can trigger potentially serious side effects, especially gastrointestinal bleeding in some individuals and in rare cases hemorrhagic stroke (bleeding within the brain). Most at risk are individuals with uncontrolled blood pressure and those regularly taking other nonsteroidal anti-inflammatory drugs (NSAIDs) or anticoagulant drugs like warfarin (Coumadin).

Thus, it is crucial that candidates for low-dose aspirin discuss the risks and benefits of aspirin therapy with a physician. Potential candidates for taking aspirin to prevent a heart attack include men 40 years and older, postmenopausal women, smokers, and people with high blood pressure, diabetes, high total or LDL cholesterol levels, low HDL cholesterol levels, or a family history of heart attacks before age 55 in men and age 65 in women. The benefit of aspirin is less certain for women without CHD than it is for men, since the studies examined by the Task Force included mostly men.

In reviewing the research data, the Task Force found that lower doses of aspirin—ranging from 75 to 160 mg taken daily or 325 mg (a standard tablet) taken every other day—were effective for primary prevention of heart disease. The analysis also revealed that the more heart attack risk factors an individual has, the more effective aspirin is in preventing a heart attack or sudden death. The Task Force concluded that the heart-protective benefits of low-dose aspirin outweigh the side effects of gastrointestinal bleeding and hemorrhagic stroke for people who have at least a 6% chance of a heart attack in the next 10 years.

After the Task Force published their recommendations, the American Heart Association released slightly different guidelines on aspirin for the primary prevention of CHD and stroke. Their position is that the benefits of aspirin outweigh the risks when the risk of a heart attack in the next 10 years is at least 10%.

NEW RESEARCH

Estrogen Alone Does Not Prevent Heart Attacks

Nearly two years after combined hormone replacement therapy with estrogen and progestin was found to increase women's risk of CHD and other diseases, new evidence from the same study dims the hope that estrogen taken alone has significant health benefits.

These latest findings from the Women's Health Initiative (WHI) show that hormone pills containing only estrogen do not protect postmenopausal women against CHD or cancer and may raise their risk of stroke. Thus, like combination therapy, estrogen replacement should not be used to prevent CHD in postmenopausal women, experts say.

The findings were based on 10,739 women age 50 to 79 who were randomly assigned to take either an estrogen replacement or a placebo over an average of nearly seven years.

Health officials stopped the study in early 2004, when it became clear that the only benefit of estrogen was a reduction in hip fractures. The therapy had no clear effect on CHD risk and was linked to a 39% increase in stroke risk.

Even though estrogen did protect against hip fracture, the overall benefits do not outweigh the risks, according to an accompanying editorial. The therapy should be used only for menopausal symptoms, and at as low a dose and for as short a time as possible.

JOURNAL OF THE AMERICAN MEDICAL ASSOCIATION
Volume 291, pages 1701 and 1769
April 14, 2004

The ABCs of Heart Attack Prevention

You can modify or treat most of the risk factors associated with a heart attack or stroke. Here is an easy-to-remember checklist of primary prevention measures for people without symptoms or a history of cardiovascular disease.

❏ **Aspirin**
Goal: Low-dose aspirin (75 to 160 mg per day) for people at elevated risk for a heart attack. Not recommended for some people, so be sure to consult with a physician before starting aspirin therapy.

❏ **Blood Pressure**
Goal: <140/90 mm Hg (optimal is <120/80 mm Hg); <130/80 mm Hg for people with diabetes or kidney disease. If you cannot reach this goal after three to nine months of lifestyle changes, you may benefit from medication.

❏ **Cholesterol**
Goal: Total cholesterol <200 mg/dL; LDL cholesterol <160 for people with no more than one risk factor; LDL <130 for those with two or more risk factors; LDL <100 (with an optional goal of <70) for some people with two or more risk factors as well as for those with diabetes, history of stroke or aortic aneurysm, peripheral arterial disease, or CHD; HDL >40; triglycerides <150. If you cannot reach LDL goal after three to nine months of dietary changes, consider drug therapy to lower LDL. Exercise, improvements in diet, and quitting smoking can help meet HDL goals.

❏ **Diet and Weight Control**
Goal: Consume a variety of fruits, vegetables, grains, low-fat or nonfat dairy products, fish, legumes, poultry, and lean meats. Saturated fats should make up <10% of total calories. If overweight, make changes in caloric intake to achieve and maintain a desirable body weight (body mass index of 18.5 to 24.9). For those who drink, limit alcohol intake (no more than two drinks a day for men, one drink a day for women).

❏ **Exercise**
Goal: Perform at least 30 minutes of moderate-intensity physical activity (such as brisk walking) on most (and preferably all) days of the week. More vigorous activity can provide additional benefits, including weight loss if caloric expenditure exceeds caloric intake.

❏ **Additional Special Goals**
• Individuals who smoke should stop completely.
• Individuals with metabolic syndrome should reach normal fasting blood glucose levels (<100 mg/dL). People with diabetes should strive for the best possible control of blood glucose levels. If diet and exercise do not adequately lower blood glucose levels, medication is usually recommended; other risk factors for CHD must be treated aggressively.

No matter which guidelines are followed, the decision whether or not to start aspirin therapy should be made in consultation with a doctor. Individuals with a history of bleeding in the gastrointestinal tract, those with uncontrolled high blood pressure, and those who take NSAIDs or anticoagulant drugs should take aspirin with caution or not at all.

Hormone Replacement Therapy and CHD

Estrogen is effective in relieving the menopausal symptoms of hot flashes and vaginal dryness. Most postmenopausal women with an intact uterus who take estrogen also take a progestin (synthetic progesterone), because progestins negate the increased risk of uterine cancer in women taking estrogen alone. This combination, usually 0.625 mg of conjugated estrogen (Premarin) and 2.5 mg of medroxyprogesterone acetate (Provera) taken daily, is called hormone replacement therapy (HRT).

Because estrogen improves both LDL and HDL cholesterol levels, it was hoped that taking estrogen might reduce the incidence of CHD. Early findings suggested that HRT reduced the incidence of CHD events in postmenopausal women. Since these findings were based on observational studies, however, the women who took HRT may have been healthier to begin with or followed more protective lifestyle measures.

Then a randomized, controlled trial called the Heart and Estrogen/Progestin Replacement Study (HERS) showed that the rates of heart attack and death due to CHD in women with known CHD were the same whether or not women took these hormones. More recently, an even larger randomized, controlled trial called the Women's Health Initiative found that after five years, women taking HRT (the study used Prempro) had a slightly increased risk of heart attacks, strokes, breast cancer, and blood clots in the lungs, compared with those taking a placebo. As a result, this portion of the Women's Health Initiative study was halted in July 2002.

Women who have had a hysterectomy can take estrogen replacement therapy (ERT)—that is, estrogen without progestin. A smaller portion of the Women's Health Initiative study assigned women to either estrogen alone or a placebo. This portion of the study was halted in February 2004, when researchers discovered that estrogen alone did not reduce the risk of heart attacks and in fact increased the risk of stroke. Estrogen alone did slightly reduce the risk of fracture, however. For more information on this study, see the sidebar on page 45.

Consequently, HRT or ERT should not be used for the prevention of heart attack and stroke and, when used to reduce the symptoms of menopause, should be taken for the shortest possible time at the smallest effective dose. Women who have had breast cancer or have a family history of early breast cancer (a mother or sister who developed the disease before age 40) should be especially cautious about using HRT or ERT for any period of time. Women with a history of breast cancer may want to consider taking tamoxifen (Nolvadex) for up to five years. Tamoxifen has beneficial effects on LDL and HDL cholesterol levels similar to those of estrogen. ∎

GLOSSARY

aneurysm—A ballooning of the wall of the heart, an artery, or a vein caused by weakening of the wall.

angina—An episode of pain, pressure, or tightness in the chest caused by an imbalance between the supply of oxygen to the heart muscle and the heart muscle's need for oxygen. Angina occurs most often during increased physical activity or emotional stress. Also called angina pectoris.

anticoagulants—Drugs that decrease the formation of blood clots by inhibiting the production of fibrin, a protein required for clots to form. Examples are heparin and warfarin (Coumadin).

antioxidants—Substances that help the body neutralize free radicals. Beta-carotene, vitamin E, and vitamin C are naturally occurring antioxidants.

antiplatelets—Drug that decrease the formation of blood clots by inhibiting the aggregation or clumping of blood cells called platelets. One example is aspirin.

aorta—The body's main artery. It transports oxygenated blood from the left ventricle of the heart to the arteries that supply the rest of the body.

arrhythmia—An abnormal heart rhythm.

atherosclerosis—An accumulation of deposits of fat and fibrous tissue, called plaques, within the walls of arteries that can narrow the arteries and reduce blood flow through them.

atria—The two upper chambers of the heart. The left atrium receives newly oxygenated blood from the lungs; the right atrium receives blood returning from the rest of the body.

body mass index (BMI)—A measurement of weight in relation to height. Calculated by multiplying weight in pounds by 704 and dividing the result by the square of height in inches. Overweight is defined as a BMI of 25 to 29.9 and obesity as a BMI of 30 and over.

c-reactive protein (CRP)—A blood marker for excessive inflammation in the walls of arteries. CRP tends to be elevated in people who develop CHD and have a heart attack.

cardiac arrest—A sudden, abrupt loss of the heart's ability to pump blood, most often as a result of ventricular fibrillation.

cardiac output—The amount of blood pumped by the heart.

cardiovascular disease—Disease affecting the heart or arterial vascular system of the body. Coronary heart disease, stroke, and peripheral arterial disease are the most common cardiovascular diseases.

cerebrovascular disease—Disease that affects arteries supplying blood to the brain.

cholesterol—A soft, waxy substance present in cells throughout the body. Deposition of cholesterol within the walls of arteries can lead to the formation of atherosclerotic plaques.

coronary artery disease—See **coronary heart disease**.

coronary heart disease (CHD)—A narrowing of the coronary arteries by atherosclerosis. Can reduce or completely block blood flow to the heart. Also called coronary artery disease.

coronary heart disease (CHD) event—Often defined as a heart attack, episode of unstable angina, or CHD-related death. Also called a coronary event.

diastolic blood pressure—The lower number in a blood pressure reading. The pressure in the arteries when the heart relaxes between beats.

echocardiography—A diagnostic test that uses ultrasound waves to visualize the heart, its valves, and the flow of blood within the heart.

electrocardiogram (ECG or EKG)—A graphical record of the heart's electrical activity obtained by applying small metal sensors to the skin. Used to detect abnormal heart rhythms and heart damage.

electron-beam computed tomography (EBCT)—A noninvasive imaging technique that reveals calcium deposits in the coronary arteries. The presence of calcium indicates atherosclerosis.

endothelium—The layer of cells that lines the walls of arteries. Injury to these cells is an important first step in the development of atherosclerosis.

estrogen replacement therapy—Use of the hormone estrogen to relieve menopausal symptoms. Not recommended for the prevention of CHD or CHD events.

exercise stress test—An electrocardiogram administered while an individual walks on a treadmill or pedals a stationary bike. Heart muscle that receives too little blood during exercise can be detected during the test.

free radicals—Chemical compounds formed during normal metabolism. They can damage cells and oxidize low-density lipoproteins, which can then be deposited in the walls of arteries.

heart attack—Tissue death caused by insufficient blood supply to a portion of the heart muscle. Technically known as myocardial infarction.

heart failure—A condition in which the heart is unable to pump enough blood to meet the needs of the body. Common signs of heart failure include shortness of

GLOSSARY—continued

breath and accumulation of fluid in the lungs, legs, and abdomen.

high-density lipoprotein (HDL)—A protein that protects against atherosclerosis by removing cholesterol deposited in artery walls.

homocysteine—An amino acid required for normal body function. High levels in the blood may promote atherosclerosis by damaging the endothelium and stimulating formation of blood clots.

hormone replacement therapy (HRT)—A combination of estrogen and progestin (a synthetic form of progesterone) used by women to relieve the symptoms of menopause. Not recommended for the prevention of CHD or CHD events.

hypertension—High blood pressure.

ischemia—An inadequate supply of blood to any part of the body. Ischemia to the heart muscle may cause chest pain.

lipoprotein—A protein that transports cholesterol and other fats in the blood.

lipoprotein(a)— A lipoprotein with a structure similar to low-density lipoprotein but containing another protein called apo(a). High levels of lipoprotein(a) are a risk factor for coronary heart disease. Also called Lp(a).

low-density lipoprotein (LDL)—A protein that transports cholesterol in the bloodstream. A major contributor to atherosclerosis.

monounsaturated fat—A fat with a single double bond that is capable of absorbing more hydrogen. Found in avocados, almonds, and olive and canola oils. Can lower LDL cholesterol levels and stabilize or raise HDL cholesterol levels when substituted for saturated fat in the diet.

multidetector computed tomography (MDCT)—A non-invasive imaging technique that reveals calcium deposits in the coronary arteries. The presence of calcium indicates atherosclerosis.

myocardial infarction—See **heart attack**.

myocardium—The muscle of the heart.

nuclear imaging—A diagnostic test that uses a special camera to trace a radioactive substance injected into a vein. The test can reveal the presence of heart damage

and help predict the risk of future heart attacks.

omega-3 fatty acids—Polyunsaturated fats found in fish and some plant foods that appear to have beneficial effects on the heart.

peripheral arterial disease—A narrowing of the arteries in the extremities, usually the legs, commonly due to atherosclerosis. Sometimes called peripheral vascular disease.

plaque—An accumulation of cholesterol-laden foam cells, smooth muscle cells, fibrous proteins, and calcium in the wall of an artery.

polyunsaturated fat—A fat containing several double bonds. Found in safflower, sunflower, and corn oils. Can lower LDL cholesterol when substituted for saturated fat in the diet.

saturated fat—A fat that contains the maximum possible amount of hydrogen atoms. Includes most animal and dairy fats and some oils, such as palm and coconut oils. A major dietary factor in raising blood cholesterol.

statins—The most popular class of cholesterol-lowering drugs. Also known as HMG-CoA reductase inhibitors, statins are the most effective medications for lowering total and LDL cholesterol levels.

systolic blood pressure—The upper number in a blood pressure reading. The pressure in the arteries when the heart is pumping blood.

trans fats—Also called trans fatty acids, these fats are formed when food manufacturers add hydrogen atoms to unsaturated fats to make them more saturated and therefore more solid and shelf-stable. Found in margarines and store-bought baked goods. Trans fats raise blood cholesterol levels.

triglyceride—A lipid (fat) that is a storage form of energy. High levels of triglycerides in the blood contribute to atherosclerosis.

ventricles—The two chambers in the lower part of the heart. The left ventricle receives blood from the left atrium and pumps it to the rest of the body; the right ventricle receives blood from the right atrium and pumps it to the lungs.

very–low-density lipoprotein (VLDL)—A protein that is the major carrier of triglycerides in the bloodstream.

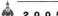

HEALTH INFORMATION ORGANIZATIONS AND SUPPORT GROUPS

American College of Cardiology
9111 Old Georgetown Rd.
Bethesda, MD 20814-1699
☎ 800-253-4636/301-897-5400
www.acc.org
Professional medical society and teaching institution that provides professional education, promotes research, offers leadership in the development of standards and guidelines, and forms health care policy.

American Dietetic Association
120 S. Riverside Plaza, Ste. 2000
Chicago, IL 60606-6995
☎ 800-366-1655/312-899-0040
www.eatright.org
Provides recorded nutrition messages, helps consumers locate registered dietitians for counseling, and provides answers to food and nutrition questions related to heart-healthy eating.

American Heart Association
7272 Greenville Ave.
Dallas, TX 75231
☎ 800-242-8721
www.americanheart.org
National health organization that provides information and public education programs on all aspects of heart disease. Check for local chapters.

Centers for Disease Control and Prevention
1600 Clifton Rd.
Atlanta, GA 30333
☎ 800-311-3435/404-639-3534
www.cdc.gov
Federal agency that develops and implements programs in chronic disease prevention. It provides fact sheets and guidelines (available printed and online) related to heart disease as well as information on state programs aimed at preventing heart disease.

National Heart, Lung, and Blood Institute Information Center
P.O. Box 30105
Bethesda, MD 20824-0105
☎ 800-575-WELL/301-592-8573
www.nhlbi.nih.gov/health/infoctr/index.htm
Branch of the National Institutes of Health that provides written information on all heart-related issues.

LEADING HOSPITALS FOR CARDIOLOGY AND HEART SURGERY

U.S. News & World Report and the National Opinion Research Center, a social-science research group at the University of Chicago, recently conducted their 15th annual nationwide survey of 8,160 board-certified physicians in 17 medical specialties. The doctors nominated the hospitals that they considered to be the best from among 6,012 U.S. medical centers. This is the current list of the best hospitals for cardiology and heart surgery, as determined by a combination of factors: doctors' recommendations from 2002, 2003, and 2004; federal death rates; and factual data regarding quality indicators, such as the ratio of registered nurses to patients and use of advanced technology. However, because the results reflect the doctors' opinions to some extent, they are partly subjective. Any institution listed is considered a leading center, and the rankings do not imply that other hospitals cannot or do not deliver excellent care.

1. Cleveland Clinic
Cleveland, OH
☎ 800-223-2273/216-444-2200
www.clevelandclinic.org

2. Mayo Clinic
Rochester, MN
☎ 507-284-2511
www.mayoclinic.org

3. Duke University Medical Center
Durham, NC
☎ 919-684-8111
www.mc.duke.edu

4. Johns Hopkins Hospital
Baltimore, MD
☎ 410-955-5000
www.hopkinsmedicine.org

5. Massachusetts General Hospital
Boston, MA
☎ 617-726-2000
www.mgh.harvard.edu

6. Brigham and Women's Hospital
Boston, MA
☎ 617-732-5500
www.brighamandwomens.org

7. New York-Presbyterian Hospital
New York, NY
☎ 212-746-5454
www.nyp.org

8. Emory University Hospital
Atlanta, GA
☎ 800-75-EMORY/
   404-778-7777
www.emoryhealthcare.org

**9. Texas Heart Institute at
St. Luke's Episcopal Hospital**
Houston, TX
☎ 800-292-2221
www.texasheartinstitute.org

10. Stanford Hospital and Clinics
Stanford, CA
☎ 650-723-4000
www.stanfordhospital.com

Source: *U.S. News & World Report,* July 12, 2004.

FISH INTAKE AND HEART DISEASE

Fish consumption has been linked to a reduced risk of coronary heart disease (CHD), but not all studies support this association, and others don't have enough statistical power to provide a definitive answer. The report reprinted here from *The American Journal of Cardiology*—an analysis of 19 studies including a total of nearly 230,000 people—suggests that eating fish regularly can indeed cut CHD risk.

The authors from Tulane University in New Orleans searched the medical literature for CHD risk studies that compared people who regularly consumed fish with those who rarely or never ate fish. They used statistical techniques to pool data from the studies and calculate the relationship between fish consumption and fatal and nonfatal CHD.

Eating fish appeared to reduce the risk of fatal CHD by about 17% and the risk of CHD in general by 14%, the researchers found. They theorize that fish may be especially effective at reducing the risk of fatal CHD because the omega-3 fatty acids contained in fish appear to have a special protective effect against sudden cardiac death by preventing abnormal heart rhythms.

The benefit appeared to be greatest for people who ate two to four servings of fish each week. A possible explanation for why people who consumed four or more servings of fish weekly benefited less than those consuming more modest amounts is that certain types of fish contain mercury, which can counteract the heart-protective power of omega-3s.

The findings also indicated that eating fish is slightly more protective for women than for men.

"These findings suggest that fish consumption may be an important component of lifestyle modification for the prevention of coronary CHD," the researchers conclude.

REPRINT

Meta-Analysis of Observational Studies on Fish Intake and Coronary Heart Disease

Seamus Paul Whelton, AB, Jiang He, MD, PhD, Paul Kieran Whelton, MD, MSc, and
Paul Muntner, PhD

Fish consumption has been associated with a lower risk of coronary heart disease (CHD) in some but not all studies. We conducted a meta-analysis of observational studies to determine if fish consumption is associated with lower fatal and total CHD. English language articles published before May 2003 were searched. In all, 19 observational studies (14 cohort and 5 case-control) in which there was a group that consumed fish on a regular basis and a comparison group that consumed little or no fish were included. With use of a standardized protocol and data extraction form, information on study design, sample size, participant characteristics, duration of follow-up, assessment of end points, and consumption of fish was abstracted. Using a random effects model, we pooled data from each study. Fish consumption versus little to no fish consumption was associated with a relative risk of 0.83 (95% confidence interval 0.76 to 0.90; $p < 0.005$) for fatal CHD and a relative risk of 0.86 (95% confidence interval 0.81 to 0.92; $p < 0.005$) for total CHD. The results indicate that fish consumption is associated with a significantly lower risk of fatal and total CHD. These findings suggest that fish consumption may be an important component of lifestyle modification for the prevention of CHD. ©2004 by Excerpta Medica, Inc.

(Am J Cardiol 2004;93:1119–1123)

A number of observational studies have examined the association between sh consumption and risk of coronary heart disease (CHD), but most of them have not had sufcient statistical power to provide convincing evidence for the presence or absence of the association. Therefore, the overall evidence for such a relation remains uncertain and controversial. Pooled results from patient studies may provide a clearer understanding of the relation between sh consumption and CHD.

METHODS

Selection of studies: A comprehensive literature search of the MEDLINE database (1966 through April 2003) was conducted using the following Medical Subject Headings (MeSH): shes, fatty acids, omega-3, sh products, sh oils, coronary disease, and myocardial infarction. In addition, a manual search of citations from relevant original studies and review articles was performed. Only studies that were published as full-length, English language manuscripts were considered. Initially, 57 articles were identied and reviewed according to predetermined selection criteria.

To be included in the analysis, studies had to have (1) been conducted in adult humans, (2) used an observational case-control or cohort study design, (3) compared a group that consumed sh on a regular basis with a group that consumed little or no sh, (4) used CHD as an outcome, and (5) reported an association in the form of a relative risk (RR), hazard ratio (HR), or odds ratio (OR) of CHD by category of sh consumption.

Nineteen studies (14 cohort and 5 case-control) that met our prestated inclusion criteria provided the data for the current meta-analysis. Major reasons for exclusion were that CHD was not reported as an end point, there were insufcient data regarding sh consumption, or the study did not use a cohort or case-control design. One included study used primary cardiac arrest as the end point. Although there are a number of possible factors that can result in primary cardiac arrest, CHD is usually an underlying cause.

Data abstraction: The data were abstracted using a standardized protocol and reporting form. The following recorded study characteristics included (1) rst investigators name, (2) publication year, (3) number of participants, (4) mean age and age range, (5) race and gender distribution of the study population, (6) type of study design (cohort or case-control), (7) definition of the end points, (8) diagnosis of the end points, (9) measure of sh intake, (10) duration of follow-up, (11) control selection for case-control studies, (12) covariables for match or adjustments in multivariate models, (13) categories of sh consumption, and (14) RR/HR/OR and the 95% condence interval (CI) for CHD associated with sh consumption.

Statistical analysis: For cohort studies, the RR or HR was used as a measure of the relation between sh consumption and CHD. For case-control studies, the OR was used as a surrogate measure of RR, because the absolute risk of CHD was low in each of the studies, a situation in which the OR should provide an accurate estimate of RR. RRs, HRs, and ORs from

From Tulane University School of Public Health and Tropical Medicine, and School of Medicine, New Orleans, Louisiana. Manuscript received September 26, 2003; revised manuscript received and accepted January 15, 2004.

Address for reprints: Jiang He, MD, PhD, Department of Epidemiology, Tulane University School of Public Health and Tropical Medicine, 1440 Canal Street, Street 20, SL-18, New Orleans, Louisiana 70112.

TABLE 1 Characteristics of 14 Cohort Studies of Fish Consumption and Risk of Coronary Heart Disease (CHD)*

Author (yr)	Location	Population Gender	Age (yrs)	CHD End Point	Events	Deaths	Outcome Definition	Follow-up (yrs)
Kromhout et al, 1985	Netherlands	852 men	40–59	Fatal		78	Ischemic heart disease[†]	20
Dolecek et al, 1991	USA	6,400 men	35–57	Fatal		175	Ischemic heart disease	6–8
Ascherio et al, 1995	USA	44,895 men	40–75	Fatal and total	1,543	264	Fatal CHD, nonfatal MI, coronary artery bypass, or angioplasty	6
Kromhout et al, 1995	Netherlands	272 men and women	64–87	Fatal		58	Ischemic heart disease	17
Salonen et al, 1995	Finland	1,833 men	42–60	Fatal and total	73	18	Ischemic heart disease	5
Rodriguez et al, 1996	USA (Hawaii)	3,310 men	45–68	Fatal			Fatal CHD	23
Daviglus et al, 1997	USA	1,822 men	40–55	Fatal		430	Ischemic heart disease	30
Pietinen et al, 1997	Finland	21,930 men	50–69	Fatal and total	1,399	635	Ischemic heart disease	5–8
Albert et al, 1998	USA	20,551 men	40–84	Fatal and total	737	308	Ischemic heart disease	11
Gillum et al, 2000	USA	8,825 men and women	22–74	Total	862		Ischemic heart disease	19
Oomen et al, 2000	Finland, Italy, Netherlands	2,738 men	50–69	Fatal		463	Ischemic heart disease	20
Yuan et al, 2001	China	18,244 men	45–64	Fatal		113	Ischemic heart disease	12
Hu et al, 2002	USA	84,688 women	30–55	Fatal and total	1,513	484	MI based on WHO criteria[‡]	16
Osler et al, 2003	Denmark	7,540 men and women	30–70	Fatal and total	491	247	Ischemic heart disease	8–18

*Total CHD includes fatal and nonfatal CHD.
[†]Ischemic heart disease: defined by ICD8/ICD9 codes 410–414.
[‡]World Health Organization (WHO) criteria: symptoms in addition to either diagnostic electrocardiographic changes or elevated cardiac enzyme levels.
MI = myocardial infarction.

each study were transformed by taking the natural logarithm, and the SE was back-calculated from the reported CIs. In 1 study, p values were used to calculate the SE of the RR.[1]

The studies included in this meta-analysis reported sh consumption using different measurement units (e.g., grams of sh per day, servings of sh per day, or grams of omega-3 consumed per day). Among the 19 studies included in the analysis, 9 reported sh consumption according to the number of servings of sh,[1–10]7 reported it as the number of grams of sh consumed,[11–17]and 3 reported it as grams of omega-3 consumed.[18–20]In consultation with a registered dietian, a serving size of sh was deemed to be 114 g (4 oz) in studies that reported grams of sh consumed. A mean value of 0.66 g of omega-3 per serving of sh was calculated using conversion values from the studies that reported grams of omega-3 consumed.[1,5,8,10,17,20] With use of these conversion factors, the quantity of sh consumed for each study was analyzed based on the number of servings per week.

Nine studies reported sh consumption as servings per week or servings per day. The value assigned to each category of sh consumption was the mean of the upper and lower bounds of that grouping. An upper bound was not reported for the highest sh consumption categories. To allocate a mean value, the group was assigned the same scale of sh consumption as the preceding group.

Fixed- and random-effect models were used to estimate pooled effects sizes. Both models yielded similar estimates. In this study, we chose to present results based on use of the random-effects model,

because a Dersimonian Q test identied signicant heterogeneity among the studies.

A series of prestated subgroup analyses were performed to examine any differences in the association between sh intake and CHD risk by covariables. The subgroups were chosen on the basis of biologic plausibility and a desire to recognize any variation attributable to differences in study design. For each subgroup, the pooled-effects estimate is reported using a random-effects model. Two studies with >75% male participants were included in the male subgroups for total CHD calculations.[14,20]

RESULTS

Characteristics of participants and study design: Characteristics for the 19 studies and their participants are presented in Tables 1 and 2. The studies published between 1985 and 2003 evaluated the experience of 228,864 participants. All of the studies were conducted in adults (aged 22 to 87 years). Nine studies included only men and 2 studies included only women, and the remaining studies included men and women (n = 8). Fish oil supplementation was reported in 1 study, but no more than 4% of the participants in this study took sh oil as a supplement. [1] Among the 8 studies for which average consumption of sh was reported, the mean intake of sh was 36 g/day or 2.2 servings per week.

A cohort design was used in 14 of the studies and a case-control design in the remaining 5. The 14 cohort studies varied in length of follow-up from 4 to 30 years (mean duration 14). The number of participants enrolled in the cohort studies ranged from 272 to

TABLE 2 Characteristics of Five Case-control Studies of Fish Consumption and Risk of Coronary Heart Disease (CHD)

Author (yr)	Location	Cases	Controls	Definition
Gramenzi et al, 1990	Italy	287 female patients hospitalized with MI	649 female patients hospitalized with an acute disorder unrelated to CHD	Hospitalization with acute MI
Siscovick et al, 1995	USA	334 men and women diagnosed with out-of-hospital primary cardiac arrest	493 male and female community controls matched for age and gender	Primary cardiac arrest
Sasazuki et al, 2001	Japan	660 men and women hospitalized with MI	1,214 male and female community controls matched for age, gender, and neighborhood	ECG/enzyme
Tavani et al, 2001	Italy	507 men and women hospitalized with MI	478 men and women hospitalized with an acute condition unrelated to CHD	Myocardial infarction based on WHO criteria*
Martinez-Gonzalez et al, 2002	Spain	171 men and women hospitalized with MI	171 men and women hospitalized with a disease unrelated to diet, and matched on gender, hospital, and time	Myocardial infarction based on WHO criteria*

*WHO criteria: symptoms in addition to either diagnostic electrocardiographic changes or elevated cardiac enzyme levels. Abbreviations as in Table 1.

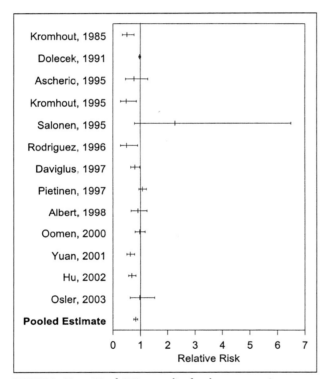

FIGURE 1. Mean RR of CHD mortality for those consuming any amount of fish versus control group in 13 cohort studies, and pooled estimate from random-effects model.

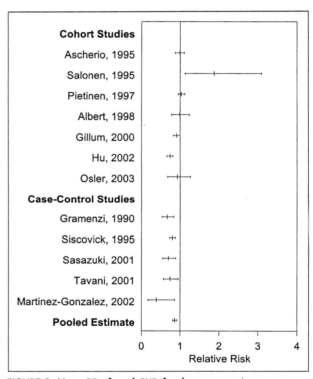

FIGURE 2. Mean RR of total CHD for those consuming any amount of fish versus control group in 6 cohort studies and 4 case-control studies, and pooled estimate from the random-effects model.

84,688 participants (mean 16,228). Among the 5 case-control studies, the number of cases ranged from 171 to 660 and the number of controls from 171 to 1,214.

Fatal and total CHD: In 6 cohort studies, sh consumption was associated with a statistically signicant reduction in fatal CHD, and in 1 cohort and 4 case-control studies, sh consumption was associated with a statistically signicant reduction in total CHD (Figures 1 and 2). The overall pooled estimate of the RR of fatal CHD for those consuming any amount of sh versus those consuming little to no sh was 0.83 (95% CI 0.76 to 0.90; p <0.005) (Table 3). The corresponding estimate for total CHD was 0.86 (95% CI 0.81 to 0.92; p <0.005).

Subgroup analysis: Table 4 summarizes the pooled estimates for sh consumption and CHD risk according to patient characteristics and study design. An inverse relation between sh consumption and fatal CHD was observed in all but 1 of the subgroups, with the caveat that this hypothesis could not be tested in case-control studies.

TABLE 3 Overall Relative Risk (RR) of Coronary Heart Disease (CHD) Associated With Fish Consumption Categorized by Level

Portions of fish per week	Fatal CHD			Total CHD		
	No. Study	RR (95% CI)	p Value	No. of Study	RR (95% CI)	p Value
Any	13	0.83 (0.76–0.90)	<0.005	12	0.86 (0.81–0.92)	<0.005
<2	9	0.83 (0.75–0.92)	<0.005	7	0.85 (0.80–0.91)	<0.005
2–<4	11	0.75 (0.62–0.92)	<0.01	9	0.83 (0.69–0.99)	<0.05
≥4	5	0.84 (0.63–1.10)	<0.15	7	0.84 (0.70–1.01)	<0.10

TABLE 4 Overall Relative Risk (RR) of Coronary Heart Disease (CHD) Associated With Any Fish Consumption According to Study Design and Characteristics of Participants

	Fatal CHD			Total CHD		
	No. Study	RR (95% CI)	p Value	No. Study	RR (95% CI)	p Value
Men	10	0.85 (0.77–0.94)	<0.01	8	0.93 (0.86–1.01)	<0.10
Women	1	0.69 (0.57–0.84)	<0.025	4	0.78 (0.71–0.87)	<0.01
Cohort	13	0.83 (0.76–0.90)	<0.005	7	0.93 (0.87–1.00)	<0.05
Case-control	0			5	0.77 (0.72–0.83)	<0.005
US	6	0.81 (0.72–0.91)	<0.01	5	0.86 (0.80–0.91)	<0.01
Non-US	7	0.82 (0.69–0.96)	<0.05	7	0.86 (0.74–1.01)	<0.10
Scandinavian	6	0.92 (0.77–1.09)	<0.20	3	1.06 (0.92–1.21)	>0.30
Non-Scandinavian	7	0.76 (0.68–0.86)	<0.005	9	0.83 (0.77–0.88)	<0.005

DISCUSSION

The present meta-analysis included 19 observational studies with 228,864 participants, representing a large and diverse population sample. Overall, the results of the study suggest that sh consumption is associated with an approximately 20% reduction in the risk of fatal CHD and a 10% reduction in total CHD. The apparent disparity in risk reduction between fatal and total CHD may merely reect much of the information for the 2 outcomes derived from different studies. Alternatively, the seemingly greater reduction in fatal CHD may be due to a special benecial effect of omega-3 fatty acids in reducing sudden cardiac death.[21] Omega-3 fatty acids have been reported to reduce the risk of sudden cardiac death by (1) increasing heart rate variability in survivors of myocardial infarction, (2) decreasing resting heart rate, and (3) reducing damage to cardiac tissue.[21]

The Diet And Reinfaction Trial (DART) is one of the few randomized controlled clinical trials that has been conducted to explore the efcacy of sh consumption in reducing the risk of CHD.[22] This secondary prevention trial was conducted in post—myocardial infarction survivors using a factorial design in which 1 group was advised to eat ≥2 portions of fatty sh per week, 1 group was encouraged to increase their consumption of dietary ber, 1 group was encouraged to reduce their intake of dietary fat and concurrently increase the ratio of the polyunsaturated to saturated fat content of their diet, and the control group was given general advice on eating a healthy diet. At the conclusion of a 2-year period of active intervention, sh consumption was observed to reduce CHD mortality risk by 30% (RR 0.70; 95% CI 0.54 to 0.92). At a subsequent evaluation, >10 years after the period of active intervention, this perceived benet was no longer apparent (RR 0.98; 95% CI 0.72 to 1.32). The investigators suggested that the lack of long-term ben-

et may have resulted from an observed reduction in sh consumption after cessation of the active intervention among the group advised to increase their intake of sh.[22] Compliance is an important challenge in long-term lifestyle modication trials and may be the primary reason that so few trials have been conducted on the efcacy of sh intake on cardiovascular disease. Although we recognize the internal validity of randomized controlled trials, observational studies allow for prolonged follow-up in more representative samples of the population.

The inverse relation that we noted between sh consumption and fatal CHD was more striking in those consuming 2 to ≤4 servings of sh per week than their counterparts who reported consuming <2 portions of sh per week. The higher RR of fatal CHD noted in those eating ≥4 servings of sh per week may have resulted from a corresponding increase in mercury consumption. Elevated blood mercury has been noted in persons who consume large quantities of sh, especially large sh (e.g., shark or swordsh), which are a known source of mercury.[16] As such, those who eat large quantities of sh are prone to consume a large amount of mercury.[23] This may result in their blood mercury concentration exceeding recommended levels, triggering an increased risk of CHD.[24] However, according to the US Food and Drug Administration, only a few varieties of commonly eaten sh contain signicant amounts of mercury.[25] Resolution of this question is unlikely until additional studies designed to investigate the inuence of mercury as a possible confounder, masking the benet of sh consumption on CHD, have been conducted.

However, it has been shown that sh from Finland have a high mercury content and this is likely true for all Scandinavian countries.[16,26] The results of our subgroup analysis show a nearly 20% reduction in fatal and total CHD for studies conducted in non-Scandinavian countries.

Our subgroup analysis suggests that sh consumption may have a slightly greater protective effect for women than for men, although the 95% CIs overlapped for men and women.

A limitation of the present analysis was its dependence on studies in which some of the comparison groups consumed sh. [6,14,15,17,27] However, inclusion of these studies would only tend to result in a more conservative estimate of the RR. As in any observational study investigating dietary factors, assessment of the exposure variable is likely to have been somewhat inaccurate, and some misclassification may have occurred in the assignment of consumption categories.

1. Ascherio A, Rimm EB, Stampfer MJ, Giovannucci EL, Willett WC. Dietary intake of marine n-3 fatty acids, sh intake, and the risk of coronary disease among men. N Engl J Med 1995;332:977—982.
2. Morris MC, Manson JE, Rosner B, Buring JE, Willett WC, Hennekens CH. Fish consumption and cardiovascular disease in the physicians health study: a prospective study. Am J Epidemiol 1995;142:166—175.
3. Gillum RF, Mussolino M, Madans JH. The relation between sh consumption, death from all causes, and incidence of coronary heart disease. the NHANES I epidemiologic follow-up study. J Clin Epidemiol 2000;53:237—244.
4. Gramenzi A, Gentile A, Fasoli M, Negri E, Parazzini F, La Vecchia C. Association between certain foods and risk of acute myocardial infarction in women. BMJ 1990;300:771—773.
5. Hu FB, Bronner L, Willett WC, Stampfer MJ, Rexrode KM, Albert CM, Hunter D, Manson JE. Fish and omega-3 fatty acid intake and risk of coronary heart disease in women. JAMA 2002;287:1815—1821.
6. Rodriguez BL, Sharp DS, Abbott RD, Burchel CM, Masaki K, Chyou PH, Huang B, Yano K, Curb JD. Fish intake may limit the increase in risk of coronary heart disease morbidity and mortality among heavy smokers. The Honolulu Heart Program. Circulation 1996;94:952—956.
7. Sasazuki S. Case-control study of nonfatal myocardial infarction in relation to selected foods in Japanese men and women. Jpn Circ J 2001;65:200—206.
8. Tavani A, Pelucchi C, Negri E, Bertuzzi M, La Vecchia C. n-3 Polyunsaturated fatty acids, sh, and nonfatal acute myocardial infarction. Circulation 2001;104:2269—2272.
9. Osler M, Andreasen AH, Hoidrup S. No inverse association between sh consumption and risk of death from all-causes, and incidence of coronary heart disease in middle-aged, Danish adults. J Clin Epidemiol 2003;56:274—279.
10. Albert CM, Hennekens CH, ODonnell CJ, Ajani UA, Carey VJ, Willett WC, Ruskin JN, Manson JE. Fish consumption and risk of sudden cardiac death. JAMA 1998;279:23—28.
11. Daviglus ML, Stamler J, Orencia AJ, Dyer AR, Liu K, Greenland P, Walsh MK, Morris D, Shekelle RB. Fish consumption and the 30-year risk of fatal myocardial infarction. N Engl J Med 1997;336:1046—1053.
12. Kromhout D, Bosschieter EB, de Lezenne Coulander C. The inverse relation between sh consumption and 20-year mortality from coronary heart disease. N Engl J Med 1985;312:1205—1209.
13. Kromhout D, Feskens EJ, Bowles CH. The protective effect of a small amount of sh on coronary heart disease mortality in an elderly population. Int J Epidemiol 1995;24:340—345.
14. Martinez-Gonzalez MA, Fernandez-Jarne E, Serrano-Martinez M, Marti A, Martinez JA, Martin-Moreno JM. Mediterranean diet and reduction in the risk of a rst acute myocardial infarction: an operational healthy dietary score. Eur J Nutr 2002;41:153—160.
15. Oomen CM, Feskens EJ, Rasanen L, Fidanza F, Nissinen AM, Menotti A, Kok FJ, Kromhout D. Fish consumption and coronary heart disease mortality in Finland, Italy, and The Netherlands. Am J Epidemiol 2000;151:999—1006.
16. Salonen JT, Seppanen K, Nyyssonen K, Korpela H, Kauhanen J, Kantola M, Tuomilehto J, Esterbauer H, Tatzber F, Salonen R. Intake of mercury from sh, lipid peroxidation, and the risk of myocardial infarction and coronary, cardiovascular, and any death in eastern Finnish men. Circulation 1995;91:645—655.
17. Yuan JM, Ross RK, Gao YT, Yu MC. Fish and shellsh consumption in relation to death from myocardial infarction among men in Shanghai, China. Am J Epidemiol 2001;154:809—816.
18. Dolecek TA, Granditis G. Dietary polyunsaturated fatty acids and mortality in the Multiple Risk Factor Intervention Trial (MRFIT). World Rev Nutr Diet 1991;66:205—216.
19. Pietinen P, Ascherio A, Korhonen P, Hartman AM, Willett WC, Albanes D, Virtamo J. Intake of fatty acids and risk of coronary heart disease in a cohort of Finnish men. The Alpha-Tocopherol, Beta-Carotene Cancer Prevention Study. Am J Epidemiol 1997;145:876—887.
20. Siscovick DS, Raghunathan TE, King I, Weinmann S, Wicklund KG, Albright J, Bovbjerg V, Arbogast P, Smith H, Kushi LH, et al. Dietary intake and cell membrane levels of long-chain n-3 polyunsaturated fatty acids and the risk of primary cardiac arrest. JAMA 1995;274:1363—1367.
21. Kris-Etherton PM, Harris WS, Appel LJ. Fish consumption, sh oil, omega-3 fatty acids, and cardiovascular disease. Circulation 2002;106:2747—2757.
22. Ness AR, Hughes J, Elwood PC, Whitley E, Smith GD, Burr ML. The long-term effect of dietary advice in men with coronary disease: follow-up of the Diet and Reinfarction trial (DART). Eur J Clin Nutr 2002;56:512—518.
23. Yoshizawa K, Rimm EB, Morris JS, Spate VL, Hsieh CC, Spiegelman D, Stampfer MJ, Willett WC. Mercury and the risk of coronary heart disease in men. N Engl J Med 2002;347:1755—1760.
24. Guallar E, Sanz-Gallardo MI, vant Veer P, Bode P, Aro A, Gomez-Aracena J, Kark JD, Riemersma RA, Martin-Moreno JM, Kok FJ. Mercury, sh oils, and the risk of myocardial infarction. N Engl J Med 2002;347:1747—1754.
25. USFDA. Mercury in sh: cause for concern?: FDA Consumer Magazine 1994.
26. Rissanen T, Voutilainen S, Nyyssonen K, Lakka TA, Salonen JT. Fish oil-derived fatty acids, docosahexaenoic acid and docosapentaenoic acid, and the risk of acute coronary events: the Kuopio ischaemic heart disease risk factor study. Circulation 2000;102:2677—2679.
27. Simonsen T, Nordoy A. Ischaemic heart disease, serum lipids and platelets in Norwegian populations with traditionally low or high sh consumption. J Intern Med Suppl 1989;225:83—89.

NOTES

NOTES

ISBN 1-933087-07-2
ISSN 1546-3672
Second Printing
Printed in the United States of America

Whelton, S.P. et al. "Meta-analysis of observational studies on fish intake and coronary heart disease." Reprinted with permission from *The American Journal of Cardiology* Vol. 93, No. 9 (May 1, 2004): 1119–1123. Copyright © 2004, Excerpta Medica.

The Johns Hopkins White Papers are published yearly by Medletter Associates, Inc.

Visit our Web site for information on Johns Hopkins Health After 50 publications, which include White Papers on specific disorders, home medical encyclopedias, consumer reference guides to drugs and medical tests, and our monthly newsletter The Johns Hopkins Medical Letter: Health After 50.
www.HopkinsAfter50.com

The Johns Hopkins White Papers

Paul Candon
Managing Editor

Catherine Richter
Senior Editor

Devon Schuyler
Consulting Editor

Kimberly Flynn
Writer/Researcher

Leslie Maltese-McGill
Copy Editor

Tim Jeffs
Art Director

Vincent Mejia
Graphic Designer

Betsy Meredith Rigo
Editorial Assistant

Robert Duckwall
Medical Illustrator

Kate Brackney
Intern

Johns Hopkins Health After 50 Publications

Rodney Friedman
Editor and Publisher

Thomas Dickey
Editorial Director

Tom Damrauer, M.L.S.
Chief of Information Resources

Jerry Loo
Product Manager

Darren Leiser
Promotions Coordinator

Joan Mullally
Head of Business Development

HYPERTENSION AND STROKE

Lawrence Appel, M.D.

and

Rafael H. Llinas, M.D.

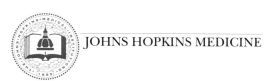
JOHNS HOPKINS MEDICINE

Dear Readers:

Hypertension is one of the most common disorders in the United States—affecting at least 65 million adults. It is also the most important risk factor for stroke and a major risk factor for heart attacks, heart failure, and kidney disease. This year's White Paper puts at your fingertips the latest findings and recommendations for the prevention and treatment of hypertension and stroke. By taking the right steps to avoid hypertension or detecting it early and treating it effectively, you can dramatically reduce your risk of stroke and other complications such as heart attacks, heart failure, and kidney disease.

Here are some of this year's highlights:

- **Over-the-counter drugs** that can raise blood pressure. (page 7)
- Find out whether you have **white coat hypertension**. (page 13)
- The newest recommendations for **salt and potassium** intake. (page 20)
- Why more people with high blood pressure should be taking **diuretics**. (page 24)
- The latest research on how certain B vitamins may **help prevent strokes**. (page 49)
- How to recognize and treat **depression** after a stroke. (page 60)
- The best time for surgery to clear **blocked carotid arteries** if you've had a stroke. (page 65)
- Long-lasting benefits: The importance of **arm rehabilitation** after a stroke. (page 68)

We hope that by learning more about these conditions, you will be able to reduce your blood pressure, stay healthy, and recover more quickly should a stroke occur.

Sincerely,

Lawrence Appel, M.D.
Professor
Departments of Medicine, Epidemiology,
  and International Health

Rafael H. Llinas, M.D.
Assistant Professor
Department of Neurology

P.S. Don't forget to visit HopkinsWhitePapers.com for the latest news on hypertension and stroke and other information that will complement your Johns Hopkins White Paper.

THE AUTHORS

Lawrence Appel, M.D., received his M.D. from the New York University School of Medicine and performed his residency at Baltimore City Hospital. He is a professor at the Johns Hopkins University School of Medicine, with adjunct appointments in the departments of epidemiology and international health (human nutrition division) of the Johns Hopkins Bloomberg School of Public Health. He is also a practicing internist.

Dr. Appel's clinical research is focused on the prevention of hypertension and cardiovascular and kidney diseases, through both nonpharmacological and pharmacological approaches. He has served on several national policy-making bodies, including the National Heart, Lung, and Blood Institute Primary Prevention of Hypertension Working Group, the Nutrition Committee of the American Heart Association, the Institute of Medicine Committee on Dietary Reference Intakes for Water, Sodium Chloride, Potassium, and Sulfate, and the U.S. Department of Agriculture/Health and Human Services Dietary Guidelines Scientific Advisory Committee.

■ ■ ■

Rafael H. Llinas, M.D., received his B.A. from Washington University in St. Louis and his M.D. from the New York University School of Medicine. He completed his residency in neurology at the Harvard Longwood Program based at the Brigham and Women's Hospital. He also completed a two-year fellowship in cerebrovascular medicine at the Beth Israel Hospital in Boston. Currently he is an assistant professor of neurology and the director of cerebrovascular neurology at the Johns Hopkins Bayview Medical Center. He also serves on the Johns Hopkins acute stroke team.

Dr. Llinas is a member of the American Heart Association stroke division and the Maryland stroke task force. His research interests include neurosonology, diffusion/perfusion imaging, the use of neuroprotective agents, and secondary stroke prevention. He has published articles in such journals as *Stroke, Neurology,* and *Progress in Cardiovascular Diseases.*

CONTENTS

Hypertension

What Is Blood Pressure? . . . . .p. 1

Causes of Hypertension . . . . .p. 4

Symptoms and Signs of Hypertension . . . . .p. 6

Classifying Blood Pressure . . . . .p. 8

      Systolic vs. Diastolic Pressure, White Coat Hypertension

Complications of Hypertension . . . . .p. 11

Prevention of Hypertension . . . . .p. 12

Diagnosis of Hypertension . . . . .p. 13

      Home Monitoring of Blood Pressure, Ambulatory Blood Pressure Monitoring,

      Medical Evaluation of Blood Pressure

Treatment of Hypertension . . . . .p. 18

      Lifestyle Modifications, Medication, The J-curve, Medical Follow-up

Stroke

The Brain's Blood Supply . . . . .p. 35

What Is a Stroke? . . . . .p. 35

Types of Stroke . . . . .p. 36

      Ischemic Stroke, Hemorrhagic Stroke

Symptoms of Stroke . . . . .p. 40

Effects of Stroke . . . . .p. 40

      The Brain Stem, Cerebellum, and Limbic System; The Cerebrum; Other Consequences

Risk Factors for Stroke . . . . .p. 43

      Risk Factors That Cannot Be Changed, Risk Factors That Can Be Changed

Prevention of Stroke . . . . .p. 48

      Antiplatelet Therapy, Anticoagulants, Carotid Endarterectomy, Angioplasty and Stents

Diagnosis of Stroke . . . . .p. 57

      Patient History, Physical Examination, Laboratory Tests, Imaging Techniques

Acute Treatment of Stroke . . . . .p. 62

      Treatment of Ischemic Stroke, Treatment of Hemorrhagic Stroke

Stroke Rehabilitation . . . . .p. 67

Chart: Antihypertensive Drugs . . . . .p. 28

Chart: Antiplatelet and Anticoagulant Drugs . . . . .p. 52

Glossary . . . . .p. 70

Health Information Organizations and Support Groups . . . . .p. 74

Leading Hospitals . . . . .p. 75

Selected Medical Journal Article . . . . .p. 76

Hypertension (high blood pressure) is one of the most prevalent disorders in the United States and the most important risk factor for stroke. Stroke is the third leading cause of death in the United States and the leading cause of disability. Because of the close relationship between hypertension and stroke, both topics are addressed in this White Paper.

Hypertension

Hypertension is diagnosed when blood pressure readings are 140/90 mm Hg or higher on at least two doctor visits. At least 65 million Americans have hypertension, and 9 out of 10 middle-aged people will eventually develop the condition. Although hypertension may not produce symptoms, it is a serious condition and is a primary cause of stroke, coronary heart disease, heart failure, kidney disease, and blindness. Fortunately, in most cases, hypertension is easily detected and usually controllable with lifestyle modifications (such as diet and exercise) and medication.

WHAT IS BLOOD PRESSURE?

Blood pressure is the amount of tension that blood exerts on the walls of blood vessels as it travels through the circulatory system. Blood does not travel through the circulatory system in a steady stream; instead, it is pushed through the blood vessels with every heartbeat. Each time the heart contracts—a period known as *systole*—blood pressure rises as more blood is forced through the arteries. Each systole is followed by a moment of relaxation, or *diastole,* when blood pressure drops as the heart refills with blood and rests before its next contraction.

Thus, pressure in the arteries rises and falls with each heartbeat. For this reason, blood pressure readings include two values: Systolic pressure, the higher number, corresponds with the peak pressure in the arteries when the heart contracts; diastolic pressure, the lower number, reflects the lowest pressure in the arteries as the heart relaxes.

Blood pressure fluctuates throughout the day under the direct influence of three parts of the body: the heart, arteries, and kidneys.

NEW RESEARCH

One Third of U.S. Adults Have Hypertension

The number of Americans with hypertension shot up during the 1990s, with nearly one third of all adults now affected by the condition, according to government researchers.

Based on data from a periodic federal health survey, the researchers estimated that in the years 1999 to 2000, at least 65 million U.S. adults had high blood pressure—an increase of roughly 30% since the period from 1988 to 1994. Overall, more women than men had hypertension, and black adults were disproportionately affected.

According to the researchers, part of the reason for the jump in hypertension cases may be that improved treatment is helping more people to avoid potentially fatal complications such as heart attack and stroke. However, they also point out that hypertension cases have risen in tandem with obesity and waning exercise rates.

Because hypertension contributes to heart disease, stroke, and kidney damage, the rising prevalence of high blood pressure bodes ill for the rates of those diseases as well, the researchers note. The findings, they conclude, underscore the need for better prevention and management of high blood pressure in the United States.

HYPERTENSION
Volume 44, page 398
October 2004

The heart can lower or raise blood pressure by varying the strength of each heartbeat. During exercise, for example, the heart beats faster and more forcefully to raise blood pressure and deliver extra oxygen and nutrients to the muscles. On the other hand, blood pressure drops as the heart slows during sleep. Small arteries are encircled by smooth muscle cells that allow these arteries to expand (dilate) or narrow (constrict). Dilation of small arteries decreases blood pressure, while constriction of these arteries increases blood pressure. The kidneys affect blood pressure by increasing or decreasing the amount of sodium and water excreted in the urine, which affects the volume of blood in the arteries.

The heart, arteries, and kidneys control blood pressure through an elaborate network of nerves and hormones. Special nerve endings (baroreceptors) in the walls of arteries monitor blood pressure. When pressure increases, the artery walls stretch and the baroreceptors signal the central nervous system to lower the pressure. Blood pressure is similarly monitored in the kidneys, specifically in the glomeruli where blood is filtered.

Three major hormones act in concert to regulate blood pressure: renin, angiotensin, and aldosterone. Renin is an enzyme produced by cells in the kidney; it acts on angiotensinogen, a protein secreted by the liver, to form angiotensin I. As blood flows through the lungs, angiotensin I is transformed into angiotensin II, which raises blood pressure by causing arteries to constrict. (Renin and angiotensinogen are also manufactured in artery walls and other organs, where they constrict blood vessels to control blood pressure locally.)

Angiotensin II also stimulates the release of aldosterone from the adrenal glands, which are located above each kidney. Aldosterone increases blood pressure by signaling the kidneys to retain sodium, which increases both the volume of blood and the amount of blood pumped by the heart. The resulting rise in blood pressure then signals the kidneys to stop secreting renin.

Other hormones also affect blood pressure. Epinephrine (adrenaline) and norepinephrine increase blood pressure in times of stress. Calcitriol (formed from dietary vitamin D) constricts small arteries, while parathyroid hormone dilates them. These two hormones are released in response to changes in the amount of calcium in the blood. However, the exact role of calcitriol and parathyroid hormone in the development of hypertension is unclear.

Atrial natriuretic factor, nitric oxide, and endothelin are additional substances involved in the regulation of blood pressure. Atrial natriuretic factor, produced by the atrium of the heart, causes the

How the Body Regulates Blood Pressure

Every tissue in the body requires a constant supply of blood to receive the oxygen and nutrients essential for metabolism and to carry away waste products. In order to meet these needs, the heart pumps blood throughout the body via a complex network of blood vessels.

Because blood must circulate through some 60,000 miles of vessels, a certain amount of force is needed to keep it moving. Blood pressure is a measurement of the force that the blood exerts on the inner walls of the large arteries—the force that maintains a continuous flow of blood.

The exact level of blood pressure required for circulation varies according to the body's demand for blood flow: In general, pressure is lower while a person is resting, and rises with increased activity or stress. These changes in blood pressure are partially governed by the heart, the kidneys, and the arteries themselves (see the illustration below). An intricate system of hormones and nerves continually monitors the body's needs and signals the heart, kidneys, and arteries to adjust the blood pressure accordingly.

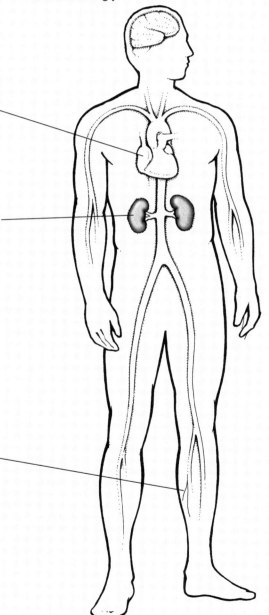

Heart
The rate and force of heart contractions can alter blood pressure: The faster and harder the heart beats, the greater the blood pressure.

Kidneys
The kidneys can alter the blood volume (amount of blood in circulation) by increasing or decreasing their excretion of sodium from the body (which adjusts the amount of water retention). The larger the blood volume, the higher the blood pressure. Plus, the kidney enzyme renin can produce hormones that constrict small arteries and cause sodium retention—which both raise blood pressure.

Small arteries
The small arteries (called arterioles) can adjust blood pressure by altering their diameter. They raise blood pressure by narrowing (constricting) and lower it by widening (dilating).

kidneys to excrete more sodium (and thus more water) and inhibits aldosterone and renin production. Nitric oxide, secreted by the endothelial cells that line blood vessel walls, relaxes smooth muscle cells and causes the arteries to dilate. Endothelin, a hormone released by endothelial cells, causes blood vessels to constrict.

Normally, this complex regulatory system allows blood pressure to rise and fall as needed while staying within a desirable range. In many people, however, abnormalities in this system lead to chronically elevated blood pressure, or hypertension.

CAUSES OF HYPERTENSION

In 90% to 95% of people, it is difficult to pinpoint the exact cause of hypertension. In these individuals, the condition is called primary hypertension. Primary hypertension often results from one or more of the following factors.

Dietary salt. Diets high in salt (sodium chloride) may raise blood pressure in two ways. One, by causing the body to retain water, salt increases blood volume and thus blood pressure. Two, salt causes vascular smooth muscle to constrict small blood vessels, which produces a greater resistance to blood flow.

Dietary potassium. A diet low in potassium tends to increase blood pressure. Conversely, increased potassium intake blunts the effects of dietary salt on blood pressure

Other dietary factors. Diets low in fruits, vegetables, and dairy products and high in fat and cholesterol raise blood pressure. In addition, overweight and obese people have higher blood pressure levels than people without weight problems. Alcohol intake beyond moderate levels (two drinks per day for men and a drink a day for women) raises blood pressure.

Metabolic syndrome. This cluster of health problems—obesity, hypertension, high triglyceride levels, low high-density lipoprotein (HDL) cholesterol levels, and elevated blood glucose (sugar) levels—occurs in about one in four Americans and in 40% of those age 60 and older. Obesity, especially a significant accumulation of fat in the abdomen, initiates the abnormalities of this syndrome by decreasing the body's ability to respond to the actions of insulin, a hormone that regulates blood glucose levels. To overcome this effect, the pancreas increases its production of insulin, and blood levels of insulin rise. Elevated blood insulin levels heighten the activity of the sympathetic nervous system and cause sodium retention by the kidneys—both of which raise blood pressure.

NEW RESEARCH

Thick Waist May Predict Blood Pressure Risk

Where people carry their weight may be more important than how much the scale says they weigh, when it comes to high blood pressure, study findings suggest.

The study of 592 Brazilian adults found that men and women who were obese based on their waistline circumference were 70% to 80% more likely than their leaner peers to develop high blood pressure over about five years. In contrast, when researchers defined obesity based on body mass index (BMI)—a measure of weight in relation to height—the link between obesity and hypertension disappeared among men.

These findings are in line with research suggesting that people who are "apple-shaped" may face a greater risk of high blood pressure, high cholesterol levels, and diabetes—even when their BMI is normal. They also add to a large body of evidence showing that abdominal obesity is a threat to overall health, the study authors note.

Considering how simple it is to measure the waistline, the authors conclude, obesity based on waist circumference—and not BMI— should be used to gauge a person's odds of developing high blood pressure. According to National Institutes of Health guidelines, a waist measurement of more than 40 inches for men or more than 35 inches for women denotes obesity.

AMERICAN JOURNAL OF HYPERTENSION
Volume 17, page 50
January 2004

Genetics. Studies of twins and other members of the same family show that primary hypertension has a genetic component. In addition, researchers have identified a number of genetic mutations that result in inherited forms of hypertension. These mutations, however, account for only a small number of cases of hypertension. Future research may identify additional mutations that are associated with more common forms of hypertension.

Lack of exercise. Physical inactivity can lead to hypertension in several ways. It increases the activity of the sympathetic nervous system, increases the stiffness of the arteries, decreases the release of hormones (such as nitric oxide) that cause arteries to dilate, and reduces the body's ability to respond to insulin.

Secondary Hypertension

When hypertension has an identifiable cause, it is called secondary hypertension. About 5% of people with hypertension fall into this category. Secondary hypertension can be caused by a number of health conditions and medications. It is important to identify secondary causes of hypertension because the resulting high blood pressure can often be cured or controlled by eliminating the underlying problem.

Kidney disorders. Kidney disease that progresses to kidney failure almost always results in hypertension owing to the excessive retention of sodium and water in the body. In addition, narrowing of the arteries that supply blood to one or both kidneys, and the resulting reduction in blood flow to the kidneys, causes a form of high blood pressure called renovascular hypertension. In this disorder, the affected kidney senses an inadequate blood supply and secretes excessive amounts of renin, which initiates a chain of events that raises blood pressure. In many people, renovascular hypertension can be cured or controlled by surgical repair of the narrowed arteries.

Adrenal tumors. Three types of adrenal tumors can cause hypertension: primary aldosteronism, Cushing's syndrome, and pheochromocytoma. In primary aldosteronism, overproduction of aldosterone leads to hypertension. In Cushing's syndrome, the tumor secretes excessive amounts of cortisone and related hormones, which raise blood pressure and cause a number of other problems. Treatment of primary aldosteronism and Cushing's syndrome is complicated and does not always lower blood pressure. In pheochromocytoma, the tumor secretes large amounts of epinephrine or norepinephrine, which can cause hypertension. Removal of the

NEW RESEARCH

Blood Pressure Rises With Age, Few Treated

According to international surveys, a substantial number of adults worldwide have hypertension. However, many don't realize they have the condition and are not being treated for their high blood pressure.

As part of their investigation, researchers reviewed surveys collected from adults in North America, Europe, Australia, Asia, and Africa. In all of these countries, the risk of hypertension gradually increased with age, and most adults had developed hypertension by age 60.

The data also revealed that more than a quarter of U.S. adults with hypertension do not realize that they have the condition. Furthermore, only half were being treated for hypertension with antihypertensive medication, and less than a third who were on antihypertensive drugs had lowered their blood pressure below 140/90 mm Hg.

These findings, the authors write, suggest that hypertension is a worldwide problem and that more effort needs to be made to prevent hypertension in the first place and to ensure that people with the condition receive appropriate treatment.

JOURNAL OF HUMAN HYPERTENSION
Volume 18, page 545
August 2004

tumor may cure the hypertension.

Other hormone problems. Over- or underproduction of thyroid hormone (hyperthyroidism or hypothyroidism, respectively), excessive release of growth hormone by a tumor in the pituitary gland, or increased blood calcium levels due to a tumor in the parathyroid gland can all cause hypertension.

Coarctation of the aorta. In this condition, a portion of the aorta narrows, resulting in hypertension in the upper body and low blood pressure in the abdomen and legs. This disorder is the most common cause of secondary hypertension in young people and can be corrected with surgery.

Sleep apnea. People with this disorder stop breathing periodically during sleep. The interruptions in breathing are the result of a temporary blockage of the airway by tissues at the back of the throat. Studies show that people with sleep apnea are more likely to develop hypertension, and the risk rises with the severity of the apnea. Fortunately, treatment of sleep apnea with continuous positive airway pressure, a device that pumps air at high pressure through the nose to keep the airway open, can significantly reduce blood pressure.

Drugs. The following prescription medications can raise blood pressure: corticosteroids such as prednisone (Deltasone and other brands); cyclosporine (Sandimmune, Neoral); tacrolimus (Prograf); epoetin (Epogen and Procrit); and nonsteroidal anti-inflammatory drugs (NSAIDs) such as indomethacin (Indocin) and celecoxib (Celebrex). Some over-the-counter remedies can also elevate blood pressure. These include pain relievers like ibuprofen (Advil, Motrin, and other brands) and naproxen (Aleve), nasal decongestants, and weight loss products containing caffeine (for a complete list of over-the-counter remedies that can elevate blood pressure, see the feature on the opposite page). Illegal drugs such as cocaine and amphetamines can increase blood pressure as well.

SYMPTOMS AND SIGNS OF HYPERTENSION

Most people with hypertension experience no symptoms, and as a result the condition may go undetected for many years. Some individuals complain of symptoms, such as headaches, but most often hypertension is discovered during a routine physical examination or, less commonly, when a patient experiences one of the complications of hypertension. These complications include transient ischemic attack (TIA), stroke, visual abnormalities, angina, heart attack, heart failure, intermittent claudication (pain in the leg

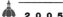
Over-the-Counter Drugs That Can Raise Blood Pressure

If you have hypertension, your doctor will avoid prescribing certain medications that are known to raise blood pressure. (See the text at left for examples of these medications.) Many people, though, are not aware that some over-the-counter medications—such as pain relievers, nasal decongestants, and weight loss products containing caffeine—can also increase blood pressure. In fact, a recent study of 51 older adults on blood pressure-lowering medication found that 37% had taken a potentially harmful pain reliever in the previous month.

Most of these over-the-counter products carry labels indicating that they are not to be used by people with high blood pressure, but not everyone reads or heeds these warnings. Some people with well controlled hypertension may be able to take these medications safely for short periods of time, but only your doctor can make that determination. In most cases, a safer treatment is available. For specific alternatives, see the chart below.

Product Type	Problem Ingredient	Brand Names	Effects	Alternatives
Decongestants (pills and syrups)	Pseudoephedrine or phenylephrine	Advil Cold & Sinus, Contac, and Sudafed (among others)	Constrict small arteries in the nose to relieve nasal congestion, but this effect occurs throughout the rest of the body as well. Constriction of arteries can elevate blood pressure.	Saline nasal sprays constrict arteries in the nose only and are safer for people with high blood pressure. Also, at least one line of cold medications (brand name Coricidin HBP) is considered safe for people with high blood pressure.
Pain relievers	Aspirin, ibuprofen, naproxen, ketoprofen	Advil, Motrin, Aleve, and Orudis KT (among others)	Cause the body to retain sodium and water, which can raise blood pressure.	Acetaminophen (Tylenol and other brands) does not affect blood pressure.
Diet pills	Caffeine	Dexatrim and Acutrim (among others)	Caffeine is a stimulant that can raise blood pressure. Diet pills used to contain phenylpropanolamine (PPA) or ephedrine, both of which also raised blood pressure but have been banned by the FDA.	None; instead, talk to your doctor about lifestyle changes (calorie restriction and an exercise program) to help you lose weight safely.
Antacids	Sodium bicarbonate	Alenic, Alka-Seltzer, Gavison, and Genaton (among others)	The sodium can raise blood pressure in some people.	Antacids with active ingredients other than sodium bicarbonate (such as calcium carbonate).

muscles associated with physical exertion), or kidney disease.

Another situation in which people may experience symptoms from hypertension is a hypertensive crisis. In a hypertensive crisis, blood pressure reaches extremely high levels (diastolic blood pressure above 120 mm Hg). This condition occurs in about 1% of people with hypertension—usually around age 40—and may be precipitated by an abrupt cessation of antihypertensive medication. There are two types of hypertensive crises: hypertensive emergency (also called malignant hypertension) and hypertensive urgency.

A hypertensive emergency produces one or more symptoms that indicate major damage is occurring to the body's organs. These symptoms include chest pain, shortness of breath, seizures, back pain, headache with confusion and blurred vision, nausea, vomiting, and unresponsiveness. When a hypertensive emergency is suspected, the affected person should not eat or drink anything and should lie down until he or she can be driven to the hospital or an ambulance arrives.

The more common form of hypertensive crisis—hypertensive urgency—does not result in symptoms indicative of major organ damage. Instead, headache and nosebleed are the two most common symptoms. Although this condition requires medical attention, treatment is not needed immediately. However, within a few hours of no treatment, a hypertensive urgency could become a hypertensive emergency.

CLASSIFYING BLOOD PRESSURE

Blood pressure levels used to be classified as optimal, normal, high-normal, and hypertension (stage 1, stage 2, and stage 3). But with the publication of the Seventh Report of the Joint National Committee on Prevention, Detection, Evaluation, and Treatment of High Blood Pressure—more commonly known as JNC 7—a new system of classifying blood pressure was adopted in 2003. This classification system has three categories: normal, prehypertension, and hypertension (stage 1 and stage 2).

Normal blood pressure. People with a blood pressure level less than 120/80 mm Hg have normal blood pressure.

Prehypertension. People with a systolic blood pressure between 120 and 139 mm Hg or a diastolic blood pressure between 80 and 89 mm Hg have a condition called prehypertension. About one in five Americans has prehypertension. These individuals are at increased risk for developing hypertension and hypertension complications such as heart attack and stroke. Lifestyle measures such as losing weight, eating a diet rich in fruits and vegetables, reducing salt intake, increasing physical activity, moderating alcohol consumption, and quitting smoking can help lower the risk (see pages 18–21 for more details). For people with both prehypertension and diabetes or kidney disease, medication may be needed to keep blood pressure below 130/80 mm Hg.

Hypertension. Individuals with a systolic blood pressure of 140 mm Hg or higher or a diastolic blood pressure of 90 mm Hg or

Evaluating and Managing Blood Pressure Levels

The JNC 7 blood pressure guidelines from the Joint National Committee on Prevention, Detection, Evaluation, and Treatment of High Blood Pressure are summarized in the table below.

To determine your blood pressure category, average your blood pressure readings from at least two doctor visits. If your systolic and diastolic blood pressures fall into different categories, use the more elevated reading. For example, an average reading of 165 mm Hg systolic and 95 mm Hg diastolic means that you have stage 2—

rather than stage 1—hypertension.

Lifestyle measures to keep blood pressure under control are recommended for all people—even those with normal blood pressure and those taking medication to manage their hypertension. Lifestyle measures include losing weight if necessary, following the Dietary Approaches to Stop Hypertension (DASH) diet, reducing salt intake, increasing physical activity, moderating alcohol consumption, and quitting smoking (see pages 18–21). Medications used to treat hypertension are listed in the table on pages 28–31.

Blood Pressure Category	Systolic Blood Pressure (mm Hg)	Diastolic Blood Pressure (mm Hg)	What To Do
Normal	<120	<80	Lifestyle measures encouraged.
Prehypertension	120–139	80–89	Lifestyle measures only. If you have diabetes or kidney disease, you may need to take medication to lower your blood pressure to less than 130/80 mm Hg.
Stage 1 hypertension	140–159	90–99	Lifestyle measures. Blood pressure medication is also required—usually a thiazide diuretic. Other types of blood pressure medication may be considered if you have heart disease, diabetes, or kidney problems or if you've had a stroke.
Stage 2 hypertension	≥160	≥100	Lifestyle measures. Also, two blood pressure medications are typically required—usually a thiazide diuretic in combination with an ACE inhibitor, angiotensin II receptor blocker, beta-blocker, or calcium channel blocker. Other combinations of blood pressure medications may be used if you have heart disease, diabetes, or kidney problems or if you've had a stroke.

higher are considered to have hypertension. Lifestyle modifications and antihypertensive medication are required to lower blood pressure and reduce the risk of hypertension-related complications. Most individuals with hypertension should aim to keep their blood pressure below 140/90 mm Hg. For those with diabetes or kidney disease, blood pressure should be maintained below 130/80 mm Hg.

Systolic vs. Diastolic Pressure

Historically, doctors focused on diastolic blood pressure for the diagnosis and treatment of hypertension. But today the focus is on both systolic and diastolic blood pressure, since systolic pressure is an important determinant of hypertension complications, particularly in people older than age 50.

In contrast to diastolic blood pressure, which tends to rise until about age 55 and then begins to fall, systolic blood pressure continues to rise with age. Previously, such elevations were thought to be a normal part of aging—caused by a gradual loss of elasticity in the arterial walls. Now, however, a substantial body of evidence shows that high systolic blood pressure with a diastolic blood pressure under 90 mm Hg carries a high risk of heart attack and stroke. In light of such findings, the JNC 7 guidelines recommend using systolic blood pressure as the standard measure for the evaluation and treatment of hypertension, especially for people age 50 and older.

Isolated systolic hypertension. A high systolic blood pressure with a normal diastolic pressure is common in older adults. In fact, 65% of people over age 60 with hypertension have a condition called isolated systolic hypertension, defined as a systolic blood pressure of 140 mm Hg or higher and a diastolic blood pressure under 90 mm Hg. Isolated systolic hypertension is associated with an increased risk of stroke, coronary heart disease, and kidney disease.

Pulse pressure. Another possible predictor of hypertension complications is pulse pressure—the difference between the systolic and diastolic blood pressures. Pulse pressure reflects the stiffness of the arteries. Researchers recently pooled the results of three major hypertension studies involving nearly 8,000 patients. They found that the higher the pulse pressure, the greater the risk of cardiovascular complications (such as heart attack and stroke) and death from any cause.

White Coat Hypertension

Some people have white coat hypertension—high blood pressure readings that are present only when they are examined by a physician or in a medical environment. Blood pressure measurements are normal when taken at home by the patient or a family member or friend. As many as 20% to 35% of people have white coat hypertension.

Whether to treat white coat hypertension with antihypertensive medication is controversial. Many (but not all) hypertension specialists believe that people with white coat hypertension who do not have other risk factors for cardiovascular disease (such as high cholesterol levels or diabetes) do not need to take medication. Instead, they should adopt lifestyle measures such as eating a healthy diet and exercising regularly. However, the general consensus is that people with white coat hypertension who have organ damage from hypertension (for example, kidney or heart disease) need treatment with medication. For more information on white coat hypertension, see the feature on page 13.

Some people experience the opposite problem to white coat hypertension: Their average daytime blood pressure is high but is normal when measured in a medical setting. Such people are unlikely to be treated for high blood pressure and therefore may miss out on the benefits of treatment.

COMPLICATIONS OF HYPERTENSION

Hypertension can damage both large and small arteries, leading to disease in the tissues and organs supplied by these damaged blood vessels. The tissues and organs most often affected by hypertension are the brain, heart, kidneys, and eyes. Fortunately, controlling blood pressure can help prevent or slow the progression of many of the complications of hypertension.

Brain. Hypertension accelerates atherosclerosis—the buildup of deposits called plaques within the walls of large arteries. If the plaques partially obstruct blood flow in an artery that leads to the brain (for example, the carotid artery), the result could be a transient ischemic attack (a ministroke in which symptoms usually subside within 5 to 20 minutes). If a blood clot forms in a plaque-containing artery, it could completely block blood flow and cause an ischemic stroke. Hypertension can also weaken arteries, resulting in a sac-like bulge (aneurysm) in the artery's wall. Rupture of an aneurysm in an artery supplying blood to the brain can result in a hemorrhagic stroke. Hypertension is also associated with lesions in the brain that can impair mental functions such as memory.

Heart. Atherosclerosis in the coronary arteries, which carry blood to the heart, can lead to a type of chest pain called angina when blood flow to the heart is insufficient. Complete blockage of a coronary artery by a blood clot results in a heart attack.

Atherosclerosis is not the only way hypertension can damage the heart. In people with hypertension, the heart works harder to pump against the higher pressures in the arteries. This excess workload thickens and increases the size of the heart's left ventricle. Called

NEW RESEARCH

Women's Heart Risks Climb With Rising Blood Pressure

For women with cardiovascular disease, the risk of heart attack and stroke rises in tandem with blood pressure, a new study finds.

High blood pressure is a well-known risk factor for cardiovascular disease, but when it comes to people with established cardiovascular disease, the relationship between blood pressure and cardiovascular events such as heart attack and stroke has been less clear.

The study of 5,218 women with cardiovascular disease—such as a history of heart attack, stroke, bypass surgery, angioplasty, or angina—found that the higher a woman's systolic blood pressure, the higher her risk of further cardiovascular events. Each 10-point increase in systolic blood pressure translated into a 9% increase in a woman's odds of suffering a heart attack or stroke, having surgery, or dying from cardiovascular complications over roughly six years.

Even women with a systolic reading of 130 to 139 mm Hg were at risk; they were 28% more likely than women with a reading between 120 and 129 mm Hg to suffer a cardiovascular complication.

According to the study authors, the findings suggest that for women with cardiovascular disease, even borderline elevations in systolic blood pressure may predict trouble—and that these women "might benefit from a lower targeted blood pressure."

CIRCULATION
Volume 109, page 1623
April 6, 2004

left ventricular hypertrophy, this condition affects 30% of people with hypertension and increases the risk of angina, heart attack, heart failure, and cardiac arrest.

Kidneys. Hypertension can damage the kidneys in two ways: by promoting atherosclerotic narrowing of the main arteries supplying the kidneys and by damaging the small arteries within the kidneys. Both can lead to progressive loss of kidney function and, eventually, kidney failure. Such kidney damage illustrates the vicious circle of hypertension: High blood pressure can lead to kidney disease and atherosclerosis; kidney disease and atherosclerosis further elevate blood pressure; and higher blood pressure causes further kidney damage.

Eyes. Persistent elevation of blood pressure can damage the tiny arteries that supply blood to the retina (the light-sensitive layer of nerve tissue that lines the back of the eye), resulting in a condition called hypertensive retinopathy. In the early stages of this disorder, the arteries in the retina thicken and narrow. Eventually, these vessels may develop blockages or begin to leak blood and fluid into the surrounding tissue. In very severe cases, the optic nerve (the nerve that carries visual impulses to the brain) may swell and cause vision loss. Hypertensive retinopathy typically evolves gradually, and many years may pass before people notice any changes in their vision.

PREVENTION OF HYPERTENSION

Prevention of any rise in blood pressure is important because organ damage can begin when blood pressure exceeds 110 mm Hg systolic or 70 mm Hg diastolic—long before hypertension is present. Preventing hypertension also eliminates the need for antihypertensive medications, which have potential side effects and can be costly. In addition, people with hypertension who successfully control their blood pressure with medication have a higher risk of hypertension complications than normotensive individuals with similar blood pressure levels. Hence, for many reasons, it is best to prevent hypertension in the first place.

The keys to preventing hypertension are weight loss, a healthy diet rich in fruits and vegetables and low in salt, regular physical activity, and moderate alcohol consumption (only for those who drink; abstainers should not begin drinking to reduce their risk of hypertension). Such lifestyle modifications can have a considerable impact. In one study, a weight loss of just 10 lbs. decreased

Should You Worry About White Coat Hypertension?

At least one in five people have blood pressure that's normal at home but elevated at the doctor's office.

Does going to a doctor's office cause you enough stress to raise your blood pressure? If so, you're not alone. Most people with hypertension have higher readings when a doctor takes their blood pressure than when they take it themselves. In fact, as many as 20% to 35% of people diagnosed with hypertension have what appear to be normal blood pressure readings at home.

This phenomenon is known as white coat hypertension (WCH). Some, but not all, experts believe that this condition can lead to unnecessary use of medication.

If your blood pressure is greater than 140/90 mm Hg on two or more separate occasions in a doctor's office, there are several ways to find out whether you have WCH.

• First, if your doctor usually measures your blood pressure, see whether it goes down when a nurse measures it—some people experience WCH only with a physician.

• Second, based on recommendations in a 2003 editorial published in *The New England Journal of Medicine,* you could get a home monitor and measure your own blood pressure twice a day for a week. You can do this while you're at home, at work, or both.

• Finally, if your average home blood pressure reading is below 135/85 mm Hg, ask your doctor whether you're a candidate for ambulatory blood pressure monitoring, in which blood pressure is repeatedly measured over a 24- to 48-hour period. Medicare started covering this technique in late 2001 to assess people with suspected WCH. An average ambulatory blood pressure reading below 130/80 mm Hg despite elevated office readings is termed WCH.

Do normal ambulatory blood pressure readings mean that antihypertensive medications aren't necessary? Several studies have suggested

that people with WCH are at higher risk for heart attack and stroke than people with normal blood pressure and should be treated with drug therapy. Other studies have found that people with WCH are no more likely to have a heart attack or stroke than people with normal blood pressure.

Until a definitive answer is reached, you should follow your doctor's advice on taking blood pressure medication. If you have no other risk factors for cardiovascular disease (such as diabetes or being a smoker) or damage to organs such as the heart, brain, or kidneys, ask your doctor whether it would be safe for you to be monitored without medication.

People with WCH, like other adults, should follow a healthy lifestyle to reduce the likelihood of heart attack and stroke. In addition, they should have repeat ambulatory blood pressure monitoring every one or two years if they are not taking medication.

the risk of hypertension by 50% in people with a systolic blood pressure between 130 and 139 mm Hg or a diastolic blood pressure between 85 and 89 mm Hg. The benefits of prevention appear to be more substantial when all of the recommended lifestyle modifications are adopted.

DIAGNOSIS OF HYPERTENSION

Hypertension is discovered most often during a routine visit to the doctor. The instrument used to evaluate blood pressure in a doctor's office is called a sphygmomanometer and typically consists of an inflating bulb, an inflatable cuff, and a mercury column gauge. Blood pressure is measured by wrapping the cuff around the upper arm and determining how much pressure is needed to compress the brachial artery—the major artery in the arm. The amount of pressure needed is equivalent to the height of the mercury in the gauge. Thus, blood pressure is expressed in millimeters of mercury, or mm Hg.

Because of concerns about mercury contamination of the environment, the Environmental Protection Agency is encouraging doctors to switch to aneroid or electronic blood pressure devices that use dial or digital gauges, respectively, to indicate blood pressure levels. Some experts are uneasy about these devices, but when used properly they can be as accurate as mercury sphygmomanometers.

Regardless of the type of device used to measure blood pressure, the following steps will help ensure accurate results. Do not smoke or consume caffeine in the 30 minutes prior to having blood pressure measured. Be seated and at rest for at least five minutes before the measurement. In addition, the results of two or more readings, taken at least one minute apart, should be averaged. Hypertension is diagnosed when the average blood pressure reading is 140/90 mm Hg or higher on at least two separate doctor visits.

Home Monitoring of Blood Pressure

Home monitoring of blood pressure can be useful in determining the presence of white coat hypertension (see pages 10–11 and the feature on page 13) and can help people with hypertension keep track of the effects of lifestyle modifications and medication on their blood pressure. Two types of monitors are available for home measurements: aneroid and electronic. Both types need to be checked annually against a standard mercury sphygmomanometer at the doctor's office to ensure continuing accuracy.

Traditionally, the best way to measure blood pressure at home has been with a manually operated aneroid monitor that consists of a cuff, bulb, and dial gauge to register blood pressure levels. A stethoscope is also required (most monitors come with one). Advantages of aneroid monitors are their accuracy, consistency, and low price ($20 to $30). Users of aneroid monitors must be able to rapidly squeeze the bulb to inflate the cuff, hear the thumping sounds of blood flow with the stethoscope, read the gauge that records the pressure, and loosen a valve to let out the air slowly. Consequently, individuals with hearing or vision problems or limited hand movement (from arthritis, for example) may not be able to use an aneroid monitor.

Electronic home monitors are improving and growing in popularity. Some types have a cuff that inflates automatically; those with manually inflated cuffs will deflate automatically. You need only

NEW RESEARCH

Home Monitoring Improves Blood Pressure Control

People with hypertension who monitor their own blood pressure at home may be more likely to keep it under control than those who have their blood pressures checked at outpatient clinics or doctors' offices, according to a new report.

The researchers performed a meta-analysis of 18 studies including a total of 1,359 people with hypertension who monitored their blood pressure at home and 1,355 others who received standard monitoring in the health care system. Patients were followed for 2 to 36 months.

Compared with people who had standard blood pressure monitoring, those who monitored their blood pressure at home had lower diastolic and systolic blood pressures and were 10% less likely to see their blood pressure climb above recommended targets.

Although the differences in blood pressure seen between the two groups were relatively small—around 2 mm Hg for both systolic and diastolic readings—they would be sufficient to significantly reduce the likelihood of hypertension complications such as stroke and heart attack in the general population, the researchers conclude. What's more, they note, home monitoring may benefit patients by helping them become more involved in managing their own blood pressure.

BMJ
Volume 329, page 145
July 17, 2004

record the numbers that appear on the digital screen. Electronic monitors are more expensive than aneroid monitors; those with automatic cuff inflation are the most expensive. Prices for electronic monitors range from about $35 to $125. The most expensive electronic monitors are not necessarily the best, and arm monitors are recommended over wrist monitors. Fingertip models are unreliable and should be avoided. A review of electronic home blood pressure monitors appeared in the June 2003 issue of *Consumer Reports*.

Ambulatory Blood Pressure Monitoring

Ambulatory blood pressure monitors automatically measure and record blood pressure over a 24- to 48-hour period. Such measurements may be useful in the diagnosis of white coat hypertension (see pages 10–11 and the feature on page 13). There is also some evidence that ambulatory monitoring may be helpful in identifying people with drug-resistant hypertension, hypotension caused by blood pressure medication, episodic hypertension, or borderline hypertension (systolic blood pressure 130 to 139 mm Hg or diastolic pressure 85 to 89 mm Hg). Ambulatory monitoring is not necessary when multiple blood pressure readings at the doctor's office are well beyond the threshold for treatment (above 140 mm Hg systolic or 90 mm Hg diastolic) or when hypertension is confirmed by home monitoring.

In ambulatory monitoring, an inflatable cuff is worn around the arm and connected to a blood pressure monitor about the size of a Walkman. The monitor is placed in a pouch that is worn at the waist in a holster. At predetermined times—typically every 15 to 30 minutes during the day and every 30 to 60 minutes during the night—the cuff inflates automatically and takes blood pressure readings that are stored in the monitor and later interpreted by a doctor. While wearing the monitor, people are asked to keep a diary of what time they awoke and went to sleep, when and what they ate, any emotions they experienced, any medications they took, and any physical activity they engaged in. This information may be helpful in explaining fluctuations in blood pressure.

The monitor is lightweight and quiet, and most people are able to sleep and carry out their normal activities while wearing it. Rarely, people may experience minor bruising, swelling, or rash. Medicare covers ambulatory blood pressure monitoring for people with suspected white coat hypertension; most private insurance companies, however, do not cover ambulatory monitoring.

NEW RESEARCH

Blood Pressure Accuracy May Be Better at Home Than Doctor's Office

Blood pressure measurements taken by patients at home may be more accurate in predicting risk of heart attack and stroke than those taken in a doctor's office, researchers report.

Nearly 5,000 patients with hypertension had their blood pressure measured several times at a physician's office. They also took their own blood pressure at home using an electronic monitor.

When researchers analyzed the home readings, they found that each 10-point increase in systolic blood pressure corresponded to a 17% increase in the risk of heart attack or stroke, while each 5-point increase in diastolic blood pressure corresponded to a 12% increase. But the same blood pressure elevations as measured in a doctor's office did not correspond to an increased risk of cardiovascular events.

Blood pressure measurements in a doctor's office may be less useful than home measurements for several reasons: First, blood pressure measured in an office setting may not reflect an individual's usual blood pressure. Second, physicians may not be measuring blood pressure accurately.

The results underscore the need to conduct additional study of the treatment and follow-up of patients who have elevated blood pressure at home but not in a doctor's office.

JOURNAL OF THE AMERICAN MEDICAL ASSOCIATION
Volume 291, page 1342
March 17, 2004

Weight Loss: A Key Player in the Fight Against Hypertension

For people who are overweight, shedding excess pounds is one of the best ways to treat high blood pressure, recent research confirms.

A number of lifestyle measures can effectively lower blood pressure in people with hypertension, as explained on pages 18–21. For people who are overweight, though, the cornerstone of lifestyle modifications should be losing excess weight. Research consistently shows that overweight people who drop pounds also drop millimeters of mercury, according to a new report. Weight loss, say the authors of the study, should be a "major component" of hypertension treatment.

Focusing on weight control is especially important given the enormous and escalating weight problem in the United States. Despite the nearly $40 billion that Americans spend each year on weight-loss programs, the nation is getting heavier. By current estimates, nearly two out of three people in the Unites States are at least overweight, with almost one in three being obese. Yet losing

weight needn't be either complicated or expensive.

What the Research Shows
The study, a meta-analysis published in *Hypertension* in 2003, combined data from 4,874 people in 25 randomized, controlled trials that tested the effects of weight loss (through diet, exercise, or both) on blood pressure. The researchers found that, on average, for every 2.2 lbs. of weight lost, blood pressure dropped by about 1/1 mm Hg. For example, people who lost about 11 lbs. had their blood pressure drop by 4.4/3.6 mm Hg.

Weight loss was especially effective at reducing blood pressure in people taking antihypertensive drugs, and people who lost weight by exercising had even greater decreases in blood pressure than those who simply cut calories. This study provides "unequivocal evidence that weight

loss makes an important contribution to the treatment of hypertension," the authors conclude.

Are You Overweight?
Before deciding to lose weight as a treatment for hypertension, you should determine, first, if you are overweight and, if so, by how much. Doctors typically use a person's body mass index (BMI) to determine if someone is overweight. To calculate your BMI, 1) multiply your weight in pounds by 704, 2) square your height in inches by multiplying the number by itself, and 3) divide the result of step 1 by the result of step 2. Use the result from step 3 and the chart at right to determine what weight category you fall into.

Losing Weight
If you need to lose weight, disregard the deluge of fad diets and over-the-counter supplements that purport to

Medical Evaluation of Blood Pressure

Proper diagnosis of hypertension requires a thorough medical history, a physical examination, and laboratory tests. Blood pressure levels determined by a doctor to be lower than 120 mm Hg systolic and 80 mm Hg diastolic should be rechecked within two years. Pressures between 120 and 139 mm Hg systolic or 80 and 89 mm Hg diastolic should be rechecked within one year.

When blood pressure levels are consistently 140/90 mm Hg or above, the next step is to determine whether the hypertension is primary or secondary. Although secondary hypertension is uncommon, secondary causes of high blood pressure should always be considered, since they are correctable in many cases and their identification may spare the patient antihypertensive medication—at least in the short term.

Precise diagnosis of a secondary cause usually requires special laboratory tests and procedures. Because these tests are expensive and inconvenient, they are not performed in everyone. Instead,

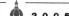

melt the pounds away magically. The most successful (and safest) strategy for weight loss is deceptively simple: expend more calories than you take in. This ideally involves both dietary calorie restriction and increased physical activity. (Prescription appetite-suppressing medication and surgery are also options, but only for a limited number of patients and only after diet and exercise have failed.)

If you are overweight or obese, a loss of 10% of your body weight over six months is a reasonable goal. To achieve this, you may need to lose 1 to 2 lbs. per week, which translates into 500 to 1,000 fewer calories than are needed daily to maintain your current weight. (Multiply your body weight in pounds by 15 to get this number.) Cutting caloric intake alone is one way to achieve this goal, but severe calorie reductions aren't recommended for older people because they can result in dangerous fluid, electrolyte, and weight shifts. Unless medically advised, daily intake should not drop below 1,200 calories in women and 1,500 calories in men.

Combining exercise with reduced calorie consumption (making sure that less than 30% of calories are from fat) is more successful than dieting alone for losing weight and keeping it off. Just 30 minutes of moderate to vigorous aerobic activity burns about 250 calories.

But there's no need to hit the ground running. Chances are that inactivity has contributed to your weight problem, and overdoing exercise will only discourage you. Ease into it. Try walking, cycling, or swimming at a comfortable pace for 30 minutes three days a week. Exercise need not take place in one contiguous spurt, either: Three 10-minute sessions will suffice. Your long-term goal should be to get at least 30 minutes of physical activity most days of the week. However, more exercise likely will be needed to keep the weight off once you have shed some pounds.

Another type of exercise—strength training—lowers overall body fat and maintains muscle mass. This improved muscle mass boosts metabolism because more energy (calories) are required to maintain muscle than fat. Include weight training or resistance-machine workouts in your exercise plan.

The Bottom Line

If you are overweight, weight loss—along with other lifestyle changes—is an excellent way not only to improve overall health but also to specifically lower blood pressure, even if you are already on antihypertensive medication. However, be sure to talk to your physician before you start any type of diet or exercise program.

Body Mass Index

Category	BMI
Underweight	<18.5
Normal weight	18.5–24.9
Overweight	25.0–24.9
Obese	≥30

they are done only when a thorough medical history and physical examination—or the results of routine laboratory tests—raise a strong suspicion for a secondary cause of hypertension. The chance that an underlying disorder is responsible for hypertension is particularly likely when lifestyle modifications and a combination of three antihypertensive medications cannot control blood pressure; blood pressure increases unexpectedly in someone whose blood pressure was previously well controlled; a hypertensive emergency occurs (see pages 7–8); blood pressure increases to greater than 180/110 mm Hg in an individual who previously had normal blood pressure; blood potassium levels drop for no particular reason; or an individual experiences headache, perspiration, and palpitations suggestive of pheochromocytoma (see pages 5–6).

A careful medical history, physical examination, and routine laboratory tests are also needed to determine whether hypertension has caused tissue or organ damage, to identify lifestyle habits that may be contributing to hypertension, and to detect the presence of additional risk factors for cardiovascular disease.

TREATMENT OF HYPERTENSION

Treatment of primary hypertension involves both lifestyle modifications and antihypertensive medications. The goal of treatment is to lower blood pressure and reduce the risk of complications from hypertension—specifically strokes, heart attacks, heart failure, and kidney disease. Most people with hypertension should aim to lower their blood pressure to less than 140/90 mm Hg. Those with diabetes or kidney disease have an even lower blood pressure goal— less than 130/80 mm Hg.

The same blood pressure goals apply to people with secondary hypertension. In these individuals, however, doctors often try to treat the underlying disorder, especially if blood pressure is difficult to control with lifestyle modifications and medications.

People experiencing a hypertensive emergency (see pages 7–8) must seek immediate medical attention and have their blood pressure lowered with intravenous antihypertensive medication in the hospital. Blood pressure is lowered gradually to avoid precipitous drops in pressure that could lead to a stroke.

Lifestyle Modifications

Lifestyle modifications are essential for both the prevention and treatment of hypertension. Lifestyle modifications proven to lower blood pressure include weight loss in people who are overweight or obese, the Dietary Approaches to Stop Hypertension (DASH) diet, reduced salt intake, increased potassium intake, regular physical activity, and moderation of alcohol consumption.

These lifestyle modifications not only help lower blood pressure, but also improve the effectiveness of antihypertensive medication and lower the risk of cardiovascular disease. Studies show that the effects of these lifestyle changes are additive, and people who adopt more of them reap the most benefits. In a recent study led by Lawrence Appel, M.D., one of the authors of this White Paper, people with prehypertension or mild hypertension who lost weight, followed the DASH diet, reduced salt and alcohol intake, and exercised regularly reduced their systolic blood pressure by an extra 4 mm Hg over a six-month period, compared with people who only received advice on these lifestyle modifications.

Weight loss. All people—whether or not they have hypertension—

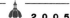

should aim for a body mass index (BMI) between 18.5 and 24.9. People with a BMI of 25 or more are considered overweight. BMI is a measure of weight in relation to height; it can be determined by multiplying weight in pounds by 704 and dividing the result by the square of height in inches. The best way to lose weight is to reduce the number of calories eaten per day while increasing physical activity. Studies show that for every 2.2 lbs. of weight lost blood pressure drops by about 1/1 mm Hg. For advice on losing weight, see the feature on pages 16–17.

DASH diet. The DASH diet is an eating plan that is rich in fruits, vegetables, and low-fat dairy products and low in saturated fat, cholesterol, and total fat. The diet also includes whole-grain products, fish, poultry, and nuts. Red meat, sweets, and sugar-containing beverages are kept to a minimum, however. Two major trials have evaluated the DASH diet.

In the first trial, people who followed the DASH diet for eight weeks reduced their blood pressure by an average of 5.5/3.0 mm Hg, compared with people who ate a typical American diet (low in fruits and vegetables and high in fat). The benefits of the DASH diet were most pronounced in people with hypertension. In these individuals, the DASH diet lowered systolic pressure by 11 mm Hg, which is similar to the level of blood pressure reduction typically achieved with a single antihypertensive drug.

In the second trial, people who combined the DASH diet with a low salt intake (1,500 mg of sodium per day) for four weeks had an average blood pressure reduction of 9/5 mm Hg, compared with people who followed a typical American diet with a high salt intake. As in the first study, the benefits were greater in people with hypertension—their systolic blood pressure dropped by an average of 12 mm Hg.

Reduced salt intake. Research indicates that, on average, blood pressure levels rise with higher intakes of salt, and limiting salt may lower systolic blood pressure by 2 to 8 mm Hg. The effects of dietary salt on blood pressure tend to be greater in blacks, middle-aged and older adults, and people with hypertension or diabetes.

The Institute of Medicine recently issued new guidelines for salt intake in adults. They set an upper limit of 2,300 mg of sodium daily, and the following minimum requirements: 1,500 mg of sodium for adults under age 50; 1,300 mg for people age 50 to 70; and 1,200 mg for those above age 70.

Salt added to foods during cooking and at the table makes up only about 10% of the sodium consumed in the typical American

NEW RESEARCH

Moderate Drinking May Benefit Men With Hypertension

Light to moderate drinking may reduce the risk of dying from cardiovascular disease in men with high blood pressure, new research reveals.

Although several studies have shown moderate alcohol consumption can cut cardiovascular disease risk in the general population, the effect of moderate to light drinking on the cardiovascular health of people with hypertension has not been clear. Heavy drinking, however, is known to increase blood pressure.

To investigate, the researchers followed 14,125 men with hypertension from the Physicians' Health Study. Compared with those who never or rarely drank, men who drank moderately (one to six alcoholic beverages each week) had a 39% lower risk of dying from cardiovascular disease, while those who drank daily cut their risk by 44%. Moderate drinkers also had a lower risk than nondrinkers of dying from any cause.

The findings don't warrant recommendations for men with hypertension to take up drinking. And for men with high blood pressure who are light to moderate alcohol drinkers (no more than two drinks a day), there is no need to drink less or to stop drinking.

ARCHIVES OF INTERNAL MEDICINE
Volume 164, page 623
March 22, 2004

New Sodium and Potassium Recommendations To Reduce Blood Pressure

Both these minerals can affect blood pressure levels, and a recent change in the recommended intakes may mean a change in your diet.

Most Americans consume too much salt, which can raise blood pressure, and too little potassium, which can help lower it. Now, 2004 dietary recommendations from the Institute of Medicine mean that even more people need to reduce the amount of salt and boost the amount of potassium they consume. Lawrence Appel, M.D., coauthor of this White Paper, headed the panel of experts who came up with the new recommendations.

Lowering Salt Intake

An elevated intake of salt is often associated with rising blood pressure levels, so lowering salt intake can have a beneficial effect on blood pressure. The U.S. government's current salt recommendation is 2,400 mg of sodium per day; the new recommendation (called the adequate intake [AI]) is much lower: 1,500 mg per day for adults under age 50. The report also recommends that adults aim for the AI but should not consume more than 2,300 mg per day (the upper limit [UL]). Because older adults usually consume fewer calories than younger people and are more susceptible to high blood pressure, the AI for this group is even lower: 1,300 mg a day for people age 50 to 70, and 1,200 mg per day for those age 71 and over.

While the new recommendations focus on sodium consumption, the primary source of sodium in the diet is salt (sodium chloride). While sodium accounts for 40% of the weight in the compound, chloride makes up the other 60%. Therefore, the new AI for sodium—1,500 mg per day—is found in 3,800 mg of table salt.

Although sodium is important for many of the body's processes, the average person needs only about 500 mg of sodium a day. The typical American consumes in excess of 4,000 mg per day, which is more than double the new AI. This high salt intake largely results from the sodium added during the processing of many foods. One study found that Americans get 77% of their daily salt intake from prepared and processed foods. For example, two slices of pizza contain almost enough sodium to achieve the AI for an entire day and may contain half of the UL for sodium per day.

Therefore, limiting salt during cooking or at the table will help but will not lower salt intake to the recommended levels. In fact, the estimates for current sodium consumption in the United States do not even include the amount of salt that people add while cooking or eating.

The U.S. Food and Drug Administration (FDA) may use the panel's recommendations to change the nutrition labels on packaged foods. For example, a canned soup that now contains 36% of the daily sodium intake would soon contain 57%, based on the new AI. However, such changes usually take several years to implement. In the meantime, read food labels carefully. Be on the lookout for the various sodium compounds that manufacturers typically add to food. These compounds include monosodium glutamate (sometimes called MSG), a

diet. A large proportion (more than 75%) comes from processed foods like cold cuts, canned vegetables, canned soups, cheeses, and snack foods. So reducing salt intake means not only avoiding the salt shaker while cooking and at meals but also reading nutrition labels and choosing foods that contain less than 140 mg of sodium per serving. For more help on lowering salt intake, see the feature above.

Potassium intake. Potassium is a mineral found in fruits, vegetables, dairy products, and beans. Increased intake of potassium has been shown to reduce blood pressure, as well as to reduce the rise in blood pressure that occurs with excessive salt consumption. According to 2004 guidelines from the Institute of Medicine, people should consume at least 4.7 g of potassium per day. To learn more about potassium, see the feature above.

seasoning often added to frozen or packaged food and used in restaurant cooking; baking soda; and baking powder. Looking for any ingredient that contains the word soda, sodium, or Na (the chemical notation for sodium) will help you identify dietary sources of sodium.

Common processed foods likely to be high in sodium include canned soups and meats; processed meats such as sausage, bacon, hot dogs, and luncheon meats; frozen dinners; and fast food. Also typically high in sodium are peanut butter and salted nuts; snack foods like potato chips; salad dressings; and preseasoned mixes.

However, food manufacturers are moving in a positive direction: for example, canned foods contain 40% less sodium than they did a few years ago, and lower-sodium versions of many foods are now available. Look for food labels that contain the following phrases: sodium free, very low sodium, low sodium, reduced sodium, no added salt, or unsalted.

Getting More Potassium

The FDA recommends 3.5 g of potassium—a mineral found in fruits and vegetables—per day for adults, but the new AI for potassium is 4.7 g per day. According to recent surveys, most people in the United States get much less than this level: American men consume approximately 2.3 to 3.2 g of potassium per day, while American women get 2.1 to 2.3 g per day. Because potassium from fruits and vegetables is considered safe, there is no upper limit for dietary potassium.

Current evidence suggests that potassium intakes at the AI level can lower blood pressure and reduce the rise in blood pressure caused by salt consumption. In addition, adequate potassium intake can reduce the risk of kidney stones and bone loss. Blacks typically have lower potassium intakes and greater risk of high blood pressure and salt sensitivity than other racial or ethnic groups. This means that blacks would benefit greatly from following the new potassium recommendations.

Food sources of potassium are recommended because part of the benefit may come from the nutrients commonly conjoined with potassium, and many studies on the health effects of potassium examined potassium as provided in foods. Potassium supplements are not recommended, as high levels can be toxic; they are also associated with gastrointestinal problems and ulcers.

Since there is no evidence that a high level of potassium from foods is dangerous in otherwise healthy people, dietary potassium is the preferred source. Good sources of potassium in the diet include bananas, spinach, cantaloupe, almonds, Brussels sprouts, mushrooms, oranges, grapefruit, potatoes, and dairy products.

High intakes of potassium—and salt substitutes, which contain potassium chloride—are not safe for people who have certain conditions (such as chronic kidney insufficiency, type 1 diabetes, end-stage kidney disease, severe heart failure, or adrenal insufficiency) or who take certain medications (such as ACE inhibitors, certain diuretics, COX-2 inhibitors, or other nonsteroidal anti-inflammatory drugs). These individuals may need lower levels of potassium than the AI and should determine this level with their physician.

Physical activity. Exercise is also important in the prevention and treatment of hypertension. Experts recommend engaging in moderate physical activity (for example, walking, bicycling, swimming, or jogging) for at least 30 minutes on most days of the week. In a recent meta-analysis of more than 50 randomized, controlled trials, regular physical activity reduced blood pressure by an average of 4/3 mm Hg. Always talk to your doctor before beginning an exercise program.

Alcohol restriction. Moderate alcohol consumption—one or two drinks a day for most men and one drink a day for women and lighter-weight men—may lower systolic blood pressure by 2 to 4 mm Hg. One drink is equivalent to 12 oz. of beer, 5 oz. of wine, or 1.5 oz. of 80-proof spirits. Nondrinkers should not begin drinking to reduce their blood pressure.

Medication

When lifestyle modifications are insufficient to lower blood pressure to goal levels, doctors add antihypertensive medications to the treatment regimen. There are 10 classes of antihypertensive drugs, and each lowers blood pressure in a different way. The best blood pressure-lowering medication(s) for a particular person depends on how severe the hypertension is and whether other health problems are present.

For people with stage 1 hypertension (140 to 159 mm Hg systolic or 90 to 99 mm Hg diastolic) who have no other health problems, a thiazide diuretic is most often prescribed along with lifestyle modifications. In the case of healthy people with stage 2 hypertension (160 mm Hg or higher systolic or 100 mm Hg or higher diastolic), a combination of two drugs is typically prescribed in addition to lifestyle modifications. The drug combination usually consists of a thiazide diuretic and an ACE inhibitor, angiotensin II receptor blocker, beta-blocker, or calcium channel blocker.

Many people with hypertension have other health conditions, and these individuals may require different or additional antihypertensive medications to control their blood pressure and manage the other health problems they might have. For example, people with angina are usually prescribed a beta-blocker or calcium channel blocker to help relieve symptoms. People who have suffered a heart attack typically take an ACE inhibitor, beta-blocker, and aldosterone blocker to prevent another heart attack. In people with severe heart failure, a combination of an ACE inhibitor, beta-blocker, angiotensin II receptor blocker, aldosterone blocker, and loop diuretic is recommended. For people who have had a stroke, taking a thiazide diuretic and an ACE inhibitor can reduce the risk of future strokes.

In people with diabetes, at least two antihypertensive medications are usually required to reach the blood pressure goal of 130/80 mm Hg. The best antihypertensive medications for people with diabetes are those that also lower the risk of diabetes complications. For example, thiazide diuretics, beta-blockers, ACE inhibitors, angiotensin II receptor blockers, and calcium channel blockers all reduce the risk of strokes and heart attacks in people with diabetes. In addition, ACE inhibitors and angiotensin II receptor blockers slow the progression of diabetic kidney disease.

People with kidney disease also have a blood pressure goal of 130/80 mm Hg, and they usually need three or more antihypertensive drugs to lower their blood pressure to this level. In these individuals, ACE inhibitors and angiotensin II receptor blockers are

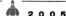

most effective in lowering blood pressure and slowing the progression of kidney disease. Because of reduced kidney function, loop diuretics rather than thiazide diuretics are commonly used.

The ten classes of antihypertensive medications are described below and in the chart on pages 28–31.

Diuretics. Often referred to as fluid or water pills, diuretics help reduce blood pressure by increasing the kidneys' excretion of sodium into the urine. These drugs also lower blood pressure by promoting the dilation of small blood vessels. There are three types of diuretics—thiazide diuretics, loop diuretics, and potassium-sparing diuretics. Each type of diuretic acts on a different site in the kidney.

Thiazide diuretics are the most commonly used diuretic. These drugs are inexpensive and need to be taken only once a day. In addition, they are at least as effective—if not more effective—than other classes of antihypertensive drugs at lowering blood pressure and reducing the risk of cardiovascular disease such as stroke and heart attack. Loop diuretics are often used in people who also have heart failure or kidney disease. Potassium-sparing diuretics are used in combination with another type of diuretic, when that diuretic results in excessive loss of potassium.

The benefits of thiazide diuretics were demonstrated in a study called ALLHAT—the Antihypertensive and Lipid-Lowering Treatment to Prevent Heart Attack Trial—published in 2002 in the *Journal of the American Medical Association.* The study looked at more than 42,000 people with hypertension who were age 55 and older and had at least one risk factor for heart disease. The participants were randomly assigned to receive either a thiazide diuretic (chlorthalidone), an ACE inhibitor (lisinopril), a calcium channel blocker (amlodipine), or an alpha-blocker (doxazosin). The researchers followed the participants for an average of five years.

The results clearly showed that the diuretic was superior to the ACE inhibitor and calcium channel blocker in terms of lowering blood pressure and preventing certain cardiovascular events. (The alpha-blocker portion of the study was stopped early because participants on this medication had a 25% increase in cardiovascular events relative to the diuretic.) People taking the diuretic had systolic blood pressures about 2 mm Hg lower than the group taking the ACE inhibitor and 1 mm Hg lower than the calcium channel blocker group. In addition, people on the diuretic had a lower risk of heart failure compared with people taking the calcium channel blocker and a lower risk of stroke, heart failure, and angina than people treated with the ACE inhibitor.

NEW RESEARCH

Race Not Key in Choosing Blood Pressure Drugs

Although studies have suggested that blacks and whites have different responses to different blood pressure medications, new research indicates race is not a good predictor of how a person will fare on a drug.

The review of 15 clinical trials over the past 20 years found that 80% to 95% of black and white patients showed similar responses to commonly used high blood pressure drugs. Although there were some differences in medication responses by race, the differences among individuals of the same race were much greater.

This, the study's author concludes, suggests that medication decisions should be based on factors such as a patient's overall health—and not race. For example, ACE inhibitors are an antihypertensive drug of choice for people with chronic kidney disease, regardless of their race.

The potential importance of race in blood pressure treatment has been suggested by evidence that, on average, white patients respond better than blacks do to ACE inhibitors and beta-blockers, while black patients fare better on diuretics and calcium channel blockers. But the new findings suggest that while there may be some small differences on average, race has "little value" in predicting how any one person will respond to any single medication.

HYPERTENSION
Volume 43, page 566
March 2004

Should You Be Taking a Diuretic?

Water pills are recommended for most people with high blood pressure, but doctors don't always prescribe them. Here's why they should.

Current treatment guidelines state that thiazide diuretics should be used as initial therapy for most patients with hypertension. But in many cases, doctors instead prescribe such drugs as ACE inhibitors, angiotensin II receptor blockers, beta-blockers, or calcium channel blockers. What is the reason for this disparity, and how do you know whether you're getting the best drug to lower your blood pressure?

What the Guidelines Say

The treatment guidelines, issued by the seventh report of the Joint National Committee on Prevention, Detection, Evaluation, and Treatment of High Blood Pressure (JNC 7) in 2003, recommend using diuretics—either alone or in combination with other drugs—as first-line therapy in all people with high blood pressure who are otherwise healthy. But in people with other health conditions,

a diuretic may not be the first choice. For example, beta-blockers or ACE inhibitors may be the preferred therapy for those with coronary heart disease or kidney disease, respectively, although diuretics may also be used. In addition, diuretics are not appropriate in people who are allergic to them or have experienced serious side effects from them. But most other people with hypertension should receive a diuretic.

The JNC 7 guidelines were based on many studies, including the Antihypertensive and Lipid-Lowering Treatment to Prevent Heart Attack Trial (ALLHAT)—the largest blood pressure drug study ever conducted. As reported in 2002 in the *Journal of the American Medical Association* (*JAMA*), the trial compared the traditional recommended therapy, thiazide diuretics, with two newer—but considerably more expensive—

medications: a calcium channel blocker and an ACE inhibitor.

Patients in all three groups fared equally well with regard to the occurrence of nonfatal heart attacks or death from coronary heart disease. The thiazide diuretic, however, was superior to the other two drugs in lowering blood pressure and reducing the risk of cardiovascular complications such as stroke and heart failure.

Differing Results

A 2003 study published in *The New England Journal of Medicine* reached a different conclusion. In it, Australian researchers concluded that initiating therapy with ACE inhibitors instead of diuretics led to fewer cardiovascular complications and deaths from any cause, despite similar reductions in blood pressure.

But there are important differences between this study—the Second

Low doses of thiazide diuretics are well tolerated. However, side effects can occur, including weakness; fatigue; malaise; sexual dysfunction; increased blood levels of glucose, triglycerides, calcium, and uric acid; and reduced blood sodium and HDL cholesterol levels. Thiazide and loop diuretics can also cause loss of potassium, which can lead to serious cardiac risks.

Beta-blockers. These drugs block the actions of epinephrine and lower blood pressure by slowing heart rate and reducing cardiac output (the amount of blood pumped by the heart). They offer the additional benefit of reducing the heart's consumption of oxygen, which can help control angina.

Potential side effects of beta-blockers include the following: wheezing in people who are sensitive to various allergens and irritants or who have preexisting lung disease; fatigue; drowsiness; malaise; depression; erectile dysfunction or decreased libido; increased blood triglyceride levels; and decreased HDL cholesterol levels. Because beta-blockers blunt the response to epinephrine, these drugs may cause problems if hypoglycemia (low blood sugar)

Annual Australian National Blood Pressure Study (ANBP2)—and the ALLHAT study. For example, ALLHAT was much larger, with about 24,000 people; ANBP2 had only 6,000 participants. ALLHAT was also better designed in that both subjects and researchers were blinded as to what drugs were being used. In addition, the results of ANBP2 were less consistent: The beneficial effect of ACE inhibitors was present in men but not in women.

Furthermore, a comprehensive meta-analysis of 42 trials recently confirmed the ALLHAT results. The meta-analysis, which was published in *JAMA* in 2003, combined data on nearly 200,000 people randomized to 7 major treatment strategies, including a placebo. It concluded that low-dose diuretics are the most effective first-line treatment for preventing cardiovascular deaths and illnesses.

The Cost Factor
In addition to being the most effective first-line treatment, diuretics are also the least expensive. The average cost of a prescription for a thiazide diuretic is less than $6, while ACE inhibitors and calcium channel blockers cost five to six times as much.

Despite these findings, many doctors continue to prescribe newer, more expensive drugs in place of diuretics. In fact, in an article published in *JAMA* in 2004, researchers found that 40% of doctors' prescriptions fell outside of the JNC 7 recommendations. The researchers theorize that doctors may choose these newer agents based on aggressive marketing campaigns, or on the basis of studies such as ANBP2 that found ACE inhibitors to be more effective than diuretics. But nationwide compliance with the JNC 7 guidelines in prescribing drugs to elderly patients with hypertension would save about $1.2 billion annually.

The Bottom Line
If you're being treated for high blood pressure and aren't taking a thiazide diuretic, ask your doctor if you should be. It may be that your doctor has selected a different drug as first-line therapy because you have a condition such as coronary heart disease, diabetes, or kidney disease, or you have had a stroke. But most people need a second drug to control blood pressure adequately. For people who aren't already taking one, that drug should usually be a thiazide diuretic.

Coexisting health conditions aren't the only factors that play a part in deciding which drug to prescribe. For example, ALLHAT found that blacks didn't respond as well as whites to ACE inhibitors. This difference may not be as significant as is commonly believed: A study published in *Hypertension* in 2004 concluded that whites and blacks respond similarly to common antihypertensive drugs about 90% of the time (see the sidebar on page 23). The potential for intolerable side effects is also a factor. So you and your doctor may need to experiment with several drugs in order to find the regimen that works best for you.

develops in people taking insulin or certain oral drugs to control their diabetes. (Epinephrine release during hypoglycemia triggers symptoms that alert people that their blood sugar is too low and that they need to take actions to increase their blood sugar.)

Beta-blockers may become less effective over time. This happens when the body compensates for the drop in blood pressure by increasing the retention of water and sodium, which causes blood pressure to rise again. Combining a beta-blocker with a diuretic may reduce this effect.

Calcium channel blockers. These drugs lower blood pressure by dilating arteries and, depending on the type of calcium channel blocker, by decreasing cardiac output as well. Like beta-blockers, calcium channel blockers help alleviate symptoms of angina. Potential side effects include headache, dizziness, flushing, leg swelling, constipation, and slow or rapid heart rate with palpitations.

Past research suggested that calcium channel blockers might increase the risk of nonfatal heart attacks and deaths due to coronary heart disease, particularly in people treated with short-acting calcium channel blockers such as nifedipine. But in the recently published ALLHAT study, people taking the calcium channel blocker amlodipine (Norvasc) were no more likely to have a heart attack or die of coronary heart disease over a five-year period than people taking the thiazide diuretic chlorthalidone (Thalitone).

However, in ALLHAT, people treated with a calcium channel blocker were 38% more likely to develop heart failure and 35% more likely to be hospitalized for heart failure, compared with people taking a diuretic. Also, other studies have found that calcium channel blockers may adversely affect kidney function, compared with ACE inhibitors. As a result, calcium channel blockers are not recommended as a first-choice treatment for hypertension and should be used cautiously in people with heart failure or kidney disease.

ACE inhibitors. ACE inhibitors decrease blood pressure by reducing the formation of angiotensin II, a potent constrictor of blood vessels. A dry cough occurs in about 25% of people using ACE inhibitors, especially in women. Uncommon adverse effects are rash and increased blood potassium levels. ACE inhibitors have no ill effects on libido or erectile function. A study comparing two commonly used ACE inhibitors, captopril (Capoten) and enalapril (Vasotec), found that captopril was associated with fewer side effects that decrease quality of life.

The Heart Outcomes Prevention Evaluation (HOPE) trial found that ACE inhibitors are appropriate for a wide range of people. The trial examined the effects of the ACE inhibitor ramipril (Altace) in more than 9,000 people with coronary heart disease, stroke, peripheral arterial disease, or diabetes and at least one other heart disease risk factor (hypertension, elevated cholesterol levels, or smoking). After five years, 14% of the participants taking ramipril had died or suffered a heart attack or stroke, compared with 18% of the patients taking a placebo. This translates into roughly 150 fewer heart attacks or strokes for every 1,000 people treated with ramipril over a four-year period. The ramipril patients were also about 30% less likely to develop diabetes.

In people with diabetes, ACE inhibitors can delay or prevent the progression of kidney disease. These medications are also beneficial in people without diabetes who have early kidney disease. In addition, a recent study found that ACE inhibitors delayed the progression of kidney disease in blacks with early evidence of kidney damage from hypertension. ACE inhibitors must be used with caution, however, when kidney disease is advanced. Furthermore, these drugs should not be used by women who are pregnant or plan to become pregnant.

Angiotensin II receptor blockers. These drugs work by interfering with the action of angiotensin II, which raises blood pressure by constricting small blood vessels and stimulating the adrenal glands to produce the sodium-retaining hormone aldosterone. The drugs may also halt the overgrowth of smooth muscle cells in blood vessel walls. In addition to their blood pressure-lowering effects, angiotensin II receptor blockers also help slow the progression of kidney disease in people with or without diabetes.

Side effects may include headache, digestive upset, and upper respiratory tract infection, although these effects occurred at about the same frequency in people taking a placebo. People who develop a cough while taking an ACE inhibitor may switch to an angiotensin II receptor blocker to eliminate this side effect. Angiotensin II receptor blockers should not be used by pregnant women or women planning a pregnancy.

Alpha-blockers. These drugs decrease blood pressure by blocking nerve impulses that constrict small arteries, thus lowering resistance to blood flow. They may cause orthostatic hypotension (lightheadedness on standing), especially in older patients, as well as weakness, fainting, drowsiness, headaches, and heart palpitations. In addition, they can lose their effectiveness over time when not used in combination with a diuretic. Alpha-blockers usually have beneficial effects on HDL cholesterol levels.

Alpha-blockers are not recommended as a first-choice therapy for hypertension. According to results from the ALLHAT study, people taking the alpha-blocker doxazosin (Cardura) had 25% more cardiovascular events and were twice as likely to be hospitalized for heart failure as people treated with a diuretic. Alpha-blockers are also prescribed for the treatment of benign prostatic hyperplasia (noncancerous enlargement of the prostate gland).

Central alpha agonists. Like alpha-blockers, these drugs lower blood pressure by blocking nerve impulses that constrict small arteries. Side effects include drowsiness, sleep disturbances, depression, dry mouth, constipation, fatigue, erectile dysfunction, and dizziness (especially in older people). These drugs should not be stopped abruptly and therefore should be taken only by people who are likely to adhere to their medication regimens. Because of a high frequency of side effects, central alpha agonists usually are used only when other medications are unable to control blood pressure adequately. In addition, central alpha agonists may become less effective over time.

NEW RESEARCH

Race Alone Can't Predict ACE Inhibitor Response

Doctors should not choose which blood pressure medication to prescribe based on a patient's race alone, according to a new study.

The researchers sought to determine how much the difference in a patient's response to the ACE inhibitor quinapril (Accupril) could be predicted by his or her race in a study of 533 black and 2,046 white individuals.

While the drug was less effective for black patients, on average, than whites, there was considerable variation within each ethnic group in terms of response, and considerable overlap in response between the two groups. And after the researchers accounted for other factors that play a role in quinapril response, the racial difference in response became much weaker.

Women, obese people, and those with lower baseline systolic blood pressure show a less dramatic response to ACE inhibitors, the researchers note, and they conclude that doctors should take such factors into account before deciding which drug to prescribe.

HYPERTENSION
Volume 43, page 1202
June 2004

Antihypertensive Drugs 2005

Drug Type	Generic Name	Brand Name	Usual Daily Dosage*	Average Retail Cost†
Diuretics	*Thiazide diuretics:*			
	chlorothiazide	Diuril	125 to 500 mg	250 mg: $7 ($6)
	chlorthalidone	Thalitone	12.5 to 25 mg	15 mg: $33 ($8)
	hydrochlorothiazide	HydroDIURIL	12.5 to 50 mg	25 mg: $7 ($5)
		Microzide	12.5 to 50 mg	12.5 mg: $24 ($15)
	indapamide	Lozol	1.25 to 2.5 mg	2.5 mg: $33 ($9)
	metolazone	Zaroxolyn	2.5 to 5 mg	5 mg: $50 ($37)
	polythiazide	Renese	2 to 4 mg	2 mg: $25
	Loop diuretics:			
	bumetanide	Bumex	0.5 to 2 mg	0.5 mg: $18 ($9)
	furosemide	Lasix	20 to 80 mg	40 mg: $10 ($5)
	torsemide	Demadex	2.5 to 10 mg	5 mg: $26 ($18)
	Potassium-sparing diuretics:			
	amiloride	Midamor	5 to 10 mg	5 mg: $19 ($15)
	spironolactone	Aldactone	25 to 50 mg	50 mg: $40 ($21)
	triamterene	Dyrenium	50 to 100 mg	50 mg: $32
Beta-blockers	acebutolol	Sectral	200 to 800 mg	200 mg: $57 ($18)
	atenolol	Tenormin	25 to 100 mg	50 mg: $39 ($8)
	betaxolol	Kerlone	5 to 20 mg	10 mg: $36 ($25)
	bisoprolol	Zebeta	2.5 to 10 mg	5 mg: $50 ($36)
	carvedilol‡	Coreg	12.5 to 50 mg	12.5 mg: $52
	labetalol‡	Normodyne	200 to 800 mg	100 mg: $21 ($12)
		Trandate	200 to 800 mg	200 mg: $28 ($15)
	metoprolol	Lopressor	50 to 100 mg	100 mg: $44 ($7)
	metoprolol, extended release	Toprol XL	50 to 100 mg	100 mg: $34
	nadolol	Corgard	40 to 120 mg	80 mg: $70 ($19)
	penbutolol	Levatol	10 to 40 mg	20 mg: $54
	pindolol	Visken	10 to 40 mg	10 mg: $46 ($15)
	propranolol	Inderal	40 to 160 mg	80 mg: $40 ($7)
	propranolol, long acting	Inderal LA	60 to 180 mg	80 mg: $46
	timolol	Blocadren	20 to 40 mg	10 mg: $20 ($10)
Calcium channel blockers	amlodipine	Norvasc	2.5 to 10 mg	5 mg: $44
	diltiazem, extended release	Cardizem CD	180 to 420 mg	120 mg: $43 ($30)
		Cardizem LA	120 to 540 mg	120 mg: $39
		Dilacor XR	180 to 420 mg	120 mg: $50 ($29)
		Tiazac	180 to 420 mg	120 mg: $40 ($31)
	felodipine	Plendil	2.5 to 20 mg	5 mg: $41
	isradipine	DynaCirc CR	2.5 to 10 mg	5 mg: $59
	nicardipine, sustained release	Cardene SR	60 to 120 mg	30 mg: $29 ($10)
	nifedipine, long acting	Adalat CC	30 to 90 mg	60 mg: $78 ($41)
		Procardia XL	30 to 90 mg	30 mg: $45 ($34)
	nisoldipine	Sular	10 to 40 mg	30 mg: $53
	verapamil, immediate release	Calan	80 to 320 mg	120 mg: $32 ($6)
		Isoptin	80 to 320 mg	120 mg: $39 ($19)
	verapamil, long acting	Calan SR	120 to 480 mg	120 mg: $40 ($19)
		Isoptin SR	120 to 480 mg	120 mg: $39 ($19)
	verapamil, controlled onset, extended release	Covera-HS	120 to 480 mg	180 mg: $46 ($11)
		Verelan PM	120 to 480 mg	100 mg: $44 ($11)

Advantages	Disadvantages
Thiazide diuretics are the first drug prescribed for most people with hypertension. These drugs can be used alone or in combination with other antihypertensive drugs, such as ACE inhibitors, angiotensin II receptor blockers, beta-blockers, and calcium channel blockers. Thiazide diuretics may make other antihypertensive drugs more effective by reversing the fluid retention that some of them cause. These drugs are also useful for people with heart failure, since they help to eliminate excess fluid from the body. The thiazide diuretic metolazone is helpful for people with impaired kidney function who do not respond to other thiazides. Loop diuretics sometimes are used for people who are not helped by thiazide diuretics, especially those with impaired kidney function. Potassium-sparing diuretics can be taken alone but generally are used in conjunction with another type of diuretic to counteract excessive potassium loss.	Thiazide diuretics may cause potassium loss, elevated triglyceride and glucose levels, decreased high-density lipoprotein (HDL, or "good") cholesterol levels, gout, weakness, erectile dysfunction, and dizziness on standing. Loop diuretics can cause dehydration, potassium loss, and changes in the acidity of the blood. Potassium-sparing diuretics can raise potassium levels, a particular danger for people who have kidney disease. Potassium-sparing diuretics should be used cautiously (if at all) in combination with ACE inhibitors or aldosterone blockers, which can also raise potassium levels.
These drugs are effective for people with hypertension who also have angina or have had a heart attack, since they can help control chest pain and reduce the risk of a second heart attack and death from any cause.	Side effects include fatigue, drowsiness, vivid dreams, loss of libido, and erectile dysfunction. These drugs may also raise triglyceride levels and lower HDL cholesterol levels. High doses may aggravate heart failure. Beta-blockers should not be taken by people with asthma. These drugs are less effective in the elderly. Abruptly stopping a beta-blocker can produce serious cardiovascular problems.
Calcium channel blockers help relieve the symptoms of angina. These drugs often lower blood pressure rapidly and effectively.	Constipation, swelling of the legs, headaches, and dizziness are possible side effects, but most people experience only mild problems, if any. Studies suggest an increased risk of heart attack in users of short-acting calcium channel blockers, but not in people taking longer-acting calcium channel blockers. However, longer-acting calcium channel blockers are associated with an increased risk of heart failure.

* These dosages represent an average range for the treatment of hypertension. The precise effective dosage varies from patient to patient and depends on many factors. Do not make any changes in your medication without consulting your doctor.
† Average price for 30 tablets or capsules (unless otherwise indicated) of the dosage strength listed. Actual price may vary. If a generic version is available, the cost is listed in parentheses. Sources: drugstore.com, eckerd.com, and walgreens.com.
‡ An alpha-blocker and beta-blocker.

Antihypertensive Drugs 2005 (continued)

Drug Type	Generic Name	Brand Name	Usual Daily Dosage*	Average Retail Cost†
ACE inhibitors	benazepril	Lotensin	10 to 40 mg	10 mg: $37 ($20)
	captopril	Capoten	25 to 100 mg	12.5 mg: $33 ($5)
	enalapril	Vasotec	2.5 to 40 mg	10 mg: $34 ($12)
	fosinopril	Monopril	10 to 40 mg	10 mg: $39 ($30)
	lisinopril	Prinivil	10 to 40 mg	10 mg: $34 ($17)
		Zestril	10 to 40 mg	10 mg: $34 ($17)
	moexipril	Univasc	7.5 to 30 mg	7.5 mg: $38 ($25)
	perindopril	Aceon	4 to 8 mg	8 mg: $52
	quinapril	Accupril	10 to 40 mg	10 mg: $36
	ramipril	Altace	2.5 to 20 mg	10 mg: $52
	trandolapril	Mavik	1 to 4 mg	4 mg: $34
Angiotensin II receptor blockers	candesartan	Atacand	8 to 32 mg	16 mg: $46
	eprosartan	Teveten	400 to 800 mg	400 mg: $36
	irbesartan	Avapro	150 to 300 mg	150 mg: $47
	losartan	Cozaar	25 to 100 mg	25 mg: $46
	olmesartan	Benicar	20 to 40 mg	20 mg: $46
	telmisartan	Micardis	20 to 80 mg	28 40-mg tablets: $51
	valsartan	Diovan	80 to 320 mg	80 mg: $48
Alpha-blockers	carvedilol‡	Coreg	12.5 to 50 mg	25 mg: $68
	doxazosin	Cardura	1 to 16 mg	2 mg: $39 ($15)
	labetalol‡	Normodyne	400 to 800 mg	100 mg: $21 ($12)
	prazosin	Minipress	2 to 20 mg	2 mg: $24 ($7)
	terazosin	Hytrin	1 to 20 mg	2 mg: $54 ($30)
Central alpha agonists	clonidine	Catapres	0.1 to 0.8 mg	0.2 mg: $45 ($6)
	clonidine patch	Catapres TTS	0.1 to 0.3 mg	12 0.1-mg patches: $150
	guanabenz	—	8 to 32 mg	(4 mg: $21)
	guanfacine	Tenex	0.5 to 2 mg	1 mg: $62 ($23)
	methyldopa	Aldomet	250 to 1,000 mg	250 mg: $12 ($7)
Peripheral-acting adrenergic antagonists	guanadrel	Hylorel	20 to 75 mg	10 mg: $56
	guanethidine	Ismelin	25 to 50 mg	10 mg: $19
Direct vasodilators	hydralazine	Apresoline	25 to 100 mg	100 mg: $26 ($7)
	minoxidil	Loniten	2.5 to 80 mg	10 mg: $60 ($17)
Aldosterone blockers	eplerenone	Inspra	50 to 100 mg	25 mg: $103

* These dosages represent an average range for the treatment of hypertension. The precise effective dosage varies from patient to patient and depends on many factors. Do not make any changes in your medication without consulting your doctor.
† Average price for 30 tablets or capsules (unless otherwise indicated) of the dosage strength listed. Actual price may vary. If a generic version is available, the cost is listed in parentheses. Sources: drugstore.com, eckerd.com, and walgreens.com.
‡ An alpha-blocker and beta-blocker.

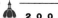

Advantages	Disadvantages
Kidney damage is slowed in people with diabetes who have mild kidney disease, even if they do not have hypertension. These drugs also slow kidney disease progression in people without diabetes. These drugs reduce the risk of death in people with heart failure and those who have had a heart attack. They also prevent heart failure after a heart attack.	Many individuals develop a dry cough. Skin rash may occur. Sense of taste may be altered. ACE inhibitors must be used with caution by those with severely impaired kidney function. These drugs should not be taken by pregnant women or women in their childbearing years (unless they are using effective contraception). On rare occasions, people experience a serious allergic reaction called angioedema, which causes the mouth to swell.
These drugs appear to have the same benefits as ACE inhibitors but with a reduced risk of dry cough and angioedema. They need to be taken only once a day.	In rare cases, these drugs may cause headache, dizziness, or fatigue. They should not be used by pregnant women or women in their childbearing years (unless they are using effective contraception).
Generally well tolerated. These drugs can reduce the symptoms of benign prostatic hyperplasia (noncancerous enlargement of the prostate gland) in men. Doxazosin and terazosin have the added benefit of raising HDL cholesterol levels.	These drugs may cause light-headedness and even fainting in older people, especially with the first dose. They may lose effectiveness over time. When used alone, doxazosin increases the risk of heart failure and stroke.
Side effects tend to be mild and to diminish with continued use. The clonidine patch requires only once-a-week dosing.	Dizziness (especially in older people), drowsiness, depression, dry mouth, constipation, sleep disturbances, and erectile dysfunction may occur. These drugs should not be stopped abruptly.
These drugs are effective for people with severe hypertension and can be combined with other classes of antihypertensive drugs for maximum benefit. Guanethidine does not cause drowsiness.	These drugs can cause diarrhea, and blood pressure may fall rapidly upon standing or with exercise.
Hydralazine can be very effective for people with severe hypertension. Minoxidil is more potent than hydralazine and is especially useful when severe hypertension is accompanied by kidney dysfunction. Combining these drugs with a beta-blocker and a diuretic greatly reduces side effects.	Hydralazine can cause a lupus-like syndrome at high doses. Minoxidil may cause unwanted hair growth. Heart palpitations and swelling of the feet or lower legs are also common.
May be used alone or in combination with other antihypertensive drugs. Works in a broad range of patients.	High blood potassium levels caused by poor kidney function are a rare but serious side effect. Less serious side effects include dizziness, fatigue, flu-like symptoms, diarrhea, and cough.

Peripheral-acting adrenergic antagonists. These medications reduce resistance to blood flow in small arteries by inhibiting the release of epinephrine and norepinephrine from nerves. Possible side effects include diarrhea and a profound drop in blood pressure when rising from a seated or reclining position or while exercising. These drugs are commonly used in people with severe hypertension.

Direct vasodilators. These drugs act directly on the smooth muscle of small arteries, causing these arteries to widen. They must be used in combination with both a diuretic and a beta-blocker to prevent fluid retention and rapid heartbeat. Excessive hair growth is an adverse side effect of minoxidil (Loniten). However, this discovery led to the development of a topical form of the drug for the treatment of baldness. Direct vasodilators are used only in people with hypertension that is difficult to control.

Aldosterone blockers. Eplerenone (Inspra) is the only drug approved in this class of antihypertensive medications. It works by blocking the activity of the hormone aldosterone. Side effects include dizziness, diarrhea, cough, fatigue, and flu-like symptoms. The drug should not be used by people with high blood potassium levels or those taking potassium supplements or potassium-sparing diuretics. People with diabetes or microalbuminuria (small amounts of protein in the urine) should avoid taking eplerenone as well.

Combination therapy. Most people with hypertension require two or more antihypertensive medications to get their blood pressure under control. Combining medications from different classes often results in greater reductions in blood pressure than using a single drug, because the actions of the drugs may complement each other. For example, diuretics reduce blood pressure by increasing the excretion of sodium and water by the kidneys. But in some people this effect stimulates the release of certain blood pressure-raising hormones to compensate for the drop in blood volume. Adding an ACE inhibitor blocks the actions of these hormones and improves blood pressure control.

Combination therapy can be achieved by taking a separate dose of each drug or using fixed-dose combination drugs (formulations of two different drugs combined in a single pill). Most fixed-dose combinations contain a thiazide diuretic (most often hydrochlorothiazide) and an ACE inhibitor, beta-blocker, angiotensin II receptor blocker, or central alpha agonist. A fixed combination of an ACE inhibitor and a calcium channel blocker is also available.

Fixed-dose combination drugs are more convenient (fewer pills to take each day) and are less expensive than taking each drug individually. Because the fixed-dose combination tends to contain smaller doses of each drug than if the drugs were taken separately, the risk of side effects may be lower as well. In some cases, one drug in the combination prevents the side effects of the other. For example, ACE inhibitors can reduce the leg swelling that often occurs with calcium channel blockers.

However, fixed-dose combinations reduce dosing flexibility—that is, the dosage of each medication in the combination cannot be varied separately. In addition, no large, long-term studies have proven that fixed-dose combinations offer any benefits over taking the two drugs separately. Therefore, fixed-dose combination drugs are most appropriate for people who have found that the combination of the two drugs effectively controls their blood pressure when taken separately at the same doses as in the combination pill.

The J-curve

A few small observational studies have suggested that people taking antihypertensive medication whose diastolic blood pressure is lowered beyond a certain point have a higher risk of heart attacks than hypertensive patients whose pressure is lowered to a lesser degree. This effect is called the J-curve phenomenon: When the number of deaths from heart attacks in people treated with antihypertensive medications is plotted against diastolic blood pressure on a graph, a line connecting the points shows an increase in deaths at the highest and lowest levels of diastolic pressure (the top of the straight part of the J and the top of the curved part of the J, respectively).

Most experts question whether a J-curve phenomenon exists, particularly in people with hypertension who do not have cardiovascular disease. The Hypertension Optimal Treatment (HOT) study, which involved 18,790 people with hypertension who had diastolic blood pressures between 100 and 105 mm Hg, showed that aggressive reduction of blood pressure to 140/85 mm Hg or lower was associated with a dramatic reduction in the risk of heart attacks. When blood pressure fell even further (for example, to 120/70 mm Hg), there was little additional benefit but also no significant additional risk, thus calling into question the J-curve phenomenon.

Medical Follow-up

People with stage 1 hypertension who are otherwise healthy are typically seen by their doctor once a month until they reach their blood pressure goal. Those with other health problems or stage 2 hypertension need to visit their doctor more frequently—every two

NEW RESEARCH

Antihypertensive Drugs Have Different Sexual Effects

Few studies have examined the effects of antihypertensive drugs on female sexual function. Now a study finds that valsartan (Diovan) may be a better choice than atenolol (Tenormin) for women concerned about their sex life.

The researchers studied 104 postmenopausal women (age 51 to 55) who were sexually active and newly diagnosed with hypertension. They were randomly assigned to receive either valsartan (an angiotensin II receptor blocker) or atenolol (a beta-blocker) for 16 weeks.

Valsartan and atenolol proved equally effective at lowering blood pressure, but the sexual effects of the drugs differed markedly according to patient questionaires. In women treated with valsartan, three aspects significantly improved: sexual desire, behavior when their partner asked for sexual relations, and sexual fantasies. In women treated with atenolol, two of those aspects got worse—desire and fantasies—and the third scored lower than with valsartan.

A possible reason for the different effects is that valsartan does not appear to affect testosterone levels, but atenolol reduces them. Research is needed on the sexual effects of thiazide diuretics, which are more commonly used than valsartan and atenolol.

AMERICAN JOURNAL OF HYPERTENSION
Volume 17, page 77
January 2004

to four weeks. At these visits, the doctor may adjust drug doses, add another drug, switch a medication if side effects are troublesome, and inquire about lifestyle modifications.

Once blood pressure is at goal or stabilizes, doctor visits are usually reduced to every three to six months, though people with other health conditions (such as diabetes or heart disease) may need to visit their doctor more often. Levels of blood sodium, potassium, and creatinine should be measured at least once or twice a year to detect any adverse effects from antihypertensive drugs and any deterioration in kidney function.

Only about a third of people with hypertension have reached the blood pressure goal of 140/90 mm Hg. One reason is that some doctors are not treating hypertension aggressively enough; another is that some people are not taking their antihypertensive medications as prescribed or are not adopting the recommended lifestyle modifications.

Poor compliance with antihypertensive therapy is understandable, considering that many people with hypertension have no or minimal symptoms yet are expected to make lifestyle modifications and take medication that may be costly or cause unpleasant side effects. Nonetheless, compliance is crucial to prevent the complications that may result from high blood pressure. On average, antihypertensive therapy is associated with a 35% to 40% lower risk of a stroke, a 20% to 25% reduced risk of a heart attack, and a 50% decrease in the risk of heart failure.

Stroke

Each year, about 700,000 people in the United States suffer a new or recurrent stroke, and about 164,000 of them die. The number of deaths from stroke rose by almost 8% from 1991 to 2001, but because the population also increased during that time, the death rate from stroke fell by about 3.5%. This fall is probably the result of more aggressive treatment of risk factors for stroke (such as hypertension), earlier diagnosis of stroke, and better medical management of the disease.

In addition to alteplase (Activase)—the first drug capable of halting a stroke in progress if administered soon enough after stroke onset—other drugs may soon be available for the emergency treatment of stroke. In addition, researchers are developing new approaches to rehabilitation, which could help people recover more fully and quickly from a stroke. Still, the best weapon against stroke is prevention. More than half of all strokes could be averted if people took the appropriate preventive steps.

THE BRAIN'S BLOOD SUPPLY

Although the brain accounts for only about 2% of the body's weight, it receives some 20% of the oxygenated and nutrient-rich blood pumped from the heart. Two pairs of arteries—the carotid arteries and the vertebral arteries—carry this large volume of blood to the brain.

The left and right carotid arteries receive blood from the heart and transport it up both sides of the front of the neck. As the two carotid arteries approach the top of the neck, each splits into an external carotid artery and an internal carotid artery. The external carotid arteries carry blood to the scalp, face, and neck, while the internal carotid arteries channel blood to the front two thirds of the brain and the eyes.

The left and right vertebral arteries run up the back of the neck, parallel to the spine. At the base of the skull, the two vertebral arteries join to form the basilar artery. Branches from the vertebral and basilar arteries bring blood to the brain stem—the lower portion of the brain near the spine—and to the rear third of the brain.

WHAT IS A STROKE?

A stroke occurs when an artery supplying blood to a portion of the brain becomes blocked or ruptures. As a result, neurons (nerve cells) in the affected area are starved of the oxygen and nutrients they need to function properly.

One reason a stroke is so dangerous is that the brain—unlike muscle or other tissues—has little or no reserve stores of energy. Consequently, when blood flow is interrupted to a part of the brain, some function may be lost in as little as four minutes. And after a few hours of interrupted blood flow, neurons cannot survive. (Areas of the brain further away from the core of the interrupted blood flow will also be affected but more slowly.)

Fortunately, the brain has some natural protection against such interruptions of blood supply—a ring of blood vessels called the circle of Willis at the base of the brain. This structure helps protect neurons by connecting the brain's front and rear blood supplies and providing alternative pathways for blood flow should a major artery become blocked or rupture.

Nerve cell damage due to a stroke is usually permanent. But despite the death of neurons, some improvement usually occurs over time as other neurons take over the functions of the neurons that were lost.

TYPES OF STROKE

There are two basic types of stroke: ischemic and hemorrhagic. Even though distinctly different mechanisms are responsible for each, hypertension increases the risk of both. Proper diagnosis of stroke type is essential for determining the best course of treatment.

Ischemic Stroke

About 88% of all strokes are ischemic, resulting from a blockage in a blood vessel leading to or in the brain. Neurons are damaged not only by the lack of oxygen and nutrients but also by a powerful chain of chemical reactions known as the ischemic (or glutamate) cascade, which leads to a buildup of toxins that further contributes to cell destruction. The degree and duration of an ischemic stroke determine whether the brain suffers temporary impairment, irreversible damage to only a few highly vulnerable neurons, or extensive neurological damage.

Cerebral thrombosis. The most common cause of ischemic stroke is cerebral thrombosis. Cerebral thrombosis occurs when a thrombus (blood clot) forms along the wall of one of the major arteries supplying the brain and completely blocks blood flow. These arteries include the carotid and vertebral arteries, which run along the front and back of the neck, respectively, as well as smaller arteries within the brain itself. Clots are most likely to develop in arteries that are already narrowed by atherosclerotic plaque—the same fatty deposits that cause coronary heart disease. The hard, rough, uneven surfaces of these plaques provide ideal sites for the formation and growth of blood clots, which may eventually completely block the already narrowed artery.

Cerebral embolism. Another possible cause of ischemic stroke is cerebral embolism. It most often occurs when part of a blood clot or a piece of atherosclerotic plaque breaks off and travels through the bloodstream (embolus) until it lodges in an artery supplying the brain and blocks blood flow. Most emboli originate in the heart or in large arteries such as the carotid artery. Emboli can also be

Imaging Techniques To Diagnose a Stroke

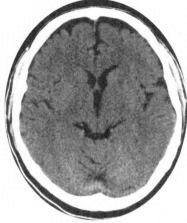

Normal CT

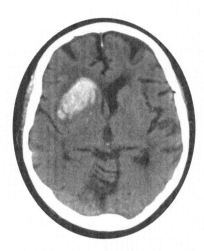

CT With Hemorrhagic Stroke

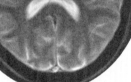

Normal MRI

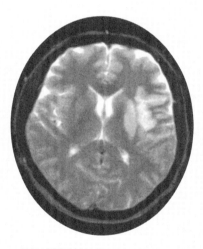

MRI With Ischemic Stroke

Computed tomography (CT) and magnetic resonance imaging (MRI) scans are the techniques most commonly used to visualize the brain when a stroke is suspected. Each has advantages and disadvantages.

In general, CT scans are best for rapidly determining whether an intracerebral or subarachnoid hemorrhage (see pages 39–40) has occurred, as well as to reveal the location and extent of any damage. MRI scans, on the other hand, provide more finely detailed images to identify smaller strokes. MRIs can also detect strokes earlier than CT scans (strokes that are visible within hours by MRI may not be visible for a few days to a week by CT), and provide better visualization of deeper parts of the brain. However, MRI scans take about 30 minutes to perform and patients must be able to remain very still through the entire procedure. CT scans, in contrast, take less than five minutes, are more readily available, and can be carried out in most hospitals.

Above are examples of the types of strokes detected most effectively by each imaging technique. The CT scan on the upper left shows a normal brain. The CT scan on the upper right reveals a hemorrhagic stroke—the irregular oval-shaped white area. (Blood appears white on a CT scan, while the brain generally appears dark.) On the lower left is an MRI scan of a normal brain. The white area in the MRI scan on the lower right indicates an ischemic stroke. This stroke would most likely not be visible by CT, since it is in the basal ganglia, which are clusters of nerve cells located deep within the brain.

composed of platelets, an air bubble, or bits of fat released from the marrow of a broken bone.

One of the most common causes of emboli is atrial fibrillation, an abnormal heart rhythm in which the atria (the upper chambers of the heart) quiver chaotically instead of contracting in a rhythmic pattern. As a result, the atria may not empty completely of blood; blood that remains in one place too long tends to stagnate and form clots. These clots can escape from the heart and travel along the increasingly narrow branches of blood vessels, ultimately lodging in an artery anywhere in the body, but usually in the brain. One third of individuals with untreated atrial fibrillation suffer a stroke during their lifetime.

People with heart muscle damage from a recent heart attack, a poorly functioning heart (for example, due to cardiomyopathy), a diseased heart valve (for example, mitral stenosis), and, possibly, atherosclerotic plaque in the aorta (the main artery emerging from the heart) also are at risk for blood clots that can break off and cause a stroke.

Lacunar strokes. Lacunar strokes are often seen in older individuals with high blood pressure. They occur when the tiny arterioles (the endmost branches of arteries) that penetrate deep into the brain become completely blocked by small emboli or atherosclerotic plaque. As a consequence of the blockages, small areas of brain tissue degenerate, leaving behind little cavities called lacunes (lakes). Because the blood vessels involved are so small, symptoms of lacunar strokes are usually mild, and diagnosis may be difficult.

Transient ischemic attacks (TIAs). TIAs are short-lived neurological deficits that result from a temporary blockage of blood flow to the brain. Most episodes subside within 5 to 20 minutes and rarely continue for more than a few hours. Because TIAs do not result in permanent neurological deficits and are almost never painful, people tend to ignore them. But TIAs are an important warning sign of an impending stroke and warrant prompt medical attention. In fact, some people have repetitive episodes of TIAs in the days or weeks before a stroke, and one third of those who experience a TIA have a stroke within five years.

Recognition and treatment of the cause of a TIA may help to prevent a stroke and its complications. For example, if carotid stenosis (narrowing of one of the carotid arteries supplying the brain) is detected, a surgical procedure called carotid endarterectomy (see pages 54–56) can be performed.

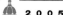

Hemorrhagic Stroke

Accounting for about 12% of all strokes, hemorrhagic strokes occur when an artery in the brain suddenly bursts and blood leaks out into the surrounding tissue. The bleeding can take place either into the brain itself (intracerebral hemorrhage) or into the space between the brain and the skull (subarachnoid hemorrhage).

Damage occurs in two ways. First, the blood supply is cut off to the parts of the brain beyond the site of the arterial rupture. Second—and posing the greatest danger—the escaped blood forms a mass that exerts excessive pressure on the brain. Blood continues to leak until it clots or until the pressure inside the skull is equal to the blood pressure in the ruptured artery.

Aneurysms—blood-filled pouches that balloon out from weak spots in a blood vessel wall—cause many hemorrhagic strokes. While some aneurysms are congenital (present at birth), they may be exacerbated or even caused by hypertension. Most strokes due to a ruptured aneurysm occur in people between the ages of 40 and 60. Aneurysms are more common in people with polycystic kidney disease (a rare inherited condition in which the kidneys contain multiple cysts) and in those with two or more close relatives with aneurysms. Magnetic resonance angiography (see page 62) can be used to detect large aneurysms.

Brain hemorrhage may also result from a congenital blood vessel defect known as an arteriovenous malformation, which is characterized by a complex, tangled web of arteries and veins. The walls of these abnormal blood vessels tend to be so thin that surges in blood pressure, or simply the wear and tear of normal blood flow, may eventually cause an arteriovenous malformation to rupture and bleed into the brain.

Intracerebral hemorrhage. Intracerebral hemorrhage is characterized by leakage of blood into tissue deep within the brain, usually the cerebrum (the part of the brain that controls higher functions such as speaking and reasoning). A tear in a small blood vessel in the brain is the primary cause of intracerebral hemorrhage; other possible causes include head injury, aneurysm, brain tumor, and use of illicit drugs such as cocaine and amphetamines. In people over age 80, a common cause of intracerebral hemorrhage is amyloid angiopathy—a weakening of blood vessels by deposits of amyloid, a starch-like substance.

Subarachnoid hemorrhage. Subarachnoid hemorrhage results from bleeding into the space between the brain and the protective arachnoid membrane that lies between the brain and the skull.

NEW RESEARCH

Treating Hypertension Cuts Hemorrhagic Stroke Risk

Blood pressure-lowering medication could prevent one in four hemorrhagic strokes among people with untreated hypertension, a new study shows.

Researchers identified 549 individuals who had suffered a hemorrhagic stroke; 322 of these strokes were intracerebral hemorrhages and 227 were subarachnoid hemorrhages. Individuals were matched by age, race, and gender to stroke-free controls.

The researchers found that people with untreated hypertension had nearly four times the risk of hemorrhagic stroke as people with normal blood pressure, while those who were taking medication for their high blood pressure had a 40% higher risk. Based on these figures, the researchers estimate that 17% to 28% of strokes in the group with untreated hypertension would have been prevented if they were on blood pressure medication.

People on Medicaid or those who paid for their own medical care were more likely to have untreated hypertension, as were men, the researchers found. They propose that "future studies of hemorrhagic stroke should include treatment or lack of treatment of hypertension in the analyses."

STROKE
Volume 35, page 1703
July 2004

Most subarachnoid hemorrhages result from a ruptured aneurysm. Head injuries, arteriovenous malformations, and other blood vessel defects also may be responsible. About 80% of subarachnoid hemorrhages occur in people age 40 to 65, 15% occur in those age 20 to 40, and 5% occur in those under age 20. Women, especially during pregnancy, are at slightly higher risk for subarachnoid hemorrhage than men.

SYMPTOMS OF STROKE

Like a heart attack, a stroke is an emergency that requires immediate medical attention. While most people know and can recognize the characteristic symptoms of a heart attack, many are unaware of the symptoms of a stroke. Moreover, when a TIA is in progress, symptoms may appear suddenly and then subside just as quickly, creating the false impression that a serious problem does not exist.

The feature on the opposite page describes the symptoms of a stroke and the appropriate steps to take if these symptoms occur. Anyone who experiences the sudden onset of any of these symptoms—even if the symptoms subside—must call 911 or go straight to the hospital. Rapid diagnosis and treatment may minimize damage to brain tissue and improve the chance of survival.

EFFECTS OF STROKE

In addition to the initial symptoms, strokes generally produce lasting neurological deficits that may impair a person's senses, motor skills, behavior, language ability, memory, or thought processes. The deficits that occur depend on which portions of the brain are damaged by the stroke (as well as on the type and severity of the stroke). Strokes can affect the following areas of the brain: the brain stem, cerebellum, limbic system, and cerebrum.

The Brain Stem, Cerebellum, and Limbic System

At the base of the brain (at the top of the spinal cord) lies the brain stem. The brain stem maintains basic life support functions—breathing, heart rate, blood pressure, and digestion. An extensive stroke affecting the brain stem is usually fatal; when patients do survive, artificial life support is often necessary. Since the brain stem also helps maintain consciousness, a major stroke in this area can result in a coma. A coma also can occur when a stroke in the cerebrum, which surrounds the brain stem, causes

Recognizing a Stroke

Like a heart attack, a stroke is an emergency that requires immediate medical attention. Since drug therapy is most likely to be effective within the first three hours of stroke onset, getting to the hospital as soon as symptoms start is essential. Listed below are the symptoms of a stroke, as well as what to do.

Symptoms of Stroke

- Sudden weakness or numbness in the face, arm, or leg on one side of the body.
- Sudden loss, blurring, or dimness of vision.
- Mental confusion, loss of memory, or sudden loss of consciousness.
- Slurred speech, loss of speech, or problems understanding others.
- Sudden, severe headache with no apparent cause.
- Unexplained dizziness, drowsiness, incoordination, or falls.
- Nausea and vomiting, especially when accompanied by any of the above symptoms.

Actions To Take

- Stay calm. Ignore any tendency to downplay a symptom; it's common for people to deny the possibility of something as serious as a stroke. Don't hesitate to take prompt action.
- Call or have someone call an ambulance. (Dial 911 in most parts of the United States.) Be sure to give your name, telephone number, and exact whereabouts.
- While waiting for the ambulance, the person suffering the stroke symptoms should be made as comfortable as possible and should not eat or drink anything other than water.
- If an ambulance cannot arrive for an extended period of time, a family member or neighbor should drive the stroke patient to the hospital. Under no circumstances should the person experiencing the stroke symptoms attempt to drive.
- Notify the stroke patient's doctor. The doctor can provide the hospital with the patient's medical history, which may be important for determining the best type of treatment.
- At the hospital, be sure to list any medical conditions the stroke patient has (such as high blood pressure), any allergies the patient has (particularly to medication), and any medications the patient is currently taking.

swelling that puts pressure on the brain stem.

Above the brain stem is the cerebellum, which controls coordination, balance, and posture. Early symptoms of a stroke in the cerebellum include dizziness, nausea, and vomiting. Later symptoms include clumsiness, shaking, or difficulty controlling certain muscles.

Above the cerebellum is a group of structures known as the limbic system. The limbic system is responsible for the primal urges and powerful emotions that ensure self-preservation: rage, terror, hunger, and sexual desire. Growth and reproductive cycles also are governed by the limbic system. Strokes in this area are rare, but when they occur, basic drives may be severely limited, or patients may lose their natural inhibitions.

The Cerebrum

Surrounding the brain stem, cerebellum, and limbic system is the cerebrum—the largest portion of the brain and a common site of strokes. The cerebrum's convoluted outer layer of gray matter, known as the cortex, is the center of conscious thought, perception, voluntary movement, and integration of all sensory input.

The cortex of the cerebrum is divided into two halves, or hemispheres, each responsible for a different set of duties. In most right-handed people, the right hemisphere specializes in spatial relationships, color perception, visual interpretation, and musical aptitude, while the left half of the brain typically oversees analytical tasks (such as mathematical computation and logical reasoning) and linguistic tasks (such as comprehending words and formulating speech). In left-handed people, the hemispheres responsible for these duties are typically reversed. One exception is speech, which usually involves both hemispheres in left-handed people.

Each hemisphere also governs movement and sensory perception on the opposite side of the body. Consequently, a stroke in the left hemisphere can result in paralysis on the right side of the body. Each hemisphere is further subdivided into four distinct sections, known as lobes. The two hemispheres constantly communicate with one another via a thick neural connecting cable known as the corpus callosum.

Frontal lobe. The frontal lobe is situated at the front of the brain, behind the brow. One of the responsibilities of this lobe is motor function—neurons in the motor cortex of the frontal lobe send signals that initiate muscle activity throughout the body. Damage to the motor cortex on one side of the brain can result in weakness or paralysis on the opposite side of the body. In addition to paralysis of the limbs and torso, muscles on one side of the face or mouth may be affected, altering the person's appearance or ability to speak clearly (a condition called dysarthria). The frontal lobe manages more abstract types of movement as well, including activities that require sequential steps. Consequently, a stroke may make it difficult or impossible to carry out a complex task, such as preparing a meal.

Expressive aphasia—difficulty in speaking, writing, or gesturing—can result when a stroke affects the frontal lobe in the dominant hemisphere (the left hemisphere of someone who is right-handed, for example). Insight, initiative, and social inhibitions are governed by the foremost portion of the frontal lobe. A stroke in this area could result in uncharacteristically impulsive or uninhibited behavior. Conversely, profound apathy, lethargy, and a lack of intentional behavior may result—a condition known as abulia.

Parietal lobe. Behind the frontal lobe is the parietal lobe, which is responsible for receiving and interpreting sensory information from all parts of the body. Common problems resulting from a stroke in the parietal lobe are sensory loss, numbness, and vision loss on the side of the body opposite from the brain damage. Damage to the highly specialized sensory cortex in the parietal lobe may result in agnosia, in which the person is unable to interpret incoming visual, auditory, or tactile stimuli, even though the senses of vision, hearing, and touch are mechanically intact and function normally.

Another common consequence of a stroke in the parietal lobe is neglect. People exhibiting neglect typically stop perceiving or acknowledging events, and even sensations, on the side of the body opposite the affected hemisphere.

Temporal lobe. The temporal lobe—situated at ear level, underneath both the parietal and frontal lobes—is dedicated to auditory perception and storage of memories. Strokes in the temporal lobe rarely cause hearing loss; however, they commonly result in language deficits known as aphasia—problems understanding speech, verbalizing thoughts, reading, or writing. Memory loss is also a common consequence of stroke in the temporal lobe. However, memory deficits may be only temporary, since the temporal lobe on the other side of the brain can eventually compensate (unless both sides of the brain have been affected by the stroke).

Occipital lobe. The occipital lobe lies at the rear of the cerebral cortex, in the back of the skull. It is dedicated entirely to the perception and interpretation of visual data delivered from the eyes via the optic nerve. A stroke on the right side of the occipital lobe causes hemianopia—blindness in the left field of vision of both eyes—rather than blindness in the left eye. An occipital lobe stroke can also result in loss of the ability to recognize and interpret visual stimuli (for example, faces).

Other Consequences

Besides the deficits described above, a stroke may produce other long-term problems, including impaired concentration, poor judgment, erratic sleep patterns, loss of libido, emotional instability, depression, and seizures. Also, immobility following a stroke may lead to aspiration pneumonia (inhalation of food and other particles into the lungs due to an inability to swallow and cough properly), bedsores, deep vein thrombosis (formation of painful blood clots in the legs), limb contractures (tightening of the muscles in the limbs), incontinence, and urinary tract infection.

RISK FACTORS FOR STROKE

A number of factors contribute to the overall chance of having a stroke. Some of these factors, such as age or race, obviously can't be modified. Fortunately, other major risk factors can be significantly

NEW RESEARCH

Western Diet Tied to Higher Stroke Risk

The more red meat and refined flour a woman eats, the more likely she is to suffer a stroke, a large new study shows.

A so-called Western diet, featuring a high intake of red and processed meats, refined grains, high-fat dairy foods, desserts, and sweets, has already been linked to coronary heart disease and colon cancer.

The current study examined data from nearly 72,000 women who were followed for up to 14 years. The researchers divided the women into two groups based on how closely their diet resembled one of two eating patterns: the Western-style diet or a prudent diet rich in vegetables, fruits, whole grains, legumes, and fish.

Among women who ate a predominantly Western diet, those who followed the most extreme form had a 58% greater risk of stroke than those who followed the most moderate form. Among those who ate a predominantly prudent diet, those who adhered to it most stringently had a 22% lower stroke risk than those who followed it least stringently.

The researchers conclude that steering clear of a Western diet and eating more fruits, vegetables, whole grains, and fish may help ward off stroke.

STROKE
Volume 35, page 2014
September 2004

reduced through lifestyle measures, medical treatment, or a combination of both. One of these modifiable risk factors is hypertension, which not only accelerates the development of atherosclerosis—the arterial narrowing that accounts for at least two thirds of all ischemic strokes—but is the most important precursor of hemorrhagic stroke.

Risk Factors That Cannot Be Changed

The following important risk factors for stroke cannot be changed. Their presence should alert people to their greater stroke risk and the need to reduce risk factors that they can change.

Age. Between the ages of 55 and 85, the risk of stroke doubles with each successive decade. Only 28% of people who suffer a stroke are younger than age 65.

Gender. Overall, the risk of stroke is approximately 25% higher in men than in women. This difference is even greater in people younger than age 65 but is nonexistent at older ages, when the protective effect of estrogen disappears after women undergo menopause. Men also have a slightly higher risk of dying of stroke than women.

Family history. Stroke risk is greater in people whose close relatives (parents or siblings) have had a stroke.

Race. Blacks have about twice the risk of death and disability from a stroke than whites. Asian-Pacific Islanders and Hispanics also are at higher risk than whites.

Prior history of stroke. People who have had a stroke are at substantial risk for having another; about 13% have another stroke within a year, and the risk of stroke in each successive year after that is 6%.

Transient ischemic attacks (TIAs). While only about 10% of strokes are preceded by TIAs, these short-lived events are a strong predictor of a full-blown stroke. A stroke is almost 10 times more likely in someone who has experienced a TIA than in someone who has not. About 36% of people who have had one or more TIAs will eventually have a stroke. Studies show that between 25% and 50% of TIAs are the result of a blood clot at a site of atherosclerotic plaque in a brain artery. Between 11% and 30% of TIAs result from emboli originating in the heart.

Accidents and other circumstances. Bone fractures, open heart surgery, the collapse of a lung (a pneumothorax), or too rapid an ascent from deep waters can result in blood clots that can lead to cerebral embolism. A violent blow to the head may

NEW RESEARCH

Age at Menopause Not a Factor In Risk of Death From Stroke

Although women who go through menopause at a relatively young age are at increased risk for coronary heart disease, a new study shows they are no more likely than others to suffer a fatal stroke.

The researchers reviewed data on 19,731 Norwegian women, 3,561 of whom died of a stroke during a 37-year period. On average, women reported undergoing menopause at about age 48. The researchers found that the 2.8% of the women who underwent menopause before age 40, as well as the 1.6% who stopped menstruating after age 55, were no more likely to die of a stroke than the other women.

The researchers conclude that "age at natural menopause is not related to stroke mortality." This may be explained by the fact that menopause has little effect on blood pressure, the most important risk factor for stroke.

STROKE
Volume 35, page 1548
July 2004

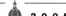

Nothing Minor About Ministrokes

A transient ischemic attack, sometimes called a ministroke, warrants the same immediate medical attention that a full-blown stroke does.

A transient ischemic attack (TIA) may not seem like an emergency. The symptoms—although nearly identical to a stroke (see the feature on page 41)—are by definition temporary, lasting no longer than 24 hours and often subsiding within 20 minutes. These so-called ministrokes are rarely painful, and people often put off seeking medical care or never consult a doctor at all about their symptoms.

But TIAs are not as benign as they may appear. Emerging evidence presented at the American Stroke Association's 27th International Stroke Conference in 2004 demonstrated that the risk of subsequent stroke and death is high among TIA patients and that hospitalization for 24 hours after a TIA may be the best course of action.

How Risky Are TIAs?
Two presentations at the conference looked at the risk of stroke and death after a TIA. The first study compared the risk of stroke, dependency, and death in TIA and stroke patients in Germany. Although stroke patients were at a higher risk in each category, patients who had a TIA still had a high likelihood of having a stroke (6%), becoming dependent on others for daily care (22%), and dying (2%) within six months of the TIA. The researchers concluded that TIAs "merit the same attention" as strokes.

The second study, conducted in California, found that nearly 6% of TIA patients experienced a stroke within 48 hours of their TIA. By three months, this percentage increased to 16%. Three years later, 30% of TIA patients had gone on to have a stroke, showing that the risk of stroke is high after a TIA, especially in the first few hours. Older patients, those with diabetes, and those with

hypertension were at a higher risk for stroke after a TIA.

Should TIA Patients Be Hospitalized?
Knowing the risks of TIAs, the California researchers conducted another study that looked at the cost-effectiveness of hospitalizing TIA patients for the first 24 hours after the event. The rationale was simple: Because TIA patients have such a high risk of stroke immediately after a TIA, if they are already in the hospital they can be given the emergency stroke drug t-PA immediately if they have a stroke. Otherwise, they may be far from medical help when a stroke occurs and not likely to receive t-PA during the short window of opportunity in which this treatment is effective.

The researchers found that 2.9% of TIA patients would have a stroke and receive t-PA if they were hospitalized compared with only 0.5% of patients not hospitalized. Hospitalizing all TIA patients for 24 hours would be cost-effective, the researchers concluded. The strategy would cost about $44,300 per quality-adjusted life-years saved. (Any intervention that costs less than $50,000 per quality-adjusted life-years saved is considered cost-effective.)

Although routine hospitalization of TIA patients is not recommended at this time, it could become standard practice if further studies bear out the result of this one. In the meantime, Rafael H. Llinas, M.D., coauthor of this White Paper, recommends people receive an inpatient or outpatient workup soon after a TIA because of the small but elevated risk of stroke within the next 48 hours.

Evaluating and Treating TIAs
Because TIAs are short-lived, they often aren't treated as emergencies—

but they should be. If you experience TIA symptoms, which are similar to stroke symptoms, call 911 or have someone drive you to the hospital, even if the symptoms go away.

At the hospital, someone will take your medical history, and you will undergo blood tests, electrocardiography, and imaging studies of the head and, possibly, carotid arteries. You can also expect to receive treatments that include those used for strokes themselves—including medications to prevent blood clots and future strokes, such as aspirin, clopidogrel (Plavix), aspirin plus dipyridamole (Aggrenox), warfarin (Coumadin), and occasionally, in specific situations, heparin.

Patients should view a TIA as a warning sign that they need to control any modifiable stroke risk factors they have (see pages 46–48). Lifestyle changes should include improving one's diet and exercising regularly, quitting smoking if you smoke, and drinking only in moderation (no more than two drinks daily for men, one for women).

Patients may also need additional medications to lower levels of blood pressure or low-density lipoprotein (LDL, or "bad") cholesterol. Those with diabetes may need medication to lower blood glucose levels. Patients with heart conditions that increase their risk of another TIA or stroke—including coronary heart disease, an abnormal heart rhythm such as atrial fibrillation, heart failure, and valvular heart disease—should receive appropriate treatment for these conditions.

Finally, for patients whose evaluation reveals a significant blockage of the carotid arteries, a surgical procedure called carotid endarterectomy (see pages 54–56) may be done to improve the flow of blood to the brain.

cause a hemorrhagic stroke. Mild kidney dysfunction also may raise the risk of stroke.

Risk Factors That Can Be Changed

The following factors raise the risk of stroke; all of them can be minimized or eliminated through lifestyle changes or medical therapy.

Hypertension. High blood pressure, the single greatest risk factor for stroke, is estimated to play a role in about 70% of all ischemic and hemorrhagic strokes. Elevations in either systolic or diastolic blood pressure increase the risk of stroke in both men and women and in people of all ages. Indeed, stroke risk is about four times greater in those with a blood pressure of 160/95 mm Hg or above than in those with a blood pressure of 140/90 mm Hg or below. A recent meta-analysis concluded that the risk of stroke was increased 10 to 12 times in people with a diastolic blood pressure of 105 mm Hg or higher compared with those with a diastolic pressure of less than 76 mm Hg.

Cigarette smoking. Smoking is an important contributor to both ischemic and hemorrhagic strokes. A recent meta-analysis found that cigarette smokers have a 50% higher risk of stroke than nonsmokers. The more cigarettes smoked, the greater the risk. Smoking appears to accelerate the progression of atherosclerosis, promote the formation of blood clots, and cause structural damage to the arteries. Also, nicotine briefly raises blood pressure after each cigarette and causes a buildup of carbon monoxide in the blood that reduces the blood's oxygen-carrying capacity and thus the amount of oxygen available to the brain. Fortunately, the increased risk of stroke associated with smoking decreases after quitting, and the risk returns to normal within five years of smoking cessation.

Diabetes. People with diabetes have a threefold higher risk of ischemic stroke than the general population. Women with diabetes are at greater risk than men. Diabetes is treatable, and evidence is growing that controlling blood sugar may lower stroke risk. Diabetes does not appear to increase the risk of hemorrhagic strokes.

Carotid stenosis. The carotid arteries in the neck supply blood to the brain. If a carotid artery becomes narrowed by the buildup of atherosclerotic plaque, blood flowing through will make an abnormal sound called a bruit. A doctor can hear this sound by placing a stethoscope over the carotid arteries in the neck. When a bruit is heard, especially in people with a history of TIA, a duplex ultrasound (see pages 60–61) is performed to determine the extent of the narrowing. Even in people without a history of TIA, a

NEW RESEARCH

Chronic Stress Drives Up Risk Of Heart Attack and Stroke

A Swedish study adds to the growing body of evidence that chronic stress contributes to heart attack and stroke.

In a study of 13,609 people (mostly men) followed for about 21 years, those reporting high levels of chronic stress at the study's outset had a 14% higher risk of heart attack or stroke than those with low stress levels. In addition, men with high levels of chronic stress had double the risk of experiencing a fatal stroke.

Because the researchers adjusted their results for factors such as cigarette smoking and sedentary lifestyle, which may increase with stress, their findings may actually underestimate the relationship between chronic stress and heart attack and stroke.

A weak relationship was seen between chronic stress and heart attack and stroke in women. The researchers note this was likely owing to the small number of women in the study and the relative rarity of heart attack and stroke in premenopausal women, rather than any protective effect of gender.

Chronic stress has been hypothesized to contribute to heart attack and stroke by producing hormones that affect blood pressure and cholesterol, and by making people more likely to smoke cigarettes and less likely to exercise.

EUROPEAN HEART JOURNAL
Volume 25, page 867
May 2004

carotid bruit suggests an increased risk of ischemic stroke since it usually indicates atherosclerotic narrowing of the carotid artery. In general, people with carotid stenosis are three times more likely to suffer a stroke than the general population.

Heart disease. Since many of the same factors contribute to both stroke and coronary heart disease, it is not surprising that the risk of stroke is doubled in those with coronary heart disease. It is uncertain whether treatment of coronary heart disease will prevent strokes, however. Other heart diseases can increase stroke risk by promoting the formation of emboli. These conditions include heart attack, heart failure (impaired ability of the heart to pump blood), valvular heart disease (damage to one or more of the heart's valves), and various abnormal heart rhythms, especially atrial fibrillation.

Alcohol abuse. Moderate alcohol consumption (two or fewer drinks per day) is associated with a reduced risk of ischemic stroke. By contrast, even moderate alcohol consumption raises the risk of hemorrhagic stroke. Habitual alcohol intake in excess of two drinks per day almost doubles the risk of stroke by producing abnormal heart rhythms, raising blood pressure, and promoting blood clot formation.

Oral contraceptives and hormone replacement therapy. Older, high-dose estrogen oral contraceptives increased the risk of stroke in women who were over age 35 and smoked cigarettes, had high blood pressure, or had a history of migraine headaches. The low-dose oral contraceptives used today are still associated with a risk of stroke, but the risk is small.

Hormone replacement therapy also increases the risk of stroke. In a randomized, controlled trial called the Women's Health Initiative, researchers discovered that postmenopausal women taking estrogen plus progestin had a 40% increased risk of stroke compared with women taking a placebo. Nearly two years later the researchers found that women taking estrogen alone also had an increased stroke risk (see the sidebar at right). Therefore, women taking hormone replacement therapy—either estrogen plus progestin or estrogen alone—for relief of menopausal symptoms should do so for the shortest time possible and at the smallest effective dose.

Drug abuse. Stimulants such as cocaine and amphetamines can cause abnormal heart rhythms, heart attack, and stroke (particularly intracerebral hemorrhage), even in young, healthy first-time users. Intravenous drug use raises the risk of cerebral embolism.

Abnormal lipid levels. High total and low-density lipoprotein (LDL, or "bad") cholesterol, elevated triglycerides, and low HDL

NEW RESEARCH

Estrogen Therapy Increases Stroke Risk in Postmenopausal Women

Nearly two years after combined hormone replacement therapy with estrogen and progestin was found to increase a women's risk of stroke and other ills, new evidence from the same study indicates that taking estrogen alone also increases stroke risk.

Health officials stopped the estrogen-only portion of the study in early 2004, when they found that estrogen increased the risk of stroke by 39% and did not protect against cancer, heart attack or heart-related deaths. Estrogen, however, did reduce the risk of hip fracture.

The study involved 10,739 women age 50 to 79 who were randomly assigned to take either an estrogen replacement or a placebo for an average of nearly seven years. Because taking estrogen without progestin increases the risk of uterine cancer, the study included only women who had had a hysterectomy.

The overall risks of estrogen use outweigh its benefits, according to the authors of an accompanying editorial. The editorialists write that estrogen-only therapy, like combined hormone replacement therapy, should not be used to prevent disease in postmenopausal women. They also write that estrogen should be taken at as low a dose and for as short a time as possible when used for the relief of menopausal symptoms.

JOURNAL OF THE AMERICAN MEDICAL ASSOCIATION
Volume 291, pages 1701 and 1769
April 14, 2004

("good") cholesterol contribute to atherosclerosis and coronary heart disease, and they are important risk factors for stroke as well. A 21-year study of more than 8,000 Israeli men found that those with HDL cholesterol levels below 35 mg/dL had a 32% greater risk of stroke than men with levels above 43 mg/dL. In addition, a study of about 1,500 New York City residents found that people with HDL cholesterol levels between 35 and 49 mg/dL had a 35% reduction in ischemic stroke risk, compared with those with HDL cholesterol levels below 35 mg/dL. Reduction of total cholesterol, LDL cholesterol, and triglyceride levels using statin drugs substantially reduces the risk of ischemic stroke (for a recent study, see the sidebar at right).

Sedentary lifestyle. Studies consistently show that regular physical activity lowers the risk of both ischemic and hemorrhagic stroke, possibly by reducing other stroke risk factors, such as obesity and hypertension. In general, people who are physically inactive are almost three times as likely to suffer a stroke than people who exercise regularly.

Obesity. Obesity increases the risk of stroke by 50% to 100%. Although obesity is associated with other risk factors for stroke, such as hypertension and diabetes, it may be an independent risk factor for stroke. Abdominal obesity (a waist circumference of greater than 40 inches in men or 35 inches in women) has an especially strong impact on diabetes and other stroke risk factors. A recent study found that abdominal obesity was a better predictor of ischemic stroke than BMI—a measure of weight in relation to height.

C-reactive protein. A newly recognized risk factor for stroke is C-reactive protein, a marker for inflammation. Research shows that people with blood levels of C-reactive protein above 3 mg/L are at increased risk for ischemic stroke, as well as for heart attack. The American Heart Association recommends that people at intermediate risk for heart attack or stroke have their CRP levels measured in addition to the usual evaluation of risk factors. CRP is measured with a simple blood test.

PREVENTION OF STROKE

The best way to prevent a stroke is to eliminate or minimize as many of the modifiable risk factors as possible. In general, this can be accomplished by losing weight (if necessary), eating a healthy diet, engaging in regular aerobic exercise, and quitting smoking.

NEW RESEARCH

Statin Drug Lowers Stroke Risk

Cholesterol-lowering drugs called statins are used primarily to reduce the risk of heart attack. But new research shows that they also appear to reduce the risk of stroke.

Researchers identified more than 20,000 people at elevated risk for stroke, including people with cerebrovascular disease, coronary heart disease, and diabetes. Study participants were randomly assigned to receive either 40 mg of the cholesterol-lowering drug simvastatin (Zocor) or a placebo daily for five years.

The researchers found that people who received simvastatin were 25% less likely than those receiving the placebo to have a stroke. When they looked only at participants who had preexisting cerebrovascular disease but not coronary heart disease, those who received simvastatin were still less likely to have a stroke.

According to the study authors, the results indicate that statin therapy should now be considered routinely for all patients at high risk for stroke, regardless of how high their initial cholesterol levels are and even if they do not have coronary heart disease.

Findings from previous studies have been mixed as to whether reducing cholesterol levels also lowers the risk of stroke, and current practice guidelines do not recommend that doctors prescribe these drugs for patients at risk for stroke.

THE LANCET
Volume 363, page 757
March 6, 2004

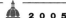

Stroke Protection Via Vitamins

Evidence is growing that some B vitamins may help prevent strokes.

If you are at high risk for a stroke, you will want to take every step you can to protect your health. In addition to the standard measures—such as lowering your blood pressure, not smoking, and exercising—some new research shows that certain B vitamins, particularly vitamin B_6, folic acid, and vitamin B_{12}, may also help lower your stroke risk.

The Role of Homocysteine
The body produces an amino acid called homocysteine, which damages the walls of blood vessels when levels are too high. Elevated levels of homocysteine are known to increase the risk of heart attack, and studies now show that they also increase the risk of stroke. Homocysteine is naturally eliminated by the body, but first it must be converted into other amino acids. Because vitamin B_6, folic acid, and vitamin B_{12} are required for this conversion, it is important to get adequate levels of these vitamins.

Research Trends
A large 2004 study in the journal *Stroke* found that elevated dietary intakes of folic acid and vitamin B_{12} are linked to a lower risk of ischemic, but not hemorrhagic, stroke. In the

study, researchers assessed the diet of 43,732 healthy men every four years from 1986 to 2000. Men with the highest intakes of folic acid in their diet were 29% less likely to have an ischemic stroke during the study than men with the lowest intakes. Dietary intakes of vitamin B_{12}, but not vitamin B_6, were also linked to a lower risk of ischemic stroke.

Another study, this one published in 2004 in the *European Journal of Clinical Investigation*, suggested that healthy people who were randomized to take supplements of vitamin B_6 (250 mg per day) and folic acid (5 mg per day) tended to have less plaque in the blood vessels leading to the brain after two years than those who took a placebo. Although the results weren't statistically significant, a larger study (this one involved only 158 people) would likely show a significant benefit, the study's authors say.

However, B vitamins may not be as protective in people who've already had a stroke. According to a 2004 study in the *Journal of the American Medical Association*, of 3,680 people who had a nondisabling stroke, supplements containing high doses of vitamin B_6, folic acid, and vitamin B_{12}

did not prevent a second stroke any better than supplements containing low doses of these vitamins (about 9% of both groups experienced a stroke after two years of treatment). This result suggests that these B vitamins may not play a role in secondary stroke risk.

Getting Your B Vitamins
To date, no randomized, controlled trial has shown that B vitamins will lower your risk of having a stroke. Consequently, the American Heart Association does not recommend that people take supplements of B vitamins to prevent stroke or coronary heart disease. However, the organization does recommend consuming five daily servings of fruits and green, leafy vegetables—which are rich in B vitamins—and only taking vitamins if diet is inadequate. Multivitamins typically contain at least the recommended levels of vitamin B_6, folic acid, and vitamin B_{12}.

Nonetheless, Raphael H. Llinas, M.D., coauthor of this White Paper, recommends taking folic acid as part of a multivitamin supplement to help prevent stroke. But he points out that taking higher doses of folic acid offers no additional protection.

Dietary Sources of Vitamin B_6, Folic Acid, and Vitamin B_{12}

Vitamin	Sources	Recommended Intake
B_6	Whole grains, bananas, beef, pork, beans, nuts, wheat germ, chicken, fish, and liver.	1.5 mg for women age 51 and older 1.7 mg for men age 51 and older
Folic acid	Leafy greens, wheat germ, liver, beans, whole and fortified grains, broccoli, and citrus fruits.	400 micrograms (mcg)
B_{12}	Liver, beef, pork, poultry, eggs, dairy products, seafood, and fortified cereals.	2.4 mcg

Medication may also be needed to control blood pressure, blood lipids, and blood glucose. In addition, antiplatelet therapy, anticoagulants, carotid endarterectomy, or angioplasty and stents may be necessary for people who have already had a stroke or TIA or are at high risk for having a stroke.

Antiplatelet Therapy

Drugs that reduce blood clot formation by inhibiting the aggregation of platelets in the blood often are prescribed to prevent ischemic strokes in people at high risk, particularly those with asymptomatic carotid bruit or a history of TIA or stroke.

Aspirin. Aspirin is by far the most widely used antiplatelet drug. A recent review of more than 100 clinical trials concluded that aspirin therapy reduces the risk of future strokes by 25% to 30% in people who have had a TIA or minor stroke. (Aspirin is not advised for stroke prevention in otherwise healthy people over age 50 who have not had a stroke or TIA.) Most stroke experts recommend an 81- to 325-mg tablet of aspirin a day to lower stroke risk. People with high blood pressure should lower it before beginning aspirin therapy: A recent study found that the benefits of aspirin in people with high blood pressure are limited mainly to those whose hypertension is under control.

Ticlopidine. Another antiplatelet drug, ticlopidine (Ticlid), is slightly more effective than aspirin in preventing strokes and is less likely to cause gastrointestinal bleeding (aspirin's primary side effect). However, ticlopidine is more costly, and 10% to 20% of people taking it have minor reactions like diarrhea or skin rash.

The most serious potential side effect of ticlopidine is a blood disorder called thrombotic thrombocytopenic purpura, which causes fever, a significant decrease in the number of platelets in the blood, neurological changes, and kidney failure. Although rare, thrombotic thrombocytopenic purpura is fatal in about 30% of cases. Ticlopidine is also associated with neutropenia (depletion of the body's infection-fighting white blood cells). Therefore, careful blood monitoring is necessary, especially in the first three months of treatment. Considering the risks and expense of ticlopidine, many experts recommend it mainly for people who cannot tolerate aspirin or who continue to have TIAs or minor strokes despite aspirin therapy.

Clopidogrel. The antiplatelet drug clopidogrel (Plavix) is another option for people at high risk for stroke. A three-year study of more than 19,000 people who had suffered a recent stroke or heart attack or had peripheral arterial disease found that 75 mg of

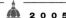

clopidogrel per day decreased the combined risk of future stroke, heart attack, or death from vascular disease by 34%, compared with a 25% risk reduction in patients taking 325 mg of aspirin a day. The risk of side effects, including rash, diarrhea, and stomach discomfort, was about the same for both drugs. The risk of thrombotic thrombocytopenic purpura appears to be lower with clopidogrel than with ticlopidine.

Dipyridamole and aspirin. In 1999, the U.S. Food and Drug Administration approved a new drug for stroke prevention for people who have experienced a previous stroke or TIA. The drug (Aggrenox) contains dipyridamole and aspirin, two antiplatelet agents. In a one-year study of about 6,600 people who had suffered a stroke, a combination of dipyridamole and aspirin was twice as effective as either drug alone in preventing a second stroke, although the overall risk of death was unaffected. Bleeding was more common in patients taking the dipyridamole-aspirin combination than in those taking aspirin alone.

Anticoagulants

Anticoagulant drugs also inhibit blood clot formation but work at a different stage in the clotting process than antiplatelets. Specifically, they interfere with the coagulation cascade and fibrin formation by hindering the activity of certain clot-promoting factors. Anticoagulants are the most effective agents for the prevention of cerebral embolisms, especially those resulting from atrial fibrillation.

People with atrial fibrillation who have other risk factors for stroke—age 75 and older, hypertension, and previous stroke or TIA—are typically treated with a long-term, low-dose regimen of anticoagulant medication, usually warfarin (Coumadin); those with no other risk factors for stroke usually are given aspirin instead. People with heart valve disorders, heart muscle damage from a heart attack, cardiomyopathy (deterioration of heart muscle), or patent foramen ovale (a hole between the left and right sides of the heart) also typically receive warfarin to reduce the risk of cerebral embolism.

Warfarin is associated with a high risk of excessive bleeding. Consequently, people taking warfarin must have regular blood tests to ensure that the dose is correct—high enough to reduce blood clotting, but not so high as to provoke bleeding. The test, called prothrombin time, measures how long it takes for blood to clot. People taking warfarin must also watch their consumption of vitamin K (from both food and dietary supplements), since higher or

NEW RESEARCH

Aspirin Offers No Added Benefit to Stroke Patients on Clopidogrel

Stroke patients who take the antiplatelet drug clopidogrel (Plavix) gain no advantage from adding aspirin to their regimen, and they are at increased risk for life-threatening bleeding, a new study shows.

Large studies have shown that clopidogrel is more effective than aspirin in preventing a second stroke. The researchers sought to determine whether combining aspirin and clopidogrel would result in even greater benefit.

The researchers randomized about 7,500 patients who had suffered an ischemic stroke or transient ischemic attack and were already taking 75 mg of clopidogrel a day to add 75 mg of aspirin or a placebo to their daily treatment regimen.

After 18 months, there was no significant difference between the two groups of patients in their likelihood of stroke, heart attack, hospitalization for ischemia, or death from vascular disease. In addition, those taking both clopidogrel and aspirin were more likely to experience life-threatening bleeding, most commonly gastrointestinal bleeding, although this did not result in a greater risk of mortality for this group.

The researchers conclude that it is not worthwhile for patients at high risk for stroke to take aspirin along with clopidogrel.

THE LANCET
Volume 364, page 331
July 24, 2004

Antiplatelet and Anticoagulant Drugs 2005

Drug Type	Generic Name	Brand Name	Average Daily Dosage*	Average Retail Cost†
Antiplatelets	aspirin	Bayer Easprin Ecotrin St. Joseph	81 to 325 mg	325 mg: $3 ($2) 975 mg: $20 81 mg: $1 ($1) 81 mg: $3 ($1)
	buffered aspirin	Ascriptin Bufferin	81 to 325 mg	325 mg: $3 ($2) 325 mg: $2 ($2)
	ticlopidine	Ticlid	500 mg	250 mg: $78 ($45)
	clopidogrel	Plavix	75 mg	75 mg: $121
	dipyridamole and aspirin	Aggrenox	400 mg dipyridamole/ 50 mg aspirin	200 mg/25 mg: $59

* These dosages represent an average range for the prevention of stroke. The precise effective dosage varies from patient to patient and depends on many factors. Do not make any changes in your medication without consulting your doctor.

† Average price for 30 tablets or capsules (unless otherwise indicated) of the dosage strength listed. Actual price may vary. If a generic version is available, the cost is listed in parentheses. Sources: drugstore.com, eckerd.com, and walgreens.com.

Advantages	Disadvantages
Aspirin is the most widely used and studied of the antiplatelets. It reduces the risk of stroke in people at high risk, for example, those who have had a previous stroke or transient ischemic attack (TIA) and those who suffer from atrial fibrillation (a heart rhythm abnormality). Aspirin helps to prevent the formation of blood clots by inhibiting the aggregation of blood components called platelets.	Common side effects of aspirin include mild stomach pain, heartburn, indigestion, nausea, and vomiting. Serious side effects include peptic ulcers and gastrointestinal bleeding. Use of aspirin with other nonsteroidal anti-inflammatory drugs (NSAIDs) or with anticoagulant drugs such as warfarin increases the risk of these serious side effects. Contact your doctor if you experience bloody or black, tarry stools; severe stomach pain; or vomiting of blood or substances that resemble coffee grounds.
Ticlopidine reduces the risk of stroke in people who have had a previous stroke or TIA. Research shows that ticlopidine is somewhat more effective than aspirin for reducing stroke risk. Like aspirin, ticlopidine prevents platelet aggregation.	Ticlopidine causes more side effects than aspirin and is generally reserved for people who cannot take aspirin or who experience strokes or TIAs while on aspirin therapy. Common side effects of ticlopidine include diarrhea, indigestion, nausea, skin rash, and mild abdominal pain. Rare but serious side effects include hepatitis and blood disorders such as thrombotic thrombocytopenic purpura and neutropenia. To reduce the risk of these serious side effects, blood tests are required every two weeks during the first three months of therapy. Contact your doctor immediately if you experience bruising or bleeding, particularly bleeding that is difficult to stop; fever, chills, or sore throat; sores, ulcers, or white spots in the mouth; dark or bloody urine; difficulty speaking; pale skin; pinpoint red spots on the skin; seizures; weakness; or yellow skin or eyes. Ticlopidine should be used with caution while taking other medications that reduce blood clotting. These medications include warfarin, aspirin, and other NSAIDs. Ticlopidine should not be taken by people with severe liver disease.
Clopidogrel reduces the risk of stroke in people who have had a previous stroke or heart attack or have other blood circulation problems that can lead to stroke. Research shows that clopidogrel is somewhat more effective than aspirin for stroke prevention. Clopidogrel is preferred over ticlopidine in people who cannot take aspirin or who have strokes or TIAs while on aspirin therapy, since the risk of thrombotic thrombocytopenic purpura is lower with clopidogrel. Clopidogrel prevents blood clot formation by inhibiting platelet aggregation.	Common side effects of clopidogrel include chest, abdominal, back, or joint pain; red or purple spots on the skin; upper respiratory infections; dizziness; flu-like symptoms; and easy bruising. Contact your doctor immediately if you experience bruising or bleeding, especially bleeding that is difficult to stop. Use of clopidogrel with aspirin or other NSAIDs can increase the risk of gastrointestinal bleeding. Clopidogrel should not be used by people with peptic ulcers.
The combination of dipyridamole and aspirin reduces the risk of stroke in people with a previous stroke or TIA. Research shows that combination therapy is more effective than aspirin alone for reducing stroke risk in people with a previous stroke; however, it is no more effective than aspirin in people who have experienced a TIA. Dipyridamole plus aspirin reduces blood clot formation by inhibiting platelet aggregation.	Common side effects of dipyridamole and aspirin include abdominal pain, nausea, vomiting, diarrhea, headache, heartburn, indigestion, and muscle or joint pain. Gastrointestinal bleeding occurs more often with combination therapy than with aspirin alone. Serious bleeding can also occur when combination therapy is taken with anticoagulant drugs (such as warfarin or heparin) or with NSAIDs. Dipyridamole and aspirin should not be used by people with severe liver or kidney disease.

Antiplatelet and Anticoagulant Drugs 2005 (continued)

Drug Type	Generic Name	Brand Name	Average Daily Dosage*	Average Retail Cost†
Anticoagulant	warfarin	Coumadin	2 to 10 mg	4 mg: $24 ($14)

* These dosages represent an average range for the prevention of stroke. The precise effective dosage varies from patient to patient and depends on many factors. Do not make any changes in your medication without consulting your doctor.

† Average price for 30 tablets or capsules (unless otherwise indicated) of the dosage strength listed. Actual price may vary. If a generic version is available, the cost is listed in parentheses. Sources: drugstore.com, eckerd.com, and walgreens.com.

lower intakes than usual can alter the drug's effectiveness. Foods rich in vitamin K include broccoli, spinach, cabbage, kale, Brussels sprouts, canola oil, and soybean oil. Many prescription and over-the-counter medications can also alter warfarin's effects, so do not change dosages or stop or start taking any medications without a doctor's permission.

Carotid Endarterectomy

When diagnostic imaging tests (see pages 59–62) reveal that one or both of the carotid arteries in the neck are substantially narrowed by atherosclerotic plaque, a condition called carotid stenosis, a surgical procedure known as carotid endarterectomy can be performed to remove the plaque. The procedure takes about two hours and usually requires two to three days of hospitalization.

Carotid endarterectomy significantly reduces the risk of stroke and TIA in some patients. However, it is not appropriate for everyone with carotid stenosis. Long-term results are best for people who have had a mild stroke or symptoms of a TIA and whose carotid arteries are severely blocked—70% or more. (Completely blocked carotid arteries cannot be reopened.) Carotid endarterectomy is not recommended for people with mild blockage (less than 30%).

For people with moderate stenosis (between 30% and 69%) who have had a minor stroke or TIA, carotid endarterectomy may be beneficial, but the degree of benefit is less than that with higher

Advantages	Disadvantages
Warfarin reduces the risk of stroke in people with atrial fibrillation, especially those with other risk factors for stroke (for example, age 75 and over, high blood pressure, and previous TIA or stroke). In these individuals, warfarin is considerably more effective than aspirin. Warfarin also is used to prevent stroke in people with heart valve disorders and cardiomyopathy (deterioration of heart muscle). Warfarin prevents strokes by hindering the activity of substances that promote blood clot formation.	Warfarin is associated with a high risk of serious bleeding. To prevent this side effect, patients must undergo regular blood tests to ensure that they are receiving the correct dose. High doses of vitamin K (found in food or dietary supplements) can decrease the effects of warfarin. Thus, foods high in vitamin K (for example, liver, broccoli, cauliflower, and green leafy vegetables) should be eaten in moderation, and you should tell your doctor about any supplements you are taking. Many medications can increase or decrease the effects of warfarin, so be sure to tell your doctor about all the medications you are using. Contact your doctor immediately if you notice any unusual bleeding or bruising. Signs of unusual bleeding include bleeding from the gums, blood in the urine, nosebleeds, pinpoint red spots on the skin, and heavy bleeding from cuts or wounds.

levels of stenosis. A trial called NASCET (North American Symptomatic Carotid Endarterectomy Trial) found that people who underwent carotid endarterectomy for 50% to 69% stenosis had a five-year stroke rate of 16%, compared with a rate of 22% in patients treated with medication alone. In addition, men appeared to benefit more than women, and overall benefits were less in patients at high risk for complications related to the procedure itself. Decisions about whether people with moderate carotid stenosis should undergo carotid endarterectomy are made on a case-by-case basis.

The most recent research suggests that carotid endarterectomy may also benefit people with no symptoms or history of stroke (that is, those with asymptomatic carotid bruit) when blockage of the carotid artery exceeds 60%. In such cases, carotid endarterectomy appears to significantly lower the risk of a first-time stroke in men, but the risk was lowered only minimally in women. (The most probable reason for this gender difference is that women are at higher risk for surgical complications because of their smaller arteries.) The reduction in risk, however, is more often for TIAs and minor strokes than for fatal or disabling strokes.

A recent review of 25 studies showed that the overall risk of death or stroke due to carotid endarterectomy was significantly lower for asymptomatic patients than for those with symptoms—3.4% vs. 5.2%. Asymptomatic patients may fare better because the same factors that prevent them from having symptoms (for example, being less prone to blood clots) make them less likely to have complications from carotid endarterectomy. Because the procedure only decreases the overall incidence of stroke in asymptomatic men from 10% to 5%, questions remain about its relative benefits and risks in such patients. These questions are more difficult to answer for women since a recent study found that women with no history of TIA or stroke had a 5.3% risk of stroke or death during hospitalization after carotid endarterectomy, while men with the same history had only a 1.6% risk.

People with coronary heart disease, uncontrolled diabetes or hypertension, advanced cancer, or serious deficits from a prior stroke may not be able to undergo carotid endarterectomy. Advanced age, however, does not rule out a person as a candidate for surgery: Studies have reported favorable results in people in their 70s and 80s. In a recent study from Australia, people age 80 and older who underwent carotid endarterectomy were 18% more likely to survive the next five years than were people of the same age in the general population.

Carotid endarterectomy nonetheless is associated with significant risks. The rate of serious complications (such as tearing the carotid artery or triggering a stroke or heart attack) varies with the medical center and the skill of the surgeon but in general ranges between 3% and 15%. By comparison, about 2% of patients have a stroke and 5% to 10% have a heart attack after bypass surgery. Experts recommend that carotid endarterectomy be done by an experienced surgeon (one that performs the procedure at least 12 times per year) and be performed at a medical center with a complication rate of no more than 3% to 4% (no more than 2% to 3% if the patient has asymptomatic carotid bruit). Getting a second opinion is strongly encouraged before undergoing carotid endarterectomy, especially for asymptomatic patients.

Angioplasty and Stents

Angioplasty involves inflating a small balloon in a blocked artery to enlarge the path for blood flow. The procedure, which was first used in patients with coronary heart disease, has been adopted to reopen partially blocked carotid arteries. Sometimes a stent—a flexible metal tube placed inside a clogged artery to keep it propped open—is implanted during angioplasty. Clinical trials are now under way to compare the results of carotid endarterectomy with those of carotid angioplasty with stenting.

To perform carotid angioplasty with stenting, a radiologist inserts a catheter into an artery in the groin and threads it up into the narrowed portion of the carotid artery. Initially, the stent is collapsed around a deflated balloon at the tip of the catheter. After inflating the balloon to widen the artery, the radiologist expands the stent until it locks in position. The stent acts as a permanent brace inside the artery. It helps maintain blood flow to the brain and may reduce the risk of ischemic stroke.

The results of research on carotid angioplasty with stenting have been mixed, and some researchers have raised concerns about the procedure. One major concern is blood clots, which may be released from the carotid artery during the procedure or form on the stent. These clots may travel to an artery in the brain and cause a stroke. Questions also remain about the long-term reliability and structural integrity of stents placed in the carotid arteries, since there is more movement in the neck than around the heart.

For now, carotid angioplasty with stenting may be a good option for high-risk patients with unstable heart conditions who are unable to withstand the rigors of carotid endarterectomy, which is a more extensive surgical procedure. Carotid angioplasty with stenting also may be useful in people who have had a prior carotid endarterectomy, neck surgery, or radiation to the neck area, which increases the risks of carotid endarterectomy.

Researchers are also studying the use of mildly radioactive stents and stents coated with anticoagulant materials or drugs. These innovations may reduce the risk of stroke after angioplasty and eventually allow more widespread use of the technique.

DIAGNOSIS OF STROKE

When a patient arrives at an emergency room with symptoms of a stroke, time is of the essence: Fast action can minimize neurological damage and even mean the difference between life and death. The doctor must rule out other potential causes of the symptoms (such as seizure, brain tumor, diabetic coma, low blood sugar, or migraine headache) and determine the type of stroke (ischemic or hemorrhagic). He or she must also identify what caused the stroke and which part or parts of the brain are affected.

Patient History

A diagnosis of stroke is suspected when a person experiences a loss of one or more brain functions and the symptoms come on

NEW RESEARCH

Clopidogrel Reduces Blood Clots During Carotid Endarterectomy

Although carotid endarterectomy is known to reduce the long-term risk of a stroke, it can produce blood clots that actually increase stroke risk immediately after the procedure. Now researchers have found that they can reduce these blood clots by administering the antiplatelet drug clopidogrel (Plavix) the night before surgery.

The study involved 100 people who needed carotid endarterectomy and were taking aspirin (150 mg per day). The researchers randomly assigned 46 of the patients to take clopidogrel 12 hours before surgery in addition to aspirin; 54 took a placebo.

The risk of having more than 20 blood clots (as detected by ultrasound) in the three hours after carotid endarterectomy was 10 times lower in the patients who received clopidogrel than in those who received a placebo. The amount of time needed for surgical incisions to close was longer in the clopidogrel group than in the placebo group, but this did not lead to increased blood loss.

The study authors conclude that clopidogrel can reduce the risk of blood clots immediately after carotid endarterectomy without increasing the risk of bleeding complications. But they did not test whether this translates to a lower chance of stroke after surgery.

CIRCULATION
Volume 109, page 1476
March 30, 2004

suddenly or become apparent on awakening, especially in a person over age 50 with vascular disease or other risk factors for stroke. Although symptoms may progress for a few hours, the condition usually stabilizes within 12 to 24 hours.

If a person with suspected stroke is conscious and able to speak, or if a family member or close friend is present, the doctor will ask questions about the patient's medical background, including any history of TIA, stroke, or recent head injury. The doctor will also ask about the symptoms: what they are, when they started, and how long they have lasted. The patient's age, sex, race, and history of other medical conditions (such as diabetes, cardiovascular disease, hypertension, hemophilia, and allergies) also are crucial, and the doctor must know if the patient is taking any medications (prescription, over the counter, or herbal) or illicit drugs.

Physical Examination
Along with the patient history, the physician will conduct a general physical examination to check breathing, pulse, blood pressure, and body temperature. The physician can listen for heart rhythm disturbances (such as atrial fibrillation) and for bruits in the carotid arteries. Close examination of the blood vessels in the eyes also is important, since it can reveal evidence of brain hemorrhage, hypertension, emboli, and other conditions related to stroke.

In addition, a neurological examination is done. The doctor will take a quick inventory of the patient's emotional status, memory, motor strength and skills, balance, gait, responsiveness to tactile stimuli, reflexes, vision, eye movements, and speech and language abilities. Deficits in any of these basic neurological functions help the doctor to determine which areas of the brain have been damaged by the stroke.

Laboratory Tests
Blood tests and urinalysis can help the physician to identify conditions—for example, low blood sugar, diabetes, high red blood cell count, an infected heart valve, or syphilis—that can mimic or lead to a stroke. Other blood tests that may help pinpoint the cause of a stroke include measurements of blood clotting, platelets, and erythrocyte sedimentation rate. High blood cholesterol levels suggest a possible cerebral thrombosis due to atherosclerosis. An electrocardiogram (ECG or EKG) can detect a heart attack or a heart rhythm abnormality—a potential cause of a cerebral embolism.

Imaging Techniques

The most definitive way to diagnose the type of stroke is to locate a blockage in a carotid artery or an artery within the brain, identify the site where damage has occurred in the brain, or detect an abnormal pool of blood within the brain tissue or the subarachnoid space. This can be accomplished with imaging techniques such as computed tomography (CT) scanning, magnetic resonance imaging (MRI), ultrasound scanning, cerebral angiography, magnetic resonance angiography (MRA), or spiral CT scanning.

Computed tomography (CT) scans. In this test, the patient lies flat on a special table while x-rays are passed through the body and sensed by a detector that rotates 360° around the patient. A computer combines all the information to create a two-dimensional, cross-sectional picture. CT scans are 10 to 20 times more sensitive than x-rays.

CT scans are most effective for rapidly determining whether an intracerebral or subarachnoid hemorrhage has occurred, as well as to reveal the location and extent of the hemorrhage. Sometimes the scans can detect aneurysms or arteriovenous malformations. However, damage inflicted by even a large ischemic stroke may not show up on a CT scan until hours or days later, and evidence of small strokes (especially those deep in the brain) may not be visible at all. Therefore, CT scans are not used in the diagnosis of ischemic stroke.

Magnetic resonance imaging (MRI). This technique requires the patient to lie still for 30 minutes or more. Magnetic fields and radio waves are used to generate a three-dimensional image of the brain. An MRI scan is more expensive than a CT scan and is not always practical because of the time required, but it provides clearer pictures and can detect smaller injuries in the brain.

Ischemic strokes may show up on an MRI scan as early as 6 to 12 hours after symptom onset. New developments in MRI technology may allow even earlier detection and the possibility of predicting the size, severity, and reversibility of neurological deficits. For instance, diffusion-weighted MRI can detect injury from an ischemic stroke within one to two hours based on alterations in water movement in the brain; perfusion-weighted MRI can show the degree of blood flow to areas in the brain. Combining diffusion and perfusion imaging may hold the key to determining which patients might benefit from thrombolytic therapy after a stroke.

According to American Heart Association guidelines, an MRI of the brain is not necessary to initiate emergency treatment of a

Dealing With Depression After a Stroke

Depression in stroke survivors usually is temporary but should not be ignored.

Depression is a frequent consequence of a stroke, affecting 35% of stroke survivors age 65 or older. In some cases, the condition is triggered by physical changes in the brain caused by the stroke. In other instances, patients become depressed as they face the stresses of dealing with physical or cognitive disabilities, loss of independence, and the challenges of rehabilitation.

Poststroke depression can seriously impede the recovery process. Depressed patients put less effort into their rehabilitation programs, and depression often exacerbates cognitive and physical problems caused by the stroke. So it's not surprising that studies have found that depressed stroke patients have poorer long-term outcomes than those who are not depressed. Depression can also adversely impact quality of life by interfering with social activities and placing a strain on relationships with family and friends.

Fortunately, depression that follows a stroke is usually temporary,

lasting less than a year in most cases. As patients begin to recover and become more independent, they feel more positive. Family and caregivers can help with depression by providing support, understanding, and encouragement. In addition, effective treatments, including psychotherapy and medication, are available.

Getting Help
The two main treatments for depression are psychotherapy and antidepressant medication, and research shows that a combination of both is more effective than either treatment alone. Moderate exercise also can improve symptoms of depression.

Psychotherapy. This treatment is an effective option for people with mild to moderate depression and may benefit a stroke survivor's relatives as well. It involves talking to a mental health professional (a psychiatrist, psychologist, psychotherapist, psychiatric social worker, or psychiatric nurse specialist) in order to identify factors, such as destructive patterns

of thinking or acting, that contribute to depression. The therapist may also help the person to learn coping skills, new patterns of behavior, stress management, and relaxation techniques. Such measures can help relieve current depression and prevent bouts in the future. A drawback, however, is that psychotherapy takes six to eight weeks to produce a noticeable improvement in symptoms.

To find a mental health professional who practices psychotherapy, ask your doctor for a referral or contact the American Psychological Association at 800-964-2000. This organization can put you in touch with your state's psychological association, which can then refer you to a psychologist in your area. You may also be able to obtain contact information for psychotherapists from a nearby hospital or your health insurance company.

Antidepressant medication. For mild to severe forms of depression, medication is effective about 70% of the time. Medication tends to

stroke. However, the organization recognizes the existence of special circumstances and recommends that decisions as to whether to perform an MRI scan in a stroke patient be made on an individual basis.

Ultrasound scanning. Ultrasound scanning uses high-frequency sound waves to generate two-dimensional images of internal body structures. Ultrasound is especially useful for determining the site of an ischemic stroke, since it allows the doctor to visualize blockages and monitor blood flow through specific arteries.

Several ultrasound techniques have been developed and each has its own advantages. Doppler ultrasound generally is used to measure how fast blood is moving through the carotid arteries; a faster flow rate indicates a site where atherosclerotic plaque has narrowed the blood vessel. (Color Doppler flow imaging is an enhancement of this technique that uses colors to indicate the speed of blood flow.)

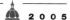

produce benefits more quickly (usually within four to six weeks) and is easier to administer than psychotherapy. Researchers believe that antidepressants work by altering levels of neurotransmitters in the brain, particularly serotonin. However, in some people, these drugs can also cause adverse effects, like weight gain and rapid heart rate. Commonly used antidepressants are considered safe and effective for stroke survivors, although all of the stroke survivor's doctors should coordinate their treatments to avoid potential drug interactions.

A primary care physician or a psychiatrist can prescribe antidepressants and determine which type is most appropriate for the stroke survivor. To find a psychiatrist, ask for a referral from your doctor or go to the American Medical Association's Web site (www.ama-assn.org), where you can search for a doctor who specializes in psychiatry. Local hospitals and your health insurance company also have listings of psychiatrists in your area.

Exercise. Many studies have demonstrated that exercise can

improve mood, and one recent report even showed that an aerobic exercise program is as effective as an antidepressant medication in the treatment of major depression in older people.

Moderate exercise appears to improve depression by decreasing stress and tension while enhancing energy. The appropriate amount and type of exercise depend on a number of factors (including fitness level, overall health, and any limitations caused by the stroke). Therefore, stroke survivors should consult their doctor before beginning an exercise program. A reasonable fitness goal in the first year after a stroke is 15 to 20 minutes of walking three times a week.

Signs of Depression

Because relatives, caregivers, and patients often attribute depressive symptoms to the stroke itself, depression is often overlooked in stroke survivors. But depression is a separate condition and should be treated. If you experience any of the following warning signs of depression or see them in a stroke survivor, a phone call to a doctor is in order:

- Changes in behavior or personality
- Significant changes in appetite or weight
- Insomnia or sleeping too much
- Agitation, irritability, rudeness, or emotional outbursts
- Constant lack of energy
- Difficulty concentrating or thinking
- Feelings of worthlessness, guilt, or helplessness
- Loss of interest and pleasure in activities formerly enjoyed
- Pessimism or hopelessness
- Depressed mood, sadness, tearfulness, or grief
- Refusal to participate in rehabilitation
- Recurrent talk of death or suicide; suicide attempts

B-mode imaging is another form of ultrasound. It provides a three-dimensional view of the carotid arteries. When combined with Doppler ultrasound, it is known as duplex scanning. Compared with CT scans, MRI scans, and other types of ultrasound scans, duplex scanning provides the most accurate images of the carotid arteries. Transcranial Doppler scanning may allow an assessment of blood flow through the arteries within the brain.

Cerebral angiography. This procedure involves the insertion of a catheter into the carotid artery and injection of an iodine-based contrast solution into the artery through the catheter. The dye helps produce a high-quality x-ray image of the blood vessels within the brain. Angiography provides more detailed information about blood vessels than other diagnostic imaging techniques, but because of the risk of complications, it is used only when noninvasive tests prove inadequate. Possible complications include a dangerous allergic reaction to the iodine in the contrast solution, reversible neurological deficits, and a stroke that results in permanent deficits. These complications occur in less than 1% of people under age 50, but their incidence rises with age and the presence of hypertension or vascular disease.

Magnetic resonance angiography (MRA). This technique is a refinement of MRI that involves the injection of a weakly magnetic contrast dye into a vein in the arm. The procedure adds about 15 minutes to a conventional MRI scan. MRA has not been perfected but is used increasingly as a screening test for blockage of large vessels. People with a normal MRA may not need to undergo cerebral angiography.

Spiral CT scanning. Spiral CT scanning (also called CT angiography) is a new method of looking at blood vessels. An iodine-based dye is injected into a vein and images of the area of interest are taken as the patient lies on a special table that slides through the scanning unit. Computer-based imaging software then isolates the blood vessels that fill with dye. The resulting image resembles that obtained from cerebral angiography and can be rotated and manipulated in three dimensions to look for aneurysms or narrowings. This technique cannot be used in people who are allergic to iodine or have kidney dysfunction.

ACUTE TREATMENT OF STROKE

Immediate emergency care for a stroke requires treatment in a hospital, where life support systems are available to maintain breathing and heart function if needed. The specific treatment received depends on whether the stroke is ischemic or hemorrhagic. In an ischemic stroke, the primary goal is to restore or at least improve blood flow to the brain; the goal in a hemorrhagic stroke is to relieve pressure on the brain and stop the bleeding.

Treatment of Ischemic Stroke

Careful monitoring and control of blood pressure are essential after an ischemic stroke. In general, elevated blood pressure is acceptable, since it promotes blood flow through the partially blocked arteries so that blood can reach the jeopardized regions of the brain. The exception is when blood pressure is so high that it is likely to damage the brain, heart, or kidneys. In such cases, it is lowered slowly. Otherwise, efforts are aimed at preventing low blood pressure (hypotension), which can limit the amount of blood reaching the brain. When low blood pressure occurs—whether due to antihypertensive drugs, dehydration, or other causes—it can be treated with intravenous saline solutions to increase blood volume and with blood pressure-raising drugs if needed.

Body temperature also must be carefully monitored and controlled, since fever can worsen damage to the brain. A study of people with stroke found that for every increase in body temperature of 2.7° F the risk of a poor outcome (death or a more severe stroke) more than doubled. In fact, deliberately lowering the body temperature of people suffering from a stroke is being examined as a treatment option.

Intravenous fluids containing glucose are usually avoided since excessive glucose in the brain may be detrimental (this practice is controversial, however). Buildup of fluid in the brain (cerebral edema) also can cause damage. Cerebral edema can be treated by limiting fluid intake and raising the head of the patient's bed to a 30° angle.

Drug therapy. Until recently, doctors could do little to intervene while an ischemic stroke was in progress. However, with the approval of the emergency stroke drug alteplase (Activase), doctors now have a specific course of action to follow for an ischemic stroke. Alteplase, which is also called tissue-type plasminogen activator (t-PA), belongs to a class of drugs known as thrombolytic ("clot-busting") agents.

Thrombolytic drugs have been used widely to treat heart attacks; prompt intravenous administration of alteplase can dissolve a clot that is blocking blood flow to the heart, thereby preventing extensive tissue damage. Some (but not all) studies have shown similar results with alteplase for strokes. But treatment with alteplase causes cerebral hemorrhage (excessive bleeding in the brain) in about 6% of stroke patients.

Early treatment with alteplase is essential. Guidelines from the American Heart Association recommend that alteplase be used only when it can be given within three hours of the onset of an ischemic stroke. If too much time has elapsed, cerebral hemorrhage may be more likely, and it may be too late to prevent brain damage.

Before receiving alteplase, all patients must have a neurological examination and a CT scan to ensure they are good candidates. Only hospitals equipped for immediate treatment of excessive bleeding should administer alteplase. In addition, alteplase cannot be used in certain individuals, including those who are having a hemorrhagic stroke, have had a stroke in the past three months,

NEW RESEARCH

Blood Pressure Drop During Stroke Associated With Poor Outcome

A sharp increase or decrease in blood pressure during a stroke may predict a poor outcome, with a significant blood pressure drop being particularly worrisome, new findings suggest.

Researchers say the findings call into question the common practice of giving patients blood pressure-lowering drugs during the acute phase of a stroke. International guidelines call for such treatment in many cases, but these guides are based on reasoning rather than evidence, according to an accompanying editorial.

The study followed 258 patients who had suffered an ischemic stroke, many of whom were treated with blood pressure medication at the hospital. Researchers found that both elevated and relatively low blood pressure were tied to an increased risk of significant brain damage or death. For every 10-point increase in systolic pressure above 180 mm Hg, the odds of having immediate or longer-term neurological damage increased; the same was true for every 10-point drop below 180 mm Hg. A fall in blood pressure of more than 20 mm Hg within a day of stroke onset was the most important predictor of a poor outcome.

If these findings are confirmed in further studies, the researchers conclude, it will be necessary to reconsider the guidelines for blood pressure treatment during a stroke.

STROKE
Volume 35, page 520
February 2004

have a blood pressure reading greater than 185/110 mm Hg, or are currently taking warfarin or heparin.

For people with stroke due to cerebral embolism, the anticoagulant drug heparin often is administered intravenously for several days to prevent new clots from forming and to keep existing clots from getting any larger. Heparin is also typically used as an immediate treatment for strokes due to severe stenosis in the carotid, vertebral, or basilar arteries (which branch off from the vertebral arteries), although its effectiveness in these situations is not clearly established. Heparin should not be given to people at risk for hemorrhage, for example, those with uncontrolled hypertension, gastrointestinal bleeding, or thrombocytopenia (a low number of blood platelets).

The anticoagulant drug warfarin often is started at the same time as heparin to treat cerebral embolism. Unlike heparin, it can be prescribed in pill form for long-term use; similar to heparin, it should not be given to people at high risk for hemorrhage. In addition, long-term use of warfarin requires careful evaluation. Although the short-term risks from warfarin are small, the chance of complications accumulates over the years. Doctors also must consider whether patients are at risk for falls, since falling and hitting the head could lead to serious bleeding in the brain.

If patients cannot be given warfarin or heparin, aspirin is the next most effective therapy to reduce the risk of future strokes. Patients who experience TIAs or new strokes while on aspirin therapy or experience intolerable side effects can be treated with other antiplatelet agents, such as dipyridamole and aspirin, clopidogrel, or ticlopidine (see pages 50–51).

Another option for the emergency treatment of an ischemic stroke is the administration of a thrombolytic drug directly into the blocked artery. A study of 180 patients looked at intra-arterial administration of a thrombolytic drug called prourokinase within six hours of the onset of an ischemic stroke. Patients received either prourokinase plus heparin or heparin alone. After three months, 40% of the people treated with prourokinase and 25% of those in the heparin-only group were able to function independently. Prourokinase did not decrease the risk of death, however, and people who received the drug had a higher rate of cerebral hemorrhage.

Patients with cerebral embolism due to atrial fibrillation may be treated with antiarrhythmic medications such as amiodarone (Cordarone) and procainamide (Procan, Pronestyl, and other brands). Also, digoxin (Lanoxin), calcium channel blockers, or beta-blockers may be given to keep the heart's ventricles (lower chambers) from responding to the rapid signals from the atria. A rapid ventricular rate can lead to poor cardiac output, low blood pressure, poor blood flow through narrowed arteries in the brain, and heart failure.

Researchers are interested in developing drugs known as cytoprotective (cell-preserving) agents, some of which are designed to prevent or halt the ischemic cascade—the chain of chemical reactions that occurs during an ischemic stroke. Studies of various cytoprotective drugs are currently under way, but the results so far have not been promising.

Surgery. Surgery is rarely part of the immediate treatment of ischemic stroke. Carotid endarterectomy (see pages 54–56), however, sometimes is performed to treat minor strokes and prevent additional ones in people with severe carotid stenosis. In the aftermath of a large ischemic stroke, the brain needs time to recover before carotid endarterectomy can be performed. In such cases, surgery may be postponed for as long as six weeks after the stroke. However, a recent study found that people who underwent carotid endarterectomy within two weeks of a stroke had a lower risk of future strokes than people who waited longer to have the surgery (see the sidebar at right). In people for whom carotid endarterectomy presents too great a risk, angioplasty with or without stenting (see pages 56–57) is being used more often.

Treatment of Hemorrhagic Stroke

Because hemorrhagic strokes often occur in association with extremely high blood pressure, the first step in treatment is to lower blood pressure to minimize the amount of bleeding from the ruptured artery. Lowering of blood pressure is done slowly, since additional brain damage can occur when blood pressure is too low.

Drug therapy. Mannitol (a type of sugar) and diuretics, which reduce fluid retention by increasing sodium and water loss in the urine, can be used to treat cerebral edema (swelling of tissues in the brain), a serious and relatively common consequence of a hemorrhagic stroke. Nimodipine (Nimotop), a calcium channel blocker, may help reduce brain damage due to vasospasm (spasm of blood vessels) in the brain. Vasospasm often occurs in the first two weeks after a subarachnoid hemorrhage; it further reduces blood flow to the brain and can be fatal.

Surgery. Surgical intervention is warranted in some cases of hemorrhagic stroke, for example, those associated with aneurysms or arteriovenous malformations in which there is a high risk of

NEW RESEARCH

Carotid Endarterectomy Most Effective Soon After TIA, Stroke

The benefits of carotid endarterectomy are greatest when performed within two weeks of a stroke or related event, recent research suggests. The procedure often is performed many weeks and even months after the stroke, which may result in no benefits at all.

Investigators identified nearly 5,900 patients who had suffered a nondisabling ischemic stroke, transient ischemic attack, or retinal blockage and had been randomized to receive either carotid endarterectomy or drug therapy. They then analyzed the risk of future strokes on the same side of the brain as the initial event and the risk of stroke or death occurring within 30 days of surgery.

The researchers found that the benefits of surgery outweighed the risks for people whose carotid arteries were blocked by 50% or more (especially in men), people age 75 and older, and those who had undergone carotid endarterectomy within two weeks of their initial stroke or related event.

According to the study authors, the procedure should ideally be performed within two weeks of a stroke. They recommend that current guidelines stating that patients should be operated on within six months should be revised based on these results.

THE LANCET
Volume 363, page 915
March 20, 2004

rebleeding. Depending on its location in the brain, an aneurysm that has leaked or ruptured can be clipped across its neck. This procedure stops blood flow into the aneurysm, thus preventing any future bleeding. A newer procedure in which a platinum coil is fed into the aneurysm, sealing it off from blood circulation, is sometimes tried in people who are unable to undergo clipping.

The risk of treating an arteriovenous malformation must be balanced against the possibility of future bleeding, which is minimal in people without symptoms. If a hemorrhage occurs, patients have about a 2% to 3% annual risk of further bleeding. When bleeding occurs from a small arteriovenous malformation, the chance of dying is about 15%. Therefore, the risk of intervention must be lower than this level; if it is not, the arteriovenous malformation usually is monitored closely and the need for treatment reconsidered if the patient's condition worsens.

The three methods of treating an arteriovenous malformation are surgical removal, embolization, and radiation therapy. Which method is used depends on the position of the arteriovenous malformation (for example, whether it is near any vital structures), its size, its accessibility, and the life expectancy of the patient. A relatively accessible arteriovenous malformation may be removed surgically, while one positioned deep within the brain might be treated with either embolization or radiation therapy.

Embolization involves passing a catheter through the arteries and into the center of the arteriovenous malformation. A "glue" is fed slowly through the catheter and injected into the arteriovenous malformation to fill it. When the glue solidifies, blood flow through the arteriovenous malformation is blocked. Embolization often is done prior to surgical removal of an arteriovenous malformation. Radiation therapy causes the abnormal blood vessels in the arteriovenous malformation to be reabsorbed by the body over a period of a few years.

Hemorrhagic strokes often result in an intracerebral hematoma—a pool of blood within the brain that damages brain cells and can increase pressure within the brain to dangerous levels. (In fact, large hematomas are usually fatal.) Emergency drainage of a hematoma, known as evacuation, can relieve the excess pressure and minimize brain damage. Sometimes, however, the hematoma is not accessible, or the release of pressure may result in further bleeding. Blood that seeps into the subarachnoid space or into the cavities within the brain known as the ventricles eventually is reabsorbed into the body. In some people, however, clotted blood

NEW RESEARCH

Stroke Doubles Risk of Dementia

Older people who have a stroke are at increased risk for dementia, according to a new analysis of data from the Framingham Study.

For the analysis, researchers identified 212 individuals who did not have dementia in 1982 and had a first stroke during the next 10 years. The control group consisted of 1,060 people who had no dementia at the study's outset and remained stroke free for 10 years afterward.

Dementia developed in 19% of people in the stroke group and 11% of the controls. After adjusting for age, sex, and educational background, having a stroke was found to double the risk of dementia. In addition, people who usually have a reduced risk of dementia—men, people with at least a high school education, and those younger than age 80—were found to be no longer at reduced risk if they had a stroke.

According to an accompanying editorial, this study suggests that treatment of stroke risk factors could prevent up to 58,000 new cases of dementia in the United States each year. In fact, the editorialist points out that the true number of people with stroke-related dementia is even higher because this study used different diagnostic criteria than other studies.

STROKE
Volume 35, page 1264
June 2004

Home Rehabilitation: A Key to Recovery

A home-based therapy program can help ready stroke survivors for outpatient care.

Although the most dramatic improvements occur in the first few weeks after a stroke, ongoing therapy is an important part of the rehabilitation process. Normally, people improve somewhat in rehabilitation after a stroke, then move from an inpatient facility (such as a hospital or rehabilitation center) to their home. It's important to continue therapy after this move: A 2004 study found that people who continued therapy after going home were 28% less likely than people who did not continue therapy to lose the ability to carry out daily tasks (such as dressing or walking).

Not everyone who leaves an inpatient facility is ready to start attending regular therapy sessions outside the home, however. Some stroke survivors may be well enough to live back at home but not mobile enough to get into a car on their own. Kelly Daley, senior physical therapist at the Johns Hopkins Outpatient Clinic, says that home-based therapy can help bridge this gap and is a temporary but valuable solution for many patients.

What Does Home-Based Therapy Involve?

In a typical home therapy situation, says Daley, the stroke survivor is sent home from an inpatient stay and needs a few visits to progress to the next level. The program usually has two components. The first is instruction in functional strengthening exercises (such as walking safely or maneuvering a wheelchair), usually done with a physical therapist. The therapist may also teach the person to use—rather than avoid—their affected body parts.

The second component is a home safety and equipment assessment. An occupational therapist may recommend installing a wheelchair ramp, widening doorways, moving rugs, or including safety rails in the bathroom.

"There's definitely something to be said for seeing how the person functions in his or her own environment," says Daley. These assessments—both of the stroke survivor and the home environment—can also help the therapists know which exercises to focus on when the time is right for an outpatient program.

A home-based therapy program is often short-lived, as the main goal is to get the person to the point where they can safely leave the house and get into a car. At that point, the person is ready for a more intensive outpatient program, which may involve a few therapy sessions a week outside the home, plus exercises to be done on their own. Learning new skills and strategies in the environment in which people will be using them the most—the home—is advantageous, but the lack of specialized physical therapy equipment greatly limits the gains that stroke survivors can make at home.

Who's a Good Candidate?

Home-based therapy is arranged by a doctor's referral. Typically, a caseworker is assigned to manage each stroke survivor's rehabilitation; the therapist who works with a stroke survivor in the inpatient facility may make a recommendation to the caseworker that home therapy would be appropriate. This recommendation is based on the stroke survivor's physical condition only, as Medicare does not consider lack of transportation to an outpatient facility a valid reason for home therapy.

Home therapy is most appropriate for people who no longer need to be in an inpatient facility but need assistance in getting around outside the home. People who mainly need physical or occupational therapy are also good candidates—speech therapists do not usually visit the home, and home nurses manage medications but do not provide therapy sessions.

interferes with this fluid resorption, leading to an excessive accumulation of fluid (called hydrocephalus or "water on the brain"). Surgery then may be needed to drain the fluid through a tube.

STROKE REHABILITATION

The process of rehabilitation after a stroke starts almost immediately after admission to the hospital and often continues for at least one to two months afterward. At first, the main goal is to reduce or prevent stroke complications, such as stiffening of the limbs and deep vein thrombosis. As the patient's condition stabilizes, the focus turns to longer-term goals of restoring mental and physical function, adapting to disability, returning to an active life, and preventing additional strokes.

Although the exact approach to rehabilitation depends on the specific loss of function caused by the stroke, it typically consists of learning strategies to overcome any deficits and performing exercises to improve range of motion in joints, strengthen weak muscles, and restore function to the greatest extent possible.

The Agency for Health Care Policy and Research has made several recommendations to help patients get the most out of rehabilitation. These include beginning rehabilitation as soon as possible after a stroke, selecting the most appropriate program (inpatient, outpatient, or home based), setting realistic goals (to avoid frustration), frequently assessing progress, and following up during the transition back to the community (when the family plays a major role). Individuals may need to accept some degree of disability, but optimal recovery depends on a combination of the following factors: the patient's determination to succeed, the support of family and friends, and the integrated efforts of specialists.

A variety of specially trained professionals are involved in the rehabilitation process. Occupational therapists teach patients new ways to perform day-to-day activities (writing, bathing, cooking, or job-related tasks) affected by their disability. Physical therapists provide instruction and exercises to help patients regain the ability to walk and move about independently, as well as to improve strength, flexibility, balance, and overall fitness. Social workers can provide information on community services available to stroke survivors and their families. Speech-language pathologists help patients regain as much of their lost swallowing ability and language skills as possible.

The eventual goal of any rehabilitation program is for the patient to return to the community, and certain steps must be taken before this transition can be made. Most patients are not fully independent when they first leave a rehabilitation program, so they and their families should be prepared to continue rehabilitation at home. In addition, the patient's home must be made ready for any special needs. It is particularly important that patients and the family members involved in their care understand what to expect and what will be required of them. Doctors and therapists can offer guidance on these issues and discuss what community services are available.

NEW RESEARCH

Exercising Arm Soon After Stroke May Aid Recovery

Putting a stroke-affected arm right back to work may improve the long-term function of the limb, according to researchers.

The study involved 100 patients whose arm function had been paralyzed by a stroke. Two to five weeks after the stroke, patients were randomly assigned to one of two groups. In the exercise group, patients were asked to sit in a rocking chair for 30 minutes each day and use the affected arm to make the chair rock back and forth. In the placebo group, patients sat in rocking chairs and were told they were receiving ultrasound stimulation to the shoulder. Therapy lasted six weeks, during which both groups also received standard rehabilitation from a physical therapist.

Researchers found that five years later, patients in the exercise group had better scores than those in the placebo group on two standard tests of arm movement and function. And the treatment appeared most effective for those whose arms had suffered the most severe stroke damage.

The investigators speculate that early, repeated stimulation of the arm—given by patients themselves rather than a therapist—helps "rewire" the brain so that arm function can be preserved despite stroke damage.

STROKE
Volume 35, page 924
April 2004

A valuable community service for caregivers is respite care, which allows caregivers to take a break from their responsibilities. Two types of respite care are available: in-home care and adult day care. In-home care involves someone coming to the stroke patient's home to provide companion services, personal care, or household help. Adult day care involves a structured program in a group setting at a community center or other facility. Program activities may include exercise, crafts, meals, discussion, and music.

Because long-term medical treatment after a stroke is complicated, one doctor should be selected to oversee the patient's care. This approach will ensure there are no gaps in treatment and allow for frequent assessments of progress and an eventual phasing out of rehabilitation when patients have progressed as far as they can. Throughout the poststroke period, all medications must be carefully monitored. For example, anticonvulsants or benzodiazepines could affect a patient's ability to participate in rehabilitation exercises and activities.

In general, the best candidates for rehabilitation have at least one significant disability (such as paralysis or aphasia), are moderately stable medically, have the physical endurance to sit up for at least one hour, and are able to learn and participate to some extent in active rehabilitation treatments. However, rehabilitation may be either unnecessary or unfeasible in some cases—for example, for patients who have no disability or are too disabled to benefit. Patients with severe disabilities may be able to begin rehabilitation after a period of rest. ■

GLOSSARY

abulia—Reduction in speech, movement, thought, and emotional reaction as a result of damage to the frontal lobe.

ACE inhibitors—Drugs that lower blood pressure by preventing the formation of angiotensin II, a hormone that causes arteries to constrict and that triggers the release of aldosterone. Also used to slow the progression of kidney disease.

agnosia—Loss of the ability to interpret incoming visual, auditory, or tactile stimuli, even though the senses of vision, hearing, and touch are mechanically intact and function normally. Results from damage to the parietal lobe.

aldosterone—A hormone released by the adrenal glands that increases blood pressure by signaling the kidneys to retain sodium, which increases blood volume.

aldosterone blockers—Drugs that lower blood pressure by interfering with the activity of the hormone aldosterone.

aldosteronism—An overproduction of aldosterone caused by a tumor or overgrowth of cells in the adrenal gland. Aldosteronism can lead to hypertension.

alpha-blockers—Drugs that decrease blood pressure by blocking nerve impulses that constrict small arteries.

alteplase—A drug used to treat heart attack and stroke that works by dissolving blood clots. Also called tissue-type plasminogen activator (t-PA).

ambulatory blood pressure monitor—A portable device that automatically measures and records blood pressure over a 24- to 48-hour period. Measurements are taken while the person goes about daily activities, as well as during sleep.

aneroid blood pressure monitor—A manually operated monitor that consists of a cuff, bulb, and dial gauge to register blood pressure levels.

aneurysm—A ballooning of the wall of a blood vessel caused by weakening of the wall.

angina—Episodes of chest pain caused by an inadequate supply of oxygen and blood to the heart. It occurs most often during physical activity. Also called angina pectoris.

angioplasty—A procedure in which a small balloon is inflated in a blocked artery to enlarge the path for blood flow.

angiotensin—A hormone that has two forms: angiotensin I and angiotensin II. The latter raises blood pressure by causing arteries to constrict and triggering the release of aldosterone.

angiotensin II receptor blockers—Drugs that help lower blood pressure by interfering with the action of angiotensin II, a hormone that causes arteries to constrict and triggers the release of aldosterone.

anticoagulants—Anticlotting drugs that work by inhibiting the formation of fibrin, a protein required for blood clot development. Examples are heparin and warfarin.

antiplatelets—Anticlotting drugs that work by inhibiting the clumping of blood cells called platelets. One example is aspirin.

aphasia—Difficulty in comprehending or producing spoken or written language. Results from damage to the frontal lobe, temporal lobe, or a part of the limbic system called the thalamus.

arteriovenous malformation—A disorder present at birth and characterized by a complex, tangled web of arteries and veins.

aspiration pneumonia—Pneumonia caused by the inhalation of food and other particles into the lungs.

atherosclerosis—The narrowing of arteries by fatty deposits (called plaques) within the artery walls that can cause a reduction in blood flow.

atrial fibrillation—A common abnormal heart rhythm in which the atria (the upper chambers of the heart) quiver chaotically instead of contracting in a rhythmic pattern.

atrial natriuretic factor—A hormone produced by the atria of the heart that helps regulate blood pressure by causing the kidneys to excrete more sodium and by inhibiting the production of aldosterone and renin.

baroreceptors—Special nerve endings in the walls of arteries that monitor blood pressure.

beta-blockers—Drugs that impede the actions of epinephrine and norepinephrine, slow heart rate, and lower blood pressure by diminishing cardiac output.

b-mode imaging—An imaging technique that uses high-frequency sound waves to produce a three-dimensional view of the carotid arteries.

brain stem—An area located at the base of the brain above the spinal cord that maintains basic life support functions such as breathing, heart rate, and blood pressure.

calcitriol—A hormone formed from dietary vitamin D that increases the absorption of calcium from the intestine and plays a role in the regulation of blood pressure by constricting small arteries.

calcium channel blockers—Drugs that lower blood pressure by dilating arteries and, in some cases, by decreasing cardiac output.

cardiac output—The amount of blood pumped by the heart.

cardiovascular disease—Disease affecting the arteries that supply blood to the heart and other organs. Coronary heart disease, stroke, and peripheral arterial disease are the most common cardiovascular diseases.

carotid arteries—Blood vessels that carry oxygenated and nutrient-rich blood from the heart to the brain. There are two carotid arteries—one on each side of the front of the neck.

carotid endarterectomy—A surgical procedure to remove plaque from the carotid arteries.

carotid stenosis—A narrowing of the carotid arteries by atherosclerotic plaque.

central alpha agonists—Drugs that lower blood pressure by blocking nerve impulses that constrict small arteries.

cerebellum—The area of the brain located above the brain stem that controls coordination, balance, and posture.

cerebral angiography—A procedure involving the injection of an iodine-based contrast solution into the bloodstream to produce high-quality x-ray images of the blood vessels within the brain.

cerebral edema—Swelling of the brain due to bleeding, trauma, stroke, or tumor.

cerebral embolism—A blockage of blood flow that occurs when part of a blood clot or a piece of atherosclerotic plaque breaks off and travels through the bloodstream until it lodges in an artery supplying blood to the brain.

cerebral thrombosis—A blockage of blood flow that occurs when a blood clot forms at the site of atherosclerotic plaque within the wall of a major artery supplying the brain. The most common cause of an ischemic stroke.

cerebrum—The largest portion of the brain. It controls conscious thought, perception, voluntary movement, and integration of sensory input.

combination therapy—A treatment approach that uses medication from two or more drug classes.

computed tomography (CT) scan—A test in which a patient lies flat on a table while x-rays are passed through the body and sensed by a rotating detector. A CT scan of the head can reveal strokes, hemorrhages, and tumors.

coronary heart disease—A narrowing of the coronary arteries by atherosclerosis. Reduces or completely blocks blood flow to the heart. Also called coronary artery disease.

Cushing's syndrome—A condition resulting from the secretion of excessive amounts of cortisone and related hormones by a tumor in the adrenal gland. A potential cause of high blood pressure.

cytoprotective drugs—A class of drugs that protect healthy tissue, for example, during an ischemic stroke.

deep vein thrombosis—The formation of a blood clot in the legs.

diabetes—A disorder characterized by abnormally high levels of glucose (sugar) in the blood.

diastolic blood pressure—The lower number in a blood pressure reading. Represents pressure in the arteries when the heart relaxes between beats.

direct vasodilators—Antihypertensive drugs that act directly on the smooth muscle of small arteries, causing them to widen.

diuretics—A class of drugs that increases loss of sodium through the kidneys, thereby increasing the production of urine and decreasing blood volume and blood pressure.

Doppler ultrasound—The use of sound waves to measure how fast blood moves through arteries, such as the carotid arteries.

electronic blood pressure monitor—A battery-operated blood pressure monitor that uses a microphone to detect blood pulses in an artery. Consists of an inflatable cuff and a gauge with a digital screen.

embolus—A blood clot or a piece of atherosclerotic plaque that travels through the bloodstream until it lodges in a narrowed vessel and blocks blood flow. The plural form is emboli.

endothelin—A hormone that causes blood vessels to constrict.

epinephrine—A hormone that increases blood pressure in response to stress. Also called adrenaline.

frontal lobe—An area at the front of the brain that deals with speech, personality, and motor function.

glomeruli—Sites in the kidneys where blood is filtered and waste products are removed.

glutamate cascade—See **ischemic cascade**.

hematoma—A mass of clotted blood that forms as a result of a ruptured blood vessel.

hemianopia—A condition, often caused by a stroke, that results in blindness on only one side of a person's field of vision in both eyes.

hemorrhagic stroke—A stroke that occurs when an artery in the brain suddenly bursts and blood leaks into the surrounding tissue.

high-density lipoprotein (HDL)—A particle in the blood that can protect against coronary heart disease by removing cholesterol from the body.

GLOSSARY—continued

hypertension—High blood pressure. Diagnosed when at least two blood pressure readings on separate occasions are 140/90 mm Hg or higher.

hypertensive crisis—A condition characterized by extremely high blood pressure levels (diastolic blood pressure above 120 mm Hg). Occurs in about 1% of people with hypertension.

hypotension—Low blood pressure. Can cause dizziness or light-headedness.

insulin—A hormone that controls the manufacture of glucose by the liver and permits muscle and fat cells to remove glucose from the blood. High blood insulin levels can cause hypertension.

intermittent claudication—Pain in the leg muscles caused by an inadequate supply of oxygen and blood to the legs. Most often occurs with walking.

intracerebral hemorrhage—Leakage of blood from a damaged blood vessel into tissues deep within the brain.

ischemia—A lack of oxygen due to a decrease in blood supply to a body organ or tissue.

ischemic cascade—A chain of chemical reactions, occurring during an ischemic stroke, that leads to a buildup of toxins and further cell destruction. Also called glutamate cascade.

ischemic stroke—A stroke resulting from the blockage of an artery supplying blood to the brain.

isolated systolic hypertension—A systolic blood pressure of 140 mm Hg or higher along with a diastolic blood pressure under 90 mm Hg. Associated with an increased risk of stroke, coronary heart disease, and kidney disease.

J-curve phenomenon—Refers to the relationship between the risk of a heart attack and blood pressure. The curve shows that those with the highest and lowest blood pressure levels are more likely to die of a heart attack than those with an intermediate blood pressure level. Many experts question whether the J-curve phenomenon actually exists.

kidneys—A pair of organs, located on the left and right sides of the abdomen, that remove waste products and excess water from the blood and produce urine.

lacunar stroke—A stroke that occurs when the tiny branches at the end of arteries in the brain become completely blocked by small emboli or atherosclerotic plaque.

left ventricular hypertrophy—A thickening of the muscular wall of the left ventricle that occurs when it must work harder to pump blood. Common in people with hypertension.

limb contracture—Consistent tightening of ligaments and tendons in the limbs.

limbic system—A group of structures in the brain responsible for primal urges and powerful emotions, for example, hunger and terror, that help ensure self-preservation.

low-density lipoprotein (LDL)—A particle that transports cholesterol in the bloodstream and is a major contributor to coronary heart disease. Its deposition in artery walls initiates plaque formation.

magnetic resonance angiography (MRA)—A technique for viewing arteries in the neck, brain, or other organs. Similar to an MRI.

magnetic resonance imaging (MRI)—A test that employs magnetic fields and radio waves to generate a three-dimensional image of a part of the body, such as the brain.

metabolic syndrome—A group of findings, including obesity, hypertension, high triglyceride levels, low HDL cholesterol levels, and elevated blood glucose levels, that is caused by a genetic predisposition to insulin resistance and an accumulation of fat in the abdomen.

motor cortex—A part of the frontal lobe of the brain. Damage to this area can result in weakness or paralysis on the opposite side of the body.

neuron—Nerve cell.

nitric oxide—A substance secreted by cells lining the walls of blood vessels that causes arteries to dilate by relaxing smooth muscle cells.

norepinephrine—A hormone that increases blood pressure in response to stress.

occipital lobe—An area of the brain at the back of the skull that is dedicated to the perception and interpretation of visual data from the eyes.

orthostatic hypotension—Abrupt drop in blood pressure on standing that causes dizziness or light-headedness. A side effect of many antihypertensive medications.

parathyroid hormone—A hormone that regulates calcium metabolism. It dilates small arteries that may play a role in the control of blood pressure.

parietal lobe—An area of the brain behind the frontal lobe that receives and interprets sensory signals from all parts of the body.

peripheral-acting adrenergic antagonists—Drugs that reduce resistance to blood flow in small arteries.

peripheral arterial disease—A narrowing of the arteries in the extremities, usually the legs. Most often due to atherosclerosis.

pheochromocytoma—A tumor in the adrenal gland

that secretes large amounts of epinephrine or norepinephrine. Can lead to hypertension.

plaque—An accumulation of cholesterol, smooth muscle cells, fibrous proteins, and calcium in artery walls.

potassium—A mineral found mainly in fruits and vegetables. Increased intake helps lower blood pressure.

prehypertension—A term used to describe people with systolic blood pressure between 120 and 139 mm Hg or diastolic blood pressure between 80 and 89 mm Hg. These individuals are at high risk for developing hypertension.

primary hypertension—Hypertension likely related to poor diet, excess weight, high salt intake, or physical inactivity. Affects 90% to 95% of people with hypertension.

pulse pressure—The difference between systolic and diastolic blood pressures. Reflects the stiffness of arteries.

renin—An enzyme produced by cells in the kidney that converts angiotensinogen to angiotensin I.

renovascular hypertension—A type of hypertension caused by a reduction in blood flow to the kidneys.

retinopathy—Damage to the retina of the eye caused by changes in the tiny blood vessels that supply the retina. The leading cause of blindness in U.S. adults.

salt—Another term for sodium chloride. One teaspoon of salt contains 2,400 mg of sodium.

secondary hypertension—Hypertension caused by another health condition or a medication. Responsible for less than 5% of cases of hypertension.

sodium—A mineral found mostly in processed foods, including salted snacks, canned soups, luncheon meats, and frozen dinners. In general, diets high in sodium cause blood pressure to rise.

sphygmomanometer—An instrument used to measure blood pressure. Consists of an inflating bulb, inflatable cuff, and gauge.

spiral computed tomography (CT) scanning—An imaging method in which an iodine-based dye is injected into the patient and a rapid CT scan is performed through the region of interest. Computer-based software then shows images of the blood vessels that fill with dye.

stent—A wire mesh tube that is inserted into an artery to help keep it open.

stroke—A sudden reduction in or loss of brain function that occurs when an artery supplying blood to a portion of the brain becomes blocked or ruptures. Neurons in the affected area are starved of the oxygen and nutrients they need to function properly.

subarachnoid hemorrhage—Leakage of blood into the space between the brain and the arachnoid membrane, the middle of three membranes that envelop the brain. Most commonly results from trauma or a ruptured aneurysm.

systolic blood pressure—The upper number in a blood pressure reading. Represents pressure in the arteries when the heart is pumping blood to the rest of the body.

temporal lobe—An area of the brain at ear level underneath the parietal and frontal lobes that is dedicated to auditory perception and storage of memories.

thrombolytic drugs—Medications that dissolve blood clots.

thrombus—A blood clot. The plural form is thrombi.

transient ischemic attack (TIA)—Short-lived neurological deficits caused by insufficient blood flow to the brain. Most episodes subside within 5 to 20 minutes.

triglyceride—A lipid (fat) in the bloodstream. Elevated levels are associated with an increased risk of coronary heart disease.

vasospasm—A constriction of blood vessels in the brain that is likely to occur in the first two weeks after a subarachnoid hemorrhage.

vertebral arteries—Blood vessels that run up the back of the neck, parallel to the spine, and carry blood to the brain stem and rear third of the brain.

white coat hypertension—High blood pressure readings that are present only when the patient's blood pressure is recorded by a physician or in a medical environment. Blood pressure is normal when taken at home by the patient, family members, or friends.

HEALTH INFORMATION ORGANIZATIONS AND SUPPORT GROUPS

American College of Cardiology
9111 Old Georgetown Rd.
Bethesda, MD 20814-1699
☎ 800-253-4636/301-897-5400
www.acc.org
Professional medical society and teaching institution that provides professional education, promotes research, offers leadership in the development of standards and guidelines, and forms health care policy.

American Heart Association
7272 Greenville Ave.
Dallas, TX 75231
☎ 800-242-8721
www.americanheart.org
National health organization that provides information and public education programs on all aspects of heart disease. Check for local chapters.

The American Occupational Therapy Association
4720 Montgomery Lane
P.O. Box 31220
Bethesda, MD 20824-1220
☎ 301-652-2682
   800-377-8555 (TDD)
www.aota.org
Provides a consumer tip sheet and information about occupational therapy services for people recovering from a stroke and their families. Also provides contact information for state associations to aid in therapist referrals.

American Physical Therapy Association
1111 N. Fairfax St.
Alexandria, VA 22314-1488
☎ 800-999-APTA/703-684-APTA
www.apta.org
National professional organization for physical therapists (PTs) that provides referrals to state PT associations.

American Society of Hypertension
148 Madison Ave., 5th Fl.
New York, NY 10016
☎ 212-696-9099
www.ash-us.org
Largest U.S. organization dedicated exclusively to hypertension and related cardiovascular disease. Organizes and conducts educational programs to promote the development of treatments for hypertension.

American Speech-Language-Hearing Association
10801 Rockville Pike
Rockville, MD 20852
☎ 800-638-8255
www.asha.org
Toll-free help line gives information on communication disorders and referrals to speech-language pathologists and audiologists around the country.

American Stroke Association
7272 Greenville Ave.
Dallas, TX 75231
☎ 888-4-STROKE
   800-553-6321 ("Warmline")
www.strokeassociation.org
A division of the American Heart Association; provides referrals to community stroke groups and information and peer counseling to survivors and caregivers. Call the "Warmline" to subscribe to their magazine, *Stroke Connection*.

HeartInfo.org—The Heart Information Network
26 Main St., 3rd Fl.
Chatham, NJ 09728
www.heartinfo.org
Educational Web site providing the latest news, advice, and self-help tools for the prevention, diagnosis, and treatment of cardiovascular disease.

Mended Hearts, Inc.
7272 Greenville Ave.
Dallas, TX 75231-4596
☎ 888-HEART-99/214-706-1442
www.mendedhearts.org
Support group for heart disease patients and their families. Call, write, or visit the Web site for information and to get in touch with other heart patients in your area.

National Aphasia Association
29 John St., #1103
New York, NY 10038
☎ 800-922-4622
www.aphasia.org
Provides educational material, a newsletter, a directory of community support groups, and a national network of volunteers who can discuss professional and social resources in their areas.

National Heart, Lung, and Blood Institute Information Center
P.O. Box 30105
Bethesda, MD 20824-0105
☎ 800-575-WELL/301-592-8573
www.nhlbi.nih.gov/health/infoctr/index.htm
Branch of the National Institutes of Health that provides written information on all heart-related issues.

National Institute of Neurological Disorders and Stroke
P.O. Box 5801
Bethesda, MD 20824
☎ 800-352-9424/301-496-5751
www.ninds.nih.gov
Leading supporter of neurological research in the United States. Provides publications about neurological disorders and a list of voluntary health agencies.

National Rehabilitation Information Center
4200 Forbes Blvd., Ste. 202
Lanham, MD 20706
☎ 800-346-2742/301-459-5900
www.naric.com
National library providing information on rehabilitation and disability, including independent living, employment, medical rehabilitation, and legislation. Makes referrals to community rehabilitation centers.

National Stroke Association
9707 E. Easter Lane
Englewood, CO 80112
☎ 800-STROKES/303-649-9299
www.stroke.org
National nonprofit organization devoting 100% of its resources to stroke. Provides education, services, and community-based activities in stroke prevention, treatment, rehabilitation, and recovery.

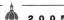

LEADING HOSPITALS

U.S. News & World Report and the National Opinion Research Center, a social-science research group at the University of Chicago, recently conducted their 15th annual nationwide survey of 8,160 board-certified physicians in 17 medical specialties. The doctors nominated the hospitals that they considered to be the best among 6,012 U.S. medical centers. This is the current list of the best hospitals for cardiology and neurology, as determined by a combination of factors: doctors'

recommendations from 2002, 2003, and 2004; federal death rates; and factual data regarding quality indicators, such as the ratio of registered nurses to patients and use of advanced technology. However, because the results reflect the doctors' opinions to some extent, they are partly subjective. Any institution listed is considered a leading center, and the rankings do not imply that other hospitals cannot or do not deliver excellent care.

NEUROLOGY AND NEUROSURGERY HOSPITALS

1. **Mayo Clinic**
Rochester, MN
☎ 507-284-2511
www.mayoclinic.org

2. **Johns Hopkins Hospital**
Baltimore, MD
☎ 410-955-5000
www.hopkinsmedicine.org

3. **Massachusetts General Hospital**
Boston, MA
☎ 617-726-2000
www.mgh.harvard.edu

4. **New York-Presbyterian Hospital**
New York, NY
☎ 212-746-5454
www.nyp.org

5. **University of California, San Francisco, Medical Center**
San Francisco, CA
☎ 888-689-UCSF/415-476-1000
www.ucsfhealth.org

6. **Cleveland Clinic**
Cleveland, OH
☎ 800-223-2273/216-444-2200
www.clevelandclinic.org

7. **Barnes-Jewish Hospital**
St. Louis, MO
☎ 314-747-3000
www.barnesjewish.org

8. **University of California, Los Angeles, Medical Center**
Los Angeles, CA
☎ 800-825-2631/310-825-9111
www.healthcare.ucla.edu

9. **St. Joseph's Hospital and Medical Center**
Phoenix, AZ
☎ 602-406-3000
www.ichosestjoes.com

10. **Methodist Hospital**
Houston, TX
☎ 713-790-3333
www.methodisthealth.com

CARDIOLOGY AND HEART SURGERY HOSPITALS

1. **Cleveland Clinic**
Cleveland, OH
☎ 800-223-2273/216-444-2200
www.clevelandclinic.org

2. **Mayo Clinic**
Rochester, MN
☎ 507-284-2511
www.mayoclinic.org

3. **Duke University Medical Center**
Durham, NC
☎ 919-684-8111
www.mc.duke.edu

4. **Johns Hopkins Hospital**
Baltimore, MD
☎ 410-955-5000
www.hopkinsmedicine.org

5. **Massachusetts General Hospital**
Boston, MA
☎ 617-726-2000
www.mgh.harvard.edu

6. **Brigham and Women's Hospital**
Boston, MA
☎ 617-732-5500
www.brighamandwomens.org

7. **New York-Presbyterian Hospital**
New York, NY
☎ 212-746-5454
www.nyp.org

8. **Emory University Hospital**
Atlanta, GA
☎ 800-75-EMORY/404-778-7777
www.emoryhealthcare.org

9. **Texas Heart Institute at St. Luke's Episcopal Hospital**
Houston, TX
☎ 800-292-2221
www.texasheartinstitute.org

10. **Stanford Hospital and Clinics**
Stanford, CA
☎ 650-723-4000
www.stanfordhospital.com

Source: *U.S. News & World Report,* July 12, 2004.

THE JOHNS HOPKINS WHITE PAPERS

Selected Medical Journal Article

EARLY STROKE TREATMENT WITH rt-PA

The more quickly a person receives anti-blood-clotting treatment after suffering a stroke, the better his or her recovery, a new analysis shows.

Recombinant tissue plasminogen activator (rt-PA) is given intravenously to treat ischemic strokes, which are caused by a blockage of blood flow in the brain. Researchers have been aware that administering rt-PA within three hours of a stroke is an effective treatment, but it has not been clear whether earlier administration is better—or whether later administration is helpful.

To investigate, the National Institute of Neurological Disorders and Stroke rt-PA Stroke Study Group, the European Cooperative Acute Stroke Study, and investigators from the ATLANTIS trial pooled findings of six clinical trials of rt-PA for stroke. Their report is reprinted here from the March 6, 2004, issue of *The Lancet.*

The six trials included a total of 2,775 patients given rt-PA or placebo within six hours of stroke onset. In the current analysis, researchers classified patients based on how quickly they received treatment and their outcome three months after stroke.

The likelihood of a good outcome increased as the time to treatment shortened, the researchers found, with the best results seen when treatment was given within 90 minutes of stroke. Their analysis suggested that the drug could continue to benefit patients if given more than three hours after stroke, but this benefit likely did not extend as far as six hours. Further research should investigate which patients will benefit from the drug when it is given later on, they note.

Association of outcome with early stroke treatment: pooled analysis of ATLANTIS, ECASS, and NINDS rt-PA stroke trials

The ATLANTIS, ECASS, and NINDS rt-PA Study Group Investigators*

Summary

Background Quick administration of intravenous recombinant tissue plasminogen activator (rt-PA) after stroke improved outcomes in previous trials. We aimed to analyse combined data for individual patients to confirm the importance of rapid treatment.

Methods We pooled common data elements from six randomised placebo-controlled trials of intravenous rt-PA. Using multivariable logistic regression we assessed the relation of the interval from stroke onset to start of treatment (OTT) on favourable 3-month outcome and on the occurrence of clinically relevant parenchymal haemorrhage.

Findings Treatment was started within 360 min of onset of stroke in 2775 patients randomly allocated to rt-PA or placebo. Median age was 68 years, median baseline National Institute of Health Stroke Scale (NIHSS) 11, and median OTT 243 min. Odds of a favourable 3-month outcome increased as OTT decreased (p=0·005). Odds were 2·8 (95% CI 1·8–4·5) for 0–90 min, 1·6 (1·1–2·2) for 91–180 min, 1·4 (1·1–1·9) for 181–270 min, and 1·2 (0·9–1·5) for 271–360 min in favour of the rt-PA group. The hazard ratio for death adjusted for baseline NIHSS was not different from 1·0 for the 0–90, 91–180, and 181–270 min intervals; for 271–360 min it was 1·45 (1·02–2·07). Haemorrhage was seen in 82 (5·9%) rt-PA patients and 15 (1·1%) controls (p<0·0001). Haemorrhage was not associated with OTT but was with rt-PA treatment (p=0·0001) and age (p=0·0002).

Interpretation The sooner that rt-PA is given to stroke patients, the greater the benefit, especially if started within 90 min. Our results suggest a potential benefit beyond 3 h, but this potential might come with some risks.

Lancet 2004; **363**: 768–74

*Details at end of report; full list online at
http://image.thelancet.com/extras/03art1122webappendix1.pdf

Correspondence to: Dr John R Marler, Associate Director, Clinical Trials, National Institute of Neurogical Disorders and Stroke, 6001 Executive Blvd, Room 2216, Rockville, MD 20852, USA

Introduction
Thrombolysis with intravenous rt-PA is effective for strokes due to acute cerebral ischaemia when given within 3 h of symptom onset. In six large, multicentre, randomised, placebo-controlled trials researchers tested the benefits of rt-PA for acute stroke within 6 h of onset.[1-5] The investigators used similar doses of rt-PA and had common outcome measures, but the maximum time allowed to start rt-PA infusion ranged from 3 to 6 h. The most appropriate interval for beginning thrombolytic treatment remains to be clarified. Better understanding of the therapeutic window for intravenous rt-PA is important because the short time currently allocated for treatment is the greatest barrier to wider application of thrombolytic therapy.

The chance of benefit from intravenous rt-PA diminishes as time elapses during the first 3 h after onset of the stroke.[6] By combining individual patients' data from six trials, we have extended this analysis to 6 h. The trials were: two National Institute of Neurological Disorders and Stroke (NINDS) trials (parts 1 and 2, 3-h window), two ECASS trials (6-h window), and two ATLANTIS trials (part A, 6-h window and part B, 5-h window). We sought to determine whether time-to-treatment with intravenous thrombolytic therapy is a critical predictor of therapeutic benefit.

Methods
Patients
The trials we analysed represent all major investigations of rt-PA for acute stroke and more than 99% of all patients treated with intravenous rt-PA in randomised controlled clinical trials of acute ischaemic stroke identified in an ongoing cumulative meta-analysis.[7] From all investigations of rt-PA identified in that meta-analysis, the results of only one small (n=27) randomised pilot feasibility trial were not included because different endpoints were used.[8] For our combined analysis, a neuroradiologist (RvK) assessed all CT scans of patients with symptomatic or asymptomatic haemorrhage within 36 h to standardise the definition of intracerebral haemorrhage across trials.

Eligibility criteria
In all six trials, inclusion was based on a clinical diagnosis of ischaemic stroke determined by a focal neurological deficit measurable on either the National Institutes of Health Stroke Scale (NIHSS)[9] for NINDS and ATLANTIS, or the Scandinavian Stroke Scale for ECASS,[10] a clearly defined time of stroke onset, and CT scan of the head that excluded haemorrhage. All investigations had strict criteria for determination of time of stroke onset. Patients who awoke with symptoms of stroke were either excluded or time of onset was defined as the time they were last awake and had no symptoms of stroke. Informed consent was obtained for all patients.

The time allowed from stroke onset to start of treatment (OTT) varied between trials. In the NINDS studies, the protocols dictated that treatment start within 3 h of onset of symptoms, and within 90 min for half the patients. Because the number of patients in the 91–180 min stratum could never exceed by more than two the number in the 0–90 min stratum, and because a permuted-block design was used, there were similar numbers of patients in both strata. In ECASS, patients were enrolled between 0–360 min from symptom onset with no stratification. Those in ATLANTIS A were enrolled from 0–360 min. ATLANTIS B initially recruited patients from 0–300 min. After the results of the NINDS trials became known, this was narrowed to 180–300 min from symptom onset.

All trials shared many exclusion criteria designed mainly to restrict the risk of bleeding. Thus, in the NINDS and ATLANTIS trials, patients were excluded if they had had stroke or serious head trauma within the preceding 3 months, major surgery within 14 days, gastrointestinal or genitourinary bleeding within 21 days, arterial puncture at a non-compressible site within 7 days, any history of intracranial haemorrhage or present symptoms suggestive of subarachnoid haemorrhage, or systolic blood pressure consistently more than 185 or diastolic more than 110 mm Hg (or patients needing aggressive treatment to lower their pressure to these levels). Patients taking oral anticoagulants, heparin within 48 h, and a raised partial thromboplastin time, and those with a prothrombin time more than 15 s or platelet count below 100 000 were also excluded. The ATLANTIS trials had slightly different allowed intervals from a previous stroke (6 weeks) and major surgery (30 days). ECASS had similar exclusions: conditions associated with gastrointestinal bleeding, trauma, surgery, or arterial puncture within 3 months; raised systolic or diastolic blood pressure; long-lasting partial thromboplastin time or prothrombin time; platelet count less than 100 000; and packed cell volume (haematocrit) less than 25.

There were no upper age limits during the later years of the NINDS part 1 trial or throughout the entire part 2 trial. ECASS and ATLANTIS excluded patients aged younger than 18 years or older than 80 years. The studies had important differences in exclusion of patients with mild or severe stroke. All investigations excluded patients who were rapidly improving. Individuals without significant deficit were excluded from NINDS parts 1 and 2 but there were no upper or lower limits of baseline NIHSS scores. In ECASS and ATLANTIS, patients with minor stroke (Scandinavian Stroke Scale >50 in ECASS, and NIHSS <4 in ATLANTIS) were excluded. Also, participants with complete hemispheric syndromes with hemiplegia and decreased consciousness or forced head and eye deviation were excluded from ECASS.

ECASS and ATLANTIS B also excluded those with extended early infarct signs on the baseline CT scan such as diffuse swelling and parenchymal hypodensity, with or without effacement of cerebral sulci in more than 33% of the middle cerebral artery territory. Detailed instructions for exclusion of such patients were provided to all of the ECASS and ATLANTIS sites. No such exclusion based on CT scan existed in the NINDS trials. To exclude possible stroke mimics, all studies excluded patients with seizure associated with stroke onset, or serum glucose below 500 mg/L or above 4000 mg/L. Patients were excluded from analysis if OTT could not be determined to be within 6 h.

Treatment

NINDS, ATLANTIS, and ECASS II gave a total intravenous study drug dose of 0·9 mg/kg bodyweight (90 mg maximum), whereas ECASS I used a total dose of 1·1 mg/kg (100 mg maximum). All studies gave 10% of the dose as a bolus during the first minute. The remainder was infused over 1 h. All trials allowed inclusion of patients who had taken antiplatelet agents before their stroke, but precluded the use of oral or intravenous anticoagulants or antiplatelet agents for the first 24 h after treatment. Specific guidelines for monitoring and treating raised blood pressure for the first 24 h after treatment were provided to all centres.

Outcome measures

The trials were similar in their outcome measures. Investigators in all studies measured NIHSS, modified Rankin Scale, and Barthel Index up to 3 months after stroke onset, calculated mortality, carefully determined the occurrence of haemorrhage with CT, and relied on clinical scales for their primary outcome measures. Measures of the Glasgow Outcome Scale and the Scandinavian Stroke Scale were not obtained in all studies and were not included. There were substantial differences between the trials in the definition of intracranial haemorrhage and in specific outcome scales and definitions of favourable outcomes that were chosen.

The trials differed in definition of primary outcome. In NINDS part 1, primary outcome was defined as the proportion of patients who improved from baseline by 4 or more points on the NIHSS scale at 24 h. In NINDS part 2, investigators assessed good outcome as low or no deficit at 90 days based on four measures (Barthel, Rankin, Glasgow Outcome, and NIHSS).[11–13] A global test statistic was used to simultaneously test for effect in all measures. ECASS I compared the median value of the Barthel and Rankin scales in the treated and control groups at 90 days. ATLANTIS A used change in NIHSS from baseline at 24 h and 30 days and the CT infarct volume at 30 days, and ATLANTIS B used the proportion at 90 days with NIHSS 0–1 as the primary outcome. The ECASS II primary endpoint was low or no deficit at 90 days with the Rankin scale.

Investigators in all studies went to great lengths to classify brain bleeding events with a central medical monitor or safety committee to review all CT scans and clinical data. The NINDS and ATLANTIS trials differentiated between symptomatic and asymptomatic intracranial haemorrhage. ECASS differentiated between four types of haemorrhagic infarction and parenchymal haemorrhage. Parenchymal hemorrhage II was defined as a dense blood clot exceeding 30% of the infarct volume with substantial space-occupying effect. Similar to the other studies, the ECASS protocol mandated CT scanning at 24 h, but also again between days 6 and 8 after stroke onset.

Statistical analysis

We focused primarily on the 3-month favourable outcome defined by three neurological function scores of modified Rankin Scale (0 or 1), Barthel Index (95 or 100), and NIHSS (0 or 1). For all three outcomes the dichotomies were chosen to represent minimal or no poststroke disability (favourable, not favourable). Of particular interest was whether the odds of a favourable outcome increased as OTT decreased (ie, whether there is an OTT by treatment interaction). We tested for this interaction with a global statistical test. We used generalised estimating equations to estimate the odds ratio, 95% CIs , and p values calculated from correlated binary outcomes in a logistic regression model.

All trials were missing one or more of these outcome measures at 90 days for some patients. A conservative algorithm assigning outcomes based on measurement made earlier than 90 days for these patients was

Potential confounders

Age (years)
Weight (kg)
Sex
Baseline diastolic blood pressure (mm Hg) at start of treatment
Baseline systolic blood pressure (mm Hg) at start of treatment
Blood glucose comcentration at baseline (mg/L)
NIHSS on admission
History of stroke or transient ischaemic attack
History of diabetes
History of angina
Previous or current atrial fibrillation
History of myocardial infarction
History of congestive heart failure
History of hypertension
On aspirin at time of index stroke

developed and applied to all investigations. If no measurements were available after baseline, the worst score for the modified Rankin Scale, NIHSS, or Barthel Index was assigned. The algorithm allowed all patients with known OTT to be included in the final intention-to-treat (ITT) analysis. 12, 11, 33, 37, 83, and 47 patients from NINDS part 1, NINDS part 2, ECASS I, ECASS II, ATLANTIS A, and ATLANTIS B, respectively, were missing one or more outcomes at 3 months based on the ITT algorithm and were given the worst outcomes. In the original report on the NINDS trials only one patient in part 1 and four in part 2 were reported as having missing outcomes. For the other 18 patients, outcomes after 90 days were available.

To obtain maximum study power to establish whether the benefit of rt-PA changes with OTT, we tested for an interaction between the two, treating OTT as a continuum in a logistic regression model, after validating the linearity of log-odds for the OTT variable. Since there might be potential confounders that mask or exaggerate the treatment by OTT interaction, the other baseline variables associated with stroke outcome from previous publications (panel) were considered for inclusion into a multivariate logistic regression model. To be a potential confounder, a variable had to be associated with either treatment or with OTT, and also associated with the outcome of interest.

To identify potential confounders, we used Spearman's correlation for testing the association between OTT and the other baseline continuous variables and likelihood-ratio tests for testing the association between treatment and the other baseline continuous or categorical variables. A

potential association was regarded as present if p≤0·2. All baseline variables with a potential association with treatment or OTT and associated with the outcome would be included into the first step multivariable model. A continuous variable as potential confounder was further tested for linearity of log-odds before inclusion in a multivariable model to determine whether transformations were needed. As a result, all continuous variables were kept as continuous and were centralised (subtracted mean and divided by SD).

Dummy variables representing a trial (NINDS, ECASS, or ATLANTIS) could not be included in the logistic regression model. Trial is collinear with OTT since OTT is defined by trial. When there is a high degree of collinearity, the logistic regression model will not converge to a solution. Trial also defines continent, ethnic background, and dose (the administered dose was higher in the ECASS I trial [planned 1·1 mg/kg] than in all others [planned 0·9 mg/kg]). Thus, these three variables were also collinear with OTT, by design, and therefore could not be considered for inclusion into the multivariate logistic regression model.

To test the consistency of treatment and OTT effect on the 3-month outcome of interest, we also did an analysis that included two-way interactions (age by NIHSS at baseline, by systolic blood pressure, and by diastolic blood pressure) taken from a previous report[14] in the final multivariate logistic regression model with their associated main effects. We used backward stepwise model selection by testing the interactions and then, if interactions were not detected, we tested main effects. Interactions with p<0·1, and their associated main effects, and main effects (cut-off p<0·05) based on the likelihood ratio statistic were retained in the final model.

The final logistic regression model was developed on the basis of only recorded data—ie, participants missing any data item were excluded. We then applied the model to the total population using the ITT approach described previously. The analyses with only observed data (n=2552) and analyses of ITT (n=2775) gave similar results; therefore ITT results are presented. Similar analytical approaches were used to study treatment and OTT effect on 3-month favourable outcomes individually, and treatment and OTT effect on modified Rankin Scale (0, 1, or 2) as defined in ECASS post-hoc analyses,[3] respectively. Analyses of recorded data and ITT datasets gave results that were much the same. Epi Info 2000 was used to do the sample size calculation, assuming α=0·05, two-sided, and power=90%. Cox regression adjusting for NIHSS at baseline was used to calculate hazard ratios for death.

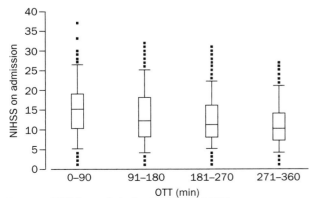

Figure 1: NIHSS on admission for different OTT
89 patients without baseline measurements for NIHSS were excluded from this analysis.

	Treatment	n	Odds ratio (95% CI)*	
			Adjusted	Unadjusted
Interval (min)				
0–90	rt-PA	161	2·81 (1·75–4·50)	1·96 (1·30–2·95)
	Placebo	150		
91–180	rt-PA	302	1·55 (1·12–2·15)	1·65 (1·23–2·22)
	Placebo	315		
181–270	rt-PA	390	1·40 (1·05–1·85)	1·34 (1·04–1·72)
	Placebo	411		
271–360	rt-PA	538	1·15 (0·90–1·47)	1·04 (0·84–1·29)
	Placebo	508		

3-month favourable outcomes include Rankin (0–1), Barthel (95–100), and NIHSS (0–1). One, eight, nine, and six patients from NINDS part I, ECASS I, ECASS II, and ATLANTIS B, respectively, were excluded from this analysis since they were randomised after 360 min or OTT was not reported. *Odds ratios calculated from global statistical approach[13] by ITT analysis. Adjusted odds ratios were calculated adjusting for age, baseline glucose concentration, baseline NIHSS, baseline diastolic blood pressure, previous hypertension, and interaction between age and baseline NIHSS.

Table 1: Odds ratio for a favourable outcome at 3 months after stroke

Role of the funding source

For the ATLANTIS trials, Genentech provided full support for the study and Genentech employees participated to some extent in study design, data collection, data analysis, and data interpretation, writing of the report, and in the decision to submit the manuscript for publication. For the ECASS trials, Boehringer Ingelheim provided full support. Employees of Boehringer Ingelheim participated in study design, in data collection, data analysis, data interpretation, writing of the report, and in the decision to submit the report for publication. For the NINDS trials, Genentech provided only the drug and additional study monitoring to ensure compliance with requirements of the US Food and Drug Administration. All support for the investigators and for data collection, analysis, and interpretation were provided by NINDS. For this combined analysis, Genentech and Boehringer Ingelheim provided data from the ATLANTIS and ECASS trials. Statistical support was provided by Boehringer Ingelheim and NINDS.

Results

The ITT analysis included 2775 patients treated at more than 300 hospitals from 18 countries. All trials included some community hospitals. Median age was 68 years, IQR 60–74 years, and 84·6% were reported as white (non-Hispanic), 9·1% as black (non-Hispanic), 2·0% as Hispanic, 0·9% as Asian, and 0·6% as being from other

ethnic backgrounds. Ethnic background was not reported for 2·8%. Median baseline NIHSS score was 11, and median OTT 243 min. 1847 patients (67%) were treated for longer than 3 h after symptom onset. Of 928 treated within 3 h, 306 (33%) were treated in trials other than NINDS. Excluded from all trials were eight patients randomised after 6 h from stroke onset and 16 patients whose OTT was not reported. Figure 1 shows the inverse correlation of baseline NIHSS with OTT.

Of 15 potential confounders related to outcome and OTT or treatment (panel), five variables and one interaction between the variables met the criteria for inclusion in the final model. The final multivariable model of favourable outcome included treatment, OTT, age, blood glucose concentrations at baseline, NIHSS on admission, baseline diastolic blood pressure, previous hypertension, interaction between age and NIHSS on admission, and interaction between OTT and treatment. Interaction between OTT and treatment remained significant (p=0·005) in the final multivariable model. In this model, the benefit from treatment increased as OTT decreased. Thus, we undertook separate analyses at four OTT periods (table 1). Figure 2 shows the odds ratios by NIHSS categories within OTT intervals. Figure 3 shows OTT by treatment interaction through estimation of global odds ratio at different times from stroke onset. Assuming a fixed value for the other variables, we plotted the global odds ratio and 95% CIs predicted by the final model for different OTT.

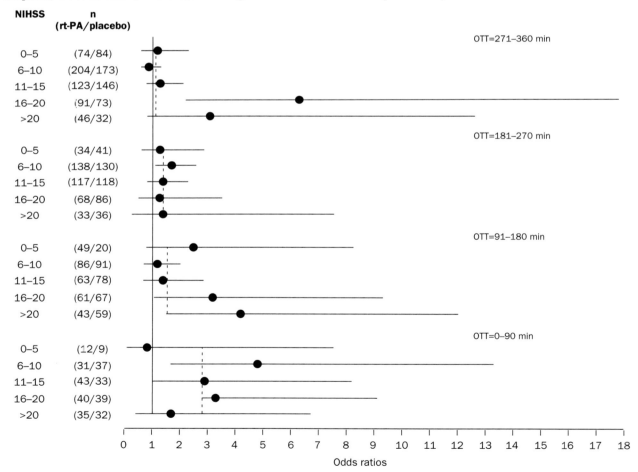

Figure 2: **Odds ratios for favourable outcome at 3 months by OTT and NIHSS category**
Odds ratios were calculated with adjustment for age, baseline glucose concentration, baseline diastolic blood pressure, and previous hypertension. The short dash lines are the overall estimates of odds ratios for each time stratum. 3-month favourable outcomes include Rankin (0–1), Barthel (95–100), and NIHSS (0–1). One, eight, nine, and six patients from NINDS part I, ECASS I, ECASS II, and ATLANTIS B, respectively, were excluded from this analysis because they were randomised after 360 min or OTT was not reported.

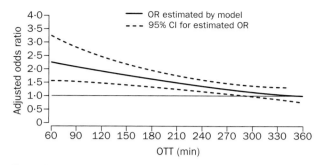

Figure 3: **Model estimating odds ratio for favourable outcome at 3 months in rt-PA-treated patients compared with controls by OTT**

Adjusted for age, baseline glucose concentration, baseline NIHSS measurement, baseline diastolic blood pressure, previous hypertension, and interaction between age and baseline NIHSS measurement.

Figure 4 shows measurements on the modified Rankin Scale at four OTT periods for placebo and rt-PA groups. After 3 months in the ITT analysis, 390 (14·0%) of 2775 patients were dead or had the worst score assigned, and 707 (25·5%) were severely disabled (modified Rankin 4–5). Fewer rt-PA patients treated within 90 min died compared with controls, but assuming all patients with missing data were alive at last follow-up the 95% CIs for the hazard ratio, adjusted for baseline NIHSS, included 1·0 (0·88, 0·54–1·46). Adjusted hazard ratios for the OTT strata 91–180 and 181–270 exceeded 1·0, but 95% CIs were not significant (1·15 [0·77–1·70]; 1·24

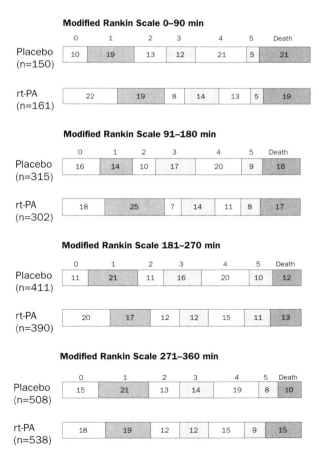

Figure 4: **Modified Rankin Scale measurement at day 90**
0–90 min, n=311; 91–180 min, n=618; 181–270 min, n=801; 270–360 min, n=1046. Values do not equal 100% because of rounding.

	Placebo		rt-PA	
	n*	Patients with parenchymal haematoma (90%, 95% CI)	n	Patients with parenchymal haematoma (90%, 95% CI)
OTT (min)				
0–90	150	0 (0, ··)	161	5 (3·1, 1·6–5·6)
91–180	315	3 (1·0, 0·4–2·0)	302	17 (5·6, 3·9–7·9)
181–270	411	7 (1·7, 1·0–2·9)	390	23 (5·9, 4·3–8·0)
271–360	508	5 (1·0, 0·5–1·8)	538	37 (6·9, 5·3–8·7)

Parenchymal haematoma is defined as a dense blood clot exceeding 30% of the infarct volume with significant space-occupying effect. *One, eight, nine, and six patients from NINDS part I, ECASS I, ECASS II, and ATLANTIS B, respectively, were excluded from this analysis because they were randomised after 360 min or OTT was not reported.

Table 2: **Frequency of parenchymal haematoma between 0 and 360 min after treatment**

[0·84–1·84]). For the OTT interval 271–360, the adjusted hazard ratio exceeded 1·0 (1·45 [1·02–2·07]).

Substantial intracerebral haemorrhage (parenchymal haematoma, type II) was seen in 5·9% of the rt-PA patients compared with 1·1% of placebo patients (p<0·0001). 59·8% of those with parenchymal haematoma died within 3 months (62·2% for rt-PA and 46·7% for placebo). Median age of patients with haematoma was 72 years (IQR 65–76). Median OTT in patients with the haematoma was 261 min (180–300), and median baseline NIHSS score was 12 (8–16). Table 2 shows the frequency of parenchymal haematoma by OTT. In the multivariate model for haematoma, including treatment, OTT, age, and NIHSS score, the OTT-treatment interaction was not significant (p=0·48). Subsequent analyses showed that the occurrence of such haematoma was associated with rt-PA treatment (p=0·0001) and age (p=0·0002), but not with OTT (p=0·71) or baseline NIHSS score (p=0·10).

Further details of results available at http://image. thelancet.com/extras/03art1122webappendix2.pdf.

Discussion

Our results confirm that rapid treatment is associated with better outcomes at 3 months. Previously, NINDS Stroke Study investigators reported that the probability of benefit from intravenous rt-PA in the combined data from the two NINDS trials diminishes as time elapses during the first 3 h after onset of the stroke.[6] Our results confirm and expand on this finding. For example, the odds ratio of a favourable outcome for patients treated with rt-PA compared with controls was 2·81 (1·75–4·50) for those treated within 90 min and 1·55 (1·12–2·15) for those treated within 91–180 min. The adjusted hazard ratio for death was not significantly different from 1·0 (HR [95% CI]) for patients treated within 0–270 min and exceeded 1·0 (1·45 [1·02–2·07]) in the interval 271–360. Our findings suggest that the beneficial effect of rt-PA might extend beyond 3 h since the odds ratio for a favourable outcome was 1·40 (1·05–1·85) for those treated within 181–270 min. However, the beneficial effect might not extend to 6 h. Our analysis did not provide strong evidence to support exclusion of patients from treatment based on their initial NIHSS for any OTT.

Definition of the limits of the treatment window for rt-PA in acute ischaemic stroke has been difficult. Based on the results of the two NINDS trials, approval for use of the drug has been restricted to within 3 h of stroke onset. Our results suggest that the benefit of rt-PA could extend beyond 3 h, a finding that is compatible with results of secondary analyses from the other rt-PA investigations.[2,3,5] Figure 3 shows that the point estimate of the odds of a

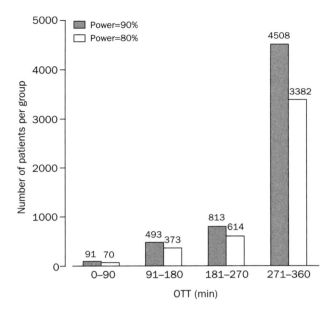

Figure 5: Sample size by OTT
Projected number of patients needed for ischaemic stroke studies of thrombolysis based on odds ratios recorded within intervals of OTT.

favourable outcome is close to 1·0 at 360 min, suggesting reduced probability of benefit beyond this time. The apparent reduction in benefit from rt-PA at later periods does not seem to be explained by an increased rate of parenchymal haematoma. We suspect that a progressive disappearance of the ischaemic penumbra is the major factor that accounts for the declining benefit with time.

Patients who continue to have potentially viable ischaemic brain tissue at later times might have substantial treatment benefits.[15,16] Our results are consistent with those from a previous trial in which investigators used transcranial doppler to correlate time to arterial recanalisation with neurological recovery at 24 h after administration of intravenous rt-PA. No individual had early complete recovery if an occlusion persisted for more than 300 min. Complete or part recanalisation of the occluded artery took place within 60 min of the start of treatment in 75% of those in whom recanalisation was seen. A third of these had recanalisation within 30 min of the start of treatment.[17] These data are also consistent with a therapeutic window from stroke symptom onset to start of intravenous rt-PA treatment of 240–270 min.

One trial, ATLANTIS B, specifically addressed the issue of the benefit or risk of such treatment within 3–5 h. This trial enrolled 79% of the participants in the 4–5 h interval and failed to show efficacy. These results are consistent with ours. In the later intervals, consistent with results from ECASS and ATLANTIS, the benefit is small in unselected patients. The sample size needed for a trial of rt-PA would vary by OTT (figure 5). Based on these power analyses, none of the individual trials that treated patients with OTT longer than 3 h had sufficient power to detect the effects of the magnitude recorded. Although these findings suggest that the therapeutic window could extend beyond 3 h, large prospective randomised trials need to confirm this idea. Additional trials are underway: IST 3 (6000 patients); ECASS III (800 patients); DIAS (630 patients); EPITHET (100 patients).

Another important finding in this study is the relation between stroke severity and time to presentation. Patients with more severe strokes arrived earlier in the emergency department, than did those whose condition was less severe (figure 1). Thus, mortality and disability are high in early treatment intervals. This trend is best seen in controls, of whom those treated earlier had greater rates of death and severe disability (modified Rankin Score 4 or 5) than did those treated in later intervals. This finding has implications for the timing of thrombolytic therapy because these patients represent those with the most to gain from treatment, since earlier treatment significantly enhances the likelihood of keeping long-term disability to a minimum. The effect of rt-PA is greatest in those treated early despite greater stroke severity.[18] This result also indicates the potential difficulties in comparing stroke treatment trials in which the time-to-treatment differs substantially, without adjustment for differences in baseline stroke severity.

The relation between time-to-treatment and effectiveness of thrombolytic therapy for stroke confirms previous findings in acute myocardial infarction. The Fibrinolytic Therapy Trialists[19] reported that the absolute difference in 30-day mortality between fibrinolytic and control therapy steadily diminished from 3·5% in patients treated at 0–1 h to 1·6% in those treated within 7–12 h. The CORE investigators[20] reported a strong relation between time-to-treatment with thrombolytic therapy and 35-day mortality. They recorded a mortality of 5·7% in individuals treated in less than 2 h and 12·5% for those treated after 6 h. The GUSTO-IIb investigators[21] reported that the time from enrolment to first balloon inflation for coronary angioplasty was a significant predictor of 30-day mortality, with 1% mortality for patients treated within 60 min and 6·4% mortality for those treated after 90 min.

Our combined analysis indicates that time-to-treatment with thrombolytic therapy is also important for acute stroke (figure 3). However, the therapeutic window for thrombolytic treatment seems to be shorter than that for acute myocardial infarction. The protocols of all trials included measures that were intended to overestimate OTT. For instance, for patients who awoke with stroke symptoms stroke onset was assumed to be at the time they were last known to be healthy. If OTT is an overestimate, the actual therapeutic window could be even shorter.

Our study is limited by differences in trial methodologies such as dose of rt-PA. The total study population was 2775, smaller than that in many acute myocardial infarction trials.[22] However, the magnitude of the differences in outcome is large compared with such trials, especially at early times. Since quicker treatment with rt-PA greatly improves the odds of a favourable outcome, particularly within 90 min, treatment without delay is paramount. Yet, doctors and other health-care personnel might take more time to begin treatment when time limits are longer.[6,23] An acute stroke intervention team can increase the speed and quality of assessment given to a stroke patient before treatment and after arrival in an emergency department. We urge setting a target of 1 h from time of presentation to intravenous treatment for patients with acute ischaemic stroke.[24] This goal could be a challenge for many institutions and might need reorganisation of resources, but it can be achieved.[25]

Our results confirm the strong association between rapid treatment and favourable outcome. Although not as effective as early treatment, our findings suggest a potential benefit from treatment after 3 h. The next step would be to identify patients who are likely to respond to treatment when they present at the later end of the suggested therapeutic interval. The success of acute stroke treatment will be dictated largely by how we use the time we have.

Writing Committee

ECASS Trials Investigators—Werner Hacke, Medical University at Heidelberg, Germany; Geoffrey Donnan, National Stroke Research Institute, Australia; Cesare Fieschi, University of Rome, Italy; Markku Kaste, Helsinki University Central Hospital, Finland; Rüdiger von Kummer, University of Technology Dresden, Germany.
NINDS rt-PA Stroke Study Group Investigators—Joseph P Broderick, University of Cincinnati Stroke Research Center; Thomas Brott, Mayo Clinic; Michael Frankel, Emory University School of Medicine; James C Grotta, University of Texas Houston Medical Center; E Clarke Haley Jr, University of Virginia Health System; Thomas Kwiatkowski, Long Island Jewish Medical Center; Steven R Levine, Mount Sinai School of Medicine; Chris Lewandowski, Henry Ford Hospital; Mei Lu, Henry Ford Health System; Patrick Lyden, University of California, San Diego Stroke Center; John R Marler, National Institute of Neurological Disorders and Stroke, Clinical Trial Group; Suresh Patel, Henry Ford Hospital; Barbara C Tilley, Medical University of South Carolina.
ATLANTIS Trial Investigators—Gregory Albers, Stanford University Medical Center Stroke Center; Thomas Brott, University of Cincinnati Medical Center; James Grotta, University of Texas Houston Medical Center.
Boehringer Ingelheim Pharmaceuticals—Erich Bluhmki, Manfred Wilhelm.
Genentech—Scott Hamilton, Stanford University School of Medicine; Corsee Sanders Genetech.

Statistical analysis

Manfred Wilhelm, Boehringer Ingelheim Pharmaceuticals, Germany; Gabi Biegert, Boehringer Ingelheim Pharmaceuticals, Germany; Yan Lin, Medical University of South Carolina.

Statistical methodology

Barbara C Tilley, Medical University of South Carolina; Manfred Wilhelm, Boehringer Ingelheim Pharmaceuticals, Germany; Mei Lu, Henry Ford Health System; Erich Bluhmki, Boehringer Ingelheim Pharmaceuticals, Germany; Scott Hamilton, Stanford University School of Medicine; Corsee Sanders, Genentech.

Contributors

All investigators made contributions to one or more of the six trials and have seen and approved the final version of the manuscript. G Albers, G Donnan, and C Fieschi did not contribute to the first draft, but did review the draft for accuracy. Two corporate sponsors, Boehringer Ingelheim and Genentech, co-operated in preparation of the document by providing access to the data from the ECASS and ATLANTIS trials for which they were the sole support.

Conflict of interest statement

Genentech provided active and placebo drug for the NINDS trials, but provided no financial support to investigators during the trials. G Albers, J P Broderick, and M Frankel (only after NINDS trials publication), C Fieschi, W Hacke, S Hamilton, M Kaste, and R von Kummer have received funding from corporate sponsors. E C Haley Jr has a Research Supply Agreement with Genentech that supplies study drug to an NIH-funded clinical trial. S Hamilton has received more than US$10 000 from one of the corporate sponsors. None of the authors has an equity or ownership interest in a corporate sponsor. G Biegert and M Wilhelm are employees of Boehringer Ingelheim.

Acknowledgments

Supported by the National Institute of Neurological Disorders and Stroke (N01-NS-02382, N01-NS-02374, N01-NS-02377, N01-NS-02381, N01-NS-02379, N01-NS-02373, N01-NS-02378, N01-NS-02376, N01-NS-02302), by Genentech (medication and some study monitoring for the NINDS studies, full support for ATLANTIS studies), and Boehringer Ingelheim (full support for ECASS studies). We thank NINDS, Genentech Inc, and Boehringer Ingelheim for making the data available for this study. Statisticians undertaking the combined analysis of the data from the six trials were provided by Boehringer Ingelheim and NINDS (N01-NS-2-2343).

References

1 The National Institute of Neurological Disorders and Stroke rt-PA Stroke Study Group. Tissue plasminogen activator for acute ischemic stroke. *N Engl J Med* 1995; **333:** 1581–87.

2 Hacke W, Kaste M, Fieschi C, et al. for the ECASS Study Group. Intravenous thrombolysis with recombinant tissue plasminogen activator for acute hemispheric stroke: the European Cooperative Acute Stroke Study (ECASS). *JAMA* 1995; **274:** 1017–25.

3 Hacke W, Kaste M, Fieschi C, et al. Randomised double-blind placebo-controlled trial of thrombolytic therapy with intravenous alteplase in acute ischaemic stroke (ECASS II). *Lancet* 1998: **352:** 1245–51.

4 Clark WM, Albers GW, Madden KP, et al. The rt-PA (alteplase) 0- to 6-hour acute stroke trial, part A (A0267g): results of a double-blind, placebo-controlled, multicenter study. *Stroke* 2000; **31:** 811–16.

5 Clark WM, Wissman S, Albers GW, et al. Recombinant tissue-type plasminogen activator (alteplase) for ischemic stroke 3 to 5 hours after symptom onset: the ATLANTIS study—a randomized controlled trial. *JAMA* 1999; **282:** 2019–26.

6 Marler JR, Tilley BC, Lu M, et al. Early stroke treatment associated with better outcome: the NINDS rt-PA Stroke Study. *Neurology* 2000; **55:** 1649–55.

7 Wardlaw JM, Sandercock PA, Berge E. Thrombolytic therapy with recombinant tissue plasminogen activator for acute ischemic stroke: where do we go from here?—a cumulative meta-analysis. *Stroke* 2003; **34:** 1437–42.

8 Haley EC Jr, Brott TG, Sheppard GL, et al. Pilot randomized trial of tissue plasminogen activator in acute ischemic stroke. *Stroke* 1993; **24:** 1000–04.

9 Brott T, Adams HP, Olinger CP, et al. Measurements of acute cerebral infarction: a clinical examination scale. *Stroke* 1989; **20:** 864–70.

10 Scandinavian Stroke Study Group. Multicenter trial of hemodilution in ischemic stroke: background and study protocol. *Stroke* 1995; **16:** 885–90.

11 Mahoney FI, Barthel DW. Functional evaluation: the Barthel Index. *Md State Med J* 1965; **14:** 61–65.

12 Van Swieten JC, Koudstaal PJ, Visser MC, Schouten HJ, van Gijn J. Interobserver agreement for the assessment of handicap in stroke patients. *Stroke* 1988; **19:** 604–07.

13 Teasdale G, Knill-Jones R, Van der Sande J. Observer variability in assessing impaired consciousness and coma. *J Neurol Neurosurg Psychiatry* 1978; **41:** 603–10.

14 The National Institute of Neurological Disorders and Stroke rt-PA Stroke Study Group. Generalized efficacy of rt-PA for acute stroke: subgroup analysis of the NINDS rt-PA stroke trial. *Stroke* 1997; **28:** 2119–25.

15 Baron JC, von Kummer R, del Zoppo GJ. Treatment of acute ischemic stroke: challenging the concept of a rigid and universal time-window. *Stroke* 1995; **26:** 2219–21.

16 Parsons MW, Barber PA, Chalk J, et al. Diffusion- and perfusion-weighted MRI response to thrombolysis in stroke. *Ann Neurol* 2002; **51:** 28–37.

17 Christou I, Alexandrov A, Burgin WS, et al. Timing of recanalization after tissue plasminogen activator therapy determined by transcranial doppler correlates with clinical recovery from ischemic stroke. *Stroke* 2000; **31:** 1812–16.

18 The NINDS t-Pa Stroke Study Group. Intracerebral hemorrhage following intravenous t-PA therapy for ischemic stroke. *Stroke* 1997; **28:** 2109–18.

19 Fibrinolytic Therapy Trialists' (FTT) Collaborative Group. Indications for fibrinolytic therapy in suspected acute myocardial infarction: collaborative overview of early mortality and major morbidity results from all randomised trials of more than 1000 patients. *Lancet* 1994; **343:** 311–22.

20 Chareonthaitawee P, Gibbons RJ, Roberts RS, et al. The impact of time to thrombolytic treatment on outcome in patients with acute myocardial infarction. *Heart* 2000; **84:** 142–48.

21 Berger PB, Ellis SG, Holmes DR, et al. Relationship between delay in performing direct coronary angioplasty and early clinical outcome in patients with acute myocardial infarction: results from the global use of strategies to open occluded arteries in acute coronary syndromes (GUSTO-IIb) trial. *Circulation* 1999; **100:** 14–20.

22 Grouppo Italiano per lo Studio della Streptokinase nell'Infarto Miocardico (GISSI). Effectiveness of intravenous thrombolytic treatment in acute myocardial infarction. *Lancet* 1986; **1:** 397–402.

23 Albers G, Bates V, Clark W, Bell R, Verro P, Hamilton S. Intravenous tissue-type plasminogen activator for treatment of acute stroke: The Standard Treatment with Alteplase to Reverse Stroke (STARS) Study. *JAMA* 2000; **283:** 1145–50.

24 Marler JR, Winters-Jones P, Emr M, eds. Proceedings of a National Symposium on Rapid Identification and Treatment of Acute Stroke; 1997. Bethesda, Maryland; National Institutes of Health, National Institute of Neurological Disorders and Stroke: 157–58.

25 Tilley BC, Lyden PD, Brott TG, et al. Total quality improvement methodology for reduction of delays between emergency department admission and treatment of acute ischemic stroke. *Arch Neurol* 1997; **54:** 1466–74.

REPRINT

NOTES

NOTES

NOTES

Copyright © 2005 Medletter Associates, Inc.

Illustrations © 2005 Medletter Associates, Inc., and Duckwall Productions

All rights reserved. No part of this White Paper may be reproduced or transmitted in any form or by any means electronic, mechanical, photocopying, recording, or otherwise, without the prior written permission of the publisher.
Please address inquiries on bulk subscriptions and permission to reproduce selections from this White Paper to
Medletter Associates, Inc., 325 Redding Road, Redding, CT 06896. The editors are interested in receiving your comments at Editors@HopkinsWhitePapers.com or the above address but regret that they cannot answer letters of any sort personally.

ISBN 1-933087-08-0
ISSN 1542-1724
Sixth Printing
Printed in the United States of America

Marler, J.R. "Association of outcome with early stroke treatment: Pooled analysis of ATLANTIS, ECASS, and NINDS rt-PA stroke trials."
Reprinted with permission from *The Lancet* Vol. 363, No. 9411 (March 6, 2004): 768–774. Copyright © 2004, The Lancet Publishing Group.

The Johns Hopkins White Papers are published yearly by Medletter Associates, Inc.

Visit our Web site for information on Johns Hopkins Health After 50 publications, which include White Papers on specific disorders, home medical encyclopedias, consumer reference guides to drugs and medical tests, and our monthly newsletter The Johns Hopkins Medical Letter: Health After 50.
www.HopkinsAfter50.com

The Johns Hopkins White Papers

Paul Candon
Managing Editor

Catherine Richter
Senior Editor

Devon Schuyler
Consulting Editor

Kimberly Flynn
Writer/Researcher

Leslie Maltese-McGill
Copy Editor

Tim Jeffs
Art Director

Vincent Mejia
Graphic Designer

Betsy Meredith Rigo
Editorial Assistant

Robert Duckwall
Medical Illustrator

Kate Brackney
Intern

Johns Hopkins Health After 50 Publications

Rodney Friedman
Editor and Publisher

Thomas Dickey
Editorial Director

Tom Damrauer, M.L.S.
Chief of Information Resources

Jerry Loo
Product Manager

Darren Leiser
Promotions Coordinator

Joan Mullally
Head of Business Development

LUNG DISORDERS

Peter B. Terry, M.D.

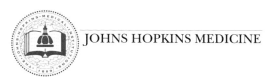JOHNS HOPKINS MEDICINE

Dear Readers:

This past year may have seemed somewhat hazardous for people with lung disorders, with researchers reporting that air fresheners and even certain asthma inhalers might worsen respiratory symptoms. But it also brought about several advances, including better treatments for lung cancer and a better way to evaluate chronic obstructive pulmonary disease (COPD).

This White Paper will give you the bottom line on these and other new findings. You will learn how the respiratory system works, and how doctors evaluate lung problems. Most important, you will gain valuable insights on how to manage such disorders as COPD, asthma, pneumonia, tuberculosis, lung cancer, and sleep apnea.

Here are some of this year's highlights:

- Why your **inhaler** for asthma or COPD may be about to change. (page 10)
- New data on the **safest painkiller** for people with asthma. (page 13)
- Important new concerns about **beta$_2$-agonist inhalers**. (pages 16 and 17)
- How **home oxygen therapy** can improve the lives of some people with COPD. (page 26)
- New research on the serious health risks of **sleep apnea**. (page 30)
- Recent findings on how certain **air fresheners** can irritate your lungs. (page 33)
- A more effective approach to **quitting smoking**. (page 43)
- The latest advances in treating **lung cancer**. (page 44)

I hope the resources provided here give you the background you need to make well-informed decisions about your health.

Sincerely,

Peter B. Terry, M.D.
Professor of Medicine
Division of Pulmonary and Critical Care Medicine
Johns Hopkins University School of Medicine

P. S. Don't forget to visit HopkinsWhitePapers.com for the latest news on lung disorders and other information that will complement your Johns Hopkins White Paper.

THE AUTHOR

Peter B. Terry, M.D., M.A., is a professor of medicine in the Division of Pulmonary and Critical Care Medicine at the Johns Hopkins University School of Medicine. He is also an associate professor in the Department of Anesthesiology/Critical Care Medicine at Johns Hopkins Hospital and an associate professor in the Department of Environmental Health Sciences at the Johns Hopkins School of Public Health.

Dr. Terry received his M.D. from St. Louis University and subsequently trained at the University of Connecticut, Johns Hopkins Hospital, and the Mayo Clinic. He has a master's degree in philosophy with a concentration in bioethics from The Kennedy Institute of Ethics at Georgetown University.

CONTENTS

Symptoms of Respiratory Disorders . . . . .p. 1

General Evaluation of Respiratory Symptoms . . . . .p. 4

General Approaches to Management . . . . .p. 10

Obstructive Diseases of the Lungs . . . . .p. 11

    Asthma . . . . .p. 12
    Chronic Obstructive Pulmonary Disease (COPD) . . . . .p. 20

Chart: Commonly Used Anti-Inflammatory Drugs . . . . .p. 14

Chart: Commonly Used Bronchodilators . . . . .p. 18

Sleep Apnea . . . . .p. 28

Interstitial Lung Disease . . . . .p. 32

Lung Cancer . . . . .p. 39

Pulmonary Embolism . . . . .p. 47

Infections . . . . .p. 51

    Acute Bronchitis . . . . .p. 51
    Influenza . . . . .p. 52
    Pneumonia . . . . .p. 55
    Tuberculosis . . . . .p. 58

Glossary . . . . .p. 63

Health Information Organizations and Support Groups .p. 65

Leading Hospitals for Lung Disorders . . . . .p. 66

Selected Medical Journal Article . . . . .p. 67

LUNG DISORDERS

Disorders of breathing (respiration) are common in the United States and are expected to increase in prevalence with the aging of the population. More than 300,000 Americans die of lung disease every year, and more than 35 million are now living with chronic lung disease. Fortunately, technological advances are producing unprecedented opportunities to prevent, diagnose, and treat respiratory disease. The result is considerable improvements in the life spans and quality of life of people who have these diseases. The topics covered in this White Paper include the following:

Asthma. Asthma is an inflammatory lung disease characterized by shortness of breath, wheezing, coughing, and tightness in the chest. It is considered an obstructive lung disease because it causes narrowing of the airways, but proper treatment can reverse the obstruction.

Chronic obstructive pulmonary disease. Chronic obstructive pulmonary disease (COPD) includes chronic bronchitis and emphysema. Like asthma, COPD is an obstructive lung disease. But the obstruction is more difficult to reverse in COPD, and there is evidence of permanent damage to the lungs.

Sleep apnea. Sleep apnea refers to temporary, recurrent breathing interruptions during sleep.

Interstitial lung disease. Interstitial lung disease refers to a group of conditions that cause extensive scarring of the tissue between the air sacs in the lungs. This tissue is called the interstitium.

Lung cancer. Lung cancer, which is most often caused by cigarette smoking, is the leading cause of cancer death in the United States.

Pulmonary embolism. A pulmonary embolism usually occurs when a blood clot from a deep vein in the leg breaks loose and blocks an artery within the lungs.

Infections. Common lung infections include acute bronchitis, influenza, bacterial pneumonia, and tuberculosis.

The purpose of this White Paper is to provide people with knowledge about the prevention and treatment of a number of common lung disorders so that they can work closely and effectively with their doctors and other health care professionals.

SYMPTOMS OF RESPIRATORY DISORDERS

Many lung disorders produce similar symptoms, which can occur alone or in combination and may worsen gradually or rapidly.

Respiratory disorders can be acute (with a short and relatively severe course) or chronic (persisting over a long time). Pneumonia and pulmonary embolism are acute lung disorders; asthma, COPD, and interstitial lung disease are chronic. Chronic lung conditions may wax and wane in severity and may worsen rapidly if a secondary problem, such as a lung infection, occurs.

Common symptoms of lung disorders include shortness of breath, coughing, noisy breathing, and chest pain. However, some people with lung disorders have only mild symptoms or none at all. In these individuals, the disorder may be detected on a chest x-ray or by a pulmonary function test during medical evaluation to rule out a pulmonary problem.

Shortness of breath. Shortness of breath (dyspnea) can dramatically compromise quality of life. The underlying cause of dyspnea is usually a mechanical problem in the lungs or diaphragm that makes breathing more difficult. Examples of mechanical problems are airway obstruction (as with asthma, COPD, and some lung cancers), increased stiffness of the lungs (as with interstitial lung disease, pneumonia, and heart failure), severe spine and rib cage abnormalities, and obesity. If left untreated, shortness of breath can lead to fatigue and weakness that may profoundly limit activities. In turn, weakness related to deconditioning (being out of shape) or musculoskeletal disease such as severe curvature of the spine may worsen shortness of breath.

Coughing. Coughing up phlegm, infectious agents, and foreign matter is one of the ways in which the lungs protect themselves. Severe coughing, however, may signal a respiratory disease. Obstructive diseases of the lungs (asthma and COPD) and lung cancer often cause a person to cough up phlegm. Yellow or green phlegm may signal an infection. Coughing up blood (hemoptysis) may suggest a benign problem such as bronchitis or a potentially life-threatening disease such as lung cancer or pulmonary embolism. Hemoptysis is a serious sign, especially in a current or former cigarette smoker. Chronic cough in an adult with a normal chest x-ray is most often the result of postnasal drip, asthma, or gastroesophageal reflux (in which stomach acid flows back into the esophagus), alone or in combination. Interstitial lung disease, bronchiectasis (persistent dilatation of the bronchi), and pneumonia, all of which produce inflammation or scarring of the lungs, also cause coughing.

Noisy breathing. Noisy breathing is an especially common sign of respiratory disease. The noise may originate from problems anywhere along the length of the airway. Abnormal sounds range from

How Obstructive Lung Diseases Disrupt Breathing

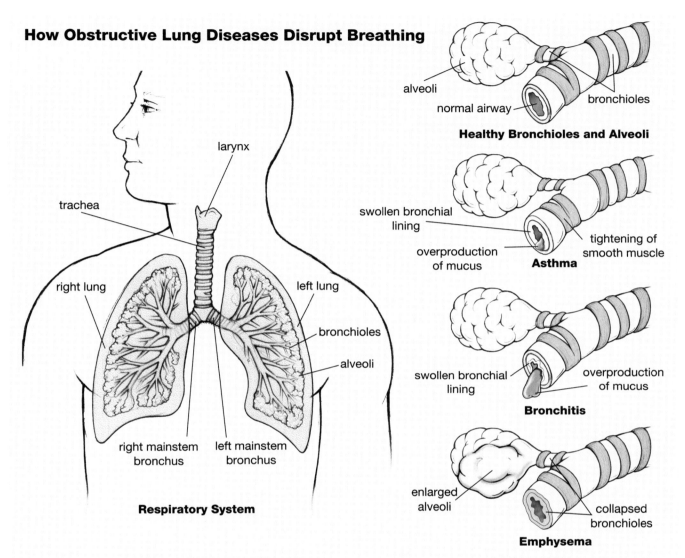

Healthy Bronchioles and Alveoli

alveoli
normal airway
bronchioles

Asthma

swollen bronchial lining
overproduction of mucus
tightening of smooth muscle

Bronchitis

swollen bronchial lining
overproduction of mucus

Emphysema

enlarged alveoli
collapsed bronchioles

larynx
trachea
right lung
left lung
bronchioles
alveoli
right mainstem bronchus
left mainstem bronchus

Respiratory System

Air enters the body through the nose and mouth. It then passes down the pharynx (throat), through the larynx (voice box), and into the trachea (windpipe), the body's largest airway. The entrance to the larynx is covered by a flap of cartilage called the epiglottis that prevents food from entering the trachea. The trachea divides into two airways, the right and left mainstem bronchi, that supply air to the lungs. The bronchi eventually branch into smaller airways called bronchioles.

The lungs have the job of supplying oxygen to the body while removing carbon dioxide from the blood. This process, called gas exchange, occurs in the alveoli (small air-filled sacs that cluster by the dozens at the end of each bronchiole). Each of the millions of alveoli in the lungs is surrounded by a thin layer of tiny blood vessels called capillaries. Oxygen from inhaled air travels through the thin walls of the alveoli and into the bloodstream via the capillaries. At the same time, carbon dioxide (a waste product that accumulates in the blood) moves from the

capillaries to the alveoli and is exhaled through the nose and mouth.

Asthma and chronic obstructive pulmonary disease (COPD), which includes chronic bronchitis and emphysema, are obstructive diseases of the lungs. These diseases narrow the airways and make breathing difficult. However, they affect the airways in slightly different ways. In asthma, the bronchial lining swells and the lungs produce an excess amount of mucus, which can obstruct the airways. Also, the smooth muscle around the bronchiole can tighten. Chronic bronchitis also involves inflammation of the bronchial lining and an overproduction of mucus; the smooth muscle around the bronchioles is often unaffected, although some people with chronic bronchitis may also have some smooth muscle tightening. In emphysema, the elasticity of the lungs is reduced and the walls between the alveoli are destroyed, causing the airways—which are normally held open by the elastic elements in the walls of the alveoli—to collapse.

a high-pitched crowing during inhalation (stridor, which occurs with croup, inflammation of the epiglottis, or tumors in the upper airway) to continuous musical sounds during exhalation (wheezing, which occurs with asthma and some other disorders). The maxim "all that wheezes is not asthma" underscores the fact that many health conditions, including laryngeal disease, heart failure, pulmonary embolism, and COPD, can cause wheezing. Repetitive loud snoring during sleep, interrupted by periods of silence in which there is no airflow, is a major sign of sleep apnea.

Chest pain. Chest pain or other discomfort has numerous causes, and determining whether the cause is a heart, esophageal, or respiratory disease is often challenging. Pain localized to one side of the chest that worsens with deep breathing, coughing, or laughing suggests pleurisy, an inflammation of the pleura (the membrane around the surface of the lungs and the inner chest wall). Pleurisy may be caused by a viral infection, pneumonia on the outer surface of the lung, pulmonary embolism, cancer, or a systemic (affecting the entire body) inflammatory disease such as systemic lupus erythematosus. Alternatively, pain worsening on inhalation may be due to a chest wall injury such as a broken rib.

Other symptoms. Respiratory illnesses also can produce some general symptoms. For example, low levels of oxygen in the blood, fragmented sleep patterns, chronic lung infections, and lung cancer can all lead to fatigue. Many people whose respiratory illness limits daily activities have particular difficulty with activities that involve the arms, such as carrying objects, showering, or performing other grooming tasks. These tasks are often more difficult than walking.

GENERAL EVALUATION OF RESPIRATORY SYMPTOMS

The first steps in the evaluation of respiratory problems involve providing a medical history and having a physical examination. These will help the doctor determine which tests, chest imaging techniques, and other studies are required.

Medical History

The doctor will ask a number of questions about current symptoms, past behaviors, occupations, toxic exposures (for example, to cigarette smoke, silica [fine dust from quartz], or asbestos), and family medical history. The presence of infections such as influenza and tuberculosis in the family or community also will be taken into account.

For example, the doctor will want to know if you have ever smoked cigarettes and whether you have inhaled any other potentially injurious agents, such as asbestos. You will need to give information about any previously diagnosed respiratory illnesses in yourself and your family. Your doctor also will ask about any allergies you may have and any medications you take. Sometimes diet pills, amiodarone (Cordarone; used to treat an irregular heart rhythm), or other medications can contribute to lung disease.

In some people, problems that seem unrelated to the lungs—such as skin rash, joint pain, and visual changes—are symptoms of a more generalized inflammatory disease with respiratory difficulty as one of its symptoms. In addition, a disease such as lung cancer can cause symptoms elsewhere in the body if it spreads (metastasizes).

Physical Examination

The physical examination for a possible lung disease includes a check of breathing rate and pattern and an assessment of how the torso moves during breathing. The way the torso moves is important because some people with lung disease use extra muscles in their abdomen, neck, and rib cage to aid in breathing. Also, reduced movement in one side of the chest might suggest disease in the lung on that side. Finally, abnormalities in the structure of the chest could be the cause of breathing difficulty.

In addition, the doctor will use his or her senses of touch and hearing to evaluate the condition. Palpating (touching) the chest wall may reveal rib fractures or other sources of chest pain. Percussion (tapping to generate sound) of the chest will help the doctor determine how far the diaphragm moves and how much the lungs inflate during respiration. A hollow sound is normal, but accentuated hollowness suggests either overinflation of the lung (as occurs in emphysema) or leakage of air into the space around the lung (pneumothorax). A dull or flat sound suggests reduced inflation of the lung (atelectasis), disease within the airspaces (such as pneumonia), or fluid within the pleural space (pleural effusion).

The doctor also will listen to breath sounds using a stethoscope, a technique called auscultation. The intensity of breath sounds is diminished in people with obstructive lung diseases, pneumonia, or pleural effusion. Wheezing and prolonged exhalation also are associated with obstructive lung diseases. Lower-pitched sounds (rhonchi) may suggest secretions within the airways. Velcro-like sounds (crackles, formerly called rales) suggest pneumonia, heart

NEW RESEARCH

Air Pollution May Hinder Kids' Lung Development

The levels of air pollution to which U.S. children are commonly exposed may stymie their lung development in adolescence, a study shows.

Researchers measured lung function in nearly 1,800 10-year-olds living in 12 California communities where air pollution was continually monitored. They found that after eight years, children who were exposed to the most air pollution—mainly from cars—had impaired lung development. For example, those exposed to the most fine particulate matter were nearly five times more likely to have impaired lung function (defined as results more than 20% lower than expected on a lung-function test) than those exposed to the least.

Because lung function typically makes substantial gains during adolescence, the findings could have implications for long-term health, according to the authors. In young adulthood, they note, impaired lung development may lead to an increased risk of respiratory conditions, such as wheezing during a viral infection; but it's later in life, when impaired lung function can be life-threatening, that the early effects of air pollution may become most evident.

The researchers write that because the pollutants examined in this study exist at similar levels in many areas, their findings probably apply to communities outside of Southern California.

THE NEW ENGLAND
JOURNAL OF MEDICINE
Volume 351, page 1057
September 9, 2004

A Cure for That Runny Nose

Allergic rhinitis can cause irritating symptoms like an itchy, runny nose and sneezing, but an array of medical treatments is available.

With some 10% to 30% of adults suffering form allergic rhinitis, the condition can seem as ubiquitous as pollen on a dry spring day. Because it is so common and causes few obvious complications, sufferers often don't seek treatment for their condition. But lifestyle changes, medication, and even allergy shots can help many people find relief.

Symptoms and Causes of Allergic Rhinitis

Allergic rhinitis is an immune response to an airborne allergen, and its symptoms occur in two phases— a response immediately upon exposure and a delayed response. Immediate symptoms include an itchy, runny nose; sneezing; and itchy, watery eyes. The main delayed symptom is nasal congestion. Patients may also experience a dry scratchy throat, chronic cough, pain or itchiness in the ear, recurrent sinus inflammation, allergic conjunctivitis (inflammation of the membranes that line the insides of the eyelids), and postnasal drip.

If untreated, allergic rhinitis may decrease quality of life even further by leading to chronic nose blowing, fatigue, sleep problems, and difficulties with learning and concentration. It may also contribute to asthma, inner ear or respiratory infections, and nasal polyps.

There are two types of allergic rhinitis: seasonal and perennial. Seasonal allergic rhinitis, sometimes called hay fever, is triggered by outdoor, seasonal allergens such as pollen from trees, grasses, and weeds as well as outdoor molds. Perennial allergic rhinitis is caused by allergens that can be in the home year-round—for example, animal dander, indoor mold, and droppings from dust mites and cockroaches. Rhinitis can also be nonallergic—in which case symptoms are caused by irritants in the air and do not involve an immune-system reaction.

How Does Your Doctor Diagnose It?

Three types of tests are commonly used to diagnose allergic rhinitis. The skin-prick test is the most common, most convenient, and least expensive. The skin is pricked with a needle containing a small amount of a potential allergen; if the skin becomes red and itchy and a patch of white swelling appears soon afterwards, the patient may be allergic to that substance.

A blood test, sometimes referred to as the radioallergosorbent test (RAST), also can be used. Blood tests are less sensitive than skin-prick tests, however, and often show abnormalities even when no allergies exist.

The least commonly used diagnostic test is an intradermal skin test, in which a small amount of antigen is injected into the skin. The test may be somewhat less comfortable than the skin-prick test, and a reaction may not occur for 15 to 20 minutes.

Treatment Strategies

Treatment for allergic rhinitis involves limiting exposure to specific allergens and often taking medication to control symptoms. Allergy shots may help those who don't respond adequately to these measures.

Limiting exposure. The first step is to try to avoid, if practical, your allergens. Steps may include keeping house and car windows closed and using air conditioning with a regularly cleaned filter system whenever possible if you are allergic to pollen; frequently dusting, vacuuming, and washing sheets and blankets to avoid dust mites; and limiting exposure to family pets to avoid pet dander. Be sure to wear a dust mask that filters out small particles while dusting or vacuuming; most other masks are of little or no use. (If you have severe indoor allergies, you should try to have someone else dust and vacuum.) For advice on limiting exposure to indoor biologicals such as mold, see the "Indoor Air Pollution" chart on pages 34–37.

Medications. Newer (second-generation) oral antihistamines (see the chart opposite) are first-line medications for mild to moderate symptoms of allergic rhinitis. These drugs are best at targeting immediate symptoms such as a runny nose, itching, and sneezing as well as allergic conjunctivitis. They may also reduce congestion. Although older (first-generation) antihistamines are similarly effective at reducing sneezing and runny nose, they are more likely to cause sedation and impaired mental performance than the newer drugs.

failure, or interstitial lung disease. A harsh "leathery" sound (rub) occasionally is heard with pneumonia or pulmonary embolism, which inflame and roughen the lining of the lungs and the rib cage.

The inhaled antihistamines also are considered first-line medical treatments for mild to moderate symptoms. They may reduce both immediate and delayed symptoms.

For patients with more severe symptoms, inhaled corticosteroids are considered first-line treatments. These nasal sprays are effective against nasal congestion and may help with a runny nose, sneezing, and itching. Many patients with severe symptoms may need both oral antihistamines and inhaled corticosteroids.

Nosebleeds are considered one of the main side effects of inhaled corticosteroids. To reduce the risk of nosebleeds, experts recommend that you direct the spray toward the outer side of your nostril rather than toward your septum. Using your left hand to spray into your right nostril and your right hand to spray into your left nostril may make this easier.

Decongestants can be used if other treatments do not adequately address congestion and often are used along with antihistamines. Leukotriene receptor antagonists sometimes are used to treat both immediate and delayed symptoms of allergic rhinitis. Intranasal cromolyn (Nasalcrom) appears to be useful in preventing symptoms but not treating them once they have occurred.

Patients whose symptoms persist despite lifestyle and medication treatment may need immunotherapy ("allergy shots"). This treatment involves a series of injections (over three to five years) of a diluted form of the patient's particular allergens. Over time, an immunity should develop to the allergens, potentially decreasing reactions. However, older patients normally are not considered good candidates for allergy shots

Drugs for the Treatment of Allergic Rhinitis

Drug Class	Drug Name
Oral antihistamines (second generation)	cetirizine (Zyrtec) desloratadine (Clarinex) fexofenadine (Allegra-D) loratadine (Claritin-D)
Oral antihistamines (first generation)	brompheniramine (Bromphen and other brands) chlorpheniramine (Chlor-Trimeton) diphenhydramine (Benadryl)
Inhaled antihistamine	azelastine (Astelin)
Intranasal corticosteroids	beclomethasone (Beconase AQ and Vancenase DS AQ) budesonide (Rhinocort) flunisolide (Nasalide, Nasarel, and other brands) fluticasone (Flonase) mometasone (Nasonex) triamcinolone (Nasacort)
Intranasal mast-cell stabilizer	cromolyn (Nasalcrom)
Leukotriene receptor antagonists	montelukast (Singulair) zafirlukast (Accolate) zileuton (Zyflo)
Intranasal decongestant	oxymetazoline (Afrin,* Dristan, and other brands) pseudoephedrine (Sudafed)†
Antihistamine plus decongestant	acrivastine and pseudoephedrine (Semprex-D) pseudoephedrine and triprolidine (Actifed and other brands)

* Afrin should not be used for more than a few days.
† Can cause blood pressure problems.

because their asthma is generally not the result of allergens.

Examination of the hands may reveal discoloration of the nail beds or clubbing of the fingers (a thickening of the fingertips and increased curvature of the fingernails). Blue nail beds suggest low levels of oxygen in the blood, while clubbing suggests lung cancer, interstitial lung disease, bronchiectasis, or other problems. Swelling of the legs and feet suggests that a heart problem may be the cause of symptoms. Heart failure can cause difficulty breathing, as can heart disease caused by high blood pressure in the lungs (cor pulmonale). Swelling in one leg suggests a blood clot, which could potentially lead to pulmonary embolism.

Laboratory Tests
Other tests can provide complementary information and are obtained on an individual basis according to the doctor's suspicions. Routine blood tests may show a low hemoglobin level (anemia), which might help explain a patient's shortness of breath or suggest a chronic condition (such as lung cancer). An elevated hemoglobin level might suggest that the body is compensating for chronically low oxygen levels. Elevated white blood cell counts might suggest lung infection or noninfectious inflammatory disease. Blood chemistry measurements reflecting the function of organs (such as the liver or kidney) or specialized tests for rheumatic disease might clarify widespread disease that also involves the lung. Samples of phlegm, when examined in a timely way by a laboratory, may reveal organisms causing lung infection or, in people with lung cancer, malignant (cancerous) cells.

Chest imaging and pulmonary function tests are two other diagnostic tools that are commonly used in people suspected of having a lung disorder. Chest imaging provides information primarily about the structure of the lungs and chest, while pulmonary function tests provide objective measures of lung function. The two tests complement each other. Exercise testing, measurement of blood bases, and sleep studies also may be required in some cases.

Chest imaging. A chest x-ray may reveal an abnormality that clearly explains the respiratory problem or may identify areas for further evaluation. Lung tumors, pneumonia, most tuberculosis cases, occupational lung diseases, emphysema, interstitial lung disease, and collections of fluid all can be seen on a chest x-ray. The current availability of chest computed tomography (CT) scans is a major advance, allowing a more detailed assessment of abnormalities than that using the chest x-ray. In addition, combination positron emission tomography (PET)/CT scans are now being used to determine the presence of lung cancer. Comparing current chest images with previous images is very important and can help to differentiate a new disease from a known condition and to see the progression of a disease over time.

Pulmonary function tests. Just as people with hypertension or diabetes need measurements of blood pressure and blood glucose, respectively, people with respiratory diseases need tests of their pulmonary function. Pulmonary function tests measure lung capacity and reveal patterns characteristic of particular diseases. A person's measurements are compared with those expected for a healthy person of the same age, height, and gender.

Commonly performed pulmonary function tests include spirometry, lung volume tests, and diffusion capacity tests. Spirometry measures the volume of air that can be exhaled and the rate of exhalation. The two most important values that spirometry measures are forced expiratory volume in one second (FEV_1) and forced vital capacity (FVC). FEV_1 measures the amount of air expelled from the lungs in the first second of a forced exhalation, while FVC is a measure of the total volume of air exhaled. These values are calculated automatically by the spirometer, along with the ratio comparing the amount of air exhaled in the first second with the total amount of air exhaled: FEV_1/FVC. Lung volume tests measure the amount of air in the lungs at different levels of inflation, and diffusion capacity testing measures how well gas moves across the membranes in the lungs.

These tests can help characterize the lung abnormality as primarily obstructive (in which the airways are narrowed), primarily restrictive (in which the ability of the lungs to expand is impaired), or a combination of the two. They also determine whether the deficit in lung function is mild, moderate, or severe. People with suspected asthma may need to be tested before and after inhaling medication to see if lung function is improved.

Exercise testing. Exercise testing using a treadmill or stationary bicycle also can be used to evaluate shortness of breath and to determine whether it is caused by a lung problem, heart disease, or deconditioning (being out of shape).

Blood gases. If the lungs are not functioning properly, the amount of oxygen and carbon dioxide in the blood (blood gases) may be affected. Blood gases can be measured by taking a sample of blood from an artery. Alternatively, pulse oximetry provides a noninvasive way to measure hemoglobin oxygen saturation (the level of oxygen in the blood). In pulse oximetry, a sensor that directs a beam of light through the tissue is placed on the fingertip or earlobe. The sensor monitors oxygen saturation by measuring the amount of light absorbed by oxygenated hemoglobin (the oxygen-carrying pigment in red blood cells).

NEW RESEARCH

Grading System Predicts Risk of Death From COPD

A group of factors considered together seems better than traditional testing at gauging the severity of chronic obstructive pulmonary disease (COPD), according to a study.

The risk of death from COPD is often judged by measuring how well a patient can force air out of the lungs. But this single measure—known as FEV_1—cannot capture the full health effects of COPD, according to the authors of the new study. They believe their findings provide a more accurate picture of the severity of patients' illness.

The study of more than 800 COPD patients found that four factors taken together—FEV_1 results, body mass index, and tests measuring patients' breathing difficulties and walking endurance—were better than FEV_1 scores alone at predicting death risk. For each one-point increase in this "grading system," the researcher report, a patient's risk of dying over the next few years grew by 34%; the risk of death specifically from respiratory causes rose 62%.

All four of these factors, the researchers note, are simple to measure, which means the grading system could be widely used. An editorial published with the report echoes that conclusion, saying that the measure "promises to be an important tool."

THE NEW ENGLAND JOURNAL OF MEDICINE
Volume 350, pages 965 and 1005
March 4, 2004

Earth-Friendly (and People-Friendly) Inhalers

Powder inhalers, nebulizers, and newer aerosols are replacing chlorofluorocarbon-driven inhalers for asthma and COPD.

Traditional inhalers for asthma and chronic obstructive pulmonary disease (COPD) are simple devices that release an aerosol spray through an L-shaped mouthpiece. But a new generation of inhalers has arrived, employing hinges and wheels, blister packs and capsules.

Why the change? Older aerosol sprays rely on chlorofluorocarbons (CFCs) to propel the medication, and although CFCs don't harm the lungs directly, they contribute to skin cancer and other health problems by depleting the Earth's ozone layer. Twenty countries banned CFCs starting in 1996 as part of the Montreal Protocol; an exception was granted for medical devices such as inhalers until suitable alternatives could be found.

The New Inhalers

Drug companies have responded to the CFC phaseout by developing a variety of new products: aerosols that use alternate propellants, hand-held mininebulizers, and dry powder inhalers.

Non-CFC aerosols. Two brands of albuterol are now available with a non-CFC propellant: Proventil HFA and Ventolin HFA. These aerosols use a propellant called hydrofluoroalkane, which is nontoxic, nonreactive, and nonflammable.

The new aerosols are so effective that the American Lung Association has petitioned the U.S. Food and Drug Administration (FDA) to remove albuterol inhalers from the list of products permitted to use CFCs. In fact, the manufacturer of Ventolin discontinued the CFC version in late 2003.

The FDA is holding off on banning CFC-propelled albuterol, however, in case manufacturing difficulties or unexpected side effects should occur with the new propellant. The FDA is also concerned about cost; generic versions of the HFA inhalers are not yet available.

Handheld mininebulizer. Premeasured vials of an ipratropium/albuterol solution (DuoNeb) are available for people with COPD to use with a nebulizer. Taking this medication involves squeezing the contents of one vial into the nebulizer reservoir and activating a compressor that turns the medication into a fine mist. The user breathes in this mist through a mouthpiece or face mask for approximately 5 to 15 minutes.

Although nebulizers are small—about the size of a pill bottle—compressors weigh 5 to 15 lbs. and must be plugged into an electrical outlet, which can make some types of travel difficult.

Sleep studies. Sleep studies (polysomnography) can be used to monitor certain body functions during sleep. Polysomnography involves electrocardiography to monitor heart rate and rhythm; electroencephalography to monitor brain waves; electromyography to monitor muscle activity; pulse oximetry to measure oxygen saturation; and measures of airflow and movements of the chest and abdomen. These studies can detect the presence, pattern, and severity of sleep-related breathing disorders (such as sleep apnea) and typically are performed in sleep laboratories.

GENERAL APPROACHES TO MANAGEMENT

Usually, the general evaluation just described provides enough information to diagnose a lung disorder and devise a management plan. Sometimes, however, the initial evaluation does not provide a definitive diagnosis. If this is the case, invasive procedures to obtain biopsy samples of cells and tissues may be necessary. For example, when fluid collects in the space around the lung, it may be sampled

Dry-powder inhalers. Most new devices for asthma and COPD are dry-powder inhalers, which are designed to release one dose of medication at a time from a blister pack or capsule. Although the medication is inhaled instead of being sprayed into the mouth, it is no less effective than aerosols. In fact, dry-powder inhalers (such as the Advair Diskus, Serevent Diskus, Foradil Aerolizer, Flovent Rotadisk, and Pulmicort Turbuhaler) are sometimes more effective than aerosols because they don't require the user to coordinate pressing the device with breathing in.

Some dry-powder inhalers are somewhat larger than aerosols but come with the medication preloaded; others are more compact but require the user to place medication capsules or packets in the device periodically or before each use.

One disadvantage of dry-powder inhalers is that excess humidity can cause the powder to clump together. To avoid this problem, the manu-

Inhalers That Use CFCs	CFC-Free Devices
AeroBid	Advair Diskus
AeroBid-M	DuoNeb
Alupent	Flovent Rotadisk
Atrovent	Foradil Aerolizer
Azmacort	Proventil HFA
Beclovent	Pulmicort Turbuhaler
Combivent	Serevent Diskus
Intal	Ventolin HFA
Maxair	
Proventil	
Tilade	
Vanceril	

facturers encase the devices in protective foil and recommend discarding them 4 to 8 weeks after opening.

Another issue is cost: Dry-powder inhalers can cost more than $100 each, and to date no generic versions are available.

To Switch or Not To Switch?

If you're still using a CFC-propelled inhaler, rest assured that the FDA will not pull it off the market until acceptable alternatives are available. But now is a good time to ask your physician about switching to a new type of inhaler. Countries such as Canada, the European Union, Australia, and Japan have all banned albuterol inhalers that contain CFCs—the United States could be next.

("tapped") with a needle (a procedure called thoracentesis). Analysis of the fluid may aid in diagnosis and treatment, while removal of the fluid might help relieve shortness of breath.

Treating someone with a respiratory illness involves weighing the risks and benefits of each treatment option and taking the patient's personal preferences into account. In some instances, the problem clears on its own or with treatment. A cure is available for many lung disorders, including many caused by infections. But for all lung disorders, a goal of treatment is to relieve symptoms.

OBSTRUCTIVE DISEASES OF THE LUNGS

Asthma and chronic obstructive pulmonary disease (COPD) are obstructive lung diseases. Obstructive lung diseases are characterized by a reduction in the diameter of the airways that obstructs airflow during exhalation. The obstruction tends to be intermittent and reversible in asthma but unremitting and less responsive to medication in COPD.

Asthma

Asthma is a chronic inflammatory disorder of the airways. It is the eighth most common chronic condition in the United States, affecting an estimated 20 million Americans. Asthma can be life threatening without proper management and prompt treatment of attacks. In 2002, more than 4,000 people—mostly elderly—died of asthma. Asthma is becoming more commonly recognized in people over the age of 65, who account for about 10% of all people with asthma. Proper treatment of asthma is especially important in older individuals, who tend to have other health problems and more frequent asthmatic symptoms.

Causes. Asthma is caused by an immune abnormality that appears to have genetic and environmental components. The characteristic features of asthma are airway inflammation and hyperreactivity of the airways, both of which lead to airflow obstruction:

- Airway inflammation involves swelling of the bronchial lining and excessive production of mucus. These problems can be worsened by a respiratory infection such as sinusitis, influenza, or a cold.
- Hyperreactive airways tend to "twitch" when exposed to allergens and other irritants.
- Airflow obstruction involves a narrowing of the airways as a result of smooth muscle contraction, swelling of the bronchial lining of the airway, and/or accumulation of excessive mucus.

Although asthma is characterized by repeated asthma attacks (in which symptoms worsen, requiring the use of medication), the inflammation may persist even when symptoms are absent and may require long-term treatment with medication.

Depending on the factors that trigger an attack, asthma sometimes is considered either extrinsic or intrinsic. However, the distinction between the two types is not always clear, and some people have both types.

In people with extrinsic asthma, which usually begins before age 30, acute episodes are initiated by exposure to a specific environmental irritant. Cigarette smoke, industrial fumes, pollen, mold, dust, animal dander or saliva, and perfumes are common environmental irritants in people with extrinsic asthma. Constriction of smooth muscles in the bronchi when exposed to such irritants can trigger an asthma attack by narrowing the airways and plugging them with sticky mucus.

Intrinsic asthma, the most common form in people who develop asthma after age 30, often is characterized by the absence of any identifiable external trigger for worsening of symptoms. However, exercise, cold or dry air, emotional stress, or gastro-esophageal reflux may trigger attacks in people with intrinsic asthma.

Symptoms. The onset of an asthma attack may be gradual or sudden. Some attacks resolve on their own, but most require medication.

Milder attacks are most common. They usually begin with tightness in the chest and a cough. Wheezing may be heard with breathing. Restlessness and difficulty sleeping may accompany these symptoms. Sometimes these mild attacks seem to improve, only to be followed by the reappearance of persistent symptoms that may require treatment in a hospital.

During severe attacks, extreme shortness of breath is accompanied by wheezing, tightness in the chest, coughing up thick phlegm, sweating, an elevated respiratory rate, and a rapid pulse. Symptoms may last for only a few minutes, particularly if treated promptly, or may persist for hours or even days despite treatment with medication. Coughing can continue for a week or longer after other acute symptoms disappear.

Diagnosis. Diagnosis during an attack usually is apparent from the symptoms, especially if the person has a history of asthma attacks. In older individuals, asthma must be distinguished from COPD and cardiac conditions such as heart failure or a heart attack. Heart failure can cause fluid to accumulate in the lungs, producing some of the same symptoms as those in asthma.

Between asthma attacks, a diagnosis may require pulmonary function tests to measure airway obstruction, an examination of mucus from the nose and lungs, and, possibly, allergy tests.

Prevention. People with asthma should avoid asthma triggers whenever possible or take preventive medications as described on pages 15–17. A handheld device called a peak flow meter measures how well air flows out of the lungs. Taking peak flow meter measurements at home is a simple and accurate way to detect worsening of lung function prior to the onset of symptoms. A person with asthma determines a "personal best" level of function; measurements below this level signal the need for more aggressive use of medications.

Treatment. People with asthma must have a plan of action in case of an attack. They should always have inhaled medication available for self-treatment. A severe attack requires taking medication immediately and quickly getting to a doctor's office or emergency

NEW RESEARCH

**Aspirin-Induced Asthma
More Common Than Thought**

New evidence suggests that one in five adults with asthma may be allergic to aspirin and similar painkillers—a problem that puts them at risk for potentially severe asthmatic reactions.

A review of 21 studies conducted since the 1970s found that 21% of asthmatic adults may be sensitive to aspirin and other nonsteroidal anti-inflammatory drugs (NSAIDs). Nearly all of the patients with so-called aspirin-induced asthma were also sensitive to the NSAIDs naproxen (Naprosyn), ibuprofen (Advil and Motrin), and diclofenac (Voltaren).

On the other hand, researchers found, few adults with aspirin-induced asthma were sensitive to acetaminophen (Tylenol)—a finding they say reinforces the current recommendation that this drug be the painkiller of choice for asthmatics.

The incidence of aspirin-induced asthma in this study was twice as high as that found in other recent research reviews. This difference, the researchers note, may arise from the fact that many people with asthma are unaware that they're sensitive to aspirin; studies that rely on patient reports rather than objective testing yield lower rates of aspirin-induced asthma.

Since people typically take over-the-counter painkillers of their own accord, the researchers stress, doctors should be sure to alert asthmatic patients to the potential for NSAID-induced attacks.

BMJ
Volume 328, page 434
February 21, 2004

Commonly Used Anti-Inflammatory Drugs 2005

Drug Type	Drug Class	Generic Name	Brand Name	Average Daily Dosage*
Inhaled	Corticosteroids, long-acting	budesonide, powder inhaler	Pulmicort Turbuhaler	1 or 2 puffs 2 times a day
		flunisolide, standard inhaler	AeroBid	2 puffs 2 times a day
		flunisolide, menthol, standard inhaler	AeroBid-M	2 puffs 2 times a day
		fluticasone, powder inhaler	Flovent	1 to 2 puffs 2 times a day
		fluticasone, powder inhaler	Flovent Rotadisk	1 to 2 puffs 2 times a day
	Corticosteroids, short-acting	beclomethasone, standard inhaler	Vanceril	2 puffs 3 or 4 times a day
		triamcinolone, standard inhaler	Azmacort	2 puffs 3 or 4 times a day or 4 puffs 2 times a day
	Respiratory inhalers, nonsteroidal	cromolyn, standard inhaler	Intal	2 puffs 4 times a day
		nedocromil, standard inhaler	Tilade	2 puffs 4 times a day
Oral	Corticosteroids, short-acting	methylprednisolone	Medrol	4 to 160 mg
		prednisone	Deltasone Sterapred	5 to 100 mg
	Leukotriene modifiers, nonsteroidal	montelukast	Singulair	10 mg
		zafirlukast	Accolate	40 mg
		zileuton	Zyflo	2,400 mg

* These dosages represent an average range for the treatment of asthma and chronic obstructive pulmonary disease. The precise effective dosage varies from patient to patient and depends on many factors. Do not make any changes in your medication without consulting your doctor.

† Average price for one device or 30 tablets or capsules of the dosage strength listed. Actual price may vary. If a generic version is available, the cost is listed in parentheses. Sources: drugstore.com, eckerd.com, and walgreens.com.

room. A milder attack may require a call or visit to the doctor if symptoms persist longer than usual after using medication. Drug therapy includes the use of bronchodilators and anti-inflammatory drugs. Bronchodilators reduce the constriction of bronchial mus-

Average Retail Price†	Possible Side Effects
1 turbuhaler: $138 7-g inhaler: $76 7-g inhaler: $76 13-g inhaler: $68 60-dose rotadisk (50 mcg/dose): $45	Side effects are not common, but can include a dry or irritated mouth or throat, cough, and hoarseness. Contact your doctor if these side effects are severe, or if you develop white spots or sores in your mouth.
16.8-g inhaler: NA 20-g inhaler: $73	Side effects are not common, but can include a dry or irritated mouth or throat, cough, and hoarseness. Contact your doctor if these side effects are severe, or if you develop white spots or sores in your mouth.
8.1-g inhaler: $54	Common side effects include throat irritation and dryness. Rare but serious side effects include difficulty swallowing; hives; itching; swelling of the face, lips, or eyelids; rash; and nosebleeds.
16.2-g inhaler: $67	There are no common side effects. Rare but serious side effects include increased wheezing, tightness or pain in the chest, and difficulty breathing.
4 mg: $36 ($15) 10 mg: $7 ($6) 5 mg: $19 ($9)	Common side effects include increased appetite, indigestion, nervousness, insomnia, greater susceptibility to infections, increased blood pressure, slowed wound healing, weight gain, easy bruising, and fluid retention. Rare but serious side effects include vision problems, frequent urination, increased thirst, rectal bleeding, blistering skin, confusion, hallucinations, paranoia, euphoria, depression, and mood swings.
10 mg: $87	Common side effects include headache. Rare but serious side effects include skin rash (indicating potentially life-threatening allergic reaction) and gastroenteritis (causing loss of appetite, nausea, vomiting, stomach upset, fever, and diarrhea).
10 mg: $40	Common side effects include headache. Rare but serious side effects include burning or prickling sensation, skin rash, and liver dysfunction (symptoms include abdominal pain, nausea, fatigue, lethargy, itching, yellow discoloration of the eyes or skin, and flu-like symptoms).
600 mg: $32	Common side effects include headache, general pain, abdominal pain, nausea, indigestion, muscle soreness, and weakness. Rare but serious side effects include liver problems causing nausea, fatigue, lethargy, skin rash or itching, yellow discoloration of the eyes or skin, flu-like symptoms, and urine that is unusually dark.

cles, while anti-inflammatories help to overcome bronchial inflammation or excessive sensitivity to irritants.

Bronchodilators. Bronchodilators, which promptly open airways by relaxing bronchial smooth muscles, are the most rapidly effective treatment for asthma attacks. They can be taken by mouth (in tablet or capsule form), but inhaled sprays usually are preferred because oral forms take longer to act and may produce more side effects. Bronchodilators can be used before activities (such as exercise or exposure to cold air) that are known to trigger asthma. This step may help to prevent an attack or make it less severe and may improve a person's ability to perform the activity.

The three types of bronchodilators are beta$_2$ agonists, anticholinergics, and methylxanthine derivatives.

Beta$_2$ agonists are the most commonly used type of bronchodilator because they work the fastest and may keep the airways open for many hours. The short-acting beta$_2$ agents—albuterol (Proventil, Ventolin), metaproterenol (Alupent), and pirbuterol (Maxair)—begin to act in about 10 minutes and last for 4 to 6 hours. Longer-acting beta$_2$ agents—salmeterol (Serevent) and formoterol (Foradil)—act within 15 to 30 minutes and continue to work for up to 12 hours.

If symptoms do not improve adequately, people may add the anticholinergic ipratropium (Atrovent), which takes effect in 15 to 30 minutes and lasts for 4 to 6 hours. Combivent, a combination of the beta$_2$ agonist albuterol and the anticholinergic ipratropium, also is available. When used excessively, beta$_2$ agonists can cause tremors and heart palpitations. They also become less effective when overused.

People who cannot tolerate beta$_2$ agonists or anticholinergics or who experience asthma symptoms at night may use one of the extended-release oral forms of the methylxanthine derivative theophylline (Theo-24, Theo-Dur, Uniphyl). Side effects of theophylline include nausea and insomnia.

Anti-inflammatory drugs. Continuous use of anti-inflammatory drugs to control chronic inflammation is a critical component of asthma therapy in those with frequent symptoms (people with mild asthma generally are not treated with anti-inflammatory drugs). The first choice of medications to counter inflammation in adults is inhaled corticosteroids, which include beclomethasone (Beclovent, Vanceril), budesonide (Pulmicort), flunisolide (AeroBid), and fluticasone (Flovent). A combination of the corticosteroid fluticasone and the long-acting beta$_2$ agonist salmeterol is also available (Advair). The most frequent side effects of inhaled corticosteroids are irritation of the throat and a yeast infection of the mouth and throat. These side effects can be reduced by rinsing the mouth (the best way to do this is to swish water around the mouth, gently gargle, and spit

NEW RESEARCH

Frequent Beta$_2$ Agonist Use May Worsen Asthma

People with asthma who use beta$_2$ agonists regularly may develop tolerance to them, and the drugs may actually worsen airway inflammation with frequent use, according to a new analysis of 22 clinical trials. The researchers looked at studies of both short- and long-acting beta$_2$ agonists and found similar effects for both types of drugs.

Guidelines recommend the short-acting form of the drug for asthma attacks, and regular use of long-acting beta$_2$ agonists as second-line treatment along with corticosteroids. But there have been concerns that beta$_2$ agonists produce tolerance, meaning they become less effective upon subsequent use.

Using beta$_2$ agonists regularly for at least one week produced tolerance, the researchers found, and people who used the drugs regularly had worse asthma control and airway inflammation than patients who took placebo. The researchers say that as-needed use of the drugs is also likely to produce tolerance and worse asthma control.

They conclude by recommending that people with asthma use beta$_2$ agonists only during asthma attacks. However, people should not stop using any asthma medication without first consulting their doctor.

ANNALS OF INTERNAL MEDICINE
Volume 140, page 802
May 18, 2004

the water out) and cleaning the inhaler after each use.

When used for long periods of time, corticosteroids also can cause osteoporosis (bone loss), high blood pressure, roundness of the face, weight gain, diabetes, cataracts, and thinning of the skin; these side effects are less common with inhaled corticosteroids because little of the medication is absorbed into the bloodstream.

Oral corticosteroids take six hours to start working and must be used at the lowest effective dose and for the shortest possible time to avoid the side effects listed previously. Also, using oral corticosteroids for more than several weeks suppresses the adrenal gland. Consequently, the medications must be discontinued slowly to allow recovery of adrenal function if used for prolonged periods.

Nonsteroidal anti-inflammatory inhaled drugs also are used in the treatment of asthma. Cromolyn (Intal) and nedocromil (Tilade), which act to prevent the release of histamine, are inhaled drugs used only for long-term prevention of asthma symptoms (not for immediate relief). The leukotriene modifiers montelukast (Singulair), zafirlukast (Accolate), and zileuton (Zyflo), which counter the actions of leukotrienes (cell products that narrow bronchi and stimulate the production of mucus), may prevent exercise-induced asthma and can enhance the action of inhaled corticosteroids. The effectiveness of these medications varies considerably from person to person.

Inhaled medications usually are administered through a device called a metered dose inhaler (MDI). An MDI delivers a highly concentrated amount of medication directly to the bronchi. Inhaled medications are less likely to produce systemic side effects than oral medications. But proper technique is important, and many people use their MDI incorrectly. People who find it difficult to use an MDI can add a spacer, an attachment that eliminates the need to release the medication and inhale simultaneously. Many people experience considerable improvement in their condition after adding a spacer. Another option is to use a device called a nebulizer, which vaporizes liquid medication into a fine mist that can be inhaled easily.

Monoclonal antibody. People age 12 and over with severe asthma related to allergies that is not adequately controlled with inhaled corticosteroids may benefit from omalizumab (Xolair), which was approved in 2003. Omalizumab, which is injected once or twice a month, decreases the body's immune response to inhaled allergens such as dust mites or animal dander by blocking the antibody IgE. The annual cost of treatment is between $5,000 and $10,000.

NEW RESEARCH

Beta₂ Agonists May Pose Heart Risks

People with asthma or chronic obstructive pulmonary disease (COPD) who take beta$_2$ agonists to improve lung function may face an increased risk of heart problems, a new study shows. Beta$_2$ agonists have effects opposite to those of beta-blockers, which are widely used to treat heart disease, so they could be anticipated to possibly harm the heart.

The researchers analyzed 33 clinical trials of beta$_2$ agonists in people with chronic obstructive lung disease. In single-dose trials, the drugs increased heart rate and reduced potassium concentration, both of which can increase the risk of abnormal heart rhythm in susceptible patients. In studies that lasted for three days to one year, people who took the drugs were more likely to have a cardiovascular event than patients on placebo. Risk was highest for developing an abnormal heart rhythm called sinus tachycardia (a fast heartbeat).

The analysis does not identify the absolute risk of taking the drug for people with lung disease, the researchers note, because it did not include studies in which no adverse events occurred. However, the researchers say, studies should be conducted to specifically investigate beta$_2$ agonist safety in patients with asthma and COPD. If patients notice an irregular or fast heartbeat or pounding in their chest associated with taking their beta$_2$ agonist, they should tell their physician.

CHEST
Volume 125, page 2309
June 2004

Commonly Used Bronchodilators 2005

Drug Type	Drug Class	Generic Name	Brand Name	Average Daily Dosage*
Inhaled	Anticholinergics, short-acting	ipratropium, standard inhaler	Atrovent	2 puffs every 4 to 6 hours
	Anticholinergics, long-acting	tiotropium, powder inhaler	Spiriva HandiHaler	1 capsule inhaled every 24 hours
	Beta$_2$ agonists, short-acting	albuterol, standard inhaler	Proventil	2 puffs every 4 to 6 hours
		albuterol, non-CFC inhaler	Proventil HFA Ventolin HFA	2 puffs every 4 to 6 hours
		metaproterenol, standard inhaler	Alupent	2 or 3 puffs every 3 to 4 hours
		pirbuterol, standard inhaler	Maxair	1 to 2 puffs every 4 to 6 hours
	Beta$_2$ agonists, long-acting	salmeterol, powder inhaler	Serevent Diskus	1 inhalation 2 times a day
		formoterol, powder inhaler	Foradil Aerolizer	1 or 2 inhalations 2 times a day
	Combination agents	albuterol and ipratropium, standard inhaler	Combivent	2 inhalation 4 times a day
		albuterol and ipratropium, nebulizer	DuoNeb	1 vial 4 to 6 times a day
		salmeterol and fluticasone, powder inhaler	Advair Diskus	1 puff 2 times a day

* These dosages represent an average range for the treatment of asthma and chronic obstructive pulmonary disease. The precise effective dosage varies from patient to patient and depends on many factors. Do not make any changes in your medication without consulting your doctor.
† Average price for one device or 30 tablets or capsules of the dosage strength listed. Actual price may vary. If a generic version is available, the cost is listed in parentheses. Sources: drugstore.com, eckerd.com, and walgreens.com.

Average Retail Price[†]	Possible Side Effects
14-g inhaler: $61

18-mcg capsules: $115 | Common side effects include dry mouth, cough, and unpleasant taste. Rare but serious side effects include persistent constipation, lower abdominal pain or bloating, wheezing or difficulty breathing, tightness in chest, severe eye pain, skin rash or hives, and swelling of the face, lips, or eyelids. |
| 17-g inhaler: $43 ($14) | Common side effects include nervousness, tremor, dizziness, headache, and insomnia. Rare but serious side effects include severe breathing difficulty (signs include persistent wheezing, coughing, shortness of breath, confusion, bluish color to lips or fingernails, and inability to speak). |
| 6.7-g inhaler: $44
18-g inhaler: $39 | |
14-g inhaler: $35	Common side effects include trouble sleeping, dry mouth, sore throat, nervousness, and restlessness. Rare but serious side effects include severe breathing difficulty (signs include persistent wheezing, coughing, shortness of breath, confusion, bluish color to lips or fingernails, and inability to speak).
14-g inhaler: $86	Common side effects include sleeping difficulty, dry mouth, sore throat, nervousness, excitability, and restlessness. Rare but serious side effects include severe breathing difficulty (signs include persistent wheezing, coughing, shortness of breath, confusion, bluish color to lips or fingernails, and inability to speak), chest pain or heaviness, irregular heartbeat, light-headedness, fainting, severe weakness, and severe headaches.
60-dose inhaler (50 mcg/dose): $89	Common side effects include headache, sore throat, and runny or stuffy nose. Rare but serious side effects include severe breathing difficulty (signs include persistent wheezing, coughing, shortness of breath, confusion, bluish color to lips or fingernails, and inability to speak), chest pain or heaviness, irregular heartbeat, light-headedness, fainting, severe weakness, and severe headache.
60-dose aerolizer (12 mcg/dose): $90	Common side effects include fast heartbeat, headache, nervousness, and trembling. Rare but serious side effects include shortness of breath, difficulty breathing, tightness in the chest, increased wheezing, swelling of the face or eyelids, and skin rash or hives.
14.7-g inhaler: $59	Common side effects include coughing, headache, and nausea. Rare but serious side effects include increased wheezing, shortness of breath, chest pain, irregular heartbeat, skin rash or hives, and swelling of the face, lips, eyelids, mouth, or throat.
60 3-mL vials: $61	There are no common side effects. Rare but serious side effects include swelling of the face, lips, eyelids, mouth, or throat, shortness of breath, increased wheezing, chest pain or discomfort, irregular heartbeat, skin rash or hives, coughing, headache, and nausea.
60-dose 100/50 diskus: $60	Common side effects include a high-pitched noise while breathing, body aches, runny or stuffy nose, coughing, dry or sore throat, fever, hoarseness, swollen glands, trouble swallowing, voice changes, and sneezing. Rare but serious side effects include difficulty breathing; shortness of breath; tightness in the chest; increased wheezing; black, tarry stools; chest pain; chills; painful or difficult urination; ulcers; white spots on lips or mouth; fatigue; burning, tingling, or numb sensation in hands and feet; abdominal pain; loss of appetite; nausea; and flu-like symptoms.

Commonly Used Bronchodilators 2005—continued

Drug Type	Drug Class	Generic Name	Brand Name	Average Daily Dosage*
Oral	Methylxanthine derivatives	theophylline, extended-release capsule, 24 hr	Theo-24	300 to 600 mg
		theophylline, extended-release tablet, 12 hr	Theo-Dur	300 to 600 mg
		theophylline, extended-release tablet, 24 hr	Uniphyl	300 to 600 mg

* These dosages represent an average range for the treatment of asthma and chronic obstructive pulmonary disease. The precise effective dosage varies from patient to patient and depends on many factors. Do not make any changes in your medication without consulting your doctor.

† Average price for one device or 30 tablets or capsules of the dosage strength listed. Actual price may vary. If a generic version is available, the cost is listed in parentheses. Sources: drugstore.com, eckerd.com, and walgreens.com.

Chronic Obstructive Pulmonary Disease (COPD)

Chronic obstructive pulmonary disease is a term that encompasses chronic bronchitis and emphysema. The symptoms of COPD develop slowly over several years and include wheezing, chronic cough with production of phlegm, and progressive shortness of breath. COPD is the fourth leading cause of death in the United States.

Emphysema is a disorder characterized by destruction of lung tissue, including its elastic fibers. By reducing the elasticity of the lungs and destroying the walls between the alveoli, emphysema leads to airway collapse and reduced airflow. More than 3 million Americans have emphysema, and more than 15,000 people die of it each year. Emphysema rates are highest for men age 65 and older.

Chronic bronchitis is a recurrent problem defined by coughing up phlegm nearly every day for at least three months of the year (for example, every winter) for two or more consecutive years. The condition reduces the diameter of the airways through a combination of bronchial inflammation and overproduction of mucus. There are more than 9 million cases of chronic bronchitis a year in the United States and more than 1,000 deaths. Chronic bronchitis is more prevalent in women than in men.

Causes. Cigarette smoking causes the vast majority of COPD cases. Cigarette smoking is thought to release proteases, enzymes that damage a protein called elastin that makes the lungs elastic. Smoking is also believed to inactivate alpha$_1$-antitrypsin, a protein produced by the liver that protects elastin from the action of proteases.

About 1 in 2,500 people worldwide have a genetic mutation that

Average Retail Price†	Possible Side Effects
100 mg: $15	Common side effects include restlessness, insomnia, loss of appetite, nervousness, irritability, and nausea. Rare but serious side effects include vomiting; trembling; confusion; rapid, irregular, or pounding pulse; chest pain; dizziness; convulsions; and skin rash.
100 mg: $21 ($14)	
400 mg: $36	

prevents the secretion of alpha₁-antitrypsin by the liver and increases the risk of developing premature emphysema, especially in smokers. Other factors that increase the likelihood of emphysema include a family history of COPD, male gender, respiratory illnesses in childhood, and occupational exposure to pollutants.

Symptoms. People with COPD typically began smoking at an early age and have a long history of a morning cough that produces phlegm. Their lung function often declines slowly over a period of many years before they seek medical advice, usually after age 50 and after noting significant shortness of breath on exertion. As COPD worsens, breathlessness begins to severely limit activities. The slow decrease in function often is punctuated by acute episodes of worsening symptoms, usually due to a viral infection with or without a bacterial infection. These acute episodes are marked by increased shortness of breath, wheezing, and a cough that produces greater-than-usual amounts of phlegm. Though acute episodes may be severe enough to be life threatening, they do not necessarily speed the rate of disease progression. COPD may also cause low levels of oxygen in the blood, which can lead to a rise in pressure in the arteries to the lungs (pulmonary hypertension). Pulmonary hypertension increases the workload of the heart's right ventricle, causing it to enlarge. At advanced stages of COPD, patients often are thin because they find eating to be tiring, and the work of breathing consumes more calories than in healthy people.

Diagnosis. People with COPD have abnormal results on spirometry testing. Spirometry testing not only indicates the presence and severity of the disorder but also predicts the prognosis.

People with COPD may appear breathless at rest and may grunt or wheeze with each exhalation. In addition, the chest often is enlarged from overinflation of the lungs. Chronic bronchitis often is accompanied by raspy breath sounds that can be heard with a stethoscope. Emphysema is characterized by diminished breath sound intensity. People who develop cor pulmonale may have enlarged neck veins, swelling of the legs (edema), and a loud second heart sound found during a heart examination, suggesting pulmonary hypertension.

A chest x-ray may show increased volume of air in the lungs and enlargement of the pulmonary arteries. Sometimes, changes also can be seen on an electrocardiogram, depending on the stage of the disease. Seeking a genetic cause by measuring levels of alpha$_1$-antitrypsin may be useful when COPD occurs in a young person or nonsmoker.

Prevention. Avoidance of cigarette smoking is the most obvious and effective way to prevent COPD. Some people with a deficiency of alpha$_1$-antitrypsin may receive some protection from weekly or twice-monthly intravenous injections of the substance, but such treatments are expensive, inconvenient, and not always effective.

Treatment. Only about half of people with COPD survive for 10 years or more after the diagnosis is made. The goals of COPD treatment are to prolong life, maintain independence, and improve comfort. These goals are achieved through a combination of lifestyle measures, medications, vaccinations, oxygen therapy, and, rarely, surgical procedures.

Lifestyle measures. The two interventions associated with improved survival in people with COPD are smoking cessation and supplemental oxygen for those who need it. Even people with advanced COPD can increase their life expectancy if they stop smoking. People with COPD should avoid exposure to other airborne toxins (including secondhand cigarette smoke), exercise as much as possible, and follow an adequate diet. People who find eating to be tiring may prefer to eat several small meals a day rather than a few large ones. Adding a liquid protein supplement to the daily diet may improve overall nutrition and help prevent weight loss. It is also important to drink plenty of fluids to avoid dehydration. People with COPD should be careful to rest when they get tired and should avoid exerting themselves when it is too hot, cold, or humid, or when air quality is poor.

Recent observations have underscored the benefits of pul-

Conserving Energy When You Have COPD

People with COPD can make daily tasks less draining.

If you have chronic obstructive pulmonary disease (COPD), you know that going about your daily routine can be exhausting. Even though activities such as bathing, grooming, and dressing require a great deal of energy, careful planning and some energy conservation can help you get through these tasks more quickly and with less effort. First, plan to bathe, groom, and dress at times when you're feeling most energetic. Second, gather all the supplies you will need before you start. For other useful tips, see the advice below:

Bathing

- Instead of standing in the shower, use a bath stool or take baths.
- Because excess humidity can make it tougher to breathe, use warm water rather than hot, leave the bathroom door open, turn on exhaust fans, and open a window whenever possible.
- If washing your hair in the shower, tub, or sink is difficult, ask someone else to do it for you.
- Using a long-handled brush or sponge can eliminate reaching to wash your back and feet.
- If you rely on oxygen, you can still use it while in the tub or shower—just drape the tube over the shower rod or side of the tub. (It's safe to remove the nasal cannula briefly while washing your face.)
- Dry off by wearing a long terry cloth robe and blotting rather than using a towel to rub yourself dry—it takes less effort.

Grooming

- Choose a simple hairstyle that doesn't require extensive blow-drying or styling.
- Conserve energy by sitting in front of a low mirror when shaving or applying makeup, rather than standing bent over the bathroom sink.
- Avoid products that are aerosolized or heavily scented, which will irritate the lungs. For example, most deodorants are available in roll-on or solid formulations, and many are also fragrance-free or unscented.
- Perfumes and colognes may also make it more difficult for you to breathe, so avoid using these products.

Dressing

- Keep your clothes—especially frequently used ones—in places that don't require you to bend or reach.
- If you're most energetic in the evenings, plan ahead and lay out tomorrow's clothes the night before.
- Avoid tight-fitting clothing that can make breathing difficult. For example, men can wear suspenders instead of belts, and women can wear camisoles or sports bras instead of regular bras.
- Don't wear socks or stockings with elastic bands, since they can restrict circulation. (Support hosiery recommended by your doctor is the exception.)
- Slip-on shoes mean you don't have to bend over to tie shoelaces. A long shoehorn (12 to 18 inches) can also make it easier to put shoes on.
- To conserve energy, stay seated as long as possible while dressing, and dress your lower half first, as it is usually more difficult. Putting your underwear inside your pants and pulling both on together may be helpful as well.

monary rehabilitation programs for people with COPD. While maintaining general strength through regular aerobic exercise is beneficial, lung exercises to strengthen the muscles used for breathing are also important. Breath training helps to control breathing rate, decrease the amount of energy required for breathing, and improve the position and function of the respiratory muscles. A respiratory therapist can help people with COPD practice the following techniques:

- Pursed-lip breathing. Inhale through your nose, and then exhale with your lips pursed in a whistling or kissing position. Each inhalation should take about two seconds and each exhalation should last about four to six seconds. It is not clear how pursed-lip breathing brings symptom relief, but it may work by keeping the airways open.

- Diaphragmatic breathing. The diaphragm is the main muscle used for normal breathing. People with COPD, however, may also use the muscles in the rib cage, neck, and abdomen to breathe. This method is less efficient than using the diaphragm. To practice using the diaphragm, lie on your back, place your hand or a small book on your abdomen, and breathe. Your hand or the book should rise on inhalation and fall on exhalation. Practice for 20 minutes twice daily. Once you have mastered this skill while lying down, try to do it while sitting up.
- Forward-bending posture. Breathing while bending slightly forward from the waist relieves symptoms for some people with severe COPD, possibly because the diaphragm has more room to expand.

Some research suggests that pulmonary rehabilitation may also increase survival, but this has not been proven.

Medications. Despite their fixed lung obstruction, many people with COPD also have some reversible airway obstruction that does respond somewhat to bronchodilators. Most commonly used are the beta$_2$ agonists and anticholinergics, which are described on page 15. The methylxanthine derivative theophylline is less effective than beta$_2$ agonists, but it may ease symptoms in about 20% of people with COPD.

If bronchodilators fail to relieve airway obstruction adequately, corticosteroids (both oral and inhaled; described on page 16) may diminish inflammation in some people. But corticosteroids are less effective for COPD than for asthma, and their side effects may be heightened in older people. Because of the difficulty in predicting who will respond to corticosteroid therapy, a carefully monitored two- to three-week trial period of oral corticosteroids is often conducted. Oral corticosteroids are discontinued promptly in people who do not benefit from them and are tapered to the lowest effective dose in people who do experience an improvement. Inhaled corticosteroids may be helpful in selected patients, and their role in the treatment of COPD continues to be assessed.

Expectorants (such as guaifenesin [gwai-FEN-uh-sin], found in Robitussin and other medications) may help to loosen mucus secretions in the airways. Antibiotics (such as tetracycline, ampicillin, erythromycin, and combinations of trimethoprim and sulfamethoxazole) are given when increased production of yellow or green phlegm signals a respiratory infection that can worsen COPD. Although moderate exacerbations of symptoms can be treated at home, severe episodes require hospitalization.

Mucus clearance devices. People with COPD who have chronic, moderate to severe mucus accumulation may benefit from a mucus clearance device. A mucus clearance device is a small handheld device shaped like a pipe. Blowing into it creates vibrations in the chest that loosen mucus and may allow medication to penetrate the lungs more easily. Some studies suggest that using a mucus clearance device before an inhaled bronchodilator can improve lung function and exercise capacity while decreasing shortness of breath in patients with COPD.

Vaccinations. People with COPD should have annual influenza vaccinations and should also receive a pneumonia vaccine about every six years to minimize the risk of acute exacerbations of their symptoms. The pneumonia vaccine protects against many forms of pneumococcal pneumonia, which is caused by the bacterium *Streptococcus pneumoniae*. This organism is only one of many causes of bacterial pneumonia.

Oxygen therapy. Supplemental oxygen can improve function and survival for people whose severely impaired lung function results in abnormally low concentrations of oxygen in the blood. For more information about home oxygen therapy, see the feature on pages 26–27.

Lung volume reduction surgery. Some people with emphysema may benefit from surgery called lung volume reduction surgery to remove diseased lung tissue. The procedure is believed to create more space in the chest cavity for the working lung tissue to expand. The procedure appears to prolong life in people who have emphysema that predominantly affects the upper lobes and low exercise capacity; Medicare started covering the procedure for these people in 2003.

Lung transplantation. Another option for people with emphysema is lung transplantation. More than 1,000 lung transplants are performed annually in the United States. About 60% of these procedures involve a single lung (unilateral), and 40% involve both lungs (bilateral). Unilateral transplants are reserved for people with emphysema or pulmonary fibrosis (chronic inflammation and progressive scarring of the walls of the alveoli); bilateral transplants are used primarily in those with cystic fibrosis (an inherited disease in infants, children, and young adults), bronchiectasis, or select emphysema patients.

The scarcity of donor lungs and the risks of the procedure make it necessary to carry out extensive evaluations to select the

NEW RESEARCH

Long-Term Corticosteroid Use Tied to Mood Problems

Depression and other mood disorders are common among people taking corticosteroids long term, a new study shows.

One- to two-week "bursts" of high-dose corticosteroid therapy are well known to cause mood problems, with mania being much more common than depression. But no previous research had been done on the mood effects of taking lower doses of the drugs over a longer period of time, as many people with asthma must.

The researchers looked at 34 people with asthma or rheumatoid arthritis (RA); 20 had taken 7.5 mg or more of prednisone daily for at least six months and 14 had not taken the drug (the control group). More people in the prednisone group than in the control group were found to have existing mania (60% vs. 7%) or depression (15% vs. none). Overall, 60% of patients on prednisone met criteria for a past or present mood disorder related to corticosteroids, with depression being the most common problem. Because of study-design limitations, these observations will need to be confirmed by others.

If you're taking long-term corticosteroid therapy and also suffer from depression, speak to your doctor about a possible link. Although you may need to remain on corticosteroids, your doctor may consider decreasing the corticosteroid dose.

ANNALS OF ALLERGY, ASTHMA & IMMUNOLOGY
Volume 92, page 500
May 2004

Using Home Oxygen Therapy for COPD

Round-the clock supplemental oxygen can improve quality of life.

Some people with COPD benefit not only from exercises, breathing techniques, and medications, but also from home oxygen therapy. Home oxygen therapy typically enhances sleep and mood, increases mental alertness and stamina, allows people to carry out daily activities more efficiently, and may prevent the development of cor pulmonale (heart disease caused by high blood pressure in the lungs) by decreasing the blood pressure in the lungs and lessening the workload of the right side of the heart. Although only a moderate percentage of COPD patients require supplemental oxygen, those who develop cor pulmonale due to low blood oxygen are especially good candidates—they have been shown to live longer if they are given supplemental oxygen.

Measurements of blood gases—the levels of oxygen, carbon dioxide, and acidity of blood taken from an artery—can help determine whether oxygen therapy would be helpful. In healthy people, the level of oxygen in the blood is usually between 75 and 95 mm Hg (millimeters of mercury, a measure of pressure). Home oxygen therapy is usually recommended for people with a resting blood oxygen level of 55 mm Hg or less. Having too little oxygen in the blood—a condition called hypoxemia—can cause symptoms such as fatigue, irritability, an inability to concentrate, breathlessness, heart problems, and fluid retention.

Oxygen level can also be measured using a noninvasive technique called oximetry. A device called an oximeter is clipped on the finger or ear and reports the oxygen saturation, which is an indirect measurement of oxygen levels in the arteries. An oximetry-measured oxygen saturation of less than 88% indicates a need for supplemental oxygen.

If oxygen therapy is recommended for you, your doctor will write a prescription detailing the flow rate (how many liters of oxygen you will breathe in per minute). Different flow rates may be prescribed for different activities, such as when you are sleeping, awake, or exercising. Using too much oxygen can slow your breathing, allowing more carbon dioxide to build up in your blood, so it's important to carefully follow the flow rates determined by your doctor.

People with COPD who require continuous oxygen therapy and use it 24 hours a day appear to have a longer life span than those who use it only while awake (15 hours per day); in turn, people who use oxygen therapy 15 hours per day have better outcomes than people who use it only while sleeping.

Home Therapy Equipment

A variety of oxygen delivery systems and oxygen conservation devices (also called oxygen concentration devices) are available, as described below. All forms of oxygen therapy are expensive; costs may be several hundred dollars a month, depending on the type of system. Oxygen concentrators are the least costly, although

their use can increase your electricity bill.

Compressed gas. Gas oxygen is stored under pressure in steel or aluminum canisters and must be purchased from a supplier. Larger canisters usually are used in the home; smaller ones are used when away from home. Normally the outflow of oxygen from the canister is constant, but some systems have an oxygen-conserving device that releases oxygen only when you inhale. When using portable canisters, learn how long each one will last so you can time your outings accordingly.

Liquid oxygen. Liquid oxygen is stored at a very cold temperature; it returns to its gaseous state when released from the container. Like compressed gas, liquid oxygen must be purchased and stored in canisters and may include an oxygen-conserving device. Liquid oxygen is more portable than compressed gas because larger amounts can be stored in smaller containers, and so it is often preferred by more active people. However, it has a limited shelf life and is more expensive than compressed gas.

Oxygen concentrators. An electric device called an oxygen concentrator can be used to extract oxygen from room air, which is about 20% oxygen. Oxygen concentrators are easier to maintain than other forms of oxygen therapy, and they may be ideal for people who spend most of their time at home. However, oxygen concentrators are not suitable for everyone. They are not portable, some of

most suitable candidates for lung transplantation. Candidates must meet disease-specific criteria for severe (end-stage) lung disease and yet be able to survive the wait for one or both donor lungs and the rigors of the operation and postoperative period. In 1998, international guidelines established an upper age limit of 64 for

them emit heat and are noisy, and the concentration of oxygen is lower than that in purchased gas or liquid oxygen. In addition, a backup source of oxygen is necessary in case of power failure.

The Delivery Method
No matter which type of oxygen therapy you use, you will need one of the following delivery systems.

In most cases, oxygen is delivered to the nose via a cannula (a two-pronged device that connects to the oxygen canister or concentrator and rests just inside your nostrils). The tubing rests on your ears or can be attached to your eyeglasses. Some people purchase eyeglass frames with a built-in cannula to make oxygen therapy somewhat less apparent. Cannulas allow you to eat and drink while still receiving oxygen.

A mask, which fits over the nose and mouth, may be better suited for someone who needs a high flow of oxygen. Also, some people who normally use a nasal cannula find a mask more effective when they have nasal congestion or irritation caused by a cold.

Some people may choose to receive oxygen directly into the lungs through a catheter inserted into a surgically created hole in the trachea (windpipe). The procedure is most appropriate for people who require a high flow of oxygen, since they often use less oxygen when it is delivered directly into the lungs. However, the catheter needs meticulous daily cleaning so that mucous does not collect on the tip of the device and block the trachea.

Using Oxygen Comfortably
Most people adjust very well to using oxygen, although a few measures may be necessary to increase comfort. Oxygen can be very drying to the body, especially to the nose. Several methods of relieving this dryness are commonly used. First, distilled water is often added to the oxygen to increase moisture, especially at higher flow rates. If your nose is still dry, you can apply an over-the-counter water-based lubricant (ask your pharmacist for a recommendation) to your nose several times a day. Also, try to inhale through your nose, rather than your mouth, which wastes oxygen and can make your mouth dry. Alternatively, if your nose is sore or uncomfortable, you can put the cannula in your mouth for two to three hours several times a day to give your nose a rest.

Using Oxygen Effectively
Oxygen can be dangerous if not used and cared for properly. It is flammable, so you—and anyone around you—should never smoke while you are using oxygen. Stay at least five feet away from open flames such as gas stoves, lighted fireplaces, and candles. Also, avoid flammable products such as aerosol sprays, paint thinners, and rubbing alcohol. Vapor rubs and petroleum jelly are also flammable and should be kept away from the oxygen canisters. Keep a fire extinguisher nearby, and tell your local fire department that oxygen is being used in the house.

If you have long tubing that allows you to move around the house, point it out to other people so they don't trip on it. Secure compressed oxygen canisters in a stand or next to something solid; if they fall over, they can be damaged and leak oxygen. Liquid oxygen canisters should be stored upright; if they fall over, the oxygen will be released, and the cold temperature can damage your skin.

When you begin home oxygen therapy, ask a representative from your medical supply company to come to your home and show you (and family members) how to use the equipment properly. You should receive specific instructions on how to clean and maintain the equipment as well.

Finally, make sure you always have access to oxygen. Order your next supply of oxygen so that it arrives before you need it. Keep your medical supply company's emergency phone numbers accessible in case of an equipment failure. And alert your electric company that you have electrical oxygen equipment in your home—you should receive priority service in the event of a power failure. If traveling, make arrangements to have oxygen available on airline flights and in your destination city or country.

When To Call Your Doctor
If you are on oxygen and develop confusion, headaches, or drowsiness, you may be getting too much oxygen and need to have your carbon dioxide levels checked. Blue fingernails or lips indicate low blood oxygen levels. Any of these symptoms should prompt an immediate call to your doctor.

unilateral and 59 for bilateral transplants. Transplants cannot be performed in people with major disease in other organs; HIV infection; cancer (other than basal or squamous cell skin cancers) diagnosed within the past two years; positive tests for hepatitis B antigen; or hepatitis C infection with liver disease. The procedure may not be suitable for people who have severe osteoporosis or are obese.

Like those who receive transplants of other solid organs, lung transplant patients are required to take medications for the rest of their life to suppress the immune system and prevent it from rejecting the transplanted lung(s). After successful transplantation, patients may experience some limitations in exercise tolerance but usually not enough to interfere with normal daily activities or adversely affect quality of life. The five-year survival rate following lung transplantation (approximately 50%) is highest in those treated for underlying emphysema and lowest in those with idiopathic pulmonary fibrosis (progressive scarring of the lungs in which the cause is unknown) or pulmonary hypertension. The most common cause of rejection, and the most dangerous complication of transplantation, is a condition called bronchiolitis obliterans, in which the bronchioles become blocked. Other common complications are infections and the side effects of the immunosuppressive drugs.

SLEEP APNEA

Sleep apnea is a disorder characterized by repeated episodes of breathing cessation (apnea) during sleep. Episodes last from 10 seconds to nearly a minute, occur throughout the night, and worsen sleep quality. Periods of apnea end with a brief partial arousal that may disrupt sleep hundreds of times a night. The resulting daytime sleepiness was made famous by Charles Dickens's description of an overweight boy in *The Pickwick Papers* who was affected by the condition. Sleep apnea is about twice as common in men as in women; a 2003 study in the *Journal of the American Medical Association* suggests that it affects about 7% of the population. An estimated 18 million Americans have clinically significant obstructive sleep apnea, and 95% of individuals with this condition remain undiagnosed and untreated.

Causes
Sleep apnea results from either a collapse and blockage of the upper airway during sleep or a central nervous system abnormality that interferes with the drive to breathe. Some people have an anatomical abnormality (such as large tonsils, excess fat in the tissues around the throat, or an enlarged tongue) that narrows the upper airway. A large neck or collar size (more than 17 inches in men or 16 inches in women) is strongly associated with sleep

apnea. Obesity, older age, weakness of the airway muscles, hypothyroidism (insufficient production of thyroid hormone), and cigarette smoking are additional risk factors. Consuming alcohol or sedatives before sleeping can further reduce the activity of the airway muscles and blunt the normal increases in breathing that occur after the fall in oxygen concentration associated with apnea.

Symptoms

The most pervasive and troublesome symptom of sleep apnea is excessive daytime sleepiness caused by poor sleep. People with sleep apnea may fall asleep during the day while reading or even while driving, so there is a major risk of motor vehicle accidents. People with sleep apnea also may suffer from memory loss and personality changes. Although loud snoring is a common manifestation of sleep apnea, snoring itself does not indicate obstructive sleep apnea.

More than half of those with sleep apnea also have high blood pressure, and their blood pressure levels do not fall during sleep as they do in most people. In fact, sleep apnea has been shown to be an independent, treatable cause of high blood pressure.

Heart rate tends to slow dramatically during periods of apnea and then rise rapidly when breathing resumes. Some evidence suggests that periods of apnea and low blood oxygen levels, along with persistently high blood pressure, increase the risk of coronary heart disease. This association is being studied.

For more information about the health risks of sleep apnea, see the feature on pages 30–31.

Diagnosis

Obtaining a sleep history is key to recognizing this common respiratory disorder. Seeking input from a person's bed partner is especially important, because the bed partner is likely to notice snoring associated with frequent periods of apnea. A definitive diagnosis usually requires the patient to spend a night in a hospital sleep laboratory to undergo sleep studies (polysomnography). Polysomnography involves monitoring brain waves to determine which stages of sleep are associated with episodes of apnea, as well as observing heart rhythms, airflow and breathing patterns, eye and leg movements, and blood oxygen levels. These expensive sleep lab studies can be replaced in some people by using a pulse oximeter to record blood oxygen levels while sleeping at home. A pulse oximeter test that shows low blood oxygen levels during sleep can aid in

NEW RESEARCH

Sleep Apnea Therapy Makes Driving Safer

Drivers with severe sleep apnea can safely take to the road within a few days of beginning a treatment with continuous positive airway pressure (CPAP), new research suggests.

Sleep apnea robs a person of a full, deep sleep, leading to daytime sleepiness, dulled reaction times, and a higher risk of traffic accidents. Research has suggested that CPAP, in which patients wear a nasal mask that delivers a continuous flow of air while they sleep, may improve patients' ability to drive.

But just how long it takes for the benefits to emerge has been unclear. The new study, of 36 adults with severe sleep apnea, found that patients' performance in computer-based driving simulator tests improved within a few days of starting CPAP. And the improvements remained—though they were beginning to fade—one week after patients stopped CPAP.

The findings, according to the authors, suggest that driving improves rapidly after patients start CPAP, and that it doesn't deteriorate after a few days without treatment. Whether a driving simulator test can accurately predict prowess on the road is not fully clear; however, the researchers note, some studies have linked test performance to accident risk.

THORAX
Volume 59, page 56
January 2004

Sleep Apnea's Multiple Health Risks

This breathing-related sleep disorder can affect your heart, your mood, and even your driving skills.

It's well established that sleep apnea—characterized by repeated episodes of breathing cessation and partial awakening during sleep—contributes to daytime fatigue. Now, experts are beginning to realize that sleep apnea can have more serious health effects as well. For example, high blood pressure, depression, and motor vehicle accidents are all more common among people with sleep apnea. However, treatment for sleep apnea (including lifestyle measures, weight loss, and continuous positive airway pressure [CPAP]) can help resolve the apnea as well as some of these related health problems.

Motor Vehicle Accidents

Research has shown that people with sleep apnea are up to nine times more likely to have an accident while driving than people without the condition. The daytime drowsiness that accompanies sleep apnea impairs their driving skills, similar to someone who has a blood alcohol level over the legal limit. But CPAP therapy for sleep apnea (see page 30) can have a quick and dramatic effect on driving ability, according to a 2004 study.

Researchers used a driving simulator to test the skills and reflexes of 36 people with sleep apnea (18 who were just beginning CPAP and a control group of 18 who were not being treated). Participants performed the 20-minute driving test 1, 3, and 7 days into a two-week CPAP trial period; then CPAP was discontinued and all participants performed the test 1, 3, and 7 days later.

Within seven days after beginning CPAP, participants improved their reaction time and ability to keep the simulated car on the road. The control group's scores did not improve, suggesting that the CPAP group's improvements were not due to growing familiarity with the simulator. After discontinuing CPAP, participants' scores remained stable during days 1 and 3 but began to worsen by day 7. This finding suggests that CPAP improves driving ability rapidly and that the benefit is not lost after a few nights of missed treatments.

Depression

The link between depression and sleep apnea has long been acknowledged, but for the first time a study has quantified the magnitude of that link in the general population. For a study published in 2003 in The Journal of Clinical Psychiatry, researchers conducted a telephone poll of nearly 19,000 Europeans and asked them questions regarding sleep quality, breathing-related sleep disorders, mental disorders, and medical conditions. The prevalence of a breathing-related sleep disorder (which includes sleep apnea and disruptive snoring) in the total pool of respondents was 4.6%; 4.3% also had major depression. More than five times as many people with depression had a breathing-related sleep disorder (18%) as people without depression (3.8%). This relationship persisted even after adjusting for breathing-related sleep disorder risk factors such as obesity and hypertension.

It is not known whether breathing-related sleep disorders lead to depression or vice versa, but both conditions share some symptoms (excessive daytime sleepiness and cognitive impairment). Some studies have suggested that CPAP may relieve depressive symptoms as well as breathing-related sleep disorders, but more research is needed to determine

the diagnosis, but a normal result does not rule out the possibility of sleep apnea.

Treatment

Lifestyle measures that may reduce sleep apnea include losing weight (for overweight and obese people), avoiding alcohol and sedatives at bedtime, quitting smoking, and sleeping on your side or in a more upright position. If hypothyroidism is present, treating it may help reduce the apnea.

If these measures are unsuccessful, continuous positive airway pressure (CPAP) may be necessary. This technique, which involves

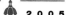

whether this is merely a placebo effect. In the meantime, the researchers suggest that people who are diagnosed with either major depression or a breathing-related sleep disorder should also be examined for the other condition.

High Blood Pressure

More than half of people with sleep apnea also have high blood pressure, and, unlike most people, their blood pressure levels do not fall during sleep. In fact, sleep apnea has been shown to be an independent, treatable cause of high blood pressure. One study found that sleep apnea increased the risk of a new diagnosis of high blood pressure four years later. The risk increased by 42% for people who had less than 5 apnea events per hour; by 103% for 5 to 15 events per hour; and by 189% for more than 15 events per hour.

This link between sleep apnea and high blood pressure appears to persist regardless of gender, age, race, and weight. Fortunately, CPAP treatment appears to treat sleep apnea as well as reduce daytime and nighttime blood pressure, according to a recent review article.

Heart Problems

Heart rate tends to slow dramatically during periods of apnea and then rise rapidly when breathing resumes. Some evidence suggests that periods of apnea and low blood oxygen levels, along with persistently high blood pressure, increase the risk of coronary heart disease. This association is being studied. Stronger associations—although not direct cause-and-effect relationships—have been found between sleep apnea and other heart-related problems, as discussed below.

Left ventricular hypertrophy. Researchers have long suspected the link between sleep apnea and left ventricular hypertrophy (a thickening of the muscular wall of the left ventricle that occurs when the heart must work harder to pump blood). Indeed, a recent study found that 88% of the participants with sleep apnea had left ventricular hypertrophy. The researchers used ultrasound to measure heart size in 25 people with severe sleep apnea. After six months, all patients who complied with CPAP therapy had a significant reduction in left ventricular hypertrophy, which is linked to cardiac-related death.

Atrial fibrillation. Similarly, sleep apnea is also linked to atrial fibrillation, an abnormal heart rhythm in which the atria (the upper chambers of the heart) quiver chaotically instead of contracting in a rhythmic pattern. Atrial fibrillation can cause blood clots and is a known cause of strokes.

A recent study found that untreated sleep apnea increases the risk that people who have had atrial fibrillation in the past will have a recurrence; the study also showed that CPAP therapy was associated with a reduced risk of recurrence. All participants had atrial fibrillation in the past and were at risk for recurrence; in addition, they had sleep apnea. Atrial fibrillation recurred in 42% of participants who were treated with CPAP, compared with 82% of participants who used CPAP either incorrectly or not at all.

Heart failure. A link also exists between sleep apnea and heart failure (the inability of the heart to pump blood efficiently). The two conditions commonly occur together, and one study suggests that as many as 37% of people with heart failure also have sleep apnea. A recent study suggests that treating sleep apnea may also have a beneficial effect on heart failure.

Researchers assigned 24 people with heart failure and sleep apnea either to continue their current medical therapy or to add CPAP therapy to their treatment regimen. After one month, the CPAP group had significant improvements in daytime blood pressures, heart rate, and heart functioning. The researchers suggest that untreated sleep apnea may prevent the heart from resting at night, placing abnormal stress on the heart.

wearing a nasal mask that delivers a steady stream of air to maintain airway pressure and keep the airways open, is effective in 80% to 90% of people. However, many people discontinue CPAP because they find the mask cumbersome or experience nasal dryness, nasal congestion, or skin irritation. Use of a humidifier or a properly fitting mask can alleviate some of these problems. Also, people may be more likely to use devices that gradually increase air pressure as they fall asleep or provide different levels of air pressure during inhalation and exhalation.

Some people benefit from a dental appliance that helps maintain an open airway by keeping the jaw and tongue in a forward position during sleep. In addition, carefully selected people who cannot tolerate CPAP may benefit from uvulopalatopharyngoplasty, a surgical procedure that increases the size of the upper airway by removing the uvula (the tag-like structure that hangs down from the back of the throat) and any excessive soft tissue surrounding it. This procedure is successful in only 40% to 50% of people, typically those with mild disease. Tonsillectomy, surgical treatment of other upper airway obstructions, and facial reconstructive procedures are helpful in some cases. In addition, a 2002 study revealed that boosting the heart rate during sleep can reduce sleep apnea; this may prove to be a practical treatment for people with pacemakers.

Finally, in 2004 the FDA approved a drug called modafanil (Provigil) to help people with sleep apnea and other sleep disorders stay awake. Modafanil was originally approved in 1998 to treat narcolepsy. The most common side effects are headache, nausea, nervousness, stuffy nose, diarrhea, back pain, anxiety, trouble sleeping, dizziness, and upset stomach.

INTERSTITIAL LUNG DISEASE

Interstitial lung disease (ILD) refers to a group of more than 200 chronic disorders that are characterized by overgrowth of cells in the interstitium (the tissue between the alveoli), varying degrees of inflammation, and scarring (fibrosis). Though many of the disorders are uncommon, taken together ILD is a frequent cause of respiratory problems and accounts for 15% of all cases seen by pulmonologists (lung specialists).

The lung scarring associated with ILD leads to stiffness that makes breathing more difficult. In addition, changes in the normal relationships between airspaces and capillaries limit the transfer of oxygen. The pace and severity of this process vary greatly from person to person.

Interstitial lung disease includes disorders such as pulmonary sarcoidosis, bronchiolitis obliterans organizing pneumonia, asbestosis, and silicosis. Pulmonary sarcoidosis is an inflammatory disease in which cell overgrowth occurs in the lungs. Bronchiolitis obliterans organizing pneumonia refers to inflammation with blockage of the bronchioles. Asbestosis and silicosis refer to damage caused by exposure to dust from asbestos and silica, respectively. Idiopathic pulmonary fibrosis is another important condition in which progressive scarring of the lung markedly compromises day-to-day function.

Causes

A variety of factors can injure the alveoli and result in ILD. Possible causes of ILD include:

- certain illegal and prescription drugs (including chemotherapy agents and cardiovascular medications);
- exposure to environmental toxins;
- infectious agents (such as viruses, bacteria, or fungi);
- substances that trigger allergic or hypersensitivity reactions (such as certain bird proteins) in susceptible persons;
- connective tissue diseases such as scleroderma, rheumatoid arthritis, and lupus, all of which can cause inflammation and scarring of organs (including the lungs); and
- the spread of cancer to the lungs from other parts of the body.

In many cases, the cause of lung injury is unknown (idiopathic).

Symptoms

Symptoms vary widely depending on the specific disease, but most people with ILD become short of breath when they exert themselves and have a persistent cough that does not produce phlegm. Fatigue, loss of appetite, and weight loss are common in many types of ILD; wheezing, chest pain, hemoptysis (coughing up blood), and fever also are possible. The course of the disease can last for several weeks, but more often the disease follows a chronic course and symptoms persist for months or years.

Diagnosis

Abnormalities on a chest x-ray may be the first evidence of ILD, but the changes often are not specific for a particular disorder.

Pulmonary function tests typically show a decrease in total lung capacity (the amount of air in the lungs after a deep inhalation). Measurements of arterial oxygen and carbon dioxide levels at rest may not be helpful for diagnosis, but seeing whether exercise causes a drop in the arterial oxygen level may be useful in first detecting the disease and following the progression of the disease or its response to treatment.

A common abnormality in people with ILD is a decrease in diffusion capacity (a pulmonary function test that measures how well gas moves across the membranes in the lungs). Like chest x-rays, however, this abnormality does not distinguish among the various underlying causes of ILD.

The results of high-resolution chest CT scans may be helpful in

NEW RESEARCH

Air Freshener By-Products Can Irritate Lungs

Chemicals emitted by plug-in air fresheners can combine with ozone to produce chemicals that irritate the lungs, a new study shows.

Fragrance chemicals contain volatile organic compounds (VOCs) that interact with ozone to produce potentially harmful by-products, which can impair lung function in healthy people and those with obstructive lung disease such as asthma and COPD.

The researchers tested emissions from a pine-scented, electrical plug-in air freshener and observed how they reacted with ozone. Outdoor air contains ozone from cars and industrial plants; indoor sources include laser printers, photocopiers, and ozone-emitting air cleaners.

The air freshener produced VOCs that reacted with ozone to create fine particles and chemicals such as formaldehyde. Concentrations of fine particles were as high as 50 micrograms (mcg) per cubic meter, "demonstrating that indoor air chemical reactions have the potential to significantly increase human exposure to fine particles." The federal standard is less than 65 mcg per cubic meter.

People can reduce exposure to harmful particles and chemicals at home by keeping ozone-producing devices such as laser printers in well-ventilated areas and limiting use of air fresheners and other products that emit VOCs.

ENVIRONMENTAL SCIENCE & TECHNOLOGY
Volume 38, page 2802
May 15, 2004

A Guide to Indoor Air Pollution

We often think of air pollution as a problem found outdoors. But indoor air pollution can be an even worse problem, especially when one considers that we spend about 90% of our time indoors. Estimates from the U.S. Environmental Protection Agency (EPA) indicate that levels of pollutants indoors can be two to five times higher than in the air outdoors. These indoor pollutants can cause symptoms ranging from mild (such as irritation of the nose) to deadly (for example, lung cancer). The chart below lists the most common indoor air pollutants and what you can do about them.

Pollutant	Sources	Health Effects
Radon	Earth and rock beneath home, well water, and building materials.	No immediate symptoms. Estimated to contribute to between 7,000 and 30,000 lung cancer deaths each year. Smokers are at elevated risk for developing radon-induced lung cancer.
Environmental tobacco smoke	Cigar, cigarette, and pipe smoke.	Eye, nose, and throat irritation; headaches; and lung cancer. May contribute to heart disease.
Biologicals	Wet or moist walls, ceilings, carpets, and furniture; poorly maintained humidifiers, dehumidifiers, and air conditioners; bedding; and household pets.	Eye, nose, and throat irritation; shortness of breath; dizziness; lethargy; fever; and digestive problems. Can cause asthma, humidifier fever, influenza, and other infectious diseases.
Carbon monoxide (CO)	Unvented kerosene and gas space heaters; leaking chimneys and furnaces; back-drafting from furnaces, gas water heaters, wood stoves, and fireplaces; gas stoves; automobile exhaust from attached garages; and environmental tobacco smoke.	At low concentrations, fatigue in healthy people and chest pain in people with heart disease. At higher concentrations, impaired vision and coordination, headaches, dizziness, confusion, and nausea. Can cause flu-like symptoms that clear up after leaving home. Fatal at very high concentrations.
Nitrogen dioxide (NO_2)	Kerosene heaters, unvented gas stoves, unvented heaters, and environmental tobacco smoke.	Eye, nose, and throat irritation.
Organic gases	Household products including paint strippers and other solvents, wood preservatives, aerosol sprays, cleansers and disinfectants, moth repellents and air fresheners, stored fuels and automotive products, hobby supplies, and dry-cleaned clothing.	Eye, nose, and throat irritation; headaches; loss of coordination; nausea; and damage to liver, kidney, and central nervous system. Some organics can cause cancer in animals; some are suspected or known to be carcinogenic in humans.

Levels in Homes	Steps To Reduce Exposure
The average indoor radon level is 1.3 picocuries per liter (pCi/L). The average outdoor levels is about 0.4 pCi/L.	• Test your home for radon—it's easy and inexpensive. • Fix your home if your radon level is 4 pCi/L or higher. • Radon levels less than 4 pCi/L still pose a risk and, in some cases, should be reduced.
Particle levels in homes without smokers or other strong particle sources are the same as, or lower than, outdoors. Homes with one or more smokers may have particle levels several times higher than outdoor levels.	• Don't smoke in your home or permit others to do so. • If smoking indoors cannot be avoided, increase ventilation in the area where smoking takes place. Open windows or use exhaust fans.
Indoor levels of pollen and fungi are lower than outdoor levels (except where indoor sources of fungi are present). Indoor levels of dust mites are higher than outdoor levels.	• Install and use fans vented to outdoors. • Vent clothes dryers to outdoors. • Clean cool-mist and ultrasonic humidifiers in accordance with manufacturer's instructions, and refill with clean water daily. • Empty water trays in air conditioners, dehumidifiers, and refrigerators frequently. • Clean and dry or remove water-damaged carpets. • Use basements as living areas only if they are leak-proof and have adequate ventilation. Use dehumidifiers, if necessary, to maintain humidity between 30% and 50%.
Average levels in homes without gas stoves vary from 0.5 to 5 parts per million (ppm). Levels near properly adjusted gas stoves are often 5 to 15 ppm, and those near poorly adjusted stoves may be 30 ppm or higher.	• Keep gas appliances properly adjusted. • Consider purchasing a vented space heater when replacing an unvented one. • Use proper fuel in kerosene space heaters. Install and use an exhaust fan vented to outdoors over gas stoves. • Open flues when fireplaces are in use. • Choose properly sized wood stoves that are certified to meed EPA emission standards. Make certain that doors on all wood stoves fit tightly. • Have a trained professional inspect, clean, and tune up central heating system (furnaces, flues, and chimneys) annually. Repair any leaks promptly. • Don't idle the car inside garage.
Average level in homes without combustion appliances is about half that of outdoors. In homes with gas stoves, kerosene heaters, or unvented gas space heaters, indoor levels often exceed outdoor levels.	• Same as those for carbon monoxide (see above).
Levels of several organics average two to five times higher indoors than outdoors. During and for several hours immediately after certain activities (such as paint stripping), levels may be 1,000 times background outdoor levels.	• Use household products according to manufacturer's directions. • Make sure you provide plenty of fresh air when using these products. • Throw away unused or little-used containers safely; buy in quantities that you will soon use.

Indoor Air Pollution (continued)

Pollutant	Sources	Health Effects
Respirable particles (small dust particles that can be inhaled deep into the lungs)	Fireplaces, wood stoves, kerosene heaters, and environmental tobacco smoke.	Eye, nose, and throat irritation; respiratory infections and bronchitis; and lung cancer. (Effects attributable to environmental tobacco smoke are listed above.)
Formaldehyde	Pressed wood products (hardwood plywood wall paneling, particleboard, fiberboard) and furniture made with these pressed-wood products; urea-formaldehyde foam insulation (UFFI); combustion sources and environmental tobacco smoke; and durable-press drapes, other textiles, and glues.	Eye, nose, and throat irritation; wheezing and coughing; fatigue; skin rash; and severe allergic reactions. May cause cancer. May also cause other effects listed under "organic gases."
Pesticides	Products used to kill household pests (insecticides, termiticides, and disinfectants) and products used on lawns and gardens that drift or are tracked inside the house.	Irritation to eye, nose, and throat; damage to the central nervous system and kidneys; and increased risk of cancer.
Asbestos	Deteriorating, damaged, or disturbed insulation, fireproofing, acoustical materials, and floor tiles.	No immediate symptoms, but long-term increased risk of chest and abdominal cancers and lung diseases. Smokers are at higher risk for developing asbestos-induced lung cancer.
Lead	Lead-based paint and contaminated soil, dust, and drinking water.	Lead affects practically all systems within the body. Lead at high levels (at or above 80 micrograms per deciliter [mcg/dL] of blood) can cause convulsions, coma, and even death. Lower levels of lead can cause adverse health effects on the central nervous system, kidneys, and blood cells. Blood lead levels as low as 10 mcg/dL can impair mental and physical development.

Adapted from: U.S. Environmental Protection Agency, "The Inside Story: A Guide to Indoor Air Quality," pp. 23–27. www.epa.gov/iaq/pubs/insidest.html

.evels in Homes	Steps To Reduce Exposure
Particle levels in homes without smoking or other strong particle sources are the same as, or lower than, outdoor levels.	• Vent all furnaces to outdoors; keep doors to rest of house open when using unvented space heaters. • Choose properly sized wood stoves certified to meet EPA emission standards; make certain that doors on all wood stoves fit tightly. • Have a trained professional inspect, clean, and tune up central heating system (furnace, flues, and chimneys) annually. Repair any leaks promptly. • Change filters on central-heating and cooling systems and air cleaners according to manufacturer's directions.
Average concentrations in older homes without UFFI are generally well below 0.1 ppm. In homes with significant amounts of new pressed-wood products, levels can be greater than 0.3 ppm.	• Use "exterior grade" pressed wood products (lower emitting because they contain phenol resins, not urea resins). • Use air conditioning and humidifiers to maintain moderate temperature and reduce humidity levels. • Increase ventilation, particularly after bringing new sources of formaldehyde into the home.
Preliminary research shows widespread presence of pesticide residue in homes.	• Use strictly according to manufacturer's directions. • Mix or dilute outdoors. • Apply only in recommended quantities. • Increase ventilation when using indoors. Take plants or pets outdoors when applying pesticides to them. • Use nonchemical methods of pest control where possible. • If you use a pest control company, select it carefully. • Do not store unneeded pesticides inside home; dispose of unwanted containers safely. • Store clothes with moth repellents in separately ventilated areas, if possible. • Keep indoor spaces clean, dry, and well ventilated to avoid pest and odor problems.
Elevated levels can occur in homes where asbestos-containing materials are damaged or disturbed.	• It is best to leave undamaged asbestos material alone if it is not likely to be disturbed. • Use trained and qualified contractors for control measures that may disturb asbestos and for cleanup. • Follow proper procedures in replacing wood stove door gaskets that may contain asbestos.
See the column to the left.	• Keep areas where children play as dust free and clean as possible. • Leave lead-based paint undisturbed if it is in good condition; do not sand or burn off paint that may contain lead. • Do not remove lead paint yourself. • Do not bring lead dust into the home. • If your work or hobby involves lead, change clothes and use doormats before entering home. • Eat a balanced diet rich in calcium and iron.

people suspected of having ILD. For example, a scan showing changes in which the severely damaged lung resembles a honeycomb on the edge of the lung may eliminate the need for a lung biopsy because it is so specific for one form of ILD.

In some cases, a specific diagnosis can be made from the examination of lung fluids obtained using bronchoalveolar lavage (washing out the lungs with a saline solution) during bronchoscopy (in which a thin, hollow, flexible tube is passed through the mouth and into the windpipe to allow viewing of the main bronchial passages).

Because different types of ILD may have similar x-ray features and result in similar decreases in lung capacity, a lung biopsy may be necessary to make a definitive diagnosis and determine the severity of the disease. Least invasive is a biopsy done through a bronchoscope. This procedure can be done on an outpatient basis, but the small size of the tissue sample often is insufficient for diagnosis. If this approach is inconclusive, an open surgical biopsy in a hospital may be necessary.

Prevention

Avoidance of potential triggers of ILD is important. For example, wearing appropriate masks and monitoring inhalational exposures in certain work environments are worthwhile precautions to take.

Treatment

Several types of ILD, notably sarcoidosis and hypersensitivity reactions, resolve on their own or respond to treatment with corticosteroids. Treatment of infections responsible for the disorder or avoidance of toxins or allergen exposures may be quite beneficial. Unfortunately, for other causes of ILD, there is no specific treatment to slow disease progression or reverse the damage that has already occurred. Further inflammation and scarring of lung tissue lead to worsening respiratory function and right heart failure (heart failure that mainly affects the right side of the heart, slowing the movement of blood through the heart). Corticosteroid treatment, which speeds the resolution of sarcoidosis, may be prescribed for symptomatic people with other forms of ILD, but it often is unsuccessful. Chemotherapy drugs such as cyclophosphamide (Cytoxan, Neosar) or azathioprine (Imuran), antifibrotic agents such as colchicine (available only in generic form), and interferon gamma have been tried in people with idiopathic pulmonary fibrosis, but an effective treatment remains elusive for this debilitating and progressive condition. Supportive care includes

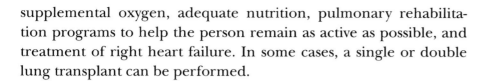

supplemental oxygen, adequate nutrition, pulmonary rehabilitation programs to help the person remain as active as possible, and treatment of right heart failure. In some cases, a single or double lung transplant can be performed.

LUNG CANCER

Lung cancer was rare before the beginning of the 20th century, but it is now the most common cause of death from cancer in both men and women in the United States; an estimated 157,200 Americans died of lung cancer in 2003. Death rates from lung cancer are high because lung cancer is difficult to treat and usually is not detected until it has already spread (metastasized). Most cases occur in people between the ages of 45 and 75 who have been exposed to cigarette smoke or other pollutants for many years. Tragically, only about 15% of people with lung cancer are alive five years after diagnosis.

Lung cancer may be primary or secondary. Primary lung cancer, which originates in the lungs, is grouped into two broad categories: small cell carcinoma (about 20% of cases) and non-small cell carcinoma (about 80%). Because small cell carcinoma spreads especially quickly and is more difficult to treat, most people with this type die within a year of diagnosis. Primary lung cancer can spread to nearly any organ. Cancer may also spread to the lungs from other sites in the body (secondary lung cancer). Such tumors usually are incurable, in which case palliative treatments are used. Palliative treatments are aimed at delaying the progression of disease, relieving pain, and limiting disease complications, rather than curing the disease.

Causes

Smoking causes an estimated 87% to 90% of lung cancer cases. Nonsmokers have only a small risk, and smokers who quit (even after smoking for years) greatly reduce their risk. One recent study provided some of the first direct evidence of how cigarette smoking leads to lung cancer. Researchers found that the body converts a substance in cigarette smoke, called benzo[a]pyrene diol epoxide (BPDE), into a potent carcinogen.

Several comprehensive reports also have concluded that passive smoking (inhaling the smoke from cigarettes smoked by others) can cause lung cancer in nonsmokers. This conclusion is based on the presence of carcinogens in the smoke coming from the end of

NEW RESEARCH

More Study Needed on Complementary Asthma Therapies

Relaxation and breathing exercises, as well as acupuncture, may help some people with asthma, but much more research must be done on complementary therapies patients are using for the condition, a new study concludes.

In the study, researchers reviewed 15 studies of complementary medicine techniques used to treat asthma. One small study found that a controlled breathing technique called buteyko breathing improved asthma patients' quality of life and reduced their medication use. Another report showed acupuncture improved immune function in people with asthma, but this improvement did not result in better lung function. A different trial found that relaxation techniques improved lung and immune function. All of the positive findings were relatively weak, and the researchers found no evidence of effectiveness for the other therapies studied.

Nevertheless, the researchers note, many people with asthma do seek out complementary and alternative therapies. More rigorous research is under way testing alternative asthma treatments, they add, and in the future doctors should have better evidence on which of these therapies will be most helpful for their patients with asthma.

JOURNAL OF ASTHMA
Volume 41, page 131
April 2004

a burning cigarette (sidestream smoke), the presence of cigarette smoke particles in the homes of smokers, detection of tobacco-smoke components in the body fluids of nonsmokers, and the 30% increased incidence of lung cancer in the nonsmoking spouses of smokers. Some data suggest that passive smoking is one of the leading causes of preventable deaths in this country, if projected deaths from lung cancer and cardiovascular disease are counted together.

Exposure to toxic substances such as radon and asbestos can also lead to lung cancer. In fact, radon is estimated to be the leading cause of lung cancer among nonsmokers and the second leading cause overall.

Radon is a colorless, odorless gas formed from radium during the decay of naturally occurring uranium in rocks and soil. Radon in the soil can pollute the air of a home by entering through cracks or other openings, usually in the basement. The incidence of lung cancer caused by radon is highest among miners of uranium and certain other substances who are exposed to high levels of radon.

Asbestos is a fibrous mineral that was used in building materials until the 1980s. Chronic exposure to asbestos can cause both lung cancer and mesothelioma, a cancer involving the pleura (the membranes that cover the lungs). The combination of asbestos exposure and cigarette smoking is especially dangerous.

Air pollution (including traffic fumes and smokestack emissions) also may contribute to lung cancer.

Symptoms

Lung cancer produces no symptoms in its early stages. Later, lung cancer patients often note symptoms of fatigue, poor appetite, and unexplained weight loss that are common to many forms of cancer. Symptoms also can result from cancer growth within the lungs or from its spread to adjacent or distant sites. Lung symptoms may include coughing up red or rust-colored phlegm, wheezing, and shortness of breath. Infection in the lung beyond an obstructed bronchus may produce a fever, and invasion of cancerous cells into the pleura or other nearby structures can produce pain in the chest, shoulders, or arms. If the cancer spreads to surrounding structures, it can also lead to hoarseness resulting from enlarged lymph nodes in the chest or neck or involvement of various nerves, such as the recurrent laryngeal nerve; difficulty swallowing, due to narrowing of the esophagus; and swelling of the neck and face from blockage of blood flow from these sites to the heart. In about 30% of patients, lung cancer causes clubbing of the fingers (a thickening of the fingertips and increased curvature of the finger-nails).

Lung cancer often spreads to the liver and bone marrow, where it can interfere with the formation of blood cells. Spread to the bones causes pain and fractures, while spread to the brain pro-duces neurological symptoms such as seizures. Small cell tumors may secrete hormones such as corticotropin or antidiuretic hor-mone. Overproduction of corticotropin stimulates excessive release of corticosteroids by the adrenal gland, leading to Cush-ing's syndrome. This syndrome produces such complications as osteoporosis, high blood pressure, and roundness of the face. Release of antidiuretic hormone results in fluid retention. Other lung cancer cell types secrete parathyroid hormone (PTH) or a PTH-like hormone. Spread of cancer to the bone and/or the PTH-like hormone trigger the release of calcium from the bone, which can lead to excessive blood levels of calcium (hypercalcemia). Hypercalcemia may cause fatigue, muscle weakness, confusion, drowsiness, and coma.

Diagnosis

About 10% of lung cancers are discovered in people with no symp-toms, usually when a chest x-ray is performed for another reason. However, the majority of lung cancers are diagnosed after a doctor requests testing for cancer based on a patient's medical history and the results of a physical examination.

Doctors usually do not recommend general screening for lung cancer in at-risk individuals (for example, smokers and former smokers). A standard chest x-ray is not sensitive enough to locate small tumors, and studies have shown that two screening meth-ods—regular chest x-rays and phlegm examinations—do not decrease the number of deaths from lung cancer.

A recently developed technology called low-radiation-dose spi-ral computed tomography (spiral CT) currently is being investigat-ed as a screening tool for lung cancer. Spiral CT generates a series of cross-sectional images of the lungs that are used to create a three-dimensional image. The radiation exposure from a spiral CT scan is slightly higher than that from a regular chest x-ray. It costs about $300, compared with $150 for the less accurate chest x-ray and $2,000 for the time-consuming positron emission tomography (PET) and magnetic resonance imaging (MRI) scans.

The advantages of spiral CT are that it is relatively inexpensive, provides clear images, and can be performed in about 20 seconds.

NEW RESEARCH

Optimism May Not Prolong Survival in Lung Cancer

Although it's commonly thought that a person's outlook can sway the course of a serious illness, a positive attitude does not appear to help lung cancer patients live longer, study findings suggest.

Researchers found no evi-dence that a high level of opti-mism before treatment prolonged survival among 179 men and women with non–small cell lung cancer. By the end of the study, which followed patients for up to 12 years, 96% had died. Those deemed optimistic at the outset—based on questionnaires about their attitudes toward life—did not differ from pessimistic patients in survival time.

According to the authors, the findings suggest that optimism provides little survival benefit, at least in lung cancer. In fact, the researchers note, encouraging patients to "be positive" may only put another burden on them and possibly make them feel responsi-ble for the outcome of their illness.

However, the authors add, even if optimism does not pro-long survival, it may help prevent depression and have other posi-tive effects on the time patients do have left. The bottom line, they conclude, is that "appropri-ate hopes," rather than unrealisti-cally sunny outlooks, should be fostered—and that when patients are feeling down, these feelings should be accepted as normal.

CANCER
Volume 100, page 1276
March 15, 2004

In addition, the majority of lung cancers detected by spiral CT appear to be in the earliest, most treatable stage. But there are disadvantages as well. Since spiral CT cannot distinguish between benign (noncancerous) and malignant (cancerous) tumors, it has a high rate of false positives, in which benign nodules are flagged as being possibly cancerous. This leads to unnecessary and risky lung biopsies and can turn a painless and relatively inexpensive test into a painful and expensive one. In fact, a recent analysis performed at Hopkins and published in the *Journal of the American Medical Association* in 2003 suggested that the procedure is not cost-effective and that the risks outweigh the benefits.

But other studies suggest that spiral CT screening for lung cancer may benefit some populations, particularly current and former smokers over age 60. In one study of 1,000 asymptomatic smokers and former smokers, the scan detected 23 early-stage cancers; standard chest x-rays missed 83% of them. Spiral CT outperformed chest x-rays on all fronts, uncovering three times as many suspicious nodules (small lumps of tissue) and four times as many cancerous tumors. Of the 27 cancerous tumors found by spiral CT scans in the study, 26 were successfully removed.

A multicenter study of spiral CT is under way to assess the rate of false-positive results and the test's impact on long-term lung cancer cure rates.

A biopsy of cancerous tissue is essential to make the diagnosis of lung cancer and to guide treatment decisions by determining the type of cancer. A biopsy sample can be obtained from the suspicious area using bronchoscopy, in which a thin, hollow, flexible tube is passed through the mouth and into the windpipe to allow viewing of the main bronchial passages. Tissue is obtained either directly from a bronchus or by passing a needle through a bronchus into adjacent tumor tissue. Alternatively, a CT-scan-guided needle biopsy through the chest wall may be used to obtain tissue from a suspicious growth within the lung. In people with suspected lung cancer, a positive result for cancer generally is reliable. A negative result does not necessarily exclude cancer, and further testing usually is necessary. This testing may include an open lung biopsy or a mediastinoscopy, in which the structures behind the breastbone in the chest cavity are examined. Sites of cancer spread—such as the lymph nodes, bone marrow, and pleura—also are suitable areas for biopsy.

Formal staging of cancer—including characteristics such as tumor size, involvement of particular lymph nodes within the chest, and presence of metastatic disease at other sites—is important for determining prognosis and selecting treatment options. Imaging procedures (for example, CT or MRI scans) are important components of this evaluation, and the recent availability of PET scans has been a major advance. While CT scans provide worthwhile anatomical information, PET scanning—in which a radioactive form of glucose (sugar) is administered to the patient—provides a metabolic assessment. Because growing tumors have high energy needs, detection of increased glucose uptake by the tumor may clarify the extent of cancer spread more accurately than CT scanning alone. An MRI provides more detailed evaluation of lung cancer that has spread to the brain.

Prevention

The best ways to prevent lung cancer are to avoid smoking and limit exposure to certain pollutants.

Smoking. Cigarette smoking is unquestionably the single greatest, controllable risk factor for lung cancer and the most common preventable cause of all premature deaths in the United States. Half of all smokers die prematurely of diseases related to smoking. While smoking cigars and pipes greatly increases the danger of cancers of the mouth, pharynx, larynx, and esophagus, the risk of lung cancer is not as high as with cigarette smoking because smoke from pipes and cigars usually is not inhaled as deeply or as frequently as cigarette smoke. The risk of lung cancer is greatest in those who start smoking at an early age and smoke the most cigarettes daily.

Because the risk of lung and other cancers gradually diminishes after smoking is discontinued, smokers can benefit from quitting at any age. The benefit of smoking cessation in reducing the risk of lung cancer becomes evident after about five years. The risk of developing lung cancer continues to decrease as the period without smoking lengthens but does not return to the level of someone who never smoked.

Radon. Many studies have examined the risk of lung cancer posed by radon in the home. Data from miners suggest that household levels of radon might account for about 15% of lung cancer deaths, an estimate supported by studies that have directly measured the risk of indoor radon. The U.S. Environmental Protection Agency (EPA) has recommended measuring radon levels in homes and reducing the levels when they exceed 4 picocuries per liter (pCi/L) over a year, a level estimated to be present in about 5% of American homes. Some critics have disagreed with this EPA recommendation,

NEW RESEARCH

Personalizing Nicotine Replacement May Help Quit Effort

Tailoring nicotine replacement therapy to smokers' personal characteristics might help more of them kick the habit, preliminary research suggests.

In a study looking at success rates with nicotine replacement nasal sprays and skin patches, certain smokers did better with sprays and others with patches. Specifically, smokers who were white, less nicotine dependent, or not obese had more success with nicotine patches (Nicoderm CQ), while minorities and smokers who were highly nicotine dependent or obese fared better on nicotine nasal spray (Nicotrol). Both methods were similarly effective: Among the 299 smokers in the study, 15% of those who used the patch and 12% who used the nicotine spray for eight weeks were able to abstain from smoking for six months.

Differences in how the therapies work may help explain the findings. For example, nicotine patches slowly increase a person's nicotine levels, while nasal sprays give a quick nicotine jolt that more closely mirrors smoking—which may explain why highly addicted smokers had more success with sprays.

Although more research is needed, the researchers conclude these findings provide "an important step" toward helping smokers and their doctors pick the nicotine replacement therapy with the best chance of helping them.

ANNALS OF INTERNAL MEDICINE
Volume 140, page 426
March 16, 2004

Advances in Treating Lung Cancer

Survival rates for lung cancer are poor, which is why developing new ways to treat the disease—or prevent it altogether—is so important.

Lung cancer is the most dangerous type of cancer, killing 85% of people within five years of diagnosis. "Lung cancer causes more deaths in women than breast and ovarian cancer combined, and more than three times more deaths in men than prostate cancer," emphasizes Julie Brahmer, M.D., an assistant professor at Hopkins's Sidney Kimmel Comprehensive Care Center.

But effective treatments for lung cancer do exist, with those that can extend survival by even a few months representing a significant advance in treatment. Treating lung cancer also can improve quality of life.

Here's an overview of the newest treatments for lung cancer, along with a look at drugs that are under development to treat or even prevent the disease.

New Combinations and Agents
Several new chemotherapy regimens for lung cancer have been developed in the last few years, and one drug has been approved.

New regimens. About 80% of lung cancers are non-small cell lung cancers. Treatment for this type of cancer usually consists of surgery followed by chemotherapy and, sometimes, radiation. In some cases, chemotherapy and radiation are used to shrink the tumor prior to surgery.

The drug cisplatin (Platinol) used to be the standard treatment for non-small cell lung cancer. Now, a second drug—such as gemcitabine (Gemzar), vinorelbine (Navelbine), paclitaxel (Taxol), or docetaxel (Taxotere)—is added to boost cisplatin's effectiveness. In addition, a less toxic drug called carboplatin (Paraplatin) sometimes is substituted for cisplatin. Like most chemotherapy regimens, these combinations usually cause temporary but severe side effects that may include nausea, vomiting, loss of appetite, hair loss, mouth sores, severe diarrhea, fatigue, and low resistance to infection.

Other regimens for non-small cell lung cancer are also being examined, such as gemcitabine (Gemzar) in combination with vinorelbine (Navelbine) or paclitaxel. Another combination that has shown promise in Japanese trials is uracil and tegafur, neither of which has been approved in the United States. The hope is that these combinations might be just as effective as older combinations, but

less toxic. Also being studied is becavizumab (Avastin), a drug that was recently approved for treating colon cancer, to see if it can extend survival when added to carboplatin and paclitaxel.

Small cell lung cancer accounts for the remaining 20% of lung cancers. Surgery is ineffective for this type of lung cancer, but chemotherapy and radiation are often used together for limited disease; chemotherapy alone is used for extensive disease.

Cisplatin plus etoposide (VePesid, Etopophos, Toposar) is usually considered the optimal chemotherapy regimen for small cell lung cancer. However, a Japanese study found that substituting irinotecan (Camptosar) for etoposide improved survival from 9.4 months to 12.8 months among people with metastatic disease (cancer that has spread beyond the lungs). Three randomized controlled trials are under way to test this finding. Researchers are also examining gemcitabine, paclitaxel, vinorelbine, and topotecan (Hycamtin) in combination with cisplatin for use in small cell lung cancer.

Gefitinib (Iressa). A new option for people with non-small cell lung

arguing that these levels of radon do not pose a significant risk and that attention should be focused on finding the homes with the highest levels. Recently, researchers estimated that reducing radon levels in all homes with readings higher than 4 pCi/L would result in 2% to 4% fewer lung cancer deaths.

To determine whether radon levels are high in your area, call your local EPA office. Taking a radon measurement in an individual house is the only way to definitively know the radon level, and several inexpensive kits are available in most hardware stores. Etched-track or electret detectors are good choices; the best of these kits take measurements over at least a three-month period.

cancer that doesn't respond to conventional chemotherapy is gefitinib, which was approved in 2003. In one study of 142 people whose tumors didn't respond to two or more types of chemotherapy, 11% had a response to gefitinib. This response lasted for at least seven months in half the people. It is unknown whether this response will translate into fewer cancer-related symptoms or longer survival. Unfortunately, attempts to boost the effectiveness of standard chemotherapy by adding gefitimib have been disappointing.

Gefitimib is taken by mouth and usually produces only minor side effects, such as diarrhea, rash, acne, and dry skin. It can also cause nausea and vomiting. Although it has several mechanisms of action, one of the ways in which it works is by blocking the activity of a tumor protein called epidermal growth factor (EGFR).

Researchers are studying other EGFR inhibitors for the treatment of non-small cell lung cancer, including erlotinib (Tarceva) and the monoclonal antibody cetuximab (Erbitux).

Novel Approaches

Two innovative approaches being tested for lung cancer treatment are vaccination and gene therapy.

Vaccination. The GVAX lung cancer vaccine is made from a patient's own tumor cells. These cells are genetically modified to secrete a hormone that stimulates the immune system to attack the tumor. In a study of 33 people with advanced non-small cell lung cancer who received the vaccine, 3 (9%) went into complete remission that lasted about a year and a half. Half the patients lived for at least a year, which is longer than the six or seven months seen in other studies with docetaxel. Two 75-person trials with the vaccine are currently being conducted.

Gene therapy. Researchers at M.D. Anderson Cancer Center and the University of Texas Southwestern have identified three tumor-suppressor genes that reduce human lung cancer growth in mice. They are hoping that by injecting the genes into a patient's lung tumor, cancer cells will die or grow more slowly.

Lung Cancer Prevention

Taking a medication to reduce the risk of cancer is a relatively new approach to cancer management. A number of agents are being tested to see if they can reduce the risk of lung cancer in people at high risk (mainly smokers and people who smoked for many years before quitting).

9-cis-retinoic acid. In a 2003 study of 177 former smokers, 9-cis-retinoic acid repaired some of the lung damage caused by smoking. This raises the possibility that 9-cis-retinoic acid, a substance related to vitamin A, might reduce the risk of lung cancer in former smokers.

Anethole dithiolethione (ADT). A recent Canadian study looked at the use of ADT, a drug used to treat dry mouth, in 101 current and former smokers with irregular growths in their lungs. Compared with a placebo, ADT halved the risk of developing new growths and progression of existing growths.

Cyclooxygenase inhibitors. A growing body of evidence indicates that the cyclooxygenase-2 (COX-2) enzyme plays a key role in lung cancer. Clinical trials are examining whether drugs that inhibit this enzyme, for example celecoxib (Celebrex), can reduce the risk of lung cancer in high-risk patients or enhance the effectiveness of chemotherapy regimens.

Other agents. Hopkins researchers are currently studying a drug called iloprost and a tea made from broccoli sprout extract in people at high risk for lung cancer, says Dr. Brahmer. To find out about more ongoing clinical trials, visit www.clinicaltrials.gov (national) or www.hopkinskimmelcancercenter.org/clinicaltrials/index.cfm (Hopkins only).

The label on the kit should say that it meets EPA requirements or is certified by the state. A state-certified contractor or one who has passed the EPA Radon Contractor Proficiency Program should be used if it is necessary to reduce radon levels in a home.

Dietary measures. Since damage of DNA by free radicals is considered one of the causes of many types of cancer, it was hoped that antioxidant supplements or an increased intake of antioxidant-rich foods might reduce the risk of lung cancer. A Scandinavian study, however, found that beta-carotene supplements increased the risk of lung cancer in cigarette smokers. Currently, no dietary measures are known to diminish the risk of lung cancer.

Treatment

The three options for treating lung cancer—surgery, chemotherapy, and radiation therapy—may be used alone or in combination. The choice of treatment depends on a number of factors, including the size and location of the tumor; whether the cancer is small cell or non-small cell; the physical condition of the patient; and whether the cancer has spread to lymph nodes or further. Because of the complexities involved with regard to treatment options, people with lung cancer should discuss their options with a multidisciplinary team of experts, which includes a pulmonologist, a thoracic surgeon, medical and radiation oncologists, and other health professionals.

Surgery. All people with lung cancer should be evaluated for possible surgery because surgery is the most effective treatment for non-small cell cancer. Resectability and operability are major considerations in deciding whether a person is a good candidate for surgery. A resectable tumor is one that can be removed in its entirety. If the tumor has spread extensively or is too close to vital structures, such as the heart or major blood vessels, it is no longer resectable. The decision that a tumor is not resectable usually is based on information from both the biopsy and scans. A tumor is considered operable if the patient is able to undergo the surgical procedure safely and can tolerate the extent of resection necessary for a cure. The patient's lung function and the presence of other diseases are key factors in determining operability.

Surgery may involve removal of a lobe (lobectomy) or an entire lung (pneumonectomy), and a hospital stay of one to two weeks usually is required. People with otherwise healthy lungs often can resume normal activities after a period of recuperation that varies based on their health status before surgery. Most people require two to six months to recover.

Chemotherapy. Chemotherapy is individualized for each patient and may involve administration of a combination of several drugs given in four to six cycles.

Possible side effects of chemotherapy include nausea and vomiting, loss of appetite, and hair loss. Reduced formation of red blood cells, white blood cells, and platelets due to the effects of these drugs on bone marrow can result in anemia, an increased risk of infection, and bleeding.

Radiation. External radiation may be the main form of treatment for people unable to tolerate surgery and for those whose cancer has spread beyond the reach of surgical removal. Radiation is administered five days a week for four to eight weeks. Radiation also may be directed to areas of cancer in the lung that cannot be removed with surgery or used to treat cancer that has spread to the brain or bones or that compresses the spinal cord. Side effects of external radiation include nausea and vomiting, local skin irritation, and fatigue.

PULMONARY EMBOLISM

A pulmonary embolus is a blockage in one or more of the arteries in the lungs. In almost all cases, it occurs when a blood clot (thrombus) originating in a deep vein in the legs, arms, or pelvis breaks loose and travels to the lungs. Depending on its size, the embolus (usually a thrombus that has broken loose) obstructs a large or small pulmonary artery within the lungs and blocks the flow of blood through that vessel. Estimates suggest that more than 600,000 people in the United States suffer a pulmonary embolism each year, and about 10% of cases are fatal. Fortunately, steps can be taken to prevent pulmonary emboli.

Pulmonary embolism varies in its severity and effects. Most dangerous is an acute, massive blood clot that blocks a main pulmonary artery and/or one of its branches. Another acute manifestation results when a small blood clot blocks a peripheral pulmonary artery (one near the surface of the lung). Some people have multiple, asymptomatic clots that block many medium-size pulmonary arteries. The network of blood vessels in the lungs is large enough to tolerate considerable amounts of obstruction, but such extensive blockage can increase the resistance to blood flow through the pulmonary arteries and eventually produce pulmonary hypertension (high blood pressure in the pulmonary arteries). Pulmonary hypertension places excessive stress on the heart's right ventricle, which pumps blood into the pulmonary arteries, potentially leading to right heart failure.

Causes
Air, amniotic fluid, or fat released from a broken bone may travel to a pulmonary artery and cause a pulmonary embolism. But the vast majority of pulmonary emboli are caused by blood clots from a deep vein in the leg, pelvis, or arm (deep vein thrombosis, or DVT). An estimated 5 million people in the United States suffer an episode of DVT annually. The condition is most common among women and older people.

A common cause of DVT is stagnation of blood flow due to immobility in bedridden people or healthy people who sit still for an extended period, such as on a long trip. Women taking oral contraceptives or hormone replacement therapy after menopause are at increased risk for DVT. People are at high risk for DVT after any major surgery, but especially after knee- or hip-replacement surgery.

A tendency for the blood to coagulate excessively (hypercoagulability) can predispose a person to DVT. The most frequent genetic abnormality that leads to hypercoagulability (present in about 5% of whites) is called factor V Leiden, which is due to a mutation in the gene for coagulation factor V. Having cancer also can cause the blood to coagulate excessively. In addition, injury to blood vessels by trauma, intravenous catheters or needles, or certain medications can cause blood clots.

Symptoms

Pulmonary emboli may produce sudden, severe shortness of breath, rapid breathing, and chest pain. Massive emboli, which often result in death within a few minutes, also may be accompanied by a feeling of impending doom, profuse sweating, loss of consciousness, a fall in blood pressure (shock), and cyanosis (a bluish color in the lips and fingertips). Peripheral emboli, which also occur abruptly and without warning, are associated with chest pain and coughing up blood (hemoptysis). People with multiple small emboli may have no symptoms for many months until they develop right heart failure with symptoms of fatigue, swelling of the ankles, weight loss, and shortness of breath.

Deep vein thrombosis can cause pain and swelling in the affected body part, and the area may be tender and feel hot to the touch. But because the condition usually occurs deep within the leg, about half the time there are no signs or symptoms. Often, DVT is discovered only when a physician looks for it in someone at high risk for the condition.

Diagnosis

Although a pulmonary embolus is suspected when symptoms occur in a person with typical findings of DVT, often there is no evidence of DVT. Large pulmonary emboli may be associated with changes that can be identified with an electrocardiogram (a recording of the electrical activity of the heart). Measurements of arterial blood gases (oxygen and carbon dioxide) may aid in making a diagnosis,

Risk Factors for Pulmonary Embolism

Pulmonary embolism is a life-threatening illness that is notoriously difficult to diagnose. But knowing the risk factors can help prevent the condition and increase the likelihood of early detection.

Most of the time pulmonary embolism is caused by a blood clot that forms in a deep vein in the leg, pelvis, or arm and then breaks loose, blocking an artery in the lungs. A number of factors increase the risk of pulmonary embolism, including modifiable factors, natural factors, factors related to women's health, medical illness, surgery, and a predisposition to abnormal clotting (thrombophilia). Not all cases of pulmonary embolism are caused by blood clots, however; other causes include fat from a broken bone or cement from a joint replacement. The chart below gives an overview of the risk factors for pulmonary embolism:

Modifiable
- Long-haul air travel
- Obesity
- Cigarette smoking
- Hypertension (high blood pressure)
- Immobility

Natural
- Increasing age

Women's health
- Oral contraceptives, including progesterone-only pills and especially third-generation pills
- Pregnancy
- Hormone replacement therapy
- Selective estrogen-receptor modulators such as raloxifene and tamoxifen

Medical illness
- Previous pulmonary embolism or deep vein thrombosis
- Cancer
- Heart failure
- Chronic obstructive pulmonary disease
- Diabetes
- Inflammatory bowel disease
- Antipsychotic drug use
- Chronic indwelling central venous catheter
- Permanent pacemaker
- Internal cardiac defibrillator
- Stroke with limb paresis (paralysis)
- Nursing-home confinement or current or repeated hospital admission
- Varicose veins

Surgical
- Trauma
- Orthopedic surgery, especially total hip replacement, total knee replacement, hip fracture surgery, knee arthroscopy
- General surgery, especially for cancer
- Gynecological and urological surgery, especially for cancer
- Neurosurgery, especially craniotomy (surgical opening of the skull) for brain tumor

Thrombophilia (an increased tendency for thrombosis)
- Factor V Leiden mutation
- Prothrombin gene mutation
- Hyperhomocysteinemia (elevated levels of homocysteine in the blood)
- Antiphospholipid antibody syndrome
- Deficiency of antithrombin III, protein C, or protein S
- High concentrations of factor VIII or XI
- Increased lipoprotein (a) levels

Nonthrombotic
- Air
- Foreign particles (e.g., hair, talc, as a consequence of intravenous drug misuse)
- Amniotic fluid
- Bone fragments, bone marrow
- Fat
- Cement

Source: Adapted from *The Lancet,* April 17, 2004, vol. 363, p. 1296.

but the results are not definitive.

Probably the most effective noninvasive test is a pulmonary isotope ventilation/perfusion (V/Q) scan. The test involves the intravenous injection of particles labeled with a radioactive substance. The particles become trapped in the small pulmonary blood vessels, and an external detector is used to locate the radioactivity. In healthy lungs, radioactivity is evenly distributed throughout the lungs. However, if a portion of the lung has had its blood supply blocked by a blood clot, there will be no radioactivity in that area. The diagnosis of a pulmonary embolus is highly unlikely when the

V/Q scan is normal.

Spiral CT scanning of the chest (see page 41) is being used increasingly to assess people with suspected pulmonary embolism. Studies to define its applications in this setting suggest that it can accurately diagnose large and medium-sized pulmonary emboli, but not small ones.

The most definitive diagnostic test is an angiogram of the pulmonary arteries—an x-ray following the injection of a contrast material into the pulmonary artery. An angiogram is an invasive procedure and is performed only when the results of other tests are insufficient to guide therapy.

Prevention

The only effective ways to prevent pulmonary emboli are to take measures to prevent the development of DVT and to recognize and treat DVT vigorously when it occurs. Steps to prevent DVT include taking frequent walks on long trips, getting out of bed as soon as possible after surgery, and using anticoagulants and other therapies (for example, pneumatic compression stockings) when possible in people who are bedridden or have had surgical procedures. People with a family history of frequent DVT should take special precautions, since they may have inherited an abnormal tendency for their blood to clot. People who have had DVT in the past also are at increased risk for a recurrence.

Treatment

During diagnostic evaluation, supportive treatment for someone with a large pulmonary embolus includes pain relief and oxygen. Administration of "clot-busting" drugs (thrombolytic agents) may dissolve the clot and restore blood flow through the blocked pulmonary artery. Surgical removal of the blood clot may be required if a patient has a large life-threatening clot and if his or her condition deteriorates during medical treatment. Thrombolytic therapy and surgery generally are reserved for people with massive clots and hemodynamic instability (shock). Most of the time, however, people with a pulmonary embolus are treated with anticoagulants—heparin and warfarin (Coumadin)—in both the short and long term. Intravenous heparin is started immediately and continued for at least five days, and oral warfarin is continued for three to six months, with close monitoring of the patient.

Anticoagulants are ineffective for preventing further emboli in some people and can be dangerous in people who are at high risk for bleeding in the head (such as people with a brain aneurysm or a vascular malformation) or have active gastrointestinal bleeding. In these instances, a sieve-like filtering device may be placed in the inferior vena cava (the vein that returns blood from the lower body to the heart) to prevent blood clots from entering the heart and lungs. Filters are also useful for people who have had recurrent bouts of pulmonary emboli. These devices become obstructed over time, but the flow of blood is not significantly affected because blood can be carried back to the heart through smaller blood vessels, called collateral vessels, that develop around the obstruction. Continued use of anticoagulants is needed because clots can still reach the lungs through these new blood vessels.

INFECTIONS

The respiratory tract has a remarkable defense system to protect against the numerous microorganisms we breathe in each day. But sometimes bacteria, viruses, or other microorganisms overwhelm this defense system and cause a respiratory infection. There are many different types of respiratory infections, but this White Paper focuses on acute bronchitis, influenza, bacterial pneumonia, and tuberculosis.

The signs and symptoms of a lung infection may overlap with those of a noninfectious lung disease and make diagnosis difficult. In fact, people with noninfectious lung diseases are at increased risk for respiratory infections, either from the lung disease itself, its treatment (for example, with corticosteroids), or a combination of both. Conversely, a respiratory infection may cause scarring of the lungs and worsening lung function that set the stage for future, recurrent episodes of lung infection.

Acute Bronchitis

Acute bronchitis refers to inflammation of the bronchi. When the bronchi are infected, they become inflamed and plugged with mucus.

Causes. Bronchitis usually is caused by a viral infection, typically a cold virus. It also can be triggered by exposure to chemical fumes, dust, smoke, or other air pollutants. Cigarette smokers and people with obstructive lung disease (such as asthma or COPD) or heart failure are at increased risk for acute bronchitis.

Symptoms. The predominant symptom of acute bronchitis is a persistent cough that may produce gray, green, or yellowish

NEW RESEARCH

Vitamin E May Help Elderly Beat Common Cold

A daily dose of vitamin E may give nursing home residents a defense against the common cold, research suggests.

The study of 617 nursing home patients found that those randomized to take a vitamin E supplement every day for a year were nearly 20% less likely to develop a cold or any upper-respiratory infections than those who took a placebo. The vitamin did not, however, guard against the potentially dangerous lung infections pneumonia and bronchitis.

In a previous study, the researchers had found that vitamin E seemed to enhance immune responses in elderly adults. It's possible, they speculate, that the vitamin may ward off viral infections, such as colds, but not bacterial infections, which frequently underlie pneumonia and other lower-respiratory illnesses.

The new study involved men and women age 65 and older at 33 nursing homes in the Boston area. Half took 200 IU of vitamin E every day in addition to a multivitamin, and the other half took a multivitamin and a placebo pill.

Further research, the authors conclude, should look at whether the vitamin battles the common cold specifically and whether the nutrient has different effects against bacterial and viral infections.

JOURNAL OF THE AMERICAN MEDICAL ASSOCIATION
Volume 292, page 828
August 18, 2004

phlegm. The cough may be preceded by a headache, fever, sore throat, or other symptoms typical of the common cold. Severe coughing bouts may produce chest pain. Other symptoms are breathing difficulties and wheezing. In healthy adults, the symptoms of bronchitis generally disappear on their own in a few days.

Diagnosis. A diagnosis is based on the signs and symptoms. A chest x-ray may be needed to rule out other lung disorders, but acute bronchitis does not produce any abnormalities that can be seen on an x-ray.

Prevention. The most important thing you can do to prevent acute bronchitis is not to smoke. In addition, you can reduce your chances of picking up a cold virus by avoiding exposure to people with respiratory infections.

Treatment. Usually, no treatment other than smoking cessation is necessary for acute bronchitis. Sometimes dextromethorphan syrup and an albuterol inhaler are used, but antibiotics and antihistamines appear to have no effect if the acute episode is due to a viral infection. However, in people with chronic pulmonary disease, such as asthma, COPD, cystic fibrosis, or interstitial lung disease, a viral infection that destroys the protective layer of cells that lines the trachea and bronchi may lead to a superimposed bacterial infection that can worsen the underlying lung disease or lead to pneumonia. In such people, an attack of acute bronchitis usually is treated with antibiotics.

Influenza

Influenza is an acute infection usually involving the upper respiratory tract. Outbreaks of influenza occur each winter and last for two to three months, producing infection in 10% to 20% of the general population. Influenza can worsen the symptoms of COPD and asthma. In addition, influenza can make a person more prone to a bacterial infection that causes pneumonia, or the influenza virus itself can cause pneumonia.

Causes. The cause of influenza is a viral infection. Influenza A virus is responsible for most of the outbreaks, causing more severe disease and more deaths than influenza B or C.

Symptoms. Influenza produces the well-recognized symptoms of the flu—headache, fever, and muscle aches that may be accompanied by chills, cough, sore throat, and weakness. Acute symptoms usually last for two to five days.

Diagnosis. A diagnosis of influenza is made when an influenza outbreak is present in the community and a person's complaints fit

Quitting Smoking: Instant Benefits

Virtually the minute you quit smoking, your health begins to improve.

The negative effects of smoking are clear: One in every three people who starts smoking will die prematurely of a smoking-related illness, the American Lung Association says, and one in every five deaths stems directly from tobacco exposure. But the good news is that it's never too late to quit smoking. The benefits of smoking cessation begin within a few minutes of your last cigarette and continue for life, even for people with lung disease.

The Risks of Smoking

Although smoking's link to lung cancer is well known, the habit is even more likely to cause a range of other illnesses. According to a 2003 survey published in *Morbidity and Mortality Weekly Report*, some 8.6 million Americans were living with a major smoking-related illness in 2000. The most common of these was chronic bronchitis (35% of cases), followed by emphysema (24%), heart attacks (19%), nonlung cancer (12%), strokes (8%), and lung cancer (1%).

The true number of people affected by smoking is probably much higher than the researchers stated because this study depended on people to report whether a doctor had ever told them they had a certain condition. People tend to underreport their own illnesses. In addition, the researchers did not look at nondebilitating conditions, such as impotence and sinusitis, that are often caused by cigarette smoking.

The Benefits of Quitting

Regardless of how long you smoked, your health begins to improve shortly after your last cigarette. And the longer you are smoke free, the greater the benefits become. The chart below lists a timeline of these health improvements.

Time Since Last Cigarette	Health Benefits
20 minutes	Elevated blood pressure levels begin to drop, and the temperature in your extremities begins to return to normal.
8 hours	You achieve normal blood levels of carbon monoxide.
1 day	Your risk of a heart attack begins to decline.
2 weeks to 3 months	Circulation improves, and lung function increases, decreasing the risk of lung infections.
1 to 9 months	Shortness of breath, sinus congestion, coughing, and fatigue improve. A few months of smoking cessation improves lung function about 5% in patients with chronic obstructive pulmonary disease (COPD), and the risk of death from COPD declines.
1 year	Your risk of having a heart attack is cut in half.
5 years	The risk of cancer in the oral cavity and esophagus is already half that of continuing smokers, and the risk continues to decline with continued cessation.
5 to 15 years	The risk of a stroke becomes similar to that of a lifelong nonsmoker.
10 years	Your risk of developing lung cancer is 30% to 50% lower than it would be had you continued to smoke, and the risk continues to decline with continued abstinence. Also, you've significantly decreased your risk of developing cancer of the bladder, cervix, esophagus, kidney, mouth, pancreas, and throat.
10 to 15 years	Your odds of dying of any cause are the same as those of someone who never smoked.
15 years	Your risk of having a heart attack is the same as a lifelong nonsmoker.

the current pattern of symptoms.

Prevention. The Centers for Disease Control and Prevention (CDC) recommends annual flu vaccinations for high-risk individuals to prevent or reduce the symptoms of influenza. This includes people age 65 and older, those with lung diseases (such as COPD and asthma), and people with certain chronic illnesses. During the 2004 flu vaccine shortage, people with these and other specific health conditions had priority over healthy people in getting the vaccine.

A needle-free influenza vaccine called FluMist that is squirted into the nostrils became available in late 2003, but this version is approved only for healthy people between the ages of 5 and 49.

In addition, the antiviral drugs amantadine (Symmetrel) and rimantadine (Flumadine) are 70% to 100% effective in preventing influenza during an outbreak when given to high-risk people who did not receive the flu vaccine.

Another antiviral drug, oseltamivir (Tamiflu), was recently approved for prevention of influenza in adults and adolescents. Not enough studies have been done in older people or those with chronic illnesses to say whether it effective in these people, but it does not appear to be harmful.

Treatment. People with influenza should get plenty of rest and drink lots of fluids. Over-the-counter products such as decongestants, antihistamines, and pain relievers may relieve symptoms. Although antibiotics may be helpful when influenza is complicated by a superimposed bacterial infection, these drugs have no impact on the influenza virus itself.

Certain prescription medications can shorten the duration of influenza if taken soon after symptoms appear. Amantadine and rimantadine can reduce symptoms by about half if administered within 48 hours of symptom onset. About 10% of people have central nervous system side effects, such as anxiety and jitters, when treated with amantadine. These problems are less common with rimantadine. Because of the side effects and inconsistent effectiveness of these drugs, the recent availability of two other antiviral therapies, oseltamivir and zanamivir (Relenza), has been an important development for people with influenza. Oseltamivir is an oral medication; zanamivir is inhaled. Use of these drugs early in the illness (within the first two days of onset of symptoms) has been associated with symptomatic improvement and a milder course of infection.

Pneumonia

Pneumonia is an infection of the air spaces (alveoli) and surrounding (interstitial) lung tissue. It is the sixth leading cause of death and the primary cause of death from infectious disease in the United States, claiming the lives of nearly 65,000 Americans in 2002. Most fatalities occur in people over the age of 65, who often have underlying disorders that increase their susceptibility to infection. Others at high risk for pneumonia include people with lung cancer or a suppressed immune system (for example, people with HIV or those who take immunosuppressive medications).

Based on x-ray findings, the types of pneumonia often are divided into those that affect a single lobe (lobar pneumonia) and those that occur as patches in several lobes (multilobar pneumonia). In addition, pneumonia may involve either one lung (unilateral) or both lungs (bilateral). Pneumonia types may be further divided on the basis of whether they involve the alveoli, interstitium, or both.

Causes. Hundreds of different microorganisms can infect the lungs. Viruses and bacteria are the most common infectious agents that cause acute pneumonia, but other organisms (such as *Mycoplasma pneumoniae, Mycobacterium tuberculosis,* fungi, and the parasite *Pneumocystis carinii*) may be responsible, especially if a person's immune defenses are compromised. Environmental exposure and the setting in which pneumonia occurs (for example, in the community, a nursing home, or a hospital) are major determinants of the type of pneumonia and the type of microorganism that most likely caused it.

The most common type of bacterial pneumonia is pneumococcal pneumonia. It is caused by the bacterium *Streptococcus pneumoniae,* which frequently is present in the throats of healthy people. It can spread from person to person (for example, by coughing) when people are in close contact with others, as is the case in military barracks, prisons, and nursing homes. Most people who develop pneumococcal pneumonia have some underlying disease. It may be an acute infection like influenza, but more often it is a chronic condition such as diabetes, alcoholism, cirrhosis, AIDS, a lung disease like chronic obstructive pulmonary disease (COPD), or a blood disorder like leukemia. Also at increased risk are cigarette smokers and individuals who are chronically malnourished or debilitated. Pneumococcal pneumonia is far more common in the elderly. For example, the number of cases per 100,000 people ranges from 20 in young adults to 280 in people over the age of 75.

Other common causes of bacterial pneumonia include *Haemo-*

NEW RESEARCH

Flu Shot Shields COPD Patients From Complications

Immunization against influenza may sharply cut the rate of flu-related acute respiratory illness in people with chronic obstructive pulmonary disease (COPD), a new study suggests.

While annual flu shots are recommended for everyone with COPD, the researchers note, few studies have investigated the effectiveness of immunization in these patients over the long term.

Among 125 patients with moderate to severe COPD given the influenza vaccine or placebo and followed for 16 months, those who had been vaccinated were much less likely to develop acute respiratory illness (ARI) related to flu, regardless of the severity of the disease, presence of other illness, age, or whether or not they smoked.

None of the patients given the vaccine required mechanical ventilation assistance because of flu-related respiratory illness, the researchers found, but all of the patients who didn't receive the vaccine and were hospitalized for ARI did require breathing help. As expected, the flu shot did not protect against non–flu-related ARI.

People with COPD should get an annual flu shot. According to an editorial accompanying the study, the report underscores the importance of getting immunized if you're at high risk for flu complications.

CHEST
Volume 125, pages 1971 and 2011
June 2004

philus influenzae (not to be confused with the influenza virus), *Legionella pneumophila* (the cause of Legionnaires' disease), *Staphylococcus aureus,* and gram-negative organisms like *Klebsiella pneumoniae, Pseudomonas aeruginosa,* and Proteus. Gram-negative and *S. aureus* pneumonias often are acquired during hospitalization and are associated with a high risk of death.

Half of all pneumonia cases are caused by viruses rather than by bacteria. Viral pneumonia most often is a complication of influenza, especially in older adults and those with other health problems. Other possible causes of viral pneumonia include parainfluenza, adenovirus, rhinovirus, herpes simplex virus, respiratory syncytial virus, hantavirus, and cytomegalovirus. Like bacterial pneumonia, a virus that causes pneumonia can spread through close contact with an infected person.

Most cases of viral pneumonia are mild and get better on their own. People at risk for more severe cases include the elderly, young children, and people with impaired immune systems (such as transplant recipients or people with HIV). People with viral pneumonia may also develop a bacterial infection, which can make their illness more serious.

Symptoms. In bacterial pneumonia, the onset of symptoms is typically abrupt. Symptoms may include a cough that produces yellow phlegm, high fever, chills, sharp chest pain precipitated by breathing or coughing, and shortness of breath. Young patients usually have increased breathing and heart rates and appear acutely ill. Many older adults have fewer symptoms, often have no fever, and experience lethargy and confusion with or without lung-related symptoms.

The early symptoms of viral pneumonia may resemble those of infection with the influenza virus: a dry cough, fever, headache, muscle pain, and weakness. Twelve to 36 hours later, people with viral pneumonia often experience increased breathlessness, worsening cough with mucus, high fever, and, possibly, blueness of the lips. People with very serious viral pneumonia may have extreme difficulty breathing.

Diagnosis. The initial diagnosis of all types of pneumonia is made from the patient's medical history, physical examination, and chest x-ray, which may show a variety of abnormalities. The organism responsible for the pneumonia may be recognized by examining the patient's phlegm under a microscope. Ideally, a phlegm sample should be obtained before treatment, but treatment should not be delayed while waiting for the phlegm to be analyzed.

Other routine laboratory tests in people with suspected pneumonia include a blood cell count, measurement of serum electrolytes, urinalysis, liver function tests, and blood cultures. In bacterial pneumonia, the white blood cell count is typically high. In contrast, the white cell count usually is low or normal in people with viral or mycoplasma pneumonia but may also be low in people with severe bacterial pneumonia.

Prevention. Although most types of bacterial pneumonia cannot be prevented, the pneumococcal vaccine is effective against 88% of the bacterial strains of *S. pneumoniae* and in preventing 60% to 70% of cases of pneumococcal pneumonia. Influenza vaccine reduces the risk of viral pneumonia.

The CDC recommends vaccination against pneumococcal pneumonia and influenza for the following people: anyone age 65 or older; people with chronic cardiovascular or lung disorders (but not those with asthma who are otherwise healthy); people with diabetes or chronic liver or kidney disease; and those with a suppressed immune system due to cancer chemotherapy or to conditions such as leukemia, multiple myeloma, or HIV.

Even people who have already had pneumococcal pneumonia should get the pneumococcal vaccine; an *S. pneumoniae* infection may confer immunity to one particular strain of the bacterium, but an infection with another strain is still possible. While the vaccine was previously given only once, a booster is now recommended every five years for people who were first vaccinated before age 65. The influenza vaccine should be given every fall, and it is safe to get at the same time as the pneumococcal vaccine.

Treatment. The treatment for pneumonia depends on the cause. Because of practical difficulties in obtaining satisfactory phlegm specimens and delays in obtaining results, antibiotic treatment often is based on the patient's characteristics, where he or she likely became infected, and the physician's suspicions about the most likely causative organism. The severity of pneumonia, the patient's general health status, and the availability of family and other caregivers to take care of the patient at home determine whether treatment requires hospitalization.

Antibiotics are the mainstay of treatment for bacterial pneumonia (as well as for some other types such as mycoplasma pneumonia), and early treatment produces the best outcomes. The antibiotic of choice depends on the type of bacteria responsible for the pneumonia. At one time, *S. pneumoniae* was highly sensitive to penicillin, but penicillin-resistant strains have become more common;

NEW RESEARCH

Prompt Antibiotics Cut Pneumonia Death Rate

Elderly pneumonia patients who get antibiotics within four hours of arriving at the hospital are less likely to die than those who must wait longer, according to a large study.

Among 13,771 Medicare patients who went to the hospital in 1998-1999 for pneumonia, those treated with antibiotics within four hours of admission were 15% less likely to die either in the hospital or during the 30 days after admission. They also had a slightly shorter hospital stay, on average. None of the patients had taken antibiotics before going to the hospital.

Pneumonia is an inflammation of the lungs, but in severe cases inflammation can spread throughout the body. Giving antibiotics to severely affected patients quickly, the study authors note, may halt this process before permanent organ damage occurs.

Overall, 61% of patients in the study received antibiotics within four hours of hospital arrival, with higher rates at smaller hospitals. Getting the drugs to all pneumonia patients quickly may be a challenge at large metropolitan hospitals, according to the researchers, but these centers could make improvements by modeling systems used at smaller hospitals.

ARCHIVES OF INTERNAL MEDICINE
Volume 164, page 637
March 22, 2004

newer antibiotics may be needed to treat highly resistant strains. In addition, because mycoplasmas and other atypical microorganisms also may cause pneumonia, and their symptoms may overlap with those of pneumonia caused by *S. pneumoniae,* combinations of antibiotics, such as a macrolide and another class of antibiotic, are generally used.

Antibiotics are not effective against viral pneumonias. Most people with viral pneumonia recover without treatment in one to three weeks. Patients may also need humidified air, supplemental oxygen, and increased fluids.

With treatment, symptom improvement usually is rapid, and the speed of recovery often depends on the patient's previous health status. For hospitalized patients with bacterial pneumonia, an early switch from intravenous to oral antibiotics as symptoms improve has been found to be safe and effective and allows earlier discharge from the hospital. The disappearance of chest x-ray abnormalities typically lags behind symptom improvement, especially in older people with multilobar pneumonia, COPD, or alcoholism.

Tuberculosis

Worldwide there are more deaths from tuberculosis (TB) than from any other single infectious disease. Recent studies show that TB is responsible for 7% of all deaths and 26% of all preventable deaths. About 95% of these deaths (and 95% of the estimated 8 million new cases of TB in 1997) occurred in developing countries.

New TB cases in the United States declined steadily between 1950 and the mid-1980s, then began to increase, and reached a peak in 1992. About 16,000 cases were diagnosed in 2000, with most new cases occurring in ethnic and racial minorities. Compared with non-Hispanic whites, the incidence of new cases is 10 times greater in blacks and 5 times greater in Hispanics and Native Americans. The number of TB cases is three times higher in urban than in rural areas and is increased in the elderly and in people with diabetes.

One probable cause for the rise in TB in recent years is the epidemic of HIV and AIDS, which greatly increases the chance that an inactive TB infection will become activated and produce clinical disease and symptoms. The rise in U.S. cases of TB also is attributable to increasing numbers of immigrants, homeless people, and drug users, all of whom are at increased risk for TB. Another major problem is the development of TB organisms that are resistant to the drugs used to treat the disease. Over the last 30 years, the prevalence of multidrug-resistant organisms has risen from 2% to

9% and is especially high in certain urban areas.

Causes. Tuberculosis infections are caused by *Mycobacterium tuberculosis*, which usually infects the lungs, but about one third of infections also involve other organs. Most often, people become infected by inhaling TB-containing microdroplets released into the air from the upper airway of a person infected with pulmonary TB. These microdroplets are released when the infected person coughs, sneezes, or speaks. Once a person becomes infected, the development of an immune response to the organism, which occurs over a 4- to 10-week period, normally reduces the extent of inflammation and causes the bacteria to become dormant. However, the organisms remain alive and can become reactivated at any time.

Symptoms. Most people have no symptoms during the stage of a TB infection when the bacteria are dormant, but some may notice a low-grade fever, sweats, and cough for a short period of time. In about 10% of people with a TB infection, the bacteria become reactivated and symptoms of active TB appear. The likelihood of developing active disease is greatest in the first year or two after infection and diminishes with the length of time following the infection. The risk of activation is especially high for those with diminished immunity due to older age, HIV or other chronic viral infections, Hodgkin's disease, leukemia, malnutrition, or treatment with immunosuppressive agents for an organ transplant or with corticosteroids for other medical problems. The risk of activation also is increased in people with silicosis, chronic kidney failure that requires dialysis, hemophilia, and diabetes. In about one third of cases, active disease results from reinfection rather than activation of latent disease. Symptoms of active disease include fever, night sweats, weight loss, and fatigue. Other manifestations depend on whether the disease remains localized to the lungs or spreads to other sites. While TB can spread to almost any site of the body, the most common sites, in decreasing order of frequency, are the lymph nodes, urogenital system, bones and joints, and linings of the brain (meninges), abdominal cavity (peritoneum), and heart (pericardium).

In the lungs, the disease most commonly occurs in the upper lobes, but it often affects the lower lobes in the elderly, in immuno-suppressed people, and in those with diabetes. Progression of the disease in the lungs may cause cough, production of bloody phlegm, and shortness of breath. Spread of TB through the blood-stream may produce myriad tiny lesions throughout both lungs—a condition known as miliary tuberculosis, because the 1- to 2-mm, yellow lung lesions resemble millet seeds. Spread to the pleura is common and may produce chest pain, fever, and pleural effusion that, if large, can cause shortness of breath.

Diagnosis. During the early infectious stage, before the onset of active disease but after the development of immunity, the presence of TB infection can be confirmed by a positive skin test, which involves injecting PPD (a purified protein from the tuberculosis bacterium) into the skin of the forearm. Most infected people will show an area of skin thickening (induration) at the injection site 48 to 72 hours later. The response to the PPD test often is blunted in people who are immunosuppressed. The PPD skin test is not as useful for the diagnosis of active disease: It is negative in about 20% of such people because of immunosuppression or severe disease, and a positive test in such individuals may only indicate a prior infection that is not active.

Once infection has progressed to active disease, the diagnosis can be strongly suspected from a chest x-ray that shows the changes in the upper lobes in the lungs, often with lesions that have a central cavity. The x-ray may also show enlargement of lymph nodes. The diagnosis is confirmed by finding the TB organism in phlegm examined under a microscope. Definitive diagnosis requires growing the organism, obtained from phlegm or other sites, in culture. These cultured bacteria are then tested for their sensitivity to various drugs. Because the TB bacteria grow so slowly, conventional culturing techniques require four to eight weeks to obtain a result; newer culture methods allow growth in two to three weeks. A diagnosis of TB requires a positive culture of bacteria from the affected site(s).

Prevention. People with active TB need to be treated so that they will not spread the infection. People in contact with TB patients can reduce their risk of contracting the infection by using masks and special lamps that kill the bacteria with ultraviolet light. Isoniazid (Laniazid, Nydrazid), also known as INH, may be used to prevent TB in people at high risk, such as those with HIV or other causes of immunosuppression. Studies also have shown a highly significant decrease in the development of active TB when people with latent infection, indicated by a positive PPD test, are treated for 6 to 12 months with daily INH.

Vaccination with an weakened strain of a bovine form of mycobacterium (BCG) once was widely advocated as a way to raise immunity to TB bacteria. Though still used in the United States in

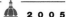

special circumstances (for example, in highly exposed health care workers), BCG vaccination is not recommended for the general population because of uncertainty about its effectiveness.

Treatment. More than half of untreated people with active disease die within five years, yet TB can be cured in almost all people infected with a TB organism that is sensitive to drugs. Treatment of TB typically involves the simultaneous use of two or more drugs to avoid the emergence of resistant strains. Before treatment is started, a complete blood count is performed and baseline tests are carried out to measure liver and kidney function. Standard treatment now involves triple drug therapy—most commonly, a combination of INH, rifampin (Rifadin, Rimactane), and pyrazinamide (available only in a generic form), either daily or three times a week, for two months. This period is followed by a four-month course of INH plus rifampin given two or three times weekly. Because INH interferes with the action of pyridoxine (vitamin B_6), supplements of the vitamin are given to people at high risk for vitamin deficiency. Ethambutol (Myambutol) or streptomycin may be added when a resistant strain is suspected. Treatment should continue for at least nine months in people whose disease has spread beyond the lungs. People who do not follow their medication regimens may be required to take their medication under observation.

During treatment, people with phlegm that contains the TB organism have regular phlegm cultures every month until the cultures are negative; repeat chest x-rays are not required in all patients. Phlegm cultures no longer contain the TB organism in about 80% of patients after two months of treatment and in virtually all patients with drug-sensitive organisms after three months. Persistence of organisms at three months is considered a treatment failure. Most people with pulmonary TB become noninfectious to others after about two weeks of treatment.

Although INH is included in nearly all regimens for the treatment of TB, about 5% of patients have adverse reactions to the medication. Of greatest concern is life-threatening liver toxicity, manifested by loss of appetite, nausea and vomiting, fatigue, weakness, jaundice, and dark urine. The risk of liver toxicity increases in older people and in people taking rifampin. Blood tests to check for liver disease are not obtained regularly during treatment but are done if the patient develops one or more of the signs of liver toxicity mentioned above. The drug INH also can cause skin rash and peripheral neuropathy (nerve damage in the hands and feet) with paresthesias (tingling sensations). Side effects of rifampin

NEW RESEARCH

Building Dampness, Mold Worsen Respiratory Problems

Indoor dampness and mold can exacerbate symptoms in people with asthma and cause breathing difficulties in healthy people, the Institute of Medicine has concluded after a review of available scientific evidence.

Damp conditions and associated problems may also be linked to asthma onset, shortness of breath, and other types of lower respiratory illness, according to the institute, a private, nonprofit group providing health policy advice to Congress.

The institute says public health initiatives must be launched to address indoor dampness and efforts should be made to change building design, construction, and maintenance to deal with the problem. Steps must also be taken to identify which strategies for coping with mold and moisture will be most effective in preventing health problems.

Laboratory and animal studies have found that molds and bacteria growing in damp indoor conditions can produce toxins and inflammation-producing substances, but there should be more research on the effects of longer-term, lower-level exposure to these particles, the institute recommends, adding that more study also is needed on the health effects of exposure to chemicals and particles released from wet building and furnishing material.

INSTITUTE OF MEDICINE: DAMP INDOOR SPACES AND HEALTH

http://national-academies.org
May 2004

include hepatitis and gastrointestinal symptoms. Blood uric acid is measured before and during treatment in people taking pyrazinamide because the drug can elevate uric acid levels and cause joint pain or gout. Visual acuity is assessed before starting ethambutol because the drug can cause optic neuritis (inflammation of the optic nerve in the eye). Streptomycin, which must be given by injection, can cause dizziness, difficulty walking, or hearing loss. ■

GLOSSARY

acute—Having a short and relatively severe course.

alpha$_1$-antitrypsin—A naturally occurring substance in the body that protects against damage to the walls of the alveoli by blocking the action of enzymes that break down proteins. A deficiency in this substance is one cause of emphysema.

alveoli—Tiny air sacs in the lungs. The walls of the alveoli contain capillaries, which absorb inhaled oxygen into the bloodstream and release carbon dioxide from the bloodstream to the lungs to be exhaled.

apnea—Cessation of breathing.

arterial blood gases—A measurement of the oxygen, carbon dioxide, and acidity of blood taken from an artery.

asthma—A disease characterized by inflammation and narrowing of the bronchi, making breathing difficult.

atelectasis—Reduced inflation of the lungs, often related to blockage of a bronchus by mucus, a tumor, or a foreign body.

blood pressure—Pressure of blood against the walls of an artery.

bronchi—Large airways in the lungs that branch from the trachea.

bronchiectasis—Persistent dilatation of the bronchi or bronchioles as the result of another disease, such as a lung infection, tumor, or cystic fibrosis.

bronchioles—Small airways in the lungs that branch from the bronchi.

bronchiolitis obliterans—Obstructive inflammation of the bronchioles.

bronchodilators—Medications that open airways by relaxing bronchial smooth muscles.

bronchoscopy—Passage of a thin, hollow, flexible tube through the mouth and windpipe to allow viewing of the main bronchial passages.

catheter—A thin, flexible tube.

chronic—Persisting over a long period.

chronic obstructive pulmonary disease (COPD)—A group of lung diseases, mainly emphysema and chronic bronchitis, characterized by an obstruction of airflow during exhalation.

cilia—Small hairs that line the bronchioles and move mucus out of the lungs with a wavelike motion.

cor pulmonale—Heart disease due to resistance of blood flow through the lungs; it often leads to right heart failure.

corticosteroids—Medications that reduce inflammation, for example, in the airways.

cyanosis—Bluish color of the skin as a result of insuffi-cient oxygen in the blood.

deep vein thrombosis—A condition caused by formation of blood clots in the deep veins of the body.

diaphragm—The muscular structure that separates the chest cavity from the abdomen. The diaphragm plays an important role in breathing.

diffusion capacity—A measurement of how well gas passes across membranes in the lungs.

dyspnea—Sensation of shortness of breath or difficulty in breathing.

emphysema—A disease in which damage to the alveoli causes the lungs to lose their elasticity. People with emphysema are unable to move adequate quantities of fresh air through their lungs.

epiglottis—A flap of cartilage in the back of the throat that prevents food from entering the trachea.

expiration—Exhalation.

fibrosis—A process by which inflamed tissue becomes scarred. Scarring in the lungs is called pulmonary fibrosis.

hemoptysis—Coughing up blood.

hypoxemia—Inadequate oxygen in the blood.

inspiration—Inhalation.

interstitial lung disease—A group of lung disorders that affect the supporting matrix of the lungs.

interstitium—The supporting matrix of the lungs, as opposed to the airways and air sacs.

larynx—Voice box.

lobe—A section of the lung; the right lung has three lobes, while the left lung has two.

lobectomy—Removal of an entire lobe of the lung.

lung volume—The amount of air in the lungs.

lung volume reduction surgery (LVRS)—A surgical procedure in which lung tissue affected by emphysema is removed.

lung volume tests—Tests to measure the amount of air in the lungs.

pharynx—Throat.

pleura—The membranes that cover the outside of the lungs and the inside wall of the chest cavity.

pleural effusion—Fluid within the pleural space.

pneumonectomy—Removal of an entire lung.

pneumonia—An infection in the lungs.

pneumothorax—Leakage of air into the space around the lung.

pulmonary artery—The blood vessel that delivers oxygen-poor blood from the right ventricle of the heart to the lungs.

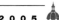

pulmonary embolism—A condition that occurs when a blood clot travels from a vein in the leg, pelvis, or arm and lodges in the pulmonary artery.

pulmonary fibrosis—Chronic inflammation and progressive scarring of the walls of the alveoli. When the cause is unknown, it is called idiopathic pulmonary fibrosis.

pulmonary function tests—A group of procedures used to evaluate the status of the lungs and to confirm the presence of certain lung disorders.

pulmonary hypertension—Abnormally high blood pressure in the arteries of the lungs.

respiration—The process of breathing; also defined as gas exchange from air to the blood and from the blood to the body's cells.

sleep apnea—Temporary cessation of breathing during sleep, often leading to daytime sleepiness.

spirometer—An instrument used in a pulmonary function test; it records the total volume and rate of air being breathed out. This test helps to diagnose or assess a lung disorder or to monitor its treatment.

spirometry—Measurement of the volume of air forcefully exhaled by the lungs as a function of time.

systemic—Affecting the body as a whole.

total lung capacity—The amount of air in the lungs after maximal inspiration.

trachea—Windpipe.

vasodilator—An agent that widens blood vessels.

ventilation—Movement of air (gases) in and out of the lungs.

x-ray—A procedure that uses invisible electromagnetic energy to produce images of bones, organs, and internal tissues.

HEALTH INFORMATION ORGANIZATIONS AND SUPPORT GROUPS

American Academy of Allergy, Asthma & Immunology
611 East Wells St.
Milwaukee, WI 53202
☎ 800-822-2762
    414-272-6071
www.aaaai.org
Offers public education on allergies and asthma through children's books, tips brochures, videos, newsletters, and a Web site. Offers referrals for allergists and immunologists. Supports asthma and allergy research through grants to medical training programs.

American Association for Respiratory Care
11030 Ables Ln.
Dallas, TX 75229
☎ 972-243-2272
www.aarc.org
Society of respiratory health professionals. Web site supplies respiratory health tips, quizzes, and links to other organizations.

American Lung Association
61 Broadway, 6th Fl.
New York, NY 10006
☎ 212-315-8700
www.lungusa.org
Oldest voluntary health organization in the United States. Funds and conducts research on all lung disorders, with a special emphasis on asthma. Institutes school and workplace educational programs; provides information on air quality and tobacco dangers.

American Thoracic Society
61 Broadway
New York, NY 10006-2747
☎ 212-315-8600
www.thoracic.org
International organization that funds research and education programs to improve patient care. Offers referrals to support groups and information on respiratory disorders. Provides educational materials and classes.

COPD-Support, Inc.
PMB 127
1940 Kings Hwy, Ste. 4
Port Charlotte, FL 33980
www.copd-support.com
On-line group offering e-mail lists, chat rooms, forums, and a newsletter for people involved with COPD. Dedicated to providing patients and caregivers with support, education, and a way to share ideas and solutions for dealing with this disorder.

The Canadian Lung Association
3 Raymond St., Ste. 300
Ottawa, ON K1R 1A3
Canada
☎ 613-569-6411
www.lung.ca
Canadian national not-for-profit health association funds medical research, provides health education and programs with a focus on lung diseases (such as asthma and COPD), tobacco, and clean air. Ten provincial Lung Associations offer programs for the one in five Canadians living with lung disease.

The National Emphysema Foundation
15 Stevens St.
Norwalk, CT 06850
www.emphysemafoundation.org
Nonprofit organization that supplies information on emphysema and other lung diseases. Web site provides articles and tips on quitting smoking. Affiliated with the Norwalk Hospital in Connecticut.

National Heart, Lung, and Blood Institute
P.O. Box 30105
Bethesda, MD 20824-0105
☎ 800-575-WELL/301-592-8573
www.nhlbi.nih.gov
Lead component of the National Institutes of Health for lung disease research; provides written information on noncancerous lung disorders (e.g., asthma, COPD, and cystic fibrosis).

National Lung Health Education Program (NLHEP)
HealthONE Center
899 Logan St., Ste. 203
Denver, CO 80203-3154
www.nlhep.org
The mission of the NLHEP is to promote the early diagnosis of COPD and related disorders through the widespread use of spirometry. "Test Your Lungs, Know Your Numbers" is the motto of the NLHEP.

LEADING HOSPITALS FOR LUNG DISORDERS

U.S. News & World Report and the National Opinion Research Center, a social-science research group at the University of Chicago, recently conducted their 15th annual nationwide survey of 8,160 board-certified physicians in 17 medical specialties. The doctors nominated the hospitals that they considered to be the best from among 6,012 U.S. medical centers. This is the current list of the best hospitals for lung disorders, as determined by a combination of factors: doctors' rec-

ommendations from 2002, 2003, and 2004; federal death rates; and factual data regarding quality indicators, such as the ratio of registered nurses to patients and use of advanced technology. However, because the results reflect the doctors' opinions to some extent, they are partly subjective. Any institution listed is considered a leading center, and the rankings do not imply that other hospitals cannot or do not deliver excellent care.

1. **National Jewish Medical and Research Center**
   Denver, CO
   ☎ 800-222-LUNG (5864)
   www.njc.org

2. **Mayo Clinic**
   Rochester, MN
   ☎ 507-284-2511
   www.mayoclinic.org

3. **Johns Hopkins Hospital**
   Baltimore, MD
   ☎ 410-955-5000
   www.hopkinsmedicine.org

4. **Massachusetts General Hospital**
   Boston, MA
   ☎ 617-726-2000
   www.mgh.harvard.edu

5. **University of California, San Francisco, Medical Center**
   San Francisco, CA
   ☎ 888-689-UCSF/415-476-1000
   www.ucsfhealth.org

6. **Barnes-Jewish Hospital**
   St. Louis, MO
   ☎ 314-747-3000
   www.barnesjewish.org

7. **Duke University Medical Center**
   Durham, NC
   ☎ 919-684-8111
   www.mc.duke.edu

8. **University of California, San Diego, Medical Center**
   San Diego, CA
   ☎ 800-926-UCSD (8273)
   www.health.ucsd.edu

9. **University of Colorado Hospital**
   Denver, CO
   ☎ 800-621-7621/303-493-8333
   www.uchsc.edu/uh

10. **University of Michigan Medical Center**
    Ann Arbor, MI
    ☎ 800-211-8181/734-936-4000
    www.med.umich.edu

Source: *U.S. News & World Report,* July 12, 2004.

MANAGING ASTHMA EXACERBATIONS

Twenty percent of people with asthma suffer frequent attacks, or exacerbations, which often require a visit to the emergency room and, in rare cases, can be fatal. In the article reprinted here from the *Journal of the American Medical Association,* Don D. Sin, M.D., and colleagues review the recent medical literature to identify the best approach to reducing or preventing exacerbations in asthma patients.

The researchers analyzed randomized controlled trials and systematic reviews published since 1980, all of which followed patients for at least three months.

For some patients with very mild asthma, using short-acting beta$_2$ agonists as needed may be enough, the researchers note. But even patients with mild disease often need inhaled corticosteroids. When used regularly, these anti-inflammatory drugs are the most effective medication for controlling asthma exacerbations and improving lung function, several well-designed clinical trials show. Inhaled corticosteroids reduce the risk of exacerbations by 55% and also improve forced expiratory volume at one second (FEV_1), a measurement of lung function.

Corticosteroids have been associated with a number of adverse effects, including osteoporosis, but proper inhaler use, employing a spacer, and rinsing the mouth after corticosteroid inhalation can help reduce system-wide exposure to the drugs, the authors note.

Patients who cannot control their asthma with low-dose corticosteroids alone may be helped by the addition of a long-acting beta$_2$ agonist, which can reduce the risk of exacerbation by another 26% compared with corticosteroids alone.

Those who are not willing or able to take corticosteroids may be helped by leukotriene pathway modifiers/receptor agonists, which are less effective but reduce the risk of exacerbation by about 40% compared with placebo. Although IgE antibodies may be useful for asthma patients with allergies and high blood levels of serum IgE, they should not be routinely prescribed to asthma patients, Dr. Sin and colleagues write.

Beyond drugs, they continue, patients should receive education on how to manage their asthma and should work to eliminate allergens in their environments. People with asthma who smoke should quit, and losing weight can help obese asthma patients to improve their lung function and ease asthma symptoms. However, the authors conclude, low-dose inhaled corticosteroids remain the mainstay of treatment for asthma patients requiring regular use of medication.

Pharmacological Management to Reduce Exacerbations in Adults With Asthma
A Systematic Review and Meta-analysis

Don D. Sin, MD, MPH

Jonathan Man, MD

Heather Sharpe, MN

Wen Qi Gan, MD, MSc

S. F. Paul Man, MD

ASTHMA IS COMMON, AFFECT-ing 5% to 12% of the adult population.[1,2] In the United States alone, asthma affects more than 200 000 adults and accounted for approximately 465 000 hospitalizations, 1.8 million emergency department visits, 10.4 million physician office visits, and 4487 deaths in 2000.[3] For largely unknown reasons, US women have a 30% higher prevalence and 40% more asthma attacks than men, and blacks have a 10% higher prevalence and 20% more asthma attacks than whites.[3] The prevalence of self-reported asthma has increased 74% over the past 2 decades,[2] with a doubling in the number of office visits and a 61% increase in asthma-related deaths.[2] The current total annual costs of asthma are $11 billion.[2-5]

Asthma is characterized clinically by repeated episodes of wheezing, breathlessness, chest tightness, and coughing, usually in the presence of variable (and reversible) airflow obstruction.[6] Most patients also demonstrate air-

See also Patient Page.

CME available online at www.jama.com.

Context Over the last 2 decades, many new pharmacological agents have been introduced to reduce the growing morbidity associated with asthma, but the long-term effects of these agents on exacerbations are unclear.

Objective To systematically review and quantitatively synthesize the long-term effects of inhaled corticosteroids, long-acting β_2 agonists, leukotriene pathway modifiers/receptor antagonists, and anti-IgE therapies on clinical outcomes and particular clinically relevant exacerbations in adult patients with chronic asthma.

Data Sources MEDLINE, EMBASE, and Cochrane databases were searched to identify relevant randomized controlled trials and systematic reviews published from January 1, 1980, to April 30, 2004. We identified additional studies by searching bibliographies of retrieved articles and contacting experts in the field.

Study Selection and Data Extraction Included trials were double-blind, had follow-up periods of at least 3 months, and contained data on exacerbations and/or forced expiratory volume in 1 second. The effects of interventions were compared with placebo, short-acting β_2 agonists, or each other.

Data Synthesis Inhaled corticosteroids were most effective, reducing exacerbations by nearly 55% compared with placebo or short-acting β_2 agonists (relative risk [RR], 0.46; 95% confidence interval [CI], 0.34-0.62; $P<.001$ for heterogeneity). Compared with placebo, the use of long-acting β_2 agonists was associated with 25% fewer exacerbations (RR, 0.75; 95% CI, 0.64-0.88; $P=.43$ for heterogeneity); when added to inhaled corticosteroids, there was a 26% reduction above that achieved by steroid monotherapy (RR, 0.74; 95% CI, 0.61-0.91; $P=.07$ for heterogeneity). Combination therapy was associated with fewer exacerbations than was increasing the dose of inhaled corticosteroids (RR, 0.86; 95% CI, 0.76-0.96; $P=.65$ for heterogeneity). Compared with placebo, leukotriene modifiers/receptor antagonists reduced exacerbations by 41% (RR, 0.59; 95% CI, 0.49-0.71; $P=.44$ for heterogeneity) but were less effective than inhaled corticosteroids (RR, 1.72; 95% CI, 1.28-2.31; $P=.91$ for heterogeneity). Use of monoclonal anti-IgE antibodies with concomitant inhaled corticosteroid therapy was associated with 45% fewer exacerbations (RR, 0.55; 95% CI, 0.45-0.66; $P=.15$ for heterogeneity).

Conclusions Inhaled corticosteroids are the single most effective therapy for adult patients with asthma. However, for those unable or unwilling to take corticosteroids, the use of leukotriene modifiers/receptor agonists appears reasonable. Long-acting β_2 agonists may be added to corticosteroids for those who remain symptomatic despite low-dose steroid therapy. Anti-IgE therapy may be considered as adjunctive therapy for young adults with asthma who have clear evidence of allergies and elevated serum IgE levels.

JAMA. 2004;292:367-376   www.jama.com

Author Affiliations and Financial Disclosures are listed at the end of this article.
Corresponding Author: Don D. Sin, MD, MPH, James Hogg iCAPTURE Center for Cardiovascular and Pulmonary Research, St Paul's Hospital, 1081 Burrard St, Vancouver, British Columbia, Canada

V6Z 1Y7
Clinical Review Section Editor: Michael S. Lauer, MD, Contributing Editor. We encourage authors to submit papers for consideration as a Clinical Review.

way hyperresponsiveness on methacholine or histamine challenge tests.[7] At the heart of asthma pathophysiology is chronic airway inflammation,[8] with infiltration of eosinophils, mast cells, and CD4[+] T lymphocytes that express T helper cell type-2 cytokines such as interleukins 4, 5, and 13, although some individuals (particularly those with very severe chronic asthma) have a predominance of neutrophils.[9,10] Airway remodeling is another characteristic feature of chronic persistent asthma, which consists of smooth muscle hypertrophy, thickening of basement membranes, increased mucus production, and denudation of airway epithelium.[8,10] Although many individuals with asthma have environmental allergies and evidence of atopy, some do not.[11] Thus, a history of allergies and atopy is helpful but cannot be relied on exclusively for diagnosing asthma.

Over the past 20 years, the basic understanding of asthma and its pathogenesis has rapidly evolved, leading to the development of novel pharmacological therapies. These include inhaled corticosteroids, long-acting β_2 agonists (LABAs), agents that affect the leukotriene pathway, combination products, and monoclonal anti-IgE therapies. While all of these therapies improve lung function to a certain extent, their long-term effects on exacerbations are less clear.

Exacerbations are one of the most important (if not the most important) end points for clinical trials in asthma because they represent periods in which patients have the greatest risk of emergency department visits, hospitalization, and even death.[12] Additionally, asthma exacerbations impose enormous amounts of emotional and financial stress, reduce quality of life, and impair the ability to work. From a societal perspective, exacerbations are the leading category of expenditures related to asthma, accounting for almost 50% of total costs.[4] Moreover, patients having frequent exacerbations (who account for approximately 20% of the total pool of those with asthma) incur 80% of the total

direct costs of asthma.[4] Prevention of exacerbations is, therefore, a central aim in asthma management.[6]

METHODS

We decided a priori to examine the effects of inhaled corticosteroids, LABAs, leukotriene pathway modifiers/receptor blockers, combination therapy with inhaled corticosteroids and LABAs, and anti-IgE therapies, because they are the most commonly used pharmacological agents for the management of adult asthma. For each of these therapies, we conducted a literature search by using MEDLINE, EMBASE, and Cochrane databases. We limited the search to English-language articles published from January 1, 1980, to April 30, 2004, reporting studies of adults (>19 years of age) in randomized clinical trials. We contacted experts to ascertain any studies that may have been missed in our initial search. As the primary purpose of this review was to ascertain the long-term effects of these therapies on rates of exacerbation, we excluded studies that did not report on exacerbations or that had a follow-up period of less than 3 months. We used the Jadad scale to adjudicate the methodologic quality of the studies.[13] We restricted the analysis to randomized clinical trials that had a score of 3 or more, complete or near-complete follow-up data, and baseline characteristics that were well balanced between the treatment and control groups. Crossover trials were excluded because these studies in general had inadequate follow-up, poor ascertainment of exacerbation data, and time-treatment interactions that were difficult to evaluate.[14] We also excluded studies that were published in abstract form only, because the methods and the results could not be fully analyzed.

Data were abstracted from each trial by 2 authors (J.M., W.Q.G.) independently using a prestandardized data abstraction form. Any discrepancies were resolved by iteration and consensus. Because we did not have access to the original patient records, we accepted the definitions for exacerbation as used by the investigators in the original stud-

ies. Although there was some heterogeneity in the way in which exacerbation was defined across the studies, most defined exacerbation as an episode requiring oral or parenteral corticosteroids, emergency visits, hospitalization, or decrease in morning peak-flow measurements of greater than 25% to 30% on 2 consecutive days.

We excluded studies that defined exacerbations exclusively as episodes requiring increased use of short-acting β_2 agonists, because LABAs and other bronchodilators may decrease the need for short-acting β_2 agonists (which is expected since β_2 agonists are themselves bronchodilators) without attenuating requirements for systemic corticosteroids or emergency visits/hospitalizations. We did not include studies in which exacerbations were reported exclusively as part of the "withdrawal" data, because the definition of an exacerbation was usually not prespecified or explicitly stated. For the inhaled corticosteroid analysis, *higher dose* was defined as doses greater than 500 μg/d of beclomethasone equivalent and at least 2-fold higher than the inhaled steroid dose contained in the comparator therapy (eg, combination of inhaled corticosteroids and a LABA).

Where possible, for each end point, we combined the results from individual studies to produce summary effect estimates. We checked for the heterogeneity of data across individual studies using the Cochran Q test. If significant heterogeneity was observed ($P\leq.10$), the DerSimonian and Laird random-effects model was used to pool the results together. In the absence of significant heterogeneity ($P>.10$), a fixed-effects model was used. To accommodate for differences in laboratory techniques of measuring values of forced expiratory volume in 1 second (FEV_1), we converted the absolute levels of FEV_1 for each study into a common unit by calculating standardized effect sizes. Standardized effect sizes were derived by dividing the mean differences in FEV_1 (from baseline to the end of the follow-up period) between those assigned to the investigational

PHARMACOLOGICAL MANAGEMENT IN ADULTS WITH ASTHMA

medication and those assigned to placebo for each study by the standard deviations (of the mean differences) from the studies.[15] As a sensitivity analysis, a weighted mean-difference technique was also used. In all cases, the data from standardized and weighted mean-difference methods produced very similar results. All analyses were conducted using Review Manager (RevMan) version 4.2 (The Cochrane Collaboration, Oxford, England).

EVIDENCE SYNTHESIS
Inhaled Corticosteroids

Randomized controlled trials have confirmed the initial observations that inhaled corticosteroids improve lung function and ameliorate patient symptoms (FIGURE 1).[16] Overall, compared with placebo or a short-acting β_2 agonists, inhaled corticosteroids reduced clinically relevant exacerbations by nearly 55% (relative risk [RR], 0.46; 95% confidence interval [CI], 0.34-0.62; $P<.001$ for heterogeneity).[17-32] Risk reduction for exacerbations was greatest in short-term studies (12 weeks' duration)[19,22,26,27] (RR, 0.34; 95% CI, 0.25-0.44), followed by medium-term studies (13-51 weeks' duration)[23,24] (RR, 0.48; 95% CI, 0.17-1.38), and least in the long-term studies ($\geq$52 weeks' duration)[17,18,20,21,25] (RR, 0.55; 95% CI, 0.38-0.80). The size of the study, on the other hand, made little difference in the results. We divided the studies into tertiles based on the sample size. Large studies (>450 participants)[21,25,27] had an RR of 0.47 (95% CI, 0.31-0.73); medium-sized studies (170-449 participants),[19,22,24,26] an RR of 0.45 (95% CI, 0.25-0.81); and small studies (<170 participants),[17,18,20,23] an RR of 0.38 (95% CI, 0.15-0.97).

We evaluated the potential modifying effects of disease severity by dividing the studies into tertiles of mean FEV_1 values at baseline. The RR reduction of exacerbations was similar across the FEV_1 tertiles (lowest FEV_1 tertile[22,26,27]: RR, 0.39; 95% CI, 0.27-0.57; middle tertile[19,21,24]: RR, 0.51; 95% CI, 0.28-0.93; highest tertile[17,18,23,25]: RR, 0.43; 95% CI, 0.24-0.75). Several studies compared higher-dose therapy (de-

fined as doses >500 µg/d of beclomethasone equivalent[33] and at least 2-fold higher than the comparator dose) with lower-dose steroid therapy. In these head-to-head comparisons, the use of higher-dose therapy was associated with fewer exacerbations compared with the lower dose (RR, 0.77; 95% CI, 0.67-0.89).[18,25,28-32]

Inhaled corticosteroids have salutary effects on FEV_1. Compared with placebo, they improved FEV_1 by approximately 330 mL (95% CI, 260-400) in the first 3 to 4 months of therapy (mean standardized estimate, 0.56 units; 95% CI, 0.45-0.66 units in favor of inhaled corticosteroids over placebo) (FIGURE 2).[19,22,26,27,34-48] There was little improvement in FEV_1 relative to that achieved with placebo beyond the first 3 months of therapy. In the trials that had at least 6 months of follow-up, the overall improvement in FEV_1 (compared with placebo) was approximately 150 mL (95% CI, 70-23; mean standardized estimate, 0.19 units; 95% CI, 0.14-0.25)[20,21,24,25,49] (Figure 2). These data suggest that the principal salutary

Figure 1. Effects of Inhaled Corticosteroids on Exacerbations

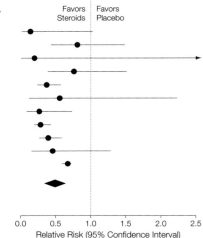

A | Inhaled Corticosteroids vs Placebo

Study	Participants, No.	Age, y, Mean (SD)	FEV, % Predicted, Mean (SD)
Juniper,[18] 1990	32	39 (14)	91 (13)
Haahtela,[17] 1991	103	38 (12)	87 (14)
Osterman,[20] 1997	75	34	NR
Nathan,[24] 1999	258	30 (12)	79 (12)
Malmstrom,[27] 1999	508	36	66 (11)
Kavuru,[22] 2000	172	37	64
Lazarus,[23] 2001	110	31 (11)	94 (9)
Nathan,[19] 2001	227	40	76
O'Byrne,[25] 2001	465	31	90 (15)
Busse,[26] 2001	227	NR	66
Pauwels,[21] 2003	7241	24 (15)	86 (14)

Pooled Summary
(RR, 0.46; 95% CI, 0.34-0.62;
Test for Heterogeneity: χ^2 = 32.15, $P<.001$)

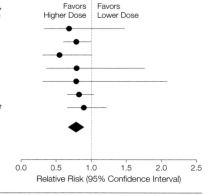

B | Higher Dose vs Lower Dose Inhaled Corticosteroids

Study	Participants, No.	Age, y, Mean (SD)	FEV, % Predicted, Mean (SD)
Hummel,[31] 1992	142	43	NR
Pauwels,[28] 1997	427	43	76
Foresi,[30] 2000	142	38 (14)	74 (11)
Lim,[32] 2000	106	40 (14)	NR
Nathan,[19] 2001	113	40	76
O'Byrne,[25] 2001	629	37	86 (17)
Ind,[29] 2003	325	45 (15)	2.3 (0.9) L†

Pooled Summary
(RR, 0.77; 95% CI, 0.67-0.89;
Test for Heterogeneity: χ^2 = 2.81, P = .83)

CI indicates confidence interval; FEV_1, forced expiratory volume in 1 second; NR, not reported/could not be ascertained; RR, relative risk.
*Missing SD values indicate that SDs were not reported.
†Except where indicated as mean FEV_1 in liters.

effects of inhaled corticosteroids on FEV_1 occur within the first 3 to 4 months of initiation of therapy.

Long-Acting β_2 Agonists

We found 13 studies (N = 3888)[50-62] that evaluated the effects of LABAs[63] on

Figure 2. Effects of Inhaled Corticosteroids on Forced Expiratory Volume in 1 Second

Study	Participants, No.	Age, y, Mean (SD)	FEV, % Predicted, Mean (SD)	
Noonan,[44] 1995	64	52	56 (13)	
Sheffer,[43] 1996	81	29	63	
Wasserman,[34] 1996	164	29	2.6 L†	
Condemi,[46] 1997	190	36	67	
Nelson,[38] 1999	75	49	61	
Bernstein,[35] 1999	144	37	75	
Galant,[37] 1999	173	30	61	
Gross,[39] 1999	230	34 (11)	67 (14)	
Kemp,[47] 1999	180	39 (13)	68 (19)	
Laviolette,[41] 1999	215	39	71 (12)	
Malmstrom,[27] 1999	508	36	66 (11)	
Fish,[48] 2000	89	52	58	
Kavuru,[22] 2000	162	37	64	
Nathan,[36] 2000	170	38	63 (9)	
Shapiro,[45] 2000	171	39	67	
Banov,[40] 2001	174	36 (12)	48 (10)	
Busse,[26] 2001	185	44	65 (17)	
Nathan,[19] 2001	112	41	76	
Meltzer,[42] 2002	184	40	NR	

Pooled Summary
(RR, 0.56; 95% CI, 0.45-0.66;
Test for Heterogeneity: χ^2 = 37.51, P = .001)

Favors Placebo — Favors Steroids

Standardized Mean Difference (SD) From Baseline
−0.6 −0.4 −0.2 0 0.2 0.4 0.6 0.8 1.0 1.2

CI indicates confidence interval; FEV_1, forced expiratory volume in 1 second; NR, not reported/could not be ascertained.
*Missing SD values indicate that SDs were not reported.
†Except where indicated as mean FEV_1 in liters.

Figure 3. Effects of Long-Acting β_2 Agonists on Exacerbations

Study	Participants, No.	Age, y, Mean (SD)	FEV, % Predicted, Mean (SD)	
Pearlman,[60] 1992	234	27 (15)	67 (9)	
D'Alonzo,[57] 1994	322	29 (12)	66 (9)	
Steffensen,[54] 1995	304	48 (14)	NR	
Van der Molen,[55] 1997	239	43 (14)	67 (16)	
Kemp,[50] 1999	506	42 (16)	63 (16)	
Lockey,[62] 1999	474	39	60	
Nathan,[52] 1999	257	30 (12)	80 (12)	
Rosenthal,[53] 1999	408	29 (11)	84 (11)	
Lazarus,[61] 2001	110	31 (11)	93 (9)	

Pooled Summary
(RR, 0.75; 95% CI, 0.64-0.88;
Test for Heterogeneity: χ^2 = 8.01, P = .43)

Favors LABA — Favors Placebo

Relative Risk (95% Confidence Interval)
0.0 0.2 0.4 0.6 0.8 1.0 1.2 1.4 1.6 1.8 2.0

CI indicates confidence interval; FEV_1, forced expiratory volume in 1 second; LABA, long-acting β_2 agonist; NR, not reported/could not be ascertained; RR, relative risk.
*Missing SD values indicate that SDs were not reported.

health outcomes in asthma. Overall, compared with placebo, the use of LABAs was associated with a 25% reduction in exacerbations (RR, 0.75; 95% CI, 0.64-0.88; P = .43 for heterogeneity) (**FIGURE 3**). Compared with regular use of short-acting β_2 agonists, the reduction in exacerbation was smaller (RR, 0.83; 95% CI, 0.67-1.05). As expected, LABAs increased FEV_1 compared with placebo (mean standardized estimate, 0.33 units; 95% CI, 0.24-0.42).

When LABAs were added to inhaled corticosteroids, exacerbations were further reduced in those who had persistent symptoms while taking low-dose corticosteroids (**FIGURE 4**). Compared with steroid monotherapy, the combination therapy with inhaled corticosteroids and LABAs was associated with a 26% reduction in exacerbations (RR, 0.74; 95% CI, 0.61-0.91; P = .07 for heterogeneity).[25,28,29,51,64-72] The addition of LABAs to inhaled corticosteroids was associated with a lower exacerbation rate than was increasing (usually doubling) the dose of inhaled corticosteroids (RR, 0.86; 95% CI, 0.76-0.96; P = .65 for heterogeneity). Combination therapy did not confer an incremental benefit beyond that achieved with steroid monotherapy in patients who were previously naive to corticosteroids.[25] Thus, in general, LABAs should be reserved for patients who continue to have symptoms despite low-dose steroid monotherapy.

These salutary effects of LABAs, however, have to be balanced against their potential long-term adverse effects.[73,74] Certain groups, such as blacks with asthma and individuals not taking regular anti-inflammatory therapies, may be particularly vulnerable.[75] Until more data are available, regular monotherapy with LABAs (in the absence of regular anti-inflammatory therapy) cannot be recommended at this time for most patients.

Leukotriene Pathway Modifiers/Receptor Antagonists

Leukotriene pathway modifiers/receptor antagonists are also effective in reducing exacerbation rates (FIGURE 5). Compared with placebo, leukotriene modifiers/receptor antagonists lowered exacerbation rates by 41% (RR, 0.59; 95% CI, 0.49-0.71; P=.44 for heterogeneity).[26,27,42,76-82] They also had a salutary effect on morning trough FEV_1 (standardized mean difference, 0.25 units; 95% CI, 0.12-0.38). However, they were inferior to inhaled corticosteroids in reducing exacerbations (RR, 1.72; 95% CI, 1.28-2.31; P=.91 for heterogeneity for leukotriene pathway modifiers/receptor antagonists vs inhaled corticorticosteroids) and in enhancing FEV_1 (mean standardized difference of 0.56 units [95% CI, 0.45-0.66] and 0.25 units [95% CI, 0.12-0.38] for leukotriene modifiers/receptor antagonists compared with placebo). Notably, the mean age of the participants of leukotriene trials was lower than that of participants in trials of LABAs and inhaled corticosteroids. We identified 3 studies comparing the efficacy of leukotriene modifiers/antagonists and LABAs as adjunctive therapy for those already taking inhaled corticosteroids (n=2662). There was some heterogeneity of data (P=.045). Overall, there was a nonsignificant trend toward improved efficacy of LABAs in reducing exacerbations (RR, 0.85; 95% CI, 0.70-1.03).[83-85]

Anti-IgE Therapies in Adults

Overall, with concomitant inhaled corticosteroid therapy, the use of recombinant monoclonal anti-IgE antibody was associated with a 45% reduction in exacerbations over the first 12 to 16 weeks of therapy (RR, 0.55; 95% CI, 0.45-0.66; P=.15 for heterogeneity).[86-89] Even in the presence of inhaled corticosteroid reduction and withdrawal, the effectiveness of monoclonal anti-IgE antibody was retained over a 12-week period (RR, 0.59; 95% CI, 0.48-0.74). Because all of these studies were performed among patients with asthma who had allergy skin test results that were positive for at least 1 or 2 perennial (and common) allergens as well as elevated serum IgE levels ($\geq$30 IU/mL), anti-IgE therapy cannot be recom-

Figure 4. Effects of Combination Therapy With Inhaled Corticosteroids and Long-Acting β_2 Agonists on Exacerbations, Compared With Higher-Dose Inhaled Corticosteroid Therapy

Study	Participants, No.	Age, y, Mean (SD)	FEV, % Predicted, Mean (SD)
Greening,[69] 1994	426	48 (16)	74 (19)
Woolcock,[71] 1996	738	44	73
Pauwels,[28] 1997	852	43	76
Van Noord,[70] 1999	274	47 (15)	72 (16)
Murray,[51] 1999	514	42 (13)	65 (10)
Matz,[65] 2001	925	37 (13)	61 (11)
Jenkins,[67] 2001	353	46	70
O'Byrne,[25] 2002	635	31	90 (15)
Ind,[29] 2003	496	45 (15)	2.3 (0.9) L†
Lalloo,[68] 2003	467	41	81

Pooled Summary
(RR, 0.86; 95% CI, 0.76-0.97;
Test for Heterogeneity: ²=6.88, P=.65)

CI indicates confidence interval; FEV_1, forced expiratory volume in 1 second; LABA, long-acting β_2 agonist; RR, relative risk.
*Missing SD values indicate that SDs were not reported.
†Except where indicated as mean FEV_1 in liters.

mended for patients with asthma who do not have these characteristics. Anti-IgE therapy also improved FEV_1, though the magnitude of the improvement was modest (weighted mean difference between anti-IgE therapy and placebo: 2.9% [95% CI, 1.3%-4.5%] of predicted FEV_1 in favor of anti-IgE therapy; or mean standardized difference of 0.18 units [95% CI, 0.07-0.29 units] in favor of anti-IgE therapy).

COMMENT

Currently, asthma is believed to be a disease of airway inflammation, caused by allergic sensitization of airways and accompanied by dysfunction of airway smooth muscle cells.[8,90] Corticosteroids are potent (but nonspecific) anti-inflammatory agents and, as such, appear to be the therapies most effective in controlling asthma symptoms and improving lung function.[91] Since airway inflammation is present even in mild disease, inhaled corticosteroids are the first-line treatments for patients who need more than an occasional inhalation of short-acting β_2 agonists.[6] In those with moderate to severe airflow impairment, higher-dose therapy appears to produce greater beneficial ef-

fects on the risk of exacerbations than does lower-dose therapy. However, the salutary effects on exacerbations should be balanced against their potential adverse effects. In a dose-dependent manner, inhaled corticosteroids have been associated with bone demineralization, osteoporosis, hip fractures, cataracts, glaucoma, skin bruising, and adrenal suppression,[92-101] although some studies have not confirmed these associations.[102-106]

The clinical trials evaluated herein were too short and underpowered to determine whether inhaled corticosteroids do indeed cause these adverse effects. Because proper inhaler technique, use of a spacer, and mouth rinsing after each actuation significantly reduce the systemic absorption of corticosteroids, patients should be educated on these safeguards.[107] Whether inhaled corticosteroids reduce mortality in asthma is uncertain. Because, fortunately, asthma deaths are relatively rare in the western world, none of the clinical trials had sufficient power to detect this end point.[108] However, several observational studies have demonstrated a protective association between therapy with inhaled corticosteroids and asthma mortality in various populations and across different jurisdictions.[109-111] It is unclear whether the provision of inhaled corticosteroids to patients who are taking oral corticosteroids after hospital or emergency department visits reduces the risk of relapses.[112] However, once oral corticosteroids are discontinued, such patients should receive inhaled corticosteroids.

In those patients whose disease remains out of control despite low-dose inhaled corticosteroid therapy, addition of a LABA appears reasonable. By themselves, LABAs have only a modest beneficial effect in reducing exacerbations. However, when given in combination with inhaled corticosteroids, the overall risk of exacerbation is reduced by approximately 26% compared with inhaled corticosteroid monotherapy. Combination therapy (with LABAs and low-dose inhaled corticosteroids) is slightly more effective than high-dose inhaled corticosteroid therapy. Monotherapy with LABAs, on the other hand, is in general best avoided because it is less effective than combination therapy or monotherapy with steroids.

For patients with mild airflow obstruction who are unwilling or unable to take inhaled corticosteroids, treatment with a leukotriene pathway modifier/receptor antagonist should be considered. These agents are less effective in reducing clinical exacerbations than monotherapy with inhaled corticosteroids. However, compared with placebo, they significantly reduce exacerbations by approximately 40%. Although these medications are generally safe and well tolerated, sporadic cases of Churg-Strauss syndrome have been associated with their use.[113-117] Whether leukotriene pathway modifiers or receptor antagonists are directly responsible for this syndrome or whether these vasculitic cases resulted from withdrawal of corticosteroids (in response to the therapeutic effects of leukotriene pathway modifiers) is uncertain.[117]

The precise role of monoclonal anti-IgE antibody therapy in the management of chronic asthma is unclear. Short-term studies have demonstrated that these medications have salutary effects on exacerbations above and beyond those achieved by inhaled corticosteroids among patients with asthma who have allergy skin test results that are positive for at least 1 or 2 perennial (and common) allergens as well as elevated serum IgE levels (≥30 IU/mL). However, as the studies have been relatively short, the long-term effects of these therapies on lung function and, more importantly, on the clinical course of patients with asthma remain uncertain. As such, they cannot be routinely recommended for most patients with asthma.

Although this review has focused on pharmacological treatment of asthma, nonpharmacological interventions are often of value in the management of chronic stable asthma. In general, treatment for asthma in adults depends on the severity of the symptoms and lung-function measurements. Either FEV_1 or peak expiratory flows should be used to assess lung function and to guide therapy. In most circumstances, FEV_1 is preferred over peak expiratory flow because the latter is more effort-dependent, demonstrates greater intra-subject and intersubject variability, and is less sensitive than FEV_1 in detecting mild airway obstruction.[118] Regardless of the device used, the overall aim is to control symptoms, preserve lung function, and maintain good quality of life using the minimum amount of medications.[6] Education aimed at self-

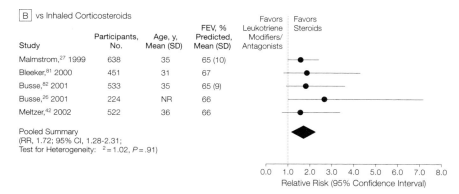

Figure 5. Effects of Leukotriene Pathway Modifiers/Receptor Antagonists on Exacerbations

A vs Placebo

Study	Participants, No.	Age, y, Mean (SD)	FEV, % Predicted, Mean (SD)
Israel,[76] 1996	401	31 (10)	60 (12)
Liu,[77] 1996	373	34	63 (13)
Reiss,[79] 1998	681	31	67 (11)
Nathan,[78] 1998	454	NR	67
Tashkin,[80] 1999	1484	31	75 (18)
Malmstrom,[27] 1999	644	35	65 (10)
Busse,[26] 2001	338	NR	66

Pooled Summary
(RR, 0.59; 95% CI, 0.49-0.71;
Test for Heterogeneity: ^{2}=5.88, P=.44)

B vs Inhaled Corticosteroids

Study	Participants, No.	Age, y, Mean (SD)	FEV, % Predicted, Mean (SD)
Malmstrom,[27] 1999	638	35	65 (10)
Bleeker,[81] 2000	451	31	67
Busse,[82] 2001	533	35	65 (9)
Busse,[26] 2001	224	NR	66
Meltzer,[42] 2002	522	36	66

Pooled Summary
(RR, 1.72; 95% CI, 1.28-2.31;
Test for Heterogeneity: ^{2}=1.02, P=.91)

CI indicates confidence interval; NR, not reported/could not be ascertained; RR, relative risk.
*Missing SD values indicate that SDs were not reported.

management is useful for most individuals with asthma.[119] Control of environment, particularly in eliminating known allergens, is recommended.[6] General measures to maintain a healthy lifestyle are strongly encouraged. Physicians should counsel their patients with asthma not to smoke, and to lose weight if overweight or obese, to improve their asthma control. Weight loss has been demonstrated to reduce symptoms and improve lung function as well as health-related quality of life in obese patients with asthma.[120,121] A proposed scheme that integrates symptoms and lung function as a guide to therapy is shown in the TABLE.

There were several important limitations to this systematic review. First, we could not evaluate whether current smoking status materially modified the effects of inhaled corticosteroids. Active smoking may directly or indirectly (through creation of oxidative reactive species) neutralize the anti-inflammatory effects of corticosteroids by inhibiting the recruitment and action of histone deacetylase, which is responsible for down-regulating expression of proinflammatory cytokines from various inflammatory cells, such as alveolar macrophages.[122] A recent study indicates that active smoking markedly attenuates the efficacy of inhaled and oral corticosteroids in stable asthma.[123] Indeed, in active smokers, even 2 weeks of oral corticosteroid therapy did not lead to significant improvements in lung function or symptom scores.[124,125] Moreover, we could not determine whether obesity, race, and other risk factors can modify treatment effects of various antiasthma medications. Large comparative studies are needed in each of these subgroups to address this important issue. Second, because the clinical trials included in this review were relatively short in duration, the long-term adverse effects of antiasthma medications could not be adequately addressed. β_2 Agonists significantly increase heart rate and decrease potassium concentrations, which may predispose susceptible individuals with asthma to cardiovascular events.[125] Several epidemiologic studies have linked the use of β_2 agonists to increased cardiovascular morbidity and mortality.[126,127] Thus, they should be used with caution in those with cardiovascular comorbid conditions. Third, we did not evaluate the usefulness of noninvasive markers for monitoring disease activity and predicting therapeutic responses in patients with asthma. Measurements of nitric oxide from exhaled gases and of inflammatory cells/cytokines from induced sputum show early promise as clinically relevant markers of airway inflammation in asthma.[128] They may be especially useful in separating asthma from other inflammatory conditions of the airway and in evaluating therapeutic responsiveness.[129] However, more work is needed to define their incremental value

Table. Proposed Guide to Asthma Therapy*

Before Treatment or Adequate Control	Step 1 Mild Intermittent Asthma	Step 2 Mild Persistent Asthma	Step 3 Moderate Persistent Asthma	Step 4 Severe Persistent Asthma
Symptoms				
Day	≤2 /wk	>2/wk, but <1/d	Daily	Continual
Night	≤2/mo	>2/mo	>1/wk	Frequent
FEV$_1$ (% of predicted) or PEF (% of personal best)	≥80	≥80	>60 to <80	≤60
PEF variability, %	≤20	20-30	>30	>30
Daily medications	No daily medication needed For treatment of infrequent adverse exacerbations, a course of systemic corticosteroids is recommended	Lower-dose inhaled corticosteroids (<500 µg/d of beclomethasone equivalent)	Preferred: low- to medium-dose inhaled corticosteroid and long-acting inhaled β$_2$ agonist Others (listed alphabetically): increased inhaled corticosteroids within medium-dose range OR low- to medium-dose inhaled corticosteroids and either leukotriene modifier or theophylline Preferred in patients with recurring severe exacerbations: increase inhaled corticosteroids within medium-dose range and add long-acting β$_2$ agonists Alternative in patients with recurring severe exacerbations: increase inhaled corticosteroids within medium-dose range and either leukotriene modifier or theophylline	Preferred: high-dose inhaled corticosteroids and long-acting β$_2$ agonists; if needed, corticosteroid tablets at 50 mg/d, with repeated attempts to reduce systemic corticosteroid For sparing of oral corticosteroid agent, see scientific review for recommendations

Abbreviations: FEV$_1$, forced expiratory volume in 1 second; PEF, peak expiratory flow.
*Modified from the National Asthma Education and Prevention Program Expert Report panel.[6] General recommendations for patients in all 4 categories: (1) smoking cessation for all smokers; (2) environmental control; self-management (including medication technique, adherence, action plan); asthma education in asthma centers; (3) short-acting β$_2$ agonist for short-term relief of symptoms as needed; use of short-acting β$_2$ agonist ≥2 times/wk indicates a need for reassessment of treatment.

above and beyond conventional measurements such as symptoms and lung function in the management of asthma. Finally, because airway inflammation in asthma is heterogeneous,[6] considerable variations in therapeutic responses can be expected among patients. Therefore, the data from the present review are not meant to replace clinical judgment or intuition; they should be used as clinical aids for practicing physicians.

In summary, there is now a wealth of evidence supporting the use of inhaled corticosteroids in low doses as first-line therapy for adult patients with asthma who require more than an occasional use of short-acting β_2 agonists for control of their disease. In those with airflow obstruction who continue to have symptoms despite low-dose steroid therapy, the addition of long-acting β_2 agonists is reasonable. Alternatively, the dose of inhaled corticosteroids may be increased, although this may be associated with increased risk of adverse effects. In relatively young patients with asthma who cannot or will not take inhaled corticosteroids, monotherapy with leukotriene pathway modifiers is effective in reducing exacerbation rates; however, these agents are less effective than monotherapy with inhaled corticosteroids.

Author Affiliations: James Hogg iCAPTURE Center for Cardiovascular and Pulmonary Research (Drs Sin, Gan, and S.F.P. Man) and Department of Medicine (Pulmonary Division) (Drs Sin, J. Man, and S.F.P. Man), University of British Columbia, Vancouver; and Department of Medicine (Pulmonary Division), University of Alberta, Edmonton (Ms Sharpe).
Financial Disclosure: Dr Sin has received grants from Merck Frosst Canada and GlaxoSmithKline, and has received fees for speaking engagements from Astra-Zeneca and GlaxoSmithKline.
Author Contributions: Dr Sin had full access to all of the data in the study and takes responsibility for the integrity of the data and the accuracy of the data analyses.
Study concept and design: Sin, S. F. P. Man.
Acquisition of data: Sin, J. Man, Sharpe, Gan.
Analysis and interpretation of data: Sin, J. Man, Sharpe, Gan, S. F. P. Man.
Drafting of the manuscript: Sin.
Critical revision of the manuscript for important intellectual content: Sin, J. Man, Sharpe, Gan, S. F. P. Man.
Statistical analysis: Sin, Gan.
Obtained funding: Sin.
Administrative, technical, or material support: Sin, J. Man, Sharpe, Gan.
Supervision: Sin.

Funding/Support: Dr Sin is supported by a Canada Research Chair (Airway Diseases) and a Michael Smith/St Paul's Hospital Foundation Professorship in chronic obstructive pulmonary disease.
Role of the Sponsors: The organizations funding this study had no role in the design and conduct of the study; in the collection, analysis, or interpretation of the data; in the preparation of the data; or in the preparation, review, or approval of the manuscript.
Additional Resources: Supplemental tables can be found at http://www.mrl.ubc.ca/sin/sin.html.

REFERENCES

1. International Study of Asthma and Allergies in Childhood (ISAAC) Steering Committee. Worldwide variation in prevalence of symptoms of asthma, allergic rhinoconjunctivitis, and atopic eczema: ISAAC. *Lancet.* 1998;351:1225-1232.
2. Mannino DM, Homa DM, Pertowski CA, et al. Surveillance for asthma—United States, 1960-1995. *MMWR CDC Surveill Summ.* 1998;47:1-27.
3. National Center for Health Statistics. Asthma prevalence, health care use and mortality, 2000-2001. Available at: http://www.cdc.gov/nchs/products/pubs/pubd/hestats/asthma/asthma.htm. Accessed January 21, 2004.
4. Weiss KB, Sullivan SD. The health economics of asthma and rhinitis, I: assessing the economic impact. *J Allergy Clin Immunol.* 2001;107:3-8.
5. Weiss KB, Sullivan SD, Lyttle CS. Trends in the cost of illness for asthma in the United States, 1985-1994. *J Allergy Clin Immunol.* 2000;106:493-499.
6. National Institutes of Health. *Global Initiative for Asthma: Global Strategy for Asthma Management and Prevention: NHLBI/WHO Workshop Report.* Bethesda, Md: National Heart, Lung, and Blood Institute; January 1995. NIH Publication 02-3659.
7. Postma DS, de Graaf-Breederveld N, Koeter GH, Sluiter HJ. The relationship between reversibility and hyperreactivity. *Eur Respir J.* 1988;1:483-485.
8. Lemanske RF Jr, Busse WW. Asthma. *JAMA.* 1997;278:1855-1873.
9. Bousquet J, Chanez P, Lacoste JY, et al. Eosinophilic inflammation in asthma. *N Engl J Med.* 1990;323:1033-1039.
10. Saetta M, Fabbri LM, Danieli D, Picotti G, Allegra L. Pathology of bronchial asthma and animal models of asthma. *Eur Respir J Suppl.* 1989;6:477s-482s.
11. Clifford RD, Howell JB, Radford M, Holgate ST. Associations between respiratory symptoms, bronchial response to methacholine, and atopy in two age groups of schoolchildren. *Arch Dis Child.* 1989;64:1133-1139.
12. Rodrigo GJ, Rodrigo C, Hall JB. Acute asthma in adults: a review. *Chest.* 2004;125:1081-1102.
13. Jadad AR, Moore RA, Carroll D, et al. Assessing the quality of reports of randomized clinical trials: is blinding necessary? *Control Clin Trials.* 1996;17:1-12.
14. Guyatt GH. Methodologic problems in clinical trials in heart failure. *J Chronic Dis.* 1985;38:353-363.
15. Curtin F, Altman DG, Elbourne D. Meta-analysis combining parallel and cross-over clinical trials, I: continuous outcomes. *Stat Med.* 2002;21:2131-2144.
16. Barnes PJ. Inhaled glucocorticoids for asthma. *N Engl J Med.* 1995;332:868-875.
17. Haahtela T, Jarvinen M, Kava T, et al. Comparison of a beta 2-agonist, terbutaline, with an inhaled corticosteroid, budesonide, in newly detected asthma. *N Engl J Med.* 1991;325:388-392.
18. Juniper EF, Kline PA, Vanzieleghem MA, Ramsdale EH, O'Byrne PM, Hargreave FE. Effect of long-term treatment with an inhaled corticosteroid (budesonide) on airway hyperresponsiveness and clinical asthma in nonsteroid-dependent asthmatics. *Am Rev Respir Dis.* 1990;142:832-836.

19. Nathan RA, Nayak AS, Graft DF, et al. Mometasone furoate: efficacy and safety in moderate asthma compared with beclomethasone dipropionate. *Ann Allergy Asthma Immunol.* 2001;86:203-210.
20. Osterman K, Carlholm M, Ekelund J, et al. Effect of 1 year daily treatment with 400 microg budesonide (Pulmicort Turbuhaler) in newly diagnosed asthmatics. *Eur Respir J.* 1997;10:2210-2215.
21. Pauwels RA, Pedersen S, Busse WW, et al. Early intervention with budesonide in mild persistent asthma: a randomised, double-blind trial. *Lancet.* 2003;361:1071-1076.
22. Kavuru M, Melamed J, Gross G, et al. Salmeterol and fluticasone propionate combined in a new powder inhalation device for the treatment of asthma: a randomized, double-blind, placebo-controlled trial. *J Allergy Clin Immunol.* 2000;105:1108-1116.
23. Lazarus SC, Boushey HA, Fahy JV, et al, Asthma Clinical Research Network for the National Heart, Lung, and Blood Institute. Long-acting beta2-agonist monotherapy vs continued therapy with inhaled corticosteroids in patients with persistent asthma: a randomized controlled trial. *JAMA.* 2001;285:2583-2593.
24. Nathan RA, Pinnas JL, Schwartz HJ, et al. A six-month, placebo-controlled comparison of the safety and efficacy of salmeterol or beclomethasone for persistent asthma. *Ann Allergy Asthma Immunol.* 1999;82:521-529.
25. O'Byrne PM, Barnes PJ, Rodriguez-Roisin R, et al. Low dose inhaled budesonide and formoterol in mild persistent asthma: the OPTIMA randomized trial. *Am J Respir Crit Care Med.* 2001;164:1392-1397.
26. Busse W, Wolfe J, Storms W, et al. Fluticasone propionate compared with zafirlukast in controlling persistent asthma: a randomized double-blind, placebo-controlled trial. *J Fam Pract.* 2001;50:595-602.
27. Malmstrom K, Rodriguez-Gomez G, Guerra J, et al, Montelukast/Beclomethasone Study Group. Oral montelukast, inhaled beclomethasone, and placebo for chronic asthma: a randomized, controlled trial. *Ann Intern Med.* 1999;130:487-495.
28. Pauwels RA, Lofdahl CG, Postma DS, et al, Formoterol and Corticosteroids Establishing Therapy (FACET) International Study Group. Effect of inhaled formoterol and budesonide on exacerbations of asthma. *N Engl J Med.* 1997;337:1405-1411.
29. Ind PW, Dal Negro R, Colman NC, Fletcher CP, Browning D, James MH. Addition of salmeterol to fluticasone propionate treatment in moderate-to-severe asthma. *Respir Med.* 2003;97:555-562.
30. Foresi A, Morelli MC, Catena E, for the Italian Study Group. Low-dose budesonide with the addition of an increased dose during exacerbations is effective in long-term asthma control. *Chest.* 2000;117:440-446.
31. Hummel S, Lehtonen L. Comparison of oral-steroid sparing by high-dose and low-dose inhaled steroid in maintenance treatment of severe asthma. *Lancet.* 1992;340:1483-1487.
32. Lim S, Jatakanon A, Gordon D, Macdonald C, Chung KF, Barnes PJ. Comparison of high dose inhaled steroids, low dose inhaled steroids plus low dose theophylline, and low dose inhaled steroids alone in chronic asthma in general practice. *Thorax.* 2000;55:837-841.
33. Boulet LP, Becker A, Berube D, Beveridge R, Ernst P, Canadian Asthma Consensus Group. Canadian Asthma Consensus Report, 1999. *CMAJ.* 1999;161(suppl 11):S1-S61.
34. Wasserman SI, Gross GN, Schoenwetter WF, et al. A 12-week dose-ranging study of fluticasone propionate powder in the treatment of asthma. *J Asthma.* 1996;33:265-274.
35. Bernstein DI, Berkowitz RB, Chervinsky P, et al. Dose-ranging study of a new steroid for asthma: mometasone furoate dry powder inhaler. *Respir Med.* 1999;93:603-612.
36. Nathan RA, Li JT, Finn A, et al. A dose-ranging study of fluticasone propionate administered once daily

via multidose powder inhaler to patients with moderate asthma. *Chest*. 2000;118:296-302.

37. Galant SP, van Bavel J, Finn A, et al. Diskus and Diskhaler: efficacy and safety of fluticasone propionate via two dry powder inhalers in subjects with mild-to-moderate persistent asthma. *Ann Allergy Asthma Immunol*. 1999;82:273-280.

38. Nelson HS, Busse WW, deBoisblanc BP, et al. Fluticasone propionate powder: oral corticosteroid-sparing effect and improved lung function and quality of life in patients with severe chronic asthma. *J Allergy Clin Immunol*. 1999;103:267-275.

39. Gross G, Thompson PJ, Chervinsky P, Vanden Burgt J. Hydrofluoroalkane-134a beclomethasone dipropionate, 400 microg, is as effective as chlorofluorocarbon beclomethasone dipropionate, 800 microg, for the treatment of moderate asthma. *Chest*. 1999; 115:343-351.

40. Banov CH, Howland WC 3rd, Lumry WR. Once-daily budesonide via Turbuhaler improves symptoms in adults with persistent asthma. *Ann Allergy Asthma Immunol*. 2001;36:627-632.

41. Laviolette M, Malmstrom K, Lu S, et al, Montelukast/Beclomethasone Additivity Group. Montelukast added to inhaled beclomethasone in treatment of asthma. *Am J Respir Crit Care Med*. 1999; 160:1862-1868.

42. Meltzer EO, Lockey RF, Friedman BF, et al, Fluticasone Propionate Clinical Research Study Group. Efficacy and safety of low-dose fluticasone propionate compared with montelukast for maintenance treatment of persistent asthma. *Mayo Clin Proc*. 2002;77:437-445.

43. Sheffer AL, LaForce C, Chervinsky P, Pearlman D, Schaberg A, Fluticasone Propionate Asthma Study Group. Fluticasone propionate aerosol: efficacy in patients with mild to moderate asthma. *J Fam Pract*. 1996; 42:369-375.

44. Noonan M, Chervinsky P, Busse WW, et al. Fluticasone propionate reduces oral prednisone use while it improves asthma control and quality of life. *Am J Respir Crit Care Med*. 1995;152:1467-1473.

45. Shapiro G, Lumry W, Wolfe J, et al. Combined salmeterol 50 microg and fluticasone propionate 250 microg in the diskus device for the treatment of asthma. *Am J Respir Crit Care Med*. 2000;161:527-534.

46. Condemi JJ, Chervinsky P, Goldstein MF, et al. Fluticasone propionate powder administered through Diskhaler versus triamcinolone acetonide aerosol administered through metered-dose inhaler in patients with persistent asthma. *J Allergy Clin Immunol*. 1997; 100:467-474.

47. Kemp J, Wanderer AA, Ramsdell J, et al. Rapid onset of control with budesonide Turbuhaler in patients with mild-to-moderate asthma. *Ann Allergy Asthma Immunol*. 1999;82:463-471.

48. Fish JE, Karpel JP, Craig TJ, et al. Inhaled mometasone furoate reduces oral prednisone requirements while improving respiratory function and health-related quality of life in patients with severe persistent asthma. *J Allergy Clin Immunol*. 2000; 106:852-860.

49. Haahtela T, Jarvinen M, Kava T, et al. Effects of reducing or discontinuing inhaled budesonide in patients with mild asthma. *N Engl J Med*. 1994;331:700-705.

50. Kemp JP, Cook DA, Incaudo GA, et al, Salmeterol Quality of Life Study Group. Salmeterol improves quality of life in patients with asthma requiring inhaled corticosteroids. *J Allergy Clin Immunol*. 1998;101:188-195.

51. Murray JJ, Church NL, Anderson WH, et al. Concurrent use of salmeterol with inhaled corticosteroids is more effective than inhaled corticosteroid dose increases. *Allergy Asthma Proc*. 1999;20:173-180.

52. Nathan RA, Pinnas JL, Schwartz HJ, et al. A six-month, placebo-controlled comparison of the safety and efficacy of salmeterol or beclomethasone for persistent asthma. *Ann Allergy Asthma Immunol*. 1999; 82:521-529.

53. Rosenthal RR, Busse WW, Kemp JP, et al. Effect of long-term salmeterol therapy compared with as-needed albuterol use on airway hyperresponsiveness. *Chest*. 1999;116:595-602.

54. Steffensen I, Faurschou P, Riska H, Rostrup J, Wegener T. Inhaled formoterol dry powder in the treatment of patients with reversible obstructive airway disease: a 3-month, placebo-controlled comparison of the efficacy and safety of formoterol and salbutamol, followed by a 12-month trial with formoterol. *Allergy*. 1995;50:657-663.

55. van der Molen T, Postma DS, Turner MO, et al, the Netherlands and Canadian Formoterol Study Investigators. Effects of the long acting beta agonist formoterol on asthma control in asthmatic patients using inhaled corticosteroids. *Thorax*. 1997;52:535-539.

56. Boulet LP, Laviolette M, Boucher S, Knight A, Hebert J, Chapman KR. A twelve-week comparison of salmeterol and salbutamol in the treatment of mild-to-moderate asthma: a Canadian multicenter study. *J Allergy Clin Immunol*. 1997;99:13-21.

57. D'Alonzo GE, Nathan RA, Henochowicz S, Morris RJ, Ratner P, Rennard SI. Salmeterol xinafoate as maintenance therapy compared with albuterol in patients with asthma. *JAMA*. 1994;271:1412-1416.

58. FitzGerald JM, Chapman KR, Della Cioppa G, et al, the Canadian FO/OD1 Study Group. Sustained bronchoprotection, bronchodilatation, and symptom control during regular formoterol use in asthma of moderate or greater severity. *J Allergy Clin Immunol*. 1999; 103:427-435.

59. Lundback B, Rawlinson DW, Palmer JB, European Study Group. Twelve month comparison of salmeterol and salbutamol as dry powder formulations in asthmatic patients. *Thorax*. 1993;48:148-153.

60. Pearlman DS, Chervinsky P, LaForce C, et al. A comparison of salmeterol with albuterol in the treatment of mild-to-moderate asthma. *N Engl J Med*. 1992; 327:1420-1425.

61. Lazarus SC, Boushey HA, Fahy JV, et al, Asthma Clinical Research Network for the National Heart, Lung, and Blood Institute. Long-acting beta2-agonist monotherapy vs continued therapy with inhaled corticosteroids in patients with persistent asthma: a randomized controlled trial. *JAMA*. 2001;285:2583-2593.

62. Lockey RF, DuBuske LM, Friedman B, Petrocella V, Cox F, Rickard K. Nocturnal asthma: effect of salmeterol on quality of life and clinical outcomes. *Chest*. 1999;115:666-673.

63. Tattersfield AE. Long-acting beta 2-agonists. *Clin Exp Allergy*. 1992;22:600-605.

64. Buhl R, Creemers JP, Vondra V, Martelli NA, Naya IP, Ekstrom T. Once-daily budesonide/formoterol in a single inhaler in adults with moderate persistent asthma. *Respir Med*. 2003;97:323-330.

65. Matz J, Emmett A, Rickard K, Kalberg C. Addition of salmeterol to low-dose fluticasone versus higher-dose fluticasone: an analysis of asthma exacerbations. *J Allergy Clin Immunol*. 2001;107:783-789.

66. Zetterstrom O, Buhl R, Mellem H, et al. Improved asthma control with budesonide/formoterol in a single inhaler, compared with budesonide alone. *Eur Respir J*. 2001;18:262-268.

67. Jenkins C, Woolcock AJ, Saarelainen P, Lundback B, James MH. Almeterol/fluticasone propionate combination therapy 50/250 microg twice daily is more effective than budesonide 800 microg twice daily in treating moderate to severe asthma. *Respir Med*. 2000; 94:715-723.

68. Lalloo UG, Malolepszy J, Kozma D, et al. Budesonide and formoterol in a single inhaler improves asthma control compared with increasing the dose of corticosteroid in adults with mild-to-moderate asthma. *Chest*. 2003;123:1480-1487.

69. Greening AP, Ind PW, Northfield M, Shaw G, Allen & Hanburys Limited UK Study Group. Added salmeterol versus higher-dose corticosteroid in asthma patients with symptoms on existing inhaled corticosteroid. *Lancet*. 1994;344:219-224.

70. van Noord JA, Schreurs AJ, Mol SJ, Mulder PG. Addition of salmeterol versus doubling the dose of fluticasone propionate in patients with mild to moderate asthma. *Thorax*. 1999;54:207-212.

71. Woolcock A, Lundback B, Ringdal N, Jacques LA. Comparison of addition of salmeterol to inhaled steroids with doubling of the dose of inhaled steroids. *Am J Respir Crit Care Med*. 1996;153:1481-1488.

72. Wallin A, Sue-Chu M, Bjermer L, et al. Effect of inhaled fluticasone with and without salmeterol on airway inflammation in asthma. *J Allergy Clin Immunol*. 2003;112:72-78.

73. Bisgaard H. Long-acting beta(2)-agonists in management of childhood asthma: a critical review of the literature. *Pediatr Pulmonol*. 2000;29:221-234.

74. Mann M, Chowdhury B, Sullivan E, Nicklas R, Anthracite R, Meyer RJ. Serious asthma exacerbations in asthmatics treated with high-dose formoterol. *Chest*. 2003;124:70-74.

75. US Food and Drug Administration. 2003 Safety Alert—Serevent (salmeterol xinafoate). Available at: http://www.fda.gov/medwatch/SAFETY/2003/serevent.htm. Accessed January 22, 2004.

76. Israel E, Cohn J, Dube L, Drazen JM, Zileuton Clinical Trial Group. Effect of treatment with zileuton, a 5-lipoxygenase inhibitor, in patients with asthma: a randomized controlled trial. *JAMA*. 1996;275:931-936.

77. Liu MC, Dube LM, Lancaster J, Zileuton Study Group. Acute and chronic effects of a 5-lipoxygenase inhibitor in asthma: a 6-month randomized multicenter trial. *J Allergy Clin Immunol*. 1996;98:859-871.

78. Nathan RA, Bernstein JA, Bielory L, et al. Zafirlukast improves asthma symptoms and quality of life in patients with moderate reversible airflow obstruction. *J Allergy Clin Immunol*. 1998;102:935-942.

79. Reiss TF, Chervinsky P, Dockhorn RJ, Shingo S, Seidenberg B, Edwards TB, Montelukast Clinical Research Study Group. Montelukast, a once-daily leukotriene receptor antagonist, in the treatment of chronic asthma: a multicenter, randomized, double-blind trial. *Arch Intern Med*. 1998;158:1213-1220.

80. Tashkin DP, Nathan RA, Howland WC, Minkwitz MC, Simonson SG, Bonuccelli CM. An evaluation of zafirlukast in the treatment of asthma with exploratory subset analyses. *J Allergy Clin Immunol*. 1999;103:246-254.

81. Bleecker ER, Welch MJ, Weinstein SF, et al. Low-dose inhaled fluticasone propionate versus oral zafirlukast in the treatment of persistent asthma. *J Allergy Clin Immunol*. 2000;105:1123-1129.

82. Busse W, Raphael GD, Galant S, et al, Fluticasone Proprionate Clinical Research Study Group. Low-dose fluticasone propionate compared with montelukast for first-line treatment of persistent asthma: a randomized clinical trial. *J Allergy Clin Immunol*. 2001;107:461-468.

83. Bjermer L, Bisgaard H, Bousquet J, et al. Montelukast and fluticasone compared with salmeterol and fluticasone in protecting against asthma exacerbation in adults: one year, double blind, randomised, comparative trial. *BMJ*. 2003;327:891.

84. Nelson HS, Nathan RA, Kalberg C, Yancey SW, Rickard KA. Comparison of inhaled salmeterol and oral zafirlukast in asthmatic patients using concomitant inhaled corticosteroids. *MedGenMed*. 2001;3:3.

85. Ringdal N, Eliraz A, Pruzinec R, et al, International Study Group. The salmeterol/fluticasone combination is more effective than fluticasone plus oral montelukast in asthma. *Respir Med*. 2003;97:234-241.

86. Busse W, Corren J, Lanier BQ, et al. Omalizumab, anti-IgE recombinant humanized monoclo-

nal antibody, for the treatment of severe allergic asthma. *J Allergy Clin Immunol.* 2001;108:184-190.

87. Soler M, Matz J, Townley R, et al. The anti-IgE antibody omalizumab reduces exacerbations and steroid requirement in allergic asthmatics. *Eur Respir J.* 2001;18:254-261.

88. Buhl R, Soler M, Matz J, et al. Omalizumab provides long-term control in patients with moderate-to-severe allergic asthma. *Eur Respir J.* 2002;20:73-78.

89. Milgrom H, Fick RB Jr, Su JQ, et al, rhuMAb-E25 Study Group. Treatment of allergic asthma with monoclonal anti-IgE antibody. *N Engl J Med.* 1999;341:1966-1973.

90. McFadden ER Jr, Gilbert IA. Asthma. *N Engl J Med.* 1992;327:1928-1937.

91. Barnes PJ, Adcock IM. How do corticosteroids work in asthma? *Ann Intern Med.* 2003;139:359-370.

92. Wong CA, Walsh LJ, Smith CJ, et al. Inhaled corticosteroid use and bone-mineral density in patients with asthma. *Lancet.* 2000;355:1399-1403.

93. Israel E, Banerjee TR, Fitzmaurice GM, et al. Effects of inhaled glucocorticoids on bone density in premenopausal women. *N Engl J Med.* 2001;345:941-947.

94. Hubbard RB, Smith CJ, Smeeth L, et al. Inhaled corticosteroids and hip fracture: a population-based case-control study. *Am J Respir Crit Care Med.* 2002;166:1563-1566.

95. van Staa TP, Leufkens HG, Cooper C. Use of inhaled corticosteroids and risk of fractures. *J Bone Miner Res.* 2001;16:581-588.

96. Cumming RG, Mitchell P, Leeder SR. Use of inhaled corticosteroids and the risk of cataracts. *N Engl J Med.* 1997;337:8-14.

97. Garbe E, Suissa S, LeLorier J. Association of inhaled corticosteroid use with cataract extraction in elderly patients. *JAMA.* 1998;280:539-544.

98. Garbe E, LeLorier J, Boivin JF, et al. Inhaled and nasal glucocorticoids and the risks of ocular hypertension or open-angle glaucoma. *JAMA.* 1997;277:722-727.

99. Mitchell P, Cumming RG, Mackey DA. Inhaled corticosteroids, family history, and risk of glaucoma. *Ophthalmology.* 1999;106:2301-2306.

100. Malo JL, Cartier A, Ghezzo H, et al. Skin bruising, adrenal function and markers of bone metabolism in asthmatics using inhaled beclomethasone and fluticasone. *Eur Respir J.* 1999;13:993-998.

101. Johnston SC. Identifying confounding by indication through blinded prospective review. *Am J Epidemiol.* 2001;154:276-284.

102. Abuekteish F, Kirkpatrick JN, Russell G. Poste-

rior subcapsular cataract and inhaled corticosteroid therapy. *Thorax.* 1995;50:674-676.

103. Simons FE, Persaud MP, Gillespie CA, et al. Absence of posterior subcapsular cataracts in young patients treated with inhaled glucocorticoids. *Lancet.* 1993;342:776-778.

104. Agertoft L, Larsen FE, Pedersen S. Posterior subcapsular cataracts, bruises and hoarseness in children with asthma receiving long-term treatment with inhaled budesonide. *Eur Respir J.* 1998;12:130-135.

105. Lau E, Mamdani M, Tu K. Inhaled or systemic corticosteroids and the risk of hospitalization for hip fracture among elderly women. *Am J Med.* 2003;114:142-145.

106. Jones A, Fay JK, Burr M, et al. Inhaled corticosteroid effects on bone metabolism in asthma and mild chronic obstructive pulmonary disease. *Cochrane Database Syst Rev.* 2002;(1):CD003537.

107. Passalacqua G, Albano M, Canonica GW, et al. Inhaled and nasal corticosteroids: safety aspects. *Allergy.* 2000;55:16-33.

108. Sears MR. Descriptive epidemiology of asthma. *Lancet.* 1997;350(suppl 2):1-4.

109. Suissa S, Ernst P, Benayoun S, Baltzan M, Cai B. Low-dose inhaled corticosteroids and the prevention of death from asthma. *N Engl J Med.* 2000;343:332-336.

110. Ishihara K, Hasegawa T, Okazaki M, et al. Long-term follow-up of patients with a history of near fatal episodes: can inhaled corticosteroids reduce the risk of death from asthma? *Intern Med.* 1995;34:77-80.

111. Sin DD, Tu JV. Inhaled corticosteroid therapy reduces the risk of rehospitalization and all-cause mortality in elderly asthmatics. *Eur Respir J.* 2001;17:380-385.

112. Rowe BH, Spooner CH, Ducharme FM, Bretzlaff JA, Bota GW. Corticosteroids for preventing relapse following acute exacerbations of asthma. *Cochrane Database Syst Rev.* 2001;(1):CD000195.

113. Green RL, Vayonis AG. Churg-Strauss syndrome after zafirlukast in two patients not receiving systemic steroid treatment. *Lancet.* 1999;353:725-726.

114. Wechsler ME, Garpestad E, Flier SR, et al. Pulmonary infiltrates, eosinophilia, and cardiomyopathy following corticosteroid withdrawal in patients with asthma receiving zafirlukast. *JAMA.* 1998;279:455-457.

115. Solans R, Bosch JA, Selva A, Orriols R, Vilardell M. Montelukast and Churg-Strauss syndrome. *Thorax.* 2002;57:183-185.

116. Guilpain P, Viallard JF, Lagarde P, et al. Churg-

Strauss syndrome in two patients receiving montelukast. *Rheumatology (Oxford).* 2002;41:535-539.

117. Wechsler ME, Finn D, Gunawardena D, et al. Churg-Strauss syndrome in patients receiving montelukast as treatment for asthma. *Chest.* 2000;117:708-713.

118. Vaughan TR, Weber RW, Tipton WR, Nelson HS. Comparison of PEFR and FEV1 in patients with varying degrees of airway obstruction: effect of modest altitude. *Chest.* 1989;95:558-562.

119. Gibson PG, Powell H, Coughlan J, et al. Self-management education and regular practitioner review for adults with asthma. *Cochrane Database Syst Rev.* 2003;(1):CD001117.

120. Stenius-Aarniala B, Poussa T, Kvarnstrom J, Gronlund EL, Ylikahri M, Mustajoki P. Immediate and long term effects of weight reduction in obese people with asthma: randomised controlled study. *BMJ.* 2000;320:827-832.

121. Hakala K, Stenius-Aarniala B, Sovijarvi A. Effects of weight loss on peak flow variability, airways obstruction, and lung volumes in obese patients with asthma. *Chest.* 2000;118:1315-1321.

122. Barnes PJ, Ito K, Adcock IM. Corticosteroid resistance in chronic obstructive pulmonary disease: inactivation of histone deacetylase. *Lancet.* 2004;363:731-733.

123. Chaudhuri R, Livingston E, McMahon AD, Thomson L, Borland W, Thomson NC. Cigarette smoking impairs the therapeutic response to oral corticosteroids in chronic asthma. *Am J Respir Crit Care Med.* 2003;168:1308-1311.

124. Chalmers GW, Macleod KJ, Little SA, et al. Influence of cigarette smoking on inhaled corticosteroid treatment in mild asthma. *Thorax.* 2002;57:226-230.

125. Salpeter SR. Cardiovascular safety of beta(2)-adrenoceptor agonist use in patients with obstructive airway disease: a systematic review. *Drugs Aging.* 2004;21:405-414.

126. Au DH, Curtis JR, Psaty BM. Risk of myocardial ischaemia and beta-adrenoceptor agonists. *Ann Med.* 2001;33:287-290.

127. Lemaitre RN, Siscovick DS, Psaty BM, et al. Inhaled beta-2 adrenergic receptor agonists and primary cardiac arrest. *Am J Med.* 2002;113:711-716.

128. Haahtela T. Assessing airway inflammation: from guessing to quantitative measurements. *Ann Med.* 2002;34:74-76.

129. Kips JC, Inman MD, Jayaram L, et al. The use of induced sputum in clinical trials. *Eur Respir J Suppl.* 2002;37:47s-50s.

ISBN 1-933087-09-9
ISSN 1542-1961
Third Printing
Printed in the United States of America

The chart on page 49 is from Goldhaber, S.Z. "Pulmonary embolism." *The Lancet* Vol. 363, No. 9417 (April 17, 2004):1295–1305. Adapted with permission from Elsevier.

Sin, D.D., Man, J., Sharpe, H., Gan, W., Man, SF. "Pharmacological management to reduce exacerbations in adults with asthma: A systematic review and meta-analysis." *Journal of the American Medical Association* Vol. 292, No. 3 (July 2004): 367–376. Copyright © 2004, American Medical Association.

The Johns Hopkins White Papers are published yearly by Medletter Associates, Inc.

Visit our Web site for information on Johns Hopkins Health After 50 publications, which include White Papers on specific disorders, home medical encyclopedias, consumer reference guides to drugs and medical tests, and our monthly newsletter The Johns Hopkins Medical Letter: Health After 50.
www.HopkinsAfter50.com

The Johns Hopkins White Papers

Paul Candon
Managing Editor

Catherine Richter
Senior Editor

Devon Schuyler
Consulting Editor

Kimberly Flynn
Writer/Researcher

Leslie Maltese-McGill
Copy Editor

Tim Jeffs
Art Director

Vincent Mejia
Graphic Designer

Betsy Meredith Rigo
Editorial Assistant

Robert Duckwall
Medical Illustrator

Kate Brackney
Intern

Johns Hopkins Health After 50 Publications

Rodney Friedman
Editor and Publisher

Thomas Dickey
Editorial Director

Tom Damrauer, M.L.S.
Chief of Information Resources

Jerry Loo
Product Manager

Darren Leiser
Promotions Coordinator

Joan Mullally
Head of Business Development

MEMORY

Peter V. Rabins, M.D., M.P.H.

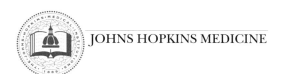

JOHNS HOPKINS MEDICINE

Dear Readers:

Nearly everyone occasionally forgets the names of movies, where they put their house keys, and even why they walked into the kitchen. So when is it time to be worried about your memory? This White Paper explains the difference between the normal memory lapses that occur with age and the signs of a more-serious memory deficit. It also reviews diagnosis and treatment of various forms of dementia, including Alzheimer's disease, vascular dementia, dementia with Lewy bodies, and frontotemporal dementia. And for people caring for a loved one with dementia, we provide advice on caregiving and the latest news on preserving your own memory.

Here are some of this year's highlights:

- The **B vitamin** that might reduce your risk of cognitive decline. (page 15)
- The 16 types of drugs that can be **hidden causes of dementia**. (pages 20–21)
- The new compound that allows visualization of **beta-amyloid deposits** in the brain. (page 23)
- **Delirium, dementia, and depression**: Three conditions that even your doctor may confuse. (pages 24–25)
- How Alzheimer's disease affects **life expectancy** in men and women. (page 27)
- The controversy over whether or not to **tell people they have dementia**. (pages 34–35)
- New study finds Alzheimer's medication to be **effective over time**. (page 41)
- When is it time for someone with dementia to **stop driving**? (pages 46–47)

I hope to empower caregivers with the knowledge and resources they need to provide the best possible quality of life for their loved ones with memory disorders.

Sincerely,

Peter Rabins MD

Peter V. Rabins, M.D., M.P.H.
Codirector
Division of Geriatric and Neuropsychiatry
Johns Hopkins University School of Medicine

P.S. Don't forget to visit HopkinsWhitePapers.com for the latest news on memory and other information that will complement your Johns Hopkins White Papers.

THE AUTHOR

Peter V. Rabins, M.D., M.P.H., received his M.D. from the Tulane University School of Medicine and his M.P.H. from the Tulane University School of Public Health. He completed his residency in psychiatry at the University of Oregon. Currently, he is codirector of the Division of Geriatric Psychiatry and Neuropsychiatry at the Johns Hopkins University School of Medicine as well as a professor of psychiatry with a joint appointment in the Department of Internal Medicine and School of Hygiene and Public Health. Dr. Rabins is serving as the principal investigator on a National Institute of Mental Health study of Alzheimer's disease in the community and a National Institute of Neurological Disorders and Stroke study of late-stage care for Alzheimer's disease patients.

Dr. Rabins has spent his career studying psychiatric disorders in the elderly. His current research includes the development of scales to measure impairment in people with severe dementia and the study of visual hallucinations in a variety of psychiatric and neurological conditions. He has published extensively in such journals as the *American Journal of Psychiatry,* the *Journal of the American Geriatrics Society,* and the *Journal of Mental Health.*

■ ■ ■

CONTENTS

The Biology of Memory .... p. 1

Age-Associated Memory Impairment .... p. 2

    Causes of Age-Associated Memory Impairment .... p. 4

    Methods To Assist Memory .... p. 5

Preventing Dementia .... p. 6

Mild Cognitive Impairment .... p. 16

Dementia .... p. 18

    Red-Flag Changes in Functioning .... p. 18

    Diagnosis of Dementia .... p. 19

Memory and Reversible Dementia .... p. 22

    Memory Loss As a Medication Side Effect .... p. 22

    Memory Loss As a Result of Depression .... p. 23

    Memory Loss Resulting From Medical Conditions .... p. 23

Memory and Irreversible Dementia .... p. 26

    Vascular Dementia .... p. 26

    Dementia With Lewy Bodies .... p. 27

    Frontotemporal Dementia .... p. 27

    Huntington's Disease .... p. 27

    Creutzfeldt-Jakob Disease .... p. 28

    Amnestic Syndrome (Amnesia) .... p. 28

    Alzheimer's Disease .... p. 29

        Degenerative changes in Alzheimer's disease .... p. 30

        Causes of Alzheimer's disease .... p. 32

        Risk factors for Alzheimer's disease .... p. 32

        Diagnosis of Alzheimer's disease .... p. 37

        Progression of Alzheimer's disease .... p. 40

        Treatment of Alzheimer's disease .... p. 40

        Investigational therapies .... p. 44

        Alternative measures .... p. 49

        Standard care for Alzheimer's disease .... p. 49

Coping With Caregiving .... p. 52

    Choosing a Nursing Home .... p. 52

Chart: Medications To Treat Alzheimer's Disease .... p. 43

Glossary .... p. 56

Health Information Organizations and Support Groups .... p. 58

Leading Hospitals for Neurology and Neurosurgery .... p. 59

Reprint .... p. 60

MEMORY

Shakespeare called memory "the warder of the brain," charged with keeping watch over an individual's personal account of being. Should this sentry begin to fail, a person's own record of self can become endangered. This is a frightening prospect for most people.

Memory loss ranges from age-associated memory impairment, which is a normal degree of forgetfulness, to dementias such as Alzheimer's disease that can profoundly affect a person's ability to function. Alzheimer's, the most common form of dementia, affects 4.5 million Americans. According to the American Academy of Neurology, 10% of people older than age 65 and nearly 50% of people older than 85 suffer from Alzheimer's disease. A 2003 study from the *Archives of Neurology* estimates that there will be 13.2 million Americans with Alzheimer's by the year 2050 if no effective prevention or cure is found.

Although Alzheimer's disease is irreversible, memory impairment resulting from other causes, such as depression or thyroid problems, can be improved with treatment. As for Alzheimer's, recent research advances should lead to improved treatments and, someday, a cure.

THE BIOLOGY OF MEMORY

Deep within the brain lies a small, S-shaped structure known as the hippocampus (Greek for "seahorse," which it resembles; see the image on page 3). This relatively small region of the brain plays a major role in the process of forging memories: It instantly evaluates incoming data from the five senses and determines whether to store or discard this new information.

But memories cannot be said to reside in the hippocampus or, for that matter, in any other specific site in the brain. Instead, memories are stored throughout the brain, especially in the cerebral cortex—the convoluted outer layer of gray matter that constitutes the "thinking" portion of the brain—as well as in the cerebellum (the fist-sized structure, located at the base of the brain beneath the cortex, that coordinates movement and balance).

During that fleeting period when the mind recognizes what the senses perceive and determines which details are important, the incoming information is said to dwell in the realm of the sensory memory. From there, data are transferred to short-term memory to be processed for immediate use and then either discarded or retained. Also known as working memory, short-term memory is sometimes equated with consciousness.

Long-term memory holds information that was learned as recently as a few minutes ago and as long ago as early childhood. For example, your name and address, what you ate for dinner last night, and the multiplication tables are all stored in long-term memory. Intentional memorization and studying can promote the transfer of information from short-term to long-term memory.

Furthermore, items that have a particular emotional impact are especially likely to earn a niche in long-term memory. (For example, nearly all people who were alive at the time remember where they were when they first heard of President Kennedy's assassination.) Indeed, it appears that the mind's ability to associate new information with other relevant information contained in long-term memory is key to both the storage of new data and the ability to recall previously stored information. The conceptual links between new and old information serve as retrieval cues; the more numerous the links and the more powerful the associations, the stronger the memory is.

Information may be difficult to recall for several reasons: It may get only as far as short-term memory and then be forgotten; it may be too similar to—or too different from—information that has already been stored; or the proper cues for retrieval may be unavailable. For example, eating similar cereals at breakfast each morning may lead people to forget which particular brand they had that day. Or remembering a person's face may not be possible until some associated fact (such as where you last saw the person) provides the necessary cue.

AGE-ASSOCIATED MEMORY IMPAIRMENT

A certain amount of forgetfulness is to be expected with age. Most people have more difficulty recalling names and words as they get older, so this is by no means symptomatic of dementia. An adage can serve to reassure those who are occasionally forgetful: "You need not worry if you forget where you put your car keys; you only need to worry if you forget what they're used for." The difference between normal forgetfulness that increases with age—known clinically as age-associated memory impairment—and serious dementia is that the former is frustrating but not disabling.

The memory lapses associated with age-associated memory

Alzheimer's Disease and Brain Shrinkage

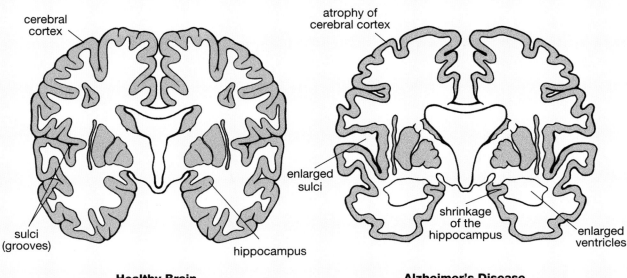

Healthy Brain

cerebral cortex

sulci (grooves)

hippocampus

Alzheimer's Disease

atrophy of cerebral cortex

enlarged sulci

shrinkage of the hippocampus

enlarged ventricles

On a microscopic level, the hallmarks of Alzheimer's disease are the plaques and tangles found between and within the brain's nerve cells. However, certain changes also are evident on the macroscopic level, when viewing the overall brain with imaging techniques or at autopsy. The illustration above compares a cross-section of a younger, healthy brain with a brain affected by Alzheimer's disease. (This is a cross-section from the middle of the brain, as if you are looking at the person from the front.)

The brain of someone with Alzheimer's disease is shrunken (atrophied) compared with a healthy brain. Specifically, the grooves in the brain (called sulci) are enlarged and the folds and bumps of brain tissue (called gyri) are atrophied. In addition, the ventricles—the spaces in the brain that are filled with cerebrospinal fluid—become larger as the surrounding tissue shrinks. Together, these changes suggest that the Alzheimer's brain has less functional tissue in some areas than the brain without dementia, a factor that may explain some impairments in cognition and behavior associated with Alzheimer's disease.

Although people without dementia can also have brain shrinkage, almost all people with Alzheimer's disease have some degree of atrophy. In Alzheimer's, shrinkage does not occur evenly throughout the brain but is con-

centrated in the frontal lobes of the brain (where behaviors such as judgment and higher levels of planning take place [not pictured]) and in the temporal lobes, particularly the hippocampus (where memories are processed; see the image). In fact, shrinkage in the outer layer of the brain is associated with an increasing number of plaques in the brain, and atrophy of the hippocampus is often associated with greater numbers of neurofibrillary tangles in this region.

Recent evidence indicates that brain atrophy—specifically in the hippocampus and adjacent internal structures of the temporal lobes—is linked directly to declines in memory. In a 2003 study from the journal *Neurology,* researchers tested the memory functioning of 55 cognitively normal people, age 60 and older, and analyzed their brain structure with magnetic imaging tests at the beginning of the study and periodically thereafter. People who had mild cognitive impairment or Alzheimer's disease at the study's end (six years later) were the most likely to have displayed the atrophy in the medial temporal lobes across the study, before memory difficulties began. This is one of the first reports to suggest that brain atrophy in people with apparently normal cognition may help predict who eventually will develop memory problems.

impairment are more likely to occur when a person is tired, sick, distracted, or under stress. Under less-stressful circumstances, the same person is usually able to remember the necessary information with ease. Indeed, studies repeatedly show that older people who do poorly on timed tests actually do as well as or better than their college-age counterparts when they are permitted to work at their own pace.

People who worry about memory loss are unlikely to suffer from a serious memory condition, while people with serious memory impairment tend to be unaware of their lapses, do not worry about them, or attribute them to other causes. However, if the memory lapses interfere with normal daily functioning, or if close friends and relatives of the individual believe that the lapses are serious, a more complex cause may be present. For more information on the differences between typical aging and more-serious memory problems, see the feature on page 7.

Causes of Age-Associated Memory Impairment

The brain contains approximately 100 billion neurons, and it is a common misconception that tens of thousands of neurons die each day. In fact, few neurons die over a person's lifetime. However, neurons do shrink, and this may explain some of the slowing of mental functioning that occurs in middle and old age. Serious memory problems occur from cell death when whole clusters of neurons are destroyed by major disorders such as a stroke or Alzheimer's disease.

In addition to neuronal shrinkage, the brain begins producing smaller quantities of many neurotransmitters starting in middle age. Brain blood flow also is reduced 15% to 20% from age 30 to 70, although this may be accounted for by neuronal shrinkage (less tissue needs less blood flow).

Other issues, such as cultural attitudes, also can contribute to the increasing frequency of memory lapses as people age. In one study, researchers compared the memory skills of two groups known for having few old-age–related stereotypes (natives of China and deaf Americans) with a third group that has numerous preconceptions about age (hearing Americans). Among these preconceptions is the notion that aging causes an inevitable decline in memory skills. The results of the study suggested a strong link between culture and memory: The first two groups were less forgetful than the third, and older Chinese participants performed as well as the younger subjects in each of these groups. Therefore, if people expect their memories to get worse, they may stop trying so hard to remember.

Other research demonstrates that the ability to remember newly acquired information depends on the same faculties used to retrieve memories from long ago—something most older people do with great ease. The implication is that a person who can still remember past events and tell interesting stories about his or her life has the faculties necessary to do the same for more recent events. This has suggested to some researchers that occasional memory lapses suggest a failure to pay attention rather than an inability to learn. Forging new memories thus depends heavily on staying interested, active, and alert.

Methods To Assist Memory

Although age-associated memory impairment is common and is not a sign of a serious neurological disorder, it can be frustrating and socially embarrassing. Although there is no way to eliminate completely the minor memory lapses that occur with age-associated memory impairment, a number of strategies can improve overall memory ability at any age.

Place commonly lost items in the same spot. If you are prone to losing certain items, such as keys or eyeglasses, choose a place to leave them, and always put them in that spot when not using them.

Write things down. If you have trouble remembering phone numbers or appointments, write them down and place the list in a conspicuous spot. Making a daily "to do" list can serve as a reminder of important tasks and obligations. In fact, the mere acts of writing notes and making lists reinforce memory.

Say words out loud. Saying "I've turned off the stove" after shutting off the stove will give you an extra verbal reminder when you later try to recall whether it is still on. Incorporating people's names into the conversation just after you have met them will serve the same purpose. For example, saying "Very nice to meet you, Jennifer" will help consolidate the memory of this name.

Use memory aids. Use a pocket notepad, personal digital assistant, wristwatch alarm, voice recorder, or other aids to help remember what you have to do or to keep track of information.

Use visual images. When learning new information, such as someone's name, create a visual image in your mind to make the information more vivid and, therefore, more memorable. For example, if you have just been introduced to a Mr. Hackman, imagine him hacking his way through a dense jungle with a

NEW RESEARCH

Bilingualism May Protect Brain Later in Life

A lifetime of speaking two languages may help keep the mind sharp into old age, a recent study suggests.

In a series of tests, researchers found that older adults who spent their lives speaking two languages—such as English and French or English and Cantonese—typically outperformed English-only participants in tests of mental speed. Because participants had similar education levels and performed comparably on tests of overall mental function, the researchers suspect that bilingualism may help keep people mentally quicker on the draw.

Bilingual adults performed better on tests looking at reaction times on computer tests. Participants had to press particular keys that corresponded with certain colors shown on the screen; in some cases, the key was on the side of the keyboard opposite to the color's screen position—a discrepancy expected to slow reaction times. It did, but less so among bilingual adults, the researchers found.

They speculate that a life spent managing two languages may help the brain retain its efficiency in controlling attention and working through complex tasks. It's unclear, they note, whether people who learn a second language but don't use it every day might see a similar benefit.

PSYCHOLOGY AND AGING
Volume 19, page 290
June 2004

machete.

Group items using mnemonics. A mnemonic is any technique used to aid in remembering. For example, when memorizing lists, names, addresses, and so on, try alphabetizing them, grouping them using an acronym (a word made from the first letters of a series of words, for example, NATO).

Another mnemonic technique is called an acrostic. Acrostics use the first letter of each item to create new words that form a sentence or phrase (for example, "Every good boy does fine" helps you remember the order of the treble-clef line notes on sheet music: E, G, B, D, F). Using rhymes ("The car is not a plane; it's parked on Main") or creating stories that connect each element to be remembered are also helpful. The more compact or meaningful the mnemonic or story, the easier it will be to remember the information.

Concentrate and relax. Many environmental stimuli compete for your attention at any given time. To remember something, you need to concentrate on the items to be remembered. Pay close attention to new information that you need to remember, and try to avoid or block out distractions. Have you ever forgotten information during a test that you know you learned well beforehand? Anxiety and stress can inhibit recall, so slow down and relax when trying to remember information. Learning a relaxation technique, such as deep breathing or muscle-relaxing exercises, may help.

Rule out other causes of memory loss. If you suspect you have memory difficulties, consult your doctor. Many medical conditions and other factors can cause reversible memory problems; these include depression, hearing or vision loss, thyroid dysfunction, certain medications, vitamin deficiencies, and stress. Treating these problems may improve memory.

PREVENTING DEMENTIA

An ever-increasing amount of research is being directed at finding ways to prevent dementia. But a treatment that only can delay the onset of dementia will still be an important step forward. Such an intervention could decrease the lifetime incidence of dementia—because many people would die of another cause before developing significant memory problems—and potentially save millions of dollars in nursing home and health care costs.

Potential strategies for preventing or delaying dementia include lowering low-density lipoprotein (LDL) cholesterol, raising high-density lipoprotein (HDL) cholesterol, decreasing blood pressure,

Everyday Forgetfulness vs. Dementia

As people age, many become concerned with "senior moments," that is, brief lapses in memory, such as forgetting a name or where you placed your keys. Such moments of forgetfulness may increase with age, a condition called age-associated memory impair-ment. But these deficits are often part of the aging process and do not necessarily indicate that a person has a more serious disease. The chart below can help you better distinguish everyday forgetfulness from the type of deficits characteristic of dementia.

Typical Age-Related Lapses	Symptoms Indicating Dementia
Independence in daily activities preserved	Person becomes dependent on others for daily living activities
Complains of memory loss but able to provide considerable detail regarding incidents of forgetfulness	May complain of memory problems only if specifically asked; unable to recall instances where memory loss was noticed by others
Person is more concerned about alleged forgetfulness than are close family members	Close family members are much more concerned about incidents of memory loss than person
Recent memory for important events, affairs, and conversations not impaired	Notable decline in memory for recent events and ability to converse
Occasional difficulty finding words	Frequent pauses and substitutions while trying to find words
Does not get lost in familiar territory; may have to pause momentarily to remember his or her way	Gets lost in familiar territory while walking or driving; may take hours to return home
Able to operate common appliances even if unwilling to learn how to operate new devices	Becomes unable to operate common appliances; unable to learn to operate even simple appliances
Maintains prior level of interpersonal social skills	Exhibits loss of interest in social activities; exhibits socially inappropriate behaviors
Normal performance on mental status examinations, taking education and culture into account	Abnormal performance on mental status examination not accounted for by education or cultural factors

Source: *Diagnosis, Management and Treatment of Dementia: A Practical Guide for Primary Care Physicians*, 1999, p. 4.

consuming antioxidants, engaging in mental and physical activity, quitting smoking, drinking alcohol only moderately, eating healthy fats while restricting unhealthy ones, maintaining a healthy body weight, preventing stroke, preventing or controlling diabetes, and taking B vitamins. (Doctors no longer consider hormone replacement therapy [HRT] for postmenopausal women to be an effective prevention.) Although none of these strategies has been proven in randomized trials to prevent or delay dementia's onset, most are nonetheless good for overall health.

LDL cholesterol. Maintaining low levels of LDL (or "bad") cholesterol may keep dementia at bay. Preliminary observations suggest that people who take statin drugs to reduce LDL cholesterol may have a reduced risk of Alzheimer's disease. In a report published in the *Archives of Neurology* in 2000 that looked at medical records of 60,000 people, those who took pravastatin (Pravachol) or lovastatin (Mevacor) had a 70% reduced rate of Alzheimer's. A report published in *The Lancet* in the same year found similar results with statins but not with other cholesterol-lowering drugs. A third report, from a 2002 issue of *Neurology*, studied 1,315 people and found that those younger than 80 years old who took statins or other cholesterol-lowering medications had a 74% lower risk of Alzheimer's than people who did not use these drugs.

However, taking medication is not the only way to lower LDL cholesterol. Exercising, consuming less saturated fat and cholesterol, losing weight if overweight, increasing intake of soluble fiber, and adding cholesterol-lowering margarines, salad dressings, and orange juices that contain plant stanols or sterols to the diet can also help lower LDL cholesterol.

HDL cholesterol. Otherwise known as "good" cholesterol, HDL cholesterol is protective against heart disease and, possibly, dementia. A 2002 Dutch report from the *Annals of Neurology* found that people with high levels of HDL cholesterol performed better on the Mini-Mental State Examination (a brief test of cognitive status) than people with low levels. The study's authors propose that HDL cholesterol may prevent the buildup of beta-amyloid in the brain or reduce inflammation, two factors that may help prevent dementia.

There are numerous ways to increase levels of good cholesterol. These include exercising, losing weight if overweight, and quitting smoking if you smoke. Certain dietary changes can also boost HDL cholesterol, including avoidance of trans fatty acids (found in packaged baked goods, commercially prepared fried foods, and most margarines) and substituting monounsaturated fats (from olive and canola oils, almonds, and avocados) for saturated fats (from animal products). A physician may also recommend medication—a statin or niacin—to increase HDL cholesterol.

Blood pressure. Hypertension—commonly known as high blood pressure—appears to be a risk factor for both Alzheimer's disease and vascular dementia. In one study of 1,449 people, those whose systolic blood pressure (the upper number in a blood pressure reading) was 160 mm Hg or higher had a 2.3-fold greater risk of developing Alzheimer's 20 years later than people whose systolic pressure was 140 mm Hg or lower. In another study, 2,418 people over age 60 with a systolic blood pressure of 140 mm Hg or above received either a blood pressure–lowering medication or a placebo. People taking the placebo were two times more likely to develop vascular dementia than those taking the medication. However, not all studies have found a link between blood pressure and the risk of dementia. The most recent guidelines state that people should keep their blood pressure below 120/80 mm Hg. This can be accomplished not only with medication but with numerous lifestyle modifications, including exercising, decreasing salt intake, not smoking, losing weight if overweight, keeping alcohol consumption moderate, and making dietary changes (specifically, eating a diet rich in fruits, vegetables, and low-fat dairy products and low in saturated fat and cholesterol).

Antioxidants. Antioxidant vitamins such as vitamins C and E are also being tested for their usefulness in protecting against Alzheimer's disease. Antioxidants neutralize free radicals, which result from normal metabolic processes in the body and cause oxidative stress. Some evidence indicates that oxidative stress contributes to the pathology of Alzheimer's disease.

A number of large, long-term correlational studies indicate that antioxidant vitamins may be beneficial in preventing dementia. For example, a 2004 study from the *Archives of Neurology* found that, among over 3,000 people age 65 and older, those who took supplements of vitamins C and E were 64% less likely to develop Alzheimer's disease over three to five years than those who did not take this combination of supplements. Nonetheless, the data have been conflicting: One recent study indicated that vitamins C and E in the diet (but not in supplements) prevented Alzheimer's disease, and another found that overall antioxidant intake (regardless of the source) in older people was not related to the risk of Alzheimer's four years later.

Even though the jury is still out, it may be beneficial to take vitamin E supplements (up to 1,000 IU daily) to forestall or prevent dementia. (Vitamin E has been shown to be effective in slowing the progression of Alzheimer's once it starts; see pages 43–44.) Be sure to consult your doctor, as high levels of vitamin E can cause bleeding in some people. The evidence that vitamin C can prevent dementia is weaker than that for vitamin E, but a large study is currently evaluating its effectiveness.

NEW RESEARCH

Blood Pressure Decline May Predict Dementia

For some elderly patients, a decline in blood pressure over time may mean a decline in mental function will soon follow, a study suggests.

Researchers found that among nearly 1,000 men and women age 75 and older, a marked drop in blood pressure over six years or less seemed to raise the risk of Alzheimer's and other forms of dementia.

For men and women who began the study with a systolic blood pressure—the top number in a blood pressure reading—below 160 mm Hg, a drop in systolic blood pressure of 15 points or more during the three to six years before diagnosis was associated with a tripling of the risk of developing dementia. A similar effect was seen in older adults who had vascular disorders such as heart disease and diabetes.

Previous research has found that people with dementia often have relatively low blood pressure. The new findings suggest that for some elderly, lowering systolic blood pressure beyond a certain point may speed the onset of dementia, according to the researchers.

It's possible, they speculate, that subtle degenerative changes in parts of the brain that regulate blood pressure may trigger a blood pressure decline that, in turn, may reduce blood flow to the brain and accelerate the already-begun degenerative process.

STROKE
Volume 35, page 1810
August 2004

Mental activity. When some people retire from their jobs, they stop engaging regularly in activities that challenge and stimulate the mind. But staying mentally active may be a key part of maintaining memory as well as other cognitive skills.

According to a 2002 study of 801 Catholic nuns, priests, and brothers published in the *Journal of the American Medical Association*, people who engaged in the highest rates of cognitively stimulating activities were 47% less likely to be diagnosed with Alzheimer's disease 4.5 years later than those reporting the lowest rates of mental activity. In addition, a study of 469 healthy people (age 75 and older), published in *The New England Journal of Medicine* in 2003, found that those who frequently engaged in leisure activities were at reduced risk for developing dementia up to 21 years later.

However, because these studies were not randomized (people chose whether or not to engage in mentally stimulating activities), no one can be entirely sure if the outcomes were the result of mental activity or some other factor. For example, people who chose to engage themselves mentally may have had more mental reserve to begin with than other people.

Nonetheless, experts recommend such activities as playing board or card games, playing a musical instrument, doing crossword puzzles, studying a foreign language, starting a new career or hobby, reading, doing volunteer work, and engaging in regular social interactions.

Physical activity. An adequate blood supply to the brain is necessary for all mental functions, including memory. Regular physical exercise helps improve blood flow to the brain and therefore facilitates better mental functioning.

A recent study from the *Journal of the American Geriatrics Society* found that exercise appears to protect one's cognitive abilities. Older people who had better aerobic capacity—meaning they were in better physical shape—at the beginning of the study were most likely to maintain their level of cognitive functioning six years later. People who were otherwise healthy but had poor aerobic capacity had worse cognitive scores after six years.

Also, the same *New England Journal of Medicine* study that found mental activity may prevent dementia also indicated that people who danced regularly had a 76% lower incidence of dementia than those who did not dance. (However, the study did not find that other forms of physical activity reduced the risk of dementia.) Dancing incorporates both physical and mental functions (for example, remembering dance steps and coordinating with a partner) that other physical activities do not—factors that may account for its benefits.

The U.S. Surgeon General and the American College of Sports Medicine recommend at least 30 minutes of moderate activity on most days of the week to stay healthy. And for people who like to exercise more, all the better: A report by the Institute of Medicine says about 60 minutes of activity a day on most days of the week helps adults maintain a healthy body weight.

Smoking. Smokers are at greater risk for mental decline than nonsmokers, and smoking cessation may reduce this risk. One study showed that current smokers over age 65 were 3.7 times more likely to experience mental decline over a one-year period than people who did not smoke or smoked only in the past. In addition, a 2003 article from the *American Journal of Public Health* showed that people who quit smoking between ages 43 and 53 were more likely to experience cognitive decline than nonsmokers; however, quitters were less likely to experience mental decline than those who continued to smoke, indicating that quitting may attenuate some of the increased risk of dementia. Smoking may impair mental function by damaging the blood vessels that supply nutrients to the brain.

Alcohol consumption. Heavy alcohol consumption can interfere with proper memory function, but people who drink moderately have a lower risk of mental decline and Alzheimer's disease than nondrinkers.

In research published in 2003 in the *Journal of the American Medical Association*, investigators reported that people who drank one to six alcoholic beverages a week had a 54% lower risk of dementia than people who never drank. People who drank less often (less than once weekly) or more often (7 to 13 drinks weekly) also appeared to have a reduced dementia risk, but this result did not reach statistical significance. However, consuming 14 or more drinks a week appeared to be linked to an increased risk of dementia. The results were similar for both Alzheimer's disease and vascular dementia, and they are in line with the findings of other recently published, large studies. But these studies are correlational, not randomized, and other factors may account for the effect.

Although no optimal level of alcohol consumption has been established, experts recommend that men consume no more than two drinks per day and women drink no more than one daily. (One drink equals 12 oz. of beer, about 5 oz. of wine, or 1.5 oz. of 80-proof liquor.) All types of alcohol—beer, wine, and liquor—appear

---

NEW RESEARCH

Walking Reduces Risk of Cognitive Decline in Men and Women

Frequent walking may reduce the risk of cognitive decline in elderly men and women, according to two recent studies. Previous studies have found an association between exercise and a reduced risk of dementia, but it was unclear whether low-intensity exercise such as walking might be protective.

For the first study, researchers asked 2,257 men without dementia how far they walked each day. None of the participants had Parkinson's disease or stroke, which would impair their ability to walk. Four to eight years later, the rate of dementia was 80% higher in those who walked the least (less than a quarter-mile a day) than in those who walked the most (more than two miles a day).

For the second study, researchers assessed levels of physical activity, including walking, in 16,466 women. Nine to 15 years later, women who got the most physical activity had a 20% lower risk of cognitive impairment than those who got the least. In addition, women who walked for at least 1.5 hours a week had less cognitive decline over a two-year period than those who walked less than 40 minutes a week.

Walking may reduce the risk of dementia by promoting blood supply to the brain.

JOURNAL OF THE AMERICAN MEDICAL ASSOCIATION
Volume 292, pages 1447 and 1454
September 22/29, 2004

to have the same effects on dementia risk. But abstainers should not start drinking to prevent dementia. The risks of excessive alcohol consumption are many, including alcoholism and accidents.

Healthy fats. Omega-3 fatty acids, a healthy type of fat, are known to reduce the risk of coronary heart disease and may also lower the risk of Alzheimer's disease. In a 2003 report from the *Archives of Neurology*, weekly consumption of fish (a good source of omega-3 fatty acids) among older people without dementia lowered the risk of developing Alzheimer's disease four years later by 60% compared with people who rarely or never ate fish. The risk was reduced by 70% for those who ate fish twice weekly. Another *Archives of Neurology* report from the same year found that the consumption of other healthy fats—omega-6 fatty acids and monounsaturated fats—was linked to a reduced risk of Alzheimer's.

In addition to being found in fish, omega-3 fatty acids are present in canola, soybeans, walnuts, and flaxseed as well as the oils of these plants. Omega-3 fatty acids are also available as supplements. Omega-6 fatty acids are found in fish, nuts, seeds, and corn, soy and safflower oils; monounsaturated fats occur in olive and canola oils, almonds, and avocados. Currently, the American Heart Association recommends two servings of fatty fish per week in addition to oils, nuts, and seeds high in omega-3 fatty acids to protect against heart disease. The results of recent studies support these recommendations for brain health, too.

Unhealthy fats. On the other hand, high intakes of unhealthy fats—specifically saturated fats and trans fatty acids—are linked to an elevated dementia risk. The aforementioned *Archives of Neurology* report that found a benefit for omega-6 polyunsaturated fats also found that people with high intakes of saturated fats (found in animal products) and trans fatty acids were twice as likely to develop Alzheimer's disease after four years as people with low intakes of these unhealthy fats. The Institute of Medicine recommends reducing trans fatty acid consumption to as little as possible. To do this, avoid foods that contain "hydrogenated" or "partially hydrogenated" oils.

Body weight. Some preliminary evidence suggests that being overweight may increase the odds of developing dementia. In a 2003 Swedish study from the *Archives of Internal Medicine*, women with a high body mass index (BMI; a ratio of weight to height) at age 70 were more likely to develop Alzheimer's disease during 18 years of follow-up than women with a low BMI. No relationship was seen between BMI and dementia in men, possibly because over-

NEW RESEARCH

Smoking May Speed Mental Decline in Elderly

Smoking may accelerate older adults' progression toward dementia, a multinational study suggests.

In three of four European studies included in the analysis, older men and women who currently smoked showed a more rapid decline in mental functioning than nonsmokers. Former smokers generally fell somewhere in between.

Smoking is a well-known risk factor for stroke, and some research suggests it contributes to dementia, including Alzheimer's disease. Experts suspect that the harm smoking wreaks on the arteries and blood circulation are to blame.

The new study included investigations in the United Kingdom, France, Denmark, and The Netherlands that followed more than 9,200 adults age 65 and older, all of whom were free from dementia at the outset. Standard tests of mental function showed that, compared with nonsmokers, current smokers showed a steeper drop in mental acuity over two years.

Only in the French study was there no association between smoking and cognitive decline. The reason is unclear, but cultural differences in smoking habits are one possibility. The authors note that before 1950, more-educated people commonly smoked, and initial evidence from the French study that smoking lowered dementia risk was explained away by higher education levels.

NEUROLOGY
Volume 62, page 920
March 23, 2004

The Insulin–Alzheimer's Link

High insulin levels might explain the increased risk for people with diabetes.

Researchers have long been interested in the link between diabetes and Alzheimer's disease. Several studies have shown that people with type 2 diabetes have an elevated risk of Alzheimer's disease compared with people without diabetes, and the risk increases further in someone taking insulin for type 2 diabetes.

Most research on the link has focused on the role that inflammation might play in both conditions, but now researchers are also looking at insulin itself. Insulin is a hormone that controls the production of glucose (sugar) by the liver and allows cells to remove glucose from the blood. One proposed theory suggests that high levels of insulin in the body lead to beta-amyloid plaques, thought by many to be a cause of Alzheimer's disease.

Recently, researchers have begun to understand that the brain, like other parts of the body, has insulin receptors and so can be affected by levels of insulin in the bloodstream. For example, a 2003 study found that memory is impaired during periods of low blood glucose levels—a common side effect of insulin therapy. This study suggests that too much insulin can affect memory in the short term; other recent research has shown that high insulin levels may affect the brain in the long run as well.

A Common Enzyme
Whether insulin might lead to increased production or decreased clearance of beta-amyloid has long been in question, but recent research suggests that it may be the latter. Two 2003 studies have suggested that the link between insulin and beta-amyloid is an enzyme that affects levels of both substances: Known as insulysin (or insulin-degrading hormone), the enzyme—in addition to having other roles within the body—clears insulin from the blood and beta-amyloid from brain tissues, according to the first study (performed in mice). However, insulysin also appears to give preferential treatment to insulin: If the insulin level is high, the enzyme will attempt to lower it, possibly leading to higher levels of beta-amyloid in the brain.

The second study, performed in humans, gave saline (placebo) or insulin injections to 16 healthy adults (age 60 to 81). All participants received insulin on one occasion and the placebo on the other, thus serving as their own control group. Two hours after each injection, the researchers measured insulin levels in the blood and spinal fluid.

As expected, participants who received insulin injections had increased levels of insulin in their spinal fluid. Surprisingly, they also had higher beta-amyloid levels in their spinal fluid than did participants who received placebo injections. This rise was seen most drastically in participants over age 70, suggesting that older adults are more vulnerable to insulin's effects on beta-amyloid levels.

If this link is proven through further research, the next step would be to find ways to lower both insulin levels in the blood and beta-amyloid levels in the brain. Some researchers are currently examining drugs that treat type 2 diabetes for this potential; diet and exercise are also under investigation.

In the meantime, people with diabetes who take insulin should continue to use this life-saving hormone; the risk of complications from untreated diabetes far outweighs any risk of memory disorders from using insulin. As always, patients should talk to their doctor about finding the optimum balance between controlling their diabetes and avoiding low blood glucose levels.

weight men don't live long enough to develop dementia. However, the study did not address whether losing weight would help prevent dementia for overweight people.

Stroke. Evidence increasingly has shown that stroke and declines in cognition are related. For example, a 2004 study in *Stroke* found that people who are at high risk for a stroke score lower on tests of cognitive function than do people with a low stroke risk.

According to the results of research called the Nun Study, having strokes may contribute to dementia symptoms in people who are susceptible to cognitive decline. In this study, 102 elderly nuns (average age 83) were evaluated for Alzheimer's- and stroke-related symptoms while they were alive, and careful examinations of their brains were made after they died. Among the nuns who had brain lesions characteristic of Alzheimer's disease, those who also had evidence of brain tissue death due to vascular disease were 11 times more likely to have shown signs of dementia when they were alive.

A 2003 report from the *Archives of Neurology* found that the risk of Alzheimer's disease was about 60% higher in older people with a history of stroke than in those who never had a stroke. In the study, 4% of people with no history of stroke developed Alzheimer's disease over seven years, compared with 5.2% of those who had experienced a stroke. The incidence of Alzheimer's in stroke victims was even higher if they also had high blood pressure, diabetes, or heart disease. The study's authors speculate that the vascular diseases that cause stroke may also contribute to Alzheimer's, or stroke may hasten the onset of Alzheimer's in people who are predisposed to dementia.

The risk of stroke can be reduced by losing excess weight, eating a healthy diet, engaging in regular aerobic exercise, and quitting smoking. Medication may also be needed to control blood pressure, cholesterol levels, and diabetes. In addition, antiplatelet therapy (such as aspirin), anticoagulants (such as warfarin [Coumadin]), or carotid endarterectomy (an operation to remove plaque from the carotid arteries, which supply blood to the brain) may be necessary for people who have already had a stroke or are at high risk for having one.

Diabetes. New research also points to a link between diabetes and the risk of cognitive decline and Alzheimer's disease. A 2004 report from the *Archives of Neurology* found that, among 824 people over age 55, those with diabetes had lower scores on many measures of cognition and a 65% greater risk of developing Alzheimer's up to nine years later than people without diabetes. For more information on the relationship between diabetes and memory, see the feature on page 13.

B vitamins. Although B vitamins have not been proven to prevent dementia, adequate levels of certain B vitamins are necessary for proper memory function.

Thiamin (Vitamin B₁). A deficiency in thiamin results in numerous health problems, including memory deficits, confusion, and difficulty walking. One of the more common causes of thiamin deficiency is alcoholism. Because alcoholics often fill up on the empty calories from alcohol, their diet lacks many essential nutri-

NEW RESEARCH

Older Diabetic Women At Risk For Mental Decline

Elderly women with type 2 diabetes may have higher-than-average odds of cognitive impairment, but blood-glucose–controlling medication may curb the risk, according to a large study.

Among nearly 19,000 women ages 70 to 81, those with type 2 diabetes had somewhat poorer scores in tests of mental functioning at the study's start. And in a group followed over the next two years, women with diabetes were more likely to show substantial cognitive decline than those without diabetes.

However, much depended on diabetes treatment. Women on oral medication to control blood glucose were similar to women without diabetes on tests of mental abilities. But those who were on insulin or no drug treatment logged worse test performances.

Poorly controlled diabetes is a major risk factor for cardiovascular disease, which is linked to cognitive decline. Research has suggested that improving blood-glucose control with oral drugs may also improve mental sharpness and possibly ward off cognitive decline.

The reason for the link between insulin treatment and poorer mental functioning is unclear. Insulin use may simply be a marker of severe diabetes. However, the growing evidence that insulin has direct effects on cognition (see the feature on page 13) means this may be relevant to dementia in people without diabetes.

BMJ
Volume 328, page 548
March 6, 2004

ents, one of the most important being thiamin. If caught in time, a thiamin deficiency can be treated with thiamin supplementation, a proper diet, and cessation of alcohol consumption (if alcoholism was the cause).

Vitamin B₆ and folic acid. Low levels of these two B vitamins can contribute to elevations in the amino acid homocysteine, which has been linked to heart attacks, strokes, and dementia. In a 2003 report from the *Annals of Neurology*, older people without dementia were more likely to experience cognitive decline over a four-year period if they had elevated blood homocysteine levels. And a 2002 report from *The New England Journal of Medicine* found that, in older people with normal cognition, the risk of both Alzheimer's disease and vascular dementia eight years later was twice as high for people with elevated homocysteine levels as it was for people with low levels. However, whether supplementation with vitamin B_6 and folic acid will prevent dementia is unknown.

Vitamin B₁₂. A deficiency in vitamin B_{12} can lead to a number of problems, including difficulties with both thinking and walking. A common correlate of vitamin B_{12} deficiency is older age. As some people get older, they don't produce enough of a substance in the stomach (called intrinsic factor) that is necessary for absorption of vitamin B_{12}. In this situation, supplements won't help; vitamin B_{12} injections are needed. A simple blood test can identify a vitamin B_{12} deficiency.

NSAIDs. Evidence first suggesting that nonsteroidal anti-inflammatory drugs (NSAIDs) may prevent Alzheimer's disease came from the observation that people with rheumatoid arthritis have a low prevalence of Alzheimer's—as much as 6 to 12 times lower than expected. Because most people with rheumatoid arthritis take NSAIDs, some experts hypothesized that these medications might provide protection against inflammation that could lead to Alzheimer's.

Other studies have also demonstrated that the risk of developing Alzheimer's disease is substantially reduced in people who have a history of using NSAIDs. In one study, the risk of developing Alzheimer's was reduced by half in those who regularly took NSAIDs—mostly ibuprofen (Advil and other brands)—compared with those who did not take these drugs. Regular use of acetaminophen (Tylenol), which is not an NSAID, did not decrease the risk of Alzheimer's. However, one recent randomized study reported at a meeting of the American College of Neuropsychopharmacology found that the now-discontinued NSAID rofecoxib (Vioxx)

NEW RESEARCH

Niacin May Protect Against Dementia

A diet rich in the B vitamin niacin may give older adults some protection from age-related mental decline and Alzheimer's disease, a study suggests.

Researchers found that among more than 3,700 older adults whom they followed for six years, those with the lowest niacin intakes had the highest risk of developing Alzheimer's. In addition, the rate of age-related decline in mental acuity was slower among men and women who consumed more niacin.

Severe deficiency in niacin (vitamin B_3) and other B vitamins, such as B_{12} and folate, is known to impair mental functioning, but there have been little data on the possible role of niacin intake in Alzheimer's risk. In this study, people who reported the higher niacin consumption from food and supplements were 40% to 70% less likely than those with the lowest intakes to develop Alzheimer's nearly six years later—regardless of factors such as age, education, genetic susceptibility, and intake of other vitamins.

Niacin is believed to be essential for maintaining DNA and nerve-cell functioning. Further research confirming that niacin protects against Alzheimer's, the authors conclude, could have "substantial public health implications."

Niacin-rich foods include meat, beans, nuts, and niacin-enriched grains and cereals.

JOURNAL OF NEUROLOGY, NEUROSURGERY AND PSYCHIATRY
Volume 75, page 1093
July 2004

was not effective in preventing people with mild cognitive impairment from developing Alzheimer's disease.

Ginkgo biloba. This dietary supplement may have antioxidant and anti-inflammatory effects on the brain. Although many marketers of ginkgo would have you believe that it effectively boosts memory, the evidence that it prevents or treats dementia is not strong, and a recent randomized study found that it does not improve memory performance in healthy people. Nonetheless, ongoing research is currently evaluating whether people randomly assigned to take ginkgo have a decreased rate of dementia.

Hormone replacement therapy. Initial evidence suggested that HRT with estrogen and progesterone protected postmenopausal women against Alzheimer's disease. However, two 2003 studies from the *Journal of the American Medical Association* found the opposite. The first report found that women randomized to take HRT were more likely to experience significant cognitive decline than those taking a placebo (7% vs. 5%). The second report found that women taking HRT were twice as likely to develop dementia as those taking a placebo. Currently, experts recommend against taking HRT to prevent dementia. A recent study suggested that estrogen alone may carry the same risks.

Other potential preventive agents. A study published in *Neurology* in 2001 found that testosterone injections improved some aspects of memory in older, healthy men. Other compounds that are being tested to improve memory or prevent or delay dementia include corticosteroids such as prednisone, colchicine (commonly used to treat gout), nicotine, and investigational drugs designed to interfere with the formation of amyloid plaques and neurofibrillary tangles.

MILD COGNITIVE IMPAIRMENT

Mild cognitive impairment falls somewhere between age-associated memory impairment and early dementia. People with mild cognitive impairment forget more than is normal for their age but do not experience other cognitive problems associated with dementia, such as becoming disoriented or confused about routine activities. They are generally able to live independently but may be less active socially.

Many experts believe that mild cognitive impairment may be an early warning sign of memory disorders later in life. In fact, studies show that 10% to 15% of people with mild cognitive

Are You at Risk for Mild Cognitive Impairment?

Somewhere along the spectrum of memory loss between age-associated memory impairment and overt dementia lies mild cognitive impairment (MCI). This diagnosis describes people who display limited cognitive impairments that neither are severe enough to be called dementia nor prevent people from living on their own. Yet people with MCI are at an increased risk for developing dementia. In fact, the condition often represents the very early stage of Alzheimer's disease.

But how common is MCI, and who is at risk for it? To answer these questions, researchers from a number of institutions, including Johns Hopkins, studied a group of 3,608 people, age 65 and older, and periodically looked for signs of memory impairment through the better part of a decade. Overall, 19% of people in this age group developed MCI during the study, the researchers reported in 2003 in the *Archives of Neurology.*

Typically, experts have considered MCI a condition that affects mainly memory but not other aspects of cognition, such as attention, concentration, visuospatial skills, or language. However, the investigators in the *Archives* study found that people with MCI had a high likelihood of having deficits in other cognitive areas in addition to memory, which could have affected how well they were able to perform daily functions, such as balancing a checkbook.

In a second study in the same publication, the same authors found that many of the demographic and genetic characteristics associated with MCI are the same as those for Alzheimer's disease. These include being older, being black, having the APOE ε4 allele, and having low levels of education (high school or less). Also, some medical conditions and procedures, particularly those that involve the heart and blood vessels, are more prevalent in the MCI population than in people without MCI (see the graph below).

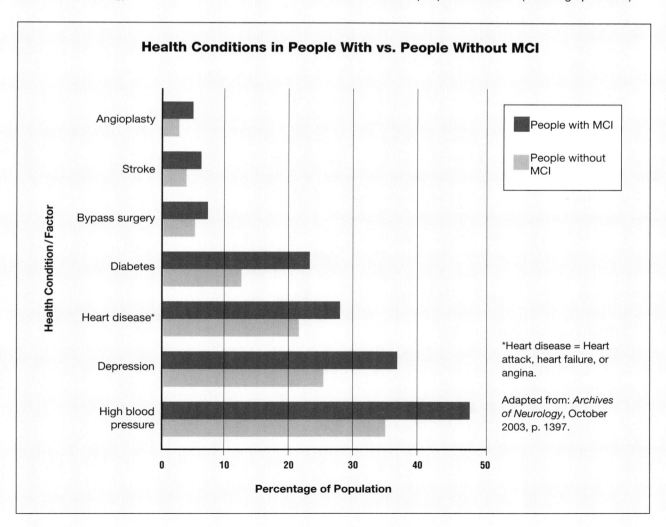

Health Conditions in People With vs. People Without MCI

People with MCI

People without MCI

*Heart disease = Heart attack, heart failure, or angina.

Adapted from: *Archives of Neurology,* October 2003, p. 1397.

impairment progress to Alzheimer's disease each year, compared with a rate of 1% to 2% a year for the general older population. And large-scale studies are currently under way to test whether therapies can halt or slow the conversion from mild cognitive impairment to Alzheimer's. By intervening at the first signs of memory trouble, researchers hope to delay Alzheimer's or prevent it altogether.

However, one such study, presented at the 9th International Conference on Alzheimer's Disease and Related Disorders in 2004, did not show a significant benefit for vitamin E or donepezil (Aricept) in slowing the development of Alzheimer's disease in people with mild cognitive impairment. Although after 18 months of treatment, patients who took donepezil had a delayed progression to Alzheimer's disease compared with those who took a placebo, by three years, people with mild cognitive impairment who took donepezil, vitamin E, or a placebo ultimately all progressed to Alzheimer's disease at the same rate.

DEMENTIA

Dementia refers to a significant intellectual decline or impairment that persists over time (often diagnosed months or even years after its onset) and affects several areas of cognition (thinking). Memory loss is a universal feature of dementia, but other functions are impaired as well—for example, abstract thinking and language.

Approximately 1% of dementia cases are reversible. In these instances, people may have a physical or psychological condition, such as an operable brain tumor, vitamin B_{12} deficiency, thyroid disease, alcoholism, or depression, that can be cured with treatment. The most common cause of reversible dementia is a toxic reaction to prescription or over-the-counter medications.

Red-Flag Changes in Functioning

According to guidelines published by the Agency for Health Care Policy and Research, a person who has difficulty with one or more of the following activities should be evaluated for dementia:

Learning and retaining new information. The person regularly misplaces objects, has trouble remembering appointments or recent conversations, or is repetitive in conversation.

Handling complex tasks. The individual has trouble with previously familiar activities, such as balancing a checkbook, cooking a meal, or other tasks that involve a complex train of thought.

Ability to reason. The person finds it difficult to respond appropriately to everyday problems, such as a flat tire. Or a previously responsible, well-adjusted person may display poor financial or social judgment.

Spatial ability and orientation. Driving and finding one's way in familiar surroundings become difficult or impossible, and the person may have problems recognizing known objects and landmarks.

Language. The ability to speak or comprehend seems impaired, and the person may have problems following or participating in conversations.

Behavior. Personality changes emerge. For example, the person appears more passive and less responsive than usual or more suspicious and irritable. Visual or auditory stimuli may be misinterpreted.

Diagnosis of Dementia

Differentiating between age-associated memory impairment and dementia resulting from a medical condition involves a process of systematic elimination. Doctors often start by looking for conditions that are most readily correctable. If these possibilities can be eliminated, then more serious, irreversible dementias—such as Alzheimer's disease—are considered. In addition, the presence of reversible disorders can complicate the irreversible forms of dementia. In these cases, diagnosing and treating concurrent depression, for example, make it possible to gain a clearer view of any conditions that may persist.

The first step in diagnosis is a thorough medical history and physical examination to identify any vision, hearing, cardiovascular, or other disorders. Although checking for these conditions might seem unnecessary, they often go unrecognized in older adults and can have an important effect on memory.

For example, heart failure (a decreased ability of the heart to pump blood) may impede mental function by reducing the amount of blood circulating to the brain. Recovering from cardiac arrest or heart bypass surgery can also affect memory. A study published in *The New England Journal of Medicine* in 2001 found that about 50% of people who undergo heart bypass surgery experience a decline in cognitive function. Furthermore, a study published in the *Journal of the American Medical Association* in 2002 found that having a newer type of heart bypass surgery called "off-pump" bypass didn't seem to reduce this risk. One theory is that some of the risk thought to be the result of surgery might actually stem from the presence of generalized vascular disease. A complete medical history is also necessary to account for any preexisting conditions, such as psychiatric

NEW RESEARCH

Blockage in Carotid Artery Linked to Cognitive Decline

Older adults with "silent" blockages in one of the large arteries supplying the brain may face an increased risk of cognitive impairment, research suggests.

The study of 4,006 adults age 65 and older found that those with substantial but asymptomatic narrowing in the left carotid artery were nearly seven times more likely than those without this narrowing to become cognitively impaired over the next five years.

The carotid artery feeds blood to the brain via two branches on either side of the neck. It's known that stroke, which usually occurs when blood flow to the brain is suddenly interrupted, can cause cognitive impairment; but it's been unclear whether the same is true of symptomless carotid-artery narrowing. The study authors hypothesized that blockages in the left carotid branch—but not the right—would raise the risk of mental decline in right-handed individuals, for whom the left side of the brain is dominant.

The 32 study participants with "high-grade" narrowing in the left carotid were more likely to see their cognitive functioning subsequently decline or to develop full-blown cognitive impairment. In contrast, there was no clear association among people with narrowing in the right carotid branch.

The authors caution, however, that it's too soon to start treating symptomless carotid-artery blockages with surgery or drugs.

ANNALS OF INTERNAL MEDICINE
Volume 140, page 237
February 17, 2004

Medications That May Impair Mental Function

Many drugs—particularly when taken at high doses or for an extended time—can cause symptoms of dementia. Older adults are most likely to experience this problem and to have it confused with a permanent memory deficit. So if a loved one is being evaluated for dementia, be sure to bring all of his or her medication bottles to the doctor's office.

Dementia caused by medication can be treated by halting the drug (if possible), switching to another one, or lowering the dosage. The following are some of the more common medications that may cause memory loss. If you are taking one of these drugs and are concerned about memory side effects, talk to your doctor before making any changes.

Drug Category	Generic Name	Brand Name
Allergy and cold medications	brompheniramine chlorpheniramine diphenhydramine pseudoephedrine	Bromfed, Bromfenex Chlor-Trimeton, Sinutab Sinus Allergy Benadryl Afrin, Sinutab, Sudafed
Antibiotics	cephalexin ciprofloxacin metronidazole ofloxacin	Biocef, Keflex Cipro Flagyl Floxin
Anticholinergic	scopolamine	Transderm-Scop
Anticonvulsants	carbamazepine phenytoin valproate	Carbatrol, Epitol, Tegretol Dilantin Depakene, Depakote
Antidepressants	amitriptyline desipramine doxepin imipramine nortriptyline	Elavil, Vanatrip Norpramin Sinequan Tofranil Pamelor
Antipsychotic drugs	chlorpromazine haloperidol	Thorazine Haldol
Cancer drugs	chlorambucil cytarabine interleukin-2 (aldesleukin)	Leukeran Cytosar-U Proleukin
Heart disease medications	amiodarone digoxin disopyramide quinidine tocainide	Cordarone Lanoxin Norpace Cardioquin, Quinidex Extentabs, Quin-Release Tonocard
High blood pressure drugs	atenolol methyldopa metoprolol nifedipine prazosin propranolol verapamil	Tenormin Aldomet Lopressor Adalat, Procardia Minipress Inderal Calan, Isoptin, Covera, Verelan

Drug Category	Generic Name	Brand Name
Immunosuppressive drugs	cyclosporine	Neoral, Sandimmune
	interferon	Infergen
Mania medication	lithium	Eskalith, Lithobid
Nausea medications	hydroxyzine	Atarax, Vistaril
	metoclopramide	Metoclopramide Intensol, Octamide, Reglan
	prochlorperazine	Compazine
	promethazine	Phenergan
Pain medications	aspirin	Anacin, Bayer, Bufferin, Easprin, ZORprin
	baclofen	Lioresal
	codeine	combined with other medications, such as aceta-minophen (Tylenol) plus codeine
	cyclobenzaprine	Flexeril
	hydrocodone	combined with other medications, such as hydrocodone and ibuprofen (Vicoprofen)
	hydrocortisone (cortisol)	Cortef, Hydrocortone, Solu-Cortef
	ibuprofen	Advil, Motrin
	indomethacin	Indocin
	meperidine	Demerol
	methocarbamol	Robaxin
	naproxen	Naprosyn
	oxycodone	OxyContin, Roxicodone
	prednisone	Deltasone, Prednicot, Prednisone Intensol, Sterapred
	propoxyphene	Darvon-N
	sulindac	Clinoril
Parkinson's disease drugs	benztropine	Cogentin
	bromocriptine	Parlodel
	entacapone	Comtan
	levodopa	Larodopa, Sinemet
	pergolide	Permax
	trihexyphenidyl	Trihexane, Trihexy-2, Trihexy-5
Sedatives	alprazolam	Xanax
	chloral hydrate	Aquachloral, Noctec
	clonazepam	Klonopin
	diazepam	Valium
	diphenhydramine	Sominex
	flurazepam	Dalmane
	lorazepam	Ativan
Ulcer/acid reflux medications	cimetidine	Tagamet HB
	ranitidine	Zantac 75

disorders, head trauma, or alcohol abuse.

Tests of mental status—for example, the Mini-Mental State Examination, the Short Test of Mental Status, or the Cognitive Capacity Screening Examination—are also given to check for any basic cognitive impairment. These tests, which take 5 to 15 minutes to complete, offer a baseline for comparison should further testing be necessary.

A history should also include an interview with a family member or close friend. Such an interview can be crucial, because someone close to the patient knows the patient's former level of functioning and therefore is able to help the physician determine whether deterioration has occurred.

The American Academy of Neurology recommends the following tests in the routine evaluation of a patient with dementia:

- complete blood cell count;
- serum electrolytes (potassium, sodium, and chloride);
- blood glucose (sugar), blood urea nitrogen, and creatinine;
- serum vitamin B_{12} levels;
- depression screening;
- liver function tests and thyroid function tests; and
- a brain scan such as computed tomography (CT) or magnetic resonance imaging (MRI).

A routine evaluation would not include single photon emission computer tomography (SPECT), genetic testing, or apolipoprotein E (APOE) genotyping. Screening for syphilis and lumbar puncture should be performed only in special circumstances.

The usefulness of positron emission tomography (PET), other genetic markers for Alzheimer's disease, and markers for Alzheimer's in cerebrospinal fluid is unknown at this time, according to the American Academy of Neurology. It is also unknown whether testing for Alzheimer's gene mutations can help in diagnosis.

MEMORY AND REVERSIBLE DEMENTIA

Memory loss can often result from things that can be controlled by the patient or physician. Medication side effects, depression, and certain medical conditions are important concerns.

Memory Loss As a Medication Side Effect

Although older adults make up only 12% of the population, they receive about 30% of all prescriptions written in the United States. Unfortunately, as people age, natural changes within the body make adverse effects more likely from medication: The kidneys may not remove drugs from the bloodstream as quickly as in younger adults, drug metabolism in the liver may be slowed, and a greater ratio of fat to muscle increases the time it takes to eliminate some drugs from the body. More important, however, is the fact that older adults take an average of more than five prescription drugs and three over-the-counter drugs at the same time. In geriatric clinics, the most common cause of reversible dementia is an adverse medication reaction.

Alcohol is the most prevalent intoxicant implicated in dementia. Fortunately, as is often the case with other drugs, the negative effects of alcohol on intellectual abilities often can be reversed with abstinence, though chronic abuse may lead to permanent damage.

For more information on medication and memory loss, see the feature on pages 20–21.

Memory Loss As a Result of Depression

Because the cognitive changes of dementia—impairment of memory, learning, attention, and concentration—can occur in people who are depressed, the diagnosis of dementia can be more difficult. In fact, depression and cognitive decline often occur together.

A person is more likely to be suffering from depression than dementia if there is a history of psychiatric illness, a rapid onset of cognitive symptoms, difficulties with sleep, or a rapid decline in the ability to perform everyday activities. (For more information on the difference among depression, dementia, and confusion [delirium], see the feature on pages 24–25.) Because depression and dementia are difficult to distinguish, it may be necessary to start antidepressant therapy and later reassess the patient for the presence of dementia.

Memory Loss Resulting From Medical Conditions

A number of medical conditions can lead to memory problems, and in some cases, treatment of the underlying illness can reverse or reduce the memory deficit. These conditions include hormonal imbalances owing to thyroid disease or Cushing's disease (overproduction of steroid hormones by the adrenal gland); infectious diseases including AIDS, syphilis, and chronic meningitis resulting from fungal infections or tuberculosis; tumors of the frontal or temporal lobe of the cerebral cortex; subdural hematomas (a collection of blood between the skull and the brain); normal-pressure hydrocephalus (caused by excess fluid in the brain); and deficien-

NEW RESEARCH

Compound Allows Visualization of Alzheimer's Brain Protein

Scientists have developed a compound that enables them to locate and quantify deposits of beta-amyloid in the brains of patients with Alzheimer's disease. The findings may help physicians diagnose Alzheimer's, evaluate the effectiveness of treatments, and develop new treatments. Currently, only an autopsy can determine definitively the presence of Alzheimer's.

The compound, Pittsburgh compound-B (PIB), is a radioactive dye that binds to the beta-amyloid protein in the brain. Researchers injected PIB into 9 healthy volunteers and 16 patients who showed signs of mild Alzheimer's and then looked into the subjects' brains using positron emission tomography.

In Alzheimer's patients, PIB collected in areas of the brain known to contain large amounts of beta amyloid, while such concentrations were not seen in healthy subjects. According to the authors, the study strongly suggests that PIB retention may be a good indicator of amyloid deposits.

An accompanying editorial noted that the study has not proven whether PIB can diagnose early Alzheimer's. Careful clinical studies will be needed for further guidance in the use of PIB.

ANNALS OF NEUROLOGY
Volume 55, pages 303 and 306
March 2004

Confused About Confusion?

Delirium, dementia, and depression all have confusion as a symptom. How do you tell the differences among them?

Confusion is a common problem in people over age 65. It may be a symptom of dementia but in some cases is the result of delirium (a temporary state of confusion) or depression. Family members and even doctors frequently have a difficult time distinguishing these three causes of confusion. But each has certain telltale features and symptoms, listed in the chart below, that health care professionals look for.

Clearing Up the Problem
A person who displays confusion should undergo a medical evaluation promptly. This evaluation may include a physical exam, mental status and neuropsychological exams, blood tests, an electroencephalogram, and a scan of the head (computed tomography or magnetic resonance imaging). The doctor also will ask family members about the timeline of symptoms,

Distinguishing Delirium From Dementia and Depression

Feature	Delirium	Dementia	Depression
Onset	sudden (hours to days), with an identifiable time of onset	gradual (months to years) with no identifiable time of onset	rapid (weeks to months)
Duration/ progression	usually hours to days; reversible with successful treatment	remainder of patient's life; typically worsens over time despite treatment	usually short term, but persistent in some people; reversible with successful treatment
Psychiatric history	often no previous psychiatric problems	often no previous psychiatric problems	usually has history of psychiatric problems, including undiagnosed episodes of depression
General deficits	displays new deficits	may try to hide any new deficits	acknowledges new deficits
Memory	rapid fluctuations; difficulty recalling recent events	memory for recent events and common knowledge slowly erodes but is relatively stable day to day; often unaware of memory loss	occasional fluctuations in performance; recognizes and is troubled by forgetfulness
Thinking	disorganized; may be sluggish or racing	difficulty with abstract ideas, word finding, calculations, judgment, recognition	fluctuating problems

changes in alertness and ability to function, the person's medical history, and any medications the person may take.

If confusion is caused by delirium, doctors need to determine the exact cause of the delirium and address it. Common causes include medications, kidney and liver failure, hypothermia, hyperthermia, infections, heart problems, stroke, and fluid (electrolyte) imbalance. Successfully treating the underlying cause should reverse the confusion. If dementia is the cause of the confusion, medication and behavioral techniques can provide some relief, but rarely is dementia reversible. Depression can be addressed with psychotherapy and antidepressant drugs.

Distinguishing Delirium from Dementia and Depression (continued)

Feature	Delirium	Dementia	Depression
Alertness/attention	inattentiveness and drowsiness a concern	usually normal; may attend to one idea for a prolonged period	generally reduced; difficulty concentrating
Language	often incoherent, rapid or slow, and slurred	often incoherent; difficulty finding correct words	slow; difficulty attending to a conversation
Answers to questions	incoherent and rambling	responds incorrectly with near misses	often responds with "I don't know"
Mood	unstable, with rapid swings	fluctuates; may show apathy, depression, or disinterest	extreme sadness, often with anxiety or irritability
Activity level	hyperactive or sluggish (may fluctuate between the two); tremors or spasms	normal at first, but decreases late in the disease	lethargic, restless, or agitated
Sleep/wake cycle	disturbed, with variations from hour to hour; sleep/wake cycles may be reversed	disturbed, often with a reversal of the day/night sleep cycle	insomnia (difficulty falling asleep or early-morning awakening) or excessive sleep
Awareness of deficit	often unaware	often unaware	often exaggerates the perceived deficits

cies of certain vitamins, especially vitamin B_{12}.

MEMORY AND IRREVERSIBLE DEMENTIA

After eliminating other causes of memory loss, physicians will consider irreversible dementias as possible diagnoses. These include Alzheimer's disease, vascular dementia, dementia with Lewy bodies, frontotemporal dementia (for example, Pick's disease), Parkinson's disease, and Huntington's disease. Other causes include infectious diseases such as Creutzfeldt-Jakob disease and AIDS.

Vascular Dementia

After Alzheimer's disease, the most common cause of memory loss is vascular dementia—a disorder often resulting from a series of tiny strokes (known as infarcts) that destroy brain cells. Each infarct may be so small that it is inconsequential alone; however, the cumulative effect of many infarcts can destroy enough brain tissue to impair memory, language, and other intellectual abilities. Symptoms often develop suddenly and involve other brain functions: Loss of bladder or bowel control (incontinence), a mask-like facial expression, and weakness or paralysis on one side of the body are thought to be noncognitive hallmarks of vascular dementia. Vascular causes account for 10% to 20% of dementia cases.

Other causes of vascular dementia include lupus and other collagen-vascular diseases (these may be at least partially reversible) as well as a major stroke. Many people suffer from vascular dementia as a result of chronic high blood pressure, diabetes, or coronary heart disease (a narrowing of the coronary arteries that jeopardizes the supply of blood to the heart). People who survive a cardiac arrest can also suffer from memory deficits.

Preventive measures can help forestall the development of dementia and prevent further deterioration. These measures can be found in the text on pages 6–16.

Cholinesterase inhibitors (see the text on pages 41–42 and the chart on page 43) and the are not approved for use in people with vascular dementia, but there is some evidence that they may be useful in these people. In a Finnish study published in *The Lancet* in 2002, researchers concluded that a medication approved to treat Alzheimer's disease—galantamine (Reminyl)—appears to be as useful for vascular dementia and Alzheimer's with cerebrovascular disease (disease of the arteries in or leading to the brain) as it is for the treatment of Alzheimer's alone. Unpublished results suggest that donepezil (Aricept) is also beneficial.

Dementia With Lewy Bodies

For more information on dementia with Lewy bodies, which sometimes occurs simultaneously with Alzheimer's or Parkinson's disease, see the feature on page 29.

Frontotemporal Dementia

Frontotemporal dementia is much less common than Alzheimer's disease and accounts for 5% of cases of dementia. It affects men and women equally, usually starting between the ages of 40 and 65. It has several forms and probably several causes, but personality changes or problems with language are usually the earliest symptoms.

Pick's disease is responsible for approximately one third of cases of frontotemporal dementia. Symptoms associated with Pick's disease include impaired initiation of plans and goal setting, personality changes, unawareness of any loss of mental function, and language difficulties (aphasia). Palilalia—compulsive repetition of a word or phrase with increasing rapidity—sometimes occurs later in the illness. The course of the disease can vary from 2 to 10 years, but its final result is death.

Recent studies suggest that five other neurological diseases that can cause dementia—corticobasal ganglionic degeneration, hippocampal sclerosis, motor neuron disease inclusion dementia, primary progressive aphasia, and progressive supranuclear palsy—have pathological similarities to frontotemporal dementia.

Huntington's Disease

Huntington's disease is a rare hereditary disorder of the central nervous system characterized by uncontrollable movement and dementia. (In the past, the disease was called Huntington's chorea, from the Greek word meaning "dance.") The illness begins gradually, usually between the ages of 30 and 40, and people can live with the disease for up to 20 years. Early signs of Huntington's disease include changes in behavior and unusual, fidgety movements. Symptoms may be mild enough for the disease to go unnoticed for several years. Eventually, however, twisting and jerking movements that spread to the entire body are followed by memory loss, confu-

NEW RESEARCH

Alzheimer's Patients' Life Expectancy Half of Norm

Older adults with Alzheimer's disease have, after diagnosis, half the life expectancy of the average American their age, the results of a study suggest.

The findings, based on data from 521 patients with Alzheimer's, also point to potential signs that a newly diagnosed patient may not live long. Among the predictors of a rapid decline were more-severe mental impairment, problems walking, a history of falls, and coexisting conditions such as heart disease and diabetes.

People differ in how they fare after an Alzheimer's diagnosis, with some worsening quickly and others living for years. Researchers say the new findings suggest ways to better predict the course of a person's disease and help patients' families plan for their care.

Looking at overall life expectancy, the investigators found that women typically lived nearly six years after an Alzheimer's diagnosis, while men lived roughly four years. After diagnosis, both men and women lived about half as long as the U.S. norm and varied according to the age at diagnosis. For example, a 70-year-old woman just diagnosed with Alzheimer's could expect to live for 8 years compared with nearly 16 years for the typical American woman her age. The corresponding figures for 70-year-old men were 4 and 9 years, respectively.

ANNALS OF INTERNAL MEDICINE
Volume 140, page 501
April 6, 2004

sion, and hallucinations.

Huntington's disease directly affects the parts of the brain that control coordination. Studies have shown a striking decrease in brain levels of the neurotransmitter gamma-aminobutyric acid (GABA), but it is unclear whether this change plays a role in the disease. In 1993, scientists identified the gene defect believed to cause Huntington's disease. The gene is dominant, meaning that children with a parent who carries the defective gene have a 50% chance of developing Huntington's disease. The discovery raises the possibility that a therapy may be developed to correct the defective gene, though currently no treatment is available. The genetic test is 100% accurate.

Creutzfeldt-Jakob Disease

Creutzfeldt-Jakob disease (CJD) is a rare, fatal brain disorder that causes a rapidly progressing dementia. The disease affects approximately 1 in 1 million people worldwide each year, including 250 to 300 Americans. It can be transmitted through infected tissue (usually transplants), be inherited, or occur with no known explanation. It typically strikes people between the ages of 50 and 70 and leads to death within a few months.

A disorder with similar symptoms appeared in England in the mid-1990s, approximately 10 years after an outbreak of bovine spongiform encephalopathy (mad cow disease) in cattle that was linked to feed that included infected animal tissue. The disorder in humans was named new variant CJD (vCJD). It has been reported in about 150 people worldwide, most of whom have been younger than age 30. All are thought to have eaten tainted beef in Europe during the epidemic of mad cow disease. The disorder progresses more slowly than classic CJD (about 14 months) but inevitably leads to death. To date no cases of vCJD have been acquired in the United States.

No treatments exist for either classic CJD or vCJD. Yet the number of cases of vCJD has declined drastically since laws have been passed banning the inclusion of animal remains in cattle feed. If a family member dies of CJD or vCJD, however, an autopsy should be performed to definitively determine the cause of death.

Amnestic Syndrome (Amnesia)

People with amnestic syndrome (amnesia) demonstrate severe memory loss but otherwise have normal intelligence. The exotic nature of the disorder—memories become hidden owing to a head injury,

Dementia With Lewy Bodies

It's a less-common form of dementia than Alzheimer's but has special considerations when it comes to treatment.

Dementia with Lewy bodies (DLB) accounts for 5% to 15% of cases of dementia. Researchers are uncertain whether it is a type of Alzheimer's or Parkinson's disease or, in fact, a separate condition. Regardless, proper diagnosis and treatment can help relieve symptoms and slow cognitive loss.

What Makes Dementia With Lewy Bodies Different?

As with Alzheimer's disease, people with DLB have cognitive impairment that worsens with time. But these individuals are more likely to experience attention problems, hallucinations, and signs of Parkinson's disease (such as shuffling gait; rigid, stooped posture; poor balance; and slowness). Falls, depression, and rapid-eye-movement sleep disorders are also typical of the condition.

No imaging tests have proven successful in differentiating DLB from Alzheimer's, but examination of the brain at autopsy reveals Lewy bodies—microscopic deposits of a protein called alpha-synuclein—throughout the brain. Most people with the disease also have plaques and tangles, although few have the quantity of tangles found in Alzheimer's. Researchers are discovering that DLB is actually far more similar to the dementia that sometimes occurs in people with Parkinson's.

Specialized Treatment

Treatment of DLB depends on the specific symptoms present. Both medication and self-care measures can be helpful.

Cholinesterase inhibitors—which include donepezil (Aricept), rivastigmine (Exelon), and galantamine (Reminyl)—help improve fluctuating cognitive impairment, visual hallucinations, apathy, anxiety, and sleep disturbances. As with Alzheimer's disease, DLB's progression is not slowed by cholinesterase inhibitors. People with DLB are prone to gastrointestinal side effects and excessive salivation (which can lead to drooling) when taking cholinesterase inhibitors.

Some doctors prescribe levodopa (Larodopa), the anti-Parkinson's disease drug, to treat motor symptoms. Because levodopa can worsen hallucinations and delusions, the lowest acceptable dose should be used.

Newer atypical antipsychotic drugs such as olanzapine (Zyprexa), quetiapine (Seroquel), and risperidone (Risperdal) can help minimize hallucinations and delusions but should be used with extreme caution to avoid marked worsening of Parkinson's-like symptoms. Older antipsychotic drugs such as haloperidol (Haldol) should be avoided altogether.

Self-care measures involve making changes in the patient's environment or behavior. Some examples are adequate lighting to reduce visual hallucinations and daytime activity to improve disordered sleep.

stroke, or encephalitis—has long fascinated scientists and the public.

The first direct evidence that structures in the medial temporal lobe (where the hippocampus is located) play an important role in memory was provided by research on a patient with amnesia. Amnesia is caused by damage to the temporal lobes resulting from an accident, severe alcoholism, prolonged low blood pressure, or viral inflammation of the brain. Brain damage from such injuries usually results in anterograde amnesia, an inability to remember anything occurring after the injury. Retrograde amnesia, a loss of memory from a time prior to the accident—such as during childhood—is uncommon.

Alzheimer's Disease

Alzheimer's disease—a progressive disorder of the brain that is characterized by deterioration of mental faculties owing to the loss of nerve cells and the connections between them—is often accompanied by changes in behavior and personality. The course of the disease is relentless, although the rates of its progress and mental decline vary from person to person. A recent study found that only half of people with Alzheimer's survive more than three years after the initial diagnosis. Earlier studies reported survival times of five to nine years. But some individuals can live for 20 years or more after diagnosis.

Degenerative changes in Alzheimer's disease. In Alzheimer's disease, nerve cells stop functioning, lose connections with each other, and ultimately die. Death of many neurons in key parts of the brain causes those areas to atrophy (shrink) and results in substantial abnormalities in memory, thinking, and behavior.

Early in the disease, destruction of neurons is particularly widespread in parts of the brain controlling memory, especially the hippocampus. This explains why memory impairment is often the first sign of Alzheimer's disease. As nerve cells in the hippocampus break down, short-term memory fails, and the ability to do familiar tasks begins to decline as well.

The other area of the brain where a great deal of damage occurs is the cerebral cortex, particularly the areas responsible for language, reasoning, perception, and judgment (the temporal, frontal, and parietal lobes). Thus, unwarranted emotional outbursts (referred to as catastrophic reactions), disturbing behaviors (such as wandering), and episodes of extreme agitation appear and become more frequent as the disease progresses.

As additional areas of the brain are affected, the person with Alzheimer's disease becomes bedridden, incontinent, totally helpless, and unresponsive to the outside world.

Plaques and tangles. Amyloid plaques and neurofibrillary tangles are the pathological hallmarks of Alzheimer's disease. Although plaques and tangles can be seen only at autopsy, these two hallmarks must be observed to make a definitive diagnosis of Alzheimer's. (Therefore, the type of dementia a person has can be diagnosed definitively only at autopsy.) It remains unclear whether these abnormal brain deposits are the cause or a byproduct of Alzheimer's, but researchers have come to understand better how plaques and tangles are formed. This improved knowledge has spawned new attempts to block the underlying process that may lead to their buildup. The success of these strategies may ultimately form the basis of prevention or treatment if these plaques and tangles are, in fact, the cause of Alzheimer's.

Amyloid plaques develop in areas of the brain that are related to memory; they are a mixture of abnormal proteins and nerve cell fragments. Their main component is beta-amyloid, a protein that breaks off from the larger amyloid precursor protein. Beta-amyloid is formed when the amyloid precursor protein that is embedded in the cell membrane is broken down for disposal. Enzymes called secretases split the protein in two and form the beta-amyloid fragment.

Researchers recently identified beta-secretase as one of the cleaving enzymes. It cuts the amyloid precursor protein in a place that causes beta-amyloid to become insoluble and deposit in the brain. Investigators suspect that blocking beta-secretase activity may prevent production of undesirable forms of beta-amyloid, and experiments are currently under way to test this hypothesis. Still a mystery, however, is what happens to the beta-amyloid segment once it separates from the amyloid precursor protein and how it might cause Alzheimer's.

Neurofibrillary tangles are the other pathological characteristic of Alzheimer's disease. Composed mostly of the protein tau, these twisted, hairlike threads are what remain after the collapse of a neuron's internal support structure, known as microtubules. In healthy neurons, microtubules act like train tracks to carry nutrients from one destination to another. Tau normally serves as the supporting "railroad ties," but in Alzheimer's, the protein becomes hopelessly twisted and disrupts the function of the microtubules. This defect clogs communication within nerve cells and eventually leads to their death.

Researchers are not sure why tau goes awry, but an enzyme called Pin1 may play an important role in keeping tau intact. When Pin1 binds to an altered tau in test-tube experiments, the protein starts to function as it should and microtubule assembly is restored. Furthermore, researchers found substantially lower levels of Pin1 in the brains of patients with Alzheimer's than in healthy subjects. The significance of these findings remains uncertain, but the presence of an enzyme such as Pin1 may help maintain or restore the proper function of tau—and prevent the formation of tangles. This possibility raises the hope that therapies might be developed to keep tau functioning and prevent Alzheimer's.

Neurotransmitters. Another characteristic of Alzheimer's disease is a reduction in the levels of certain neurotransmitters that are necessary for healthy brain function. The cholinergic neurons in the brain produce acetylcholine, a neurotransmitter crucial to

NEW RESEARCH

Alzheimer's-Related Gene May Raise Vulnerability to B$_{12}$ Deficiency

People who carry a particular gene variant linked to Alzheimer's may be more susceptible to the mental effects of vitamin B$_{12}$ deficiency, according to researchers.

The gene variation in question is APOE ε4, and scientists have known that this form of the APOE gene may increase a person's risk of Alzheimer's. Deficiencies in B$_{12}$ and another B vitamin, folate, are known to impair mental function, but whether the gene variant affects a person's vulnerability to these nutritional deficiencies has been unclear.

In the new study, researchers gave memory tests to 167 adults age 75 and older who were free from dementia. They found that participants who carried the APOE ε4 allele and had low B$_{12}$ stores performed more poorly than others on the most demanding test, in which they were quickly shown a series of unrelated words and then given two minutes to recall as many words as possible. A similar trend was seen with lower folate levels, but the effect was not statistically significant.

The findings, the researchers conclude, "confirm that there is good reason" to consider B$_{12}$ and folate supplements as part of older adults' health regimen, and suggest that APOE ε4 carriers may particularly benefit. This seems to be especially true if their vitamin B$_{12}$ or folate blood levels are low.

NEUROPSYCHOLOGY
Volume 18, page 362
April 2004

memory and learning. These neurons are plentiful in the hippocampus and the cerebral cortex—two regions of the brain most ravaged by Alzheimer's. (As is true for plaques and tangles, it is not known whether neuronal loss in these parts of the brain is a cause or an effect of Alzheimer's.) As the disease progresses, acetylcholine levels drop dramatically and dementia becomes more pronounced. Levels of serotonin, norepinephrine, somatostatin, and GABA—neurotransmitters involved in many brain functions—are diminished in almost half of people with Alzheimer's. Such imbalances may lead to insomnia, depression, aggression, and mood or personality changes.

Causes of Alzheimer's disease. Despite tremendous advances in the understanding of Alzheimer's disease, scientists have yet to pinpoint a true cause of the disorder. The leading theory is that Alzheimer's disease is caused by an accumulation of insoluble fragments of beta-amyloid.

Risk factors for Alzheimer's disease. Risk factors increase the likelihood that an individual will develop Alzheimer's disease but are not thought to directly induce it. The distinction between cause and risk factor is sometimes unclear because the biology of the disease is not fully understood.

Risk factors for Alzheimer's include older age, being female, genetics, the presence of a specific form ($\varepsilon4$) of the gene that makes a protein called apolipoprotein E, elevated levels of lipoprotein(a), cardiovascular disorders (such as high blood pressure, high blood cholesterol, and heart attack), and Down syndrome. Head injury and depression are possible risk factors for Alzheimer's.

Older age. Older age is the strongest risk factor for Alzheimer's disease. The likelihood of developing the disease doubles every five years beginning at age 65. The risk is .25% per year at age 65, 1% a year at age 75, 2% at age 80, and 7% to 8% at age 90. It is unclear how age contributes to Alzheimer's disease. There is some evidence that the number of new cases begins to drop off around age 90, but the reason for this is unknown.

Female gender. Most researchers now agree that women are at higher risk for developing Alzheimer's disease than men. In the past, the issue was confused by the fact that women live seven to eight years longer than men on average, and this placed them at higher risk because of older age. Why women are at higher risk is not clear. Researchers are studying whether decreased estrogen levels (which occurs after menopause) or some other factor is responsible.

Genetics. Heredity plays a significant role in Alzheimer's disease. A handful of Alzheimer's patients (fewer than 2%) have the disease as a result of a defective gene. In these families, Alzheimer's is carried as a dominant trait (which means that half of the offspring will inherit the abnormal gene) on one of three separate chromosomes—1, 14, and 21. However, in other families, genetic predisposition is found both in Alzheimer's patients and in their relatives who exhibit no Alzheimer's symptoms. Therefore, environmental risk factors probably combine with a person's genetic makeup either to increase the chances that he or she will develop Alzheimer's or to cause the disease to begin earlier in life. In one study of identical twins, who share exactly the same genetic material, the age of onset of Alzheimer's varied by as much as 15 years. By studying people from different ethnic, racial, and social groups, scientists may discover the full range of additional risk factors. These findings, in turn, could provide new insights into what triggers the disease.

Apolipoprotein E. A number of studies have focused on a protein called apolipoprotein E (APOE), which appears to play a role in the formation of amyloid plaques. APOE is one of the lipoproteins that carry cholesterol and other fats in the blood. The gene that directs the production of APOE is located on chromosome 19. It exists in three different versions, known as alleles—APOE ε2, APOE ε3, and APOE ε4. Every person carries two APOE genes, one inherited from each parent. A person can therefore have any one of six combinations of these alleles: either a mixed set (for example, ε2/ε4) or a matched pair (for example, ε4/ε4).

Different alleles appear to confer different risks for the development of Alzheimer's disease. People who inherit the relatively rare APOE ε2 appear to be at lower risk for Alzheimer's than others, and if they do develop the disease, the age of onset is usually later. APOE ε3 is the most common variety (half the general population is ε3/ε3); researchers believe this allele plays a neutral role in Alzheimer's. APOE ε4, however, is linked with an increased risk or earlier onset of Alzheimer's. Individuals with at least one copy of APOE ε4 have a three times greater risk of developing Alzheimer's than those with no APOE ε4. A person with two copies of APOE ε4 (approximately 3% of the white population) has a 50% chance of developing Alzheimer's by age 80.

How APOE ε4 increases a person's susceptibility to Alzheimer's disease is not yet known. For some reason, APOE ε4 appears to speed up the Alzheimer's process and lower the age of onset of the disease. The average age when Alzheimer's symptoms arise is 84 in

NEW RESEARCH

Genes May Strongly Influence Memory

Genes may play a vital role in whether a person has a "good" memory, a study of Alzheimer's-affected families suggests.

Researchers found that in 266 families, most of whom had two or more relatives with Alzheimer's disease, heritability seemed to strongly influence performance on memory tests. Finding out which genes are at work might also help pinpoint the genes involved in Alzheimer's, according to the study authors. APOE and other genes are likely involved.

The study included 1,036 members of Alzheimer's—or mild cognitive impairment—affected families, mostly from the Dominican Republic and Puerto Rico. All took standard tests of memory, reasoning, language skills, and visuospatial abilities. The authors found that when it came to certain types of memory, heritability appeared key in a person's test score, even with other factors—such as age, education, and overall intelligence scores—taken into account. In one test in which participants had to remember a list of words they had learned a short time before, heritability explained 60% of the variance on participants' test scores.

It's possible, the researchers note, that genes lack such sway in families without a history of Alzheimer's. They say further research will "genetically dissect" the roots of Alzheimer's disease as well as memory functions unrelated to the illness.

NEUROLOGY
Volume 62, page 414
February 10, 2004

Should Patients Be Told They Have Alzheimer's Disease?

Some are glad to know the cause of their memory problems; others can't accept it.

Most Americans expect that their doctor will inform them of all medical findings and that they will be able to make their own decisions about their health care. Alzheimer's disease, however, presents two unique problems in informing patients that they have a disease. First, many patients are unaware that they have a memory problem and, even when informed, are not able to understand or accept this fact. Second, since memory is impaired in all patients with Alzheimer's disease, they often cannot remember the medical information once they have been told.

What, then, should doctors and caregivers tell patients with Alzheimer's disease? The American Medical Association recommends telling a person that he or she has the disease "if at all possible"—which means taking into account the degree of remaining cognitive function. A recent study, however, indicates that doctors are far more likely to give the diagnosis to a family member than to the person with Alzheimer's disease. Researchers surveyed 57 family members of people with dementia and found that 93% had been given the diagnosis by the doctor, but only 49% of patients had been told. Of the patients who were told, 46% took the news well, and 51% reacted poorly. However, family members still overwhelmingly thought that a person diagnosed with dementia should be told the truth (72%).

Peter V. Rabins, M.D., M.P.H, author of this White Paper, believes in full disclosure. "Since it is customary and desirable to be honest with patients regarding their health status," he says, "I believe it appropriate to indicate to everyone, at the time of assessment, that a problem with memory is present."

What To Expect

Some patients respond by denying the problem ("There's nothing wrong with my memory" or "I might have a little trouble, but I'm like everyone else my age"). If a patient reacts in this manner, it might be best to drop the issue because such remarks imply that individuals are unable to appreciate the fact that they have a memory problem, often because the disease has impaired their capacity to perceive that such a problem exists.

If the person resists accepting the fact that he or she has Alzheimer's disease, there is little benefit in forcing the issue, says Dr. Rabins. "The reason most patients are unaware of the fact that they have Alzheimer's disease is an intrinsic part of the disease itself—that is, the disease in some way blocks an individual's ability to understand or appreciate any mental deficits," he points out.

those with no copies of APOE ε4, 75 in those with one copy, and 68 in those with two copies. Increased risk, however, does not guarantee illness, and the presence or absence of APOE ε4 in a blood sample cannot predict who will get Alzheimer's. A person can have APOE ε4 and never get the disease. For example, a woman in the Nun Study who died at age 107 had one copy of the APOE ε4 allele but was highly functional when she died.

Lipoprotein(a). A protein known as lipoprotein(a) may play a role in encouraging the APOE protein to bind to and enter neurons. In a 2000 study of 284 people with Alzheimer's disease, elevated levels of lipoprotein(a) increased the risk of late-onset Alzheimer's among carriers of the APOE ε4 allele. In people over age 80, those with the APOE ε4 allele and high levels of lipoprotein(a) had a six times greater risk of Alzheimer's than those with lower levels. Conversely, high levels of lipoprotein(a) reduced the risk of Alzheimer's by 60% in noncarriers of the APOE ε4 allele who were over age 80.

On the other hand, some patients benefit from being informed. Many do not react to the news by giving up; instead, a clear diagnosis can actually be reassuring—the patient knows that a physical illness is causing the memory problems. The amount of information that patients can comprehend about their diagnosis and prognosis depends on the stage of their illness. But just putting a name to their problem is helpful for many people.

If a person has not written a will or executed an advance directive, for example, then he or she can take this opportunity to do so. Because cognitive decline is inevitable with Alzheimer's disease, it is important that these tasks be done as early as possible in the illness. Other business, financial, or personal issues can also be addressed while the person with Alzheimer's disease still has the capacity to make informed decisions. In addition, people with mild Alzheimer's can still make valuable contributions: For example, herb

grower Thomas DeBaggio, diagnosed with Alzheimer's at age 57, responded to his diagnosis by writing two memoirs, including the well-received *Losing My Mind: An Intimate Look at Life with Alzheimer's.*

Also at issue is access to clinical trials of investigational treatments. Although family members can give consent for people with dementia, it is preferable for the person to give this consent in advance.

Having the Conversation
If you are a family member who has been told of your loved one's diagnosis, you need to decide whether and how to share this news with the patient. If you decide to tell the person about the diagnosis, take some time to plan your approach and to anticipate the person's reactions:
• Choose your setting carefully. A conference, consisting of you, other caregivers, the doctor, and the patient may be helpful for some people; others may respond better to a one-on-one conversation. If you

fear the patient might direct anger at you, ask his or her doctor to deliver the diagnosis.
• Confusion, anger, and denial are common reactions. If they occur, don't try to argue with or convince the person—further detailed discussion likely will not be helpful.
• Don't be surprised if the person already suspects that he or she has Alzheimer's disease.
• Provide as much information as the patient is able to understand, especially about symptoms, medications, and upcoming lifestyle changes.
• Watch for signs of sadness, anger, frustration, or anxiety, and let the patient know that these are understandable feelings and you are open to discussing his or her needs and emotions.
• Finally, reassure the person that you, the doctor, and other caregivers will continue to provide help and support.

Other genes. Studies show that abnormal genes on three different chromosomes—the amyloid precursor protein gene on chromosome 21, the presenilin-1 (PS-1) gene on chromosome 14, and the presenilin-2 (PS-2) gene on chromosome 1—may be directly linked to Alzheimer's disease. However, these alterations are uncommon. A defective amyloid precursor protein gene, for instance, has been found in only 25 families worldwide. Passed down from either parent, these genetic abnormalities account for fewer than 10% of early-onset (before age 60) cases of inherited Alzheimer's. People with an altered amyloid precursor protein gene usually develop Alzheimer's between 40 and 65 years of age. Individuals who carry a PS-1 mutation may show signs of Alzheimer's as early as age 30, while people with PS-2 alterations get the disease anywhere from age 40 to 90. Though these three mutations affect only a small number of families, a person carrying one of them will inevitably develop Alzheimer's if he or she lives long enough.

Cardiovascular disease. Numerous risk factors for cardiovascular disease also appear to be risk factors for Alzheimer's disease. These include elevated LDL cholesterol, low HDL cholesterol, high blood pressure, smoking, excessive fat consumption, and excess body weight. (For more information on how these risk factors relate to dementia, see the text on pages 8–9 and 12–13).

Down syndrome. People with Down syndrome have three to five times the risk of Alzheimer's disease as people in the general population. The faulty cell division that causes Down syndrome appears to contribute to Alzheimer's as well.

Head injury. Scientists are divided over the role of head injury in the development of Alzheimer's disease. Although some studies have shown that a head injury makes a person more likely to develop Alzheimer's later in life, other reports have demonstrated no such association. Further research has shown that head injuries do not increase the incidence of Alzheimer's but may cause people who are already susceptible to the disease to develop it earlier.

Depression. Two recent studies suggest that experiencing negative emotions such as depression makes a person more susceptible to Alzheimer's disease later in life. The first study, from a 2003 issue of the *Archives of Neurology*, found that those who experienced depression in midlife were 71% more likely to develop Alzheimer's disease in older age than those who never experienced significant depressive symptoms. A second 2003 report, from the journal *Neurology*, found that older people who reported experiencing more "negative emotional states" across their lifetime were twice as likely to later develop Alzheimer's as those who were not prone to distress. However, no evidence yet suggests that treating depression will lower the risk of developing Alzheimer's.

Other possible risk factors. Other conditions that have been considered possible triggers of Alzheimer's disease, but for which no good evidence supports a causal relationship, are immune-system malfunctions, endocrine (hormonal) disorders, slow-acting viruses or bacteria, vitamin deficiencies, exposure to electromagnetic fields, and accumulation of metals such as zinc, copper, iron, and aluminum in the body.

Much publicity followed the discovery of a possible link between aluminum and Alzheimer's disease when researchers observed larger-than-expected amounts of the metal in the brains of some people who died of Alzheimer's. Worried that aluminum might somehow promote the disease, many people began to throw away cans, cookware, cosmetics, antacids, antiperspirants, and other items containing the metal. However, studies of people who were exposed to large quantities of aluminum revealed no increased incidence of dementia. Most likely, the deposition of aluminum in brain tissue is a result—not a cause—of the factors that underlie the dementia. (Incidentally, more aluminum leaches into soft drinks from glass bottles—which contain approximately 1% aluminum—than from aluminum cans, which are coated with a thin layer of plastic.)

Diagnosis of Alzheimer's disease. Although only an autopsy can definitively prove the presence of Alzheimer's disease, the clinical diagnosis is usually accurate. The current approach for establishing the cause of memory loss involves both eliminating some potential causes and finding confirmatory support for others. Once other conditions—such as depression, Huntington's disease, or hypothyroidism—have been ruled out as causes of dementia, the diagnosis of Alzheimer's is made on the accumulation of data from the patient's history, mental status exams, and interviews with the patient, family members, and friends over a period of several weeks. Diagnoses based on such clinical features are accurate about 90% of the time. Criteria for the diagnosis of Alzheimer's from the *Diagnostic and Statistical Manual of Mental Disorders* require the presence of memory impairment and at least one other cognitive deficit (such as difficulty communicating) that is severe enough to affect social or job functioning. Also, the decline must be gradual. Laboratory and imaging studies can provide information needed to diagnose many non-Alzheimer's dementias.

Laboratory tests. Two laboratory tests called the ADmark Assays are available to aid in the diagnosis of Alzheimer's disease. One of these assays measures beta-amyloid and tau protein in the cerebrospinal fluid (requiring a spinal tap). Its use is currently discouraged because it is about as accurate as a careful clinical assessment, which needs to be carried out anyway.

The other assay is for the APOE genotype; it bases the *probability* that a person's dementia stems from Alzheimer's disease on whether APOE ε4 alleles are present (because some individuals with this allele will never develop Alzheimer's). This test is not part of routine evaluation of people with dementia.

Some people without dementia request an assay for the APOE genotype, but this is discouraged for several reasons. Most important, the presence of an ε4 allele only indicates that the person is at increased risk for developing Alzheimer's disease, not that the person will develop Alzheimer's. Furthermore, according to a panel of experts assembled by the National Institutes of Health, testing for

NEW RESEARCH

Depression May Spur Mental Decline in Old Age

Older adults with depressive symptoms may show a quicker mental decline over time than others, study findings suggest.

Depression and cognitive decline often coexist, but whether depressive symptoms are in some cases a risk factor for impaired cognition is unclear. In this study, people age 65 and up took standard tests of mental function and depressive symptoms two or three times over an average of five years.

The study of nearly 4,400 older people found that the more depressive symptoms participants had initially, the faster their rate of mental decline. Those who reported 4 symptoms of depression on a 10-item scale at the study's start declined 20% faster than those who were free from depression.

It's possible that chronic depression affects the hippocampus and other brain structures in a way that increases their vulnerability to the degenerative changes. However, according to an accompanying editorial, it remains uncertain whether depression is a cause of mental decline or the result of an underlying brain disease. The author notes that most depression studies, including the present one, rely on "simplistic" measures of depressive symptoms and cannot capture the complexity of the disorder—including its connection to an array of health problems that may affect mental decline.

JOURNAL OF NEUROLOGY, NEUROSURGERY AND PSYCHIATRY
Volume 75, pages 5 and 126
January 2004

the APOE ε4 gene should not be performed because there is presently no cure for Alzheimer's and no recommended treatment to lower the risk of developing it. In addition, knowledge of the gene's presence could produce unnecessary anxiety in the individual and lead to discrimination by employers or health insurance companies.

The reaction to atropine eyedrops was widely reported as a useful screening test, but it is ineffective in identifying early Alzheimer's disease.

Imaging studies. CT and MRI scans are used to examine brain structure or function and rule out other possible causes of mental impairment. The routine use of PET and SPECT is not recommended at this time because it is unclear that they are helpful when the diagnosis is in doubt.

A CT scan uses an x-ray method that makes hundreds of images while rotating 360° around the area that is being studied. A computer processes these images to produce two-dimensional cross-sectional images of the area—like slices from a loaf of bread. This technique can rule out some causes of dementia other than Alzheimer's disease—such as stroke, brain tumor, brain abscess, or hydrocephalus (fluid in the brain). However, specific structures such as the hippocampus cannot be visualized. A CT scan can identify enlargement of the lower portions of the lateral ventricles—chambers in the brain that contain and circulate cerebrospinal fluid (see the illustration on page 3). Enlargement of these portions of the lateral ventricles, which are adjacent to the hippocampus, indirectly suggests a decrease in the volume of the hippocampus. In clinical studies, this technique has detected 75% to 95% of people with Alzheimer's. However, the likelihood of hippocampal atrophy increases in older patients—even in healthy people—and reduces the specificity of the test.

MRI also can detect atrophy and ventricular enlargement. Like CT, this technique forms two-dimensional, cross-sectional images of the brain. But MRI uses a powerful magnet rather than x-rays to capture the images. Because it is based on the amount of water in a given tissue, MRI provides a more refined visualization of the brain and, therefore, better resolution.

A promising development in imaging is functional MRI, which looks not only at the structure of the brain, but also at the metabolic processes taking place within it at the time of the scan. For example, functional MRI can detect changes in brain activity that occur as different areas of the brain are stimulated—through memory

NEW RESEARCH

Brain Scan May Help Differentiate Causes of Dementia

A brain scan that snaps a picture of blood flow in the brain may help distinguish Alzheimer's disease from other causes of dementia, according to researchers.

Right now, doctors diagnose "probable" Alzheimer's based on symptoms, because only an autopsy of the brain can prove the presence of the disease. But with researchers working on medications aimed at hindering Alzheimer's progression, finding a noninvasive way to separate Alzheimer's from other dementias has become increasingly important.

They used single-photon emission computed tomography (SPECT) to view blood flow in a brain region called the posterior cingulate in healthy elderly adults and those with either Alzheimer's disease or frontotemporal dementia. Scientists have suggested that people with Alzheimer's have reduced blood flow in the posterior cingulate.

In this study, 16 of 20 patients with proven Alzheimer's showed such effects on brain scans compared with only 1 of the patients with proven frontotemporal disease, whose condition was later diagnosed as probable Alzheimer's.

Although the posterior cingulate "sign" did not capture all of the Alzheimer's cases in this study, the researchers conclude that it may eventually help differentiate the illness from frontotemporal disease. However, what the study did not determine is whether SPECT scans can detect early Alzheimer's.

JOURNAL OF NUCLEAR MEDICINE
Volume 45, page 771
May 2004

Tracking Dementia via Behavior

Standardized tests such as the Mini-Mental State Examination are useful tools for monitoring the progress of cognitive impairment in patients with Alzheimer's disease. But over time, patients also suffer from a variety of noncognitive symptoms, including behavioral problems and physical disabilities. Tracking such symptoms is a valuable way to evaluate a patient's condition and needs.

Caregivers should take note of any new or worsened behavioral or physical problems and report them to the doctor at each visit. In addition, caregivers can provide the doctor with more detailed information by completing the Functional Dementia Scale, a 20-item questionnaire reprinted below.

Circle one rating for each item.

	None or little of the time	Some of the time	Good part of the time	Most or all of the time
1. Has difficulty in completing simple tasks on own (e.g., dressing, bathing, arithmetic).	1	2	3	4
2. Spends time either sitting or in apparently purposeless activity.	1	2	3	4
3. Wanders at night or needs to be restrained to prevent wandering.	1	2	3	4
4. Hears things that are not there.	1	2	3	4
5. Requires supervision or assistance in eating.	1	2	3	4
6. Loses things.	1	2	3	4
7. Appearance is disorderly if left to own devices.	1	2	3	4
8. Moans.	1	2	3	4
9. Cannot control bowel function.	1	2	3	4
10. Threatens to harm others.	1	2	3	4
11. Cannot control bladder function.	1	2	3	4
12. Needs to be watched so does not injure self (e.g., by careless smoking, leaving the stove on, falling).	1	2	3	4
13. Destructive (e.g., breaks furniture, throws food trays, tears up magazines).	1	2	3	4
14. Shouts or yells.	1	2	3	4
15. Accuses others of doing him/her bodily harm or stealing his/her possessions when the accusations are not true.	1	2	3	4
16. Is unaware of limitations posed by illness.	1	2	3	4
17. Becomes confused and does not know where he/she is.	1	2	3	4
18. Has trouble remembering.	1	2	3	4
19. Has sudden changes of mood (e.g., gets upset, is angered, or cries easily).	1	2	3	4
20. If left alone, wanders aimlessly during day or needs to be restrained to prevent wandering.	1	2	3	4

Source: *Journal of Family Practice,* March 1983.

Total Score _____

tests or mathematical tasks, for example. Such images, which show the structure and the metabolic function of the brain, were formerly possible only with a combination of either CT or MRI and another technique—usually PET or SPECT scanning. Functional MRI might become an effective diagnostic tool for Alzheimer's. Detecting functional abnormalities—which may precede atrophy—can allow earlier diagnosis, and early treatment might prevent or slow the progression of Alzheimer's.

PET and SPECT imaging examines how the brain is working metabolically by assessing how much of a radioactive tracer is taken up by brain cells. An exciting experimental technique involves using radioactively expelled compounds to measure how much beta-amyloid is in the brain. If this measurement is accurate, it could become the standard diagnostic test.

Progression of Alzheimer's disease. Alzheimer's disease advances slowly through three symptomatic stages, ranging from mild forgetfulness to severe dementia.

Symptoms of the first stage include impaired memory of recent events, faulty judgment, and poor insight. People may forget important appointments, recent family events, and highly publicized news items. Other symptoms include losing or misplacing possessions, repetition of questions or statements, and minor or occasional disorientation.

As the disease progresses into the second stage, memory problems grow worse and basic self-care skills begin to decline. Patients have trouble expressing themselves verbally or in writing and may be unable to perform everyday activities such as dressing, bathing, using a knife or fork, or brushing their teeth. They may also suffer from delusions or hallucinations.

In the third stage, almost all capacity for reasoning is lost. Patients end up completely dependent on others for their care. The disorder eventually becomes so debilitating that most patients cannot walk or feed themselves, and patients become susceptible to other diseases. Lung and urinary tract infections are common. Pneumonia is the most frequent cause of death.

Treatment of Alzheimer's disease. As of yet, no treatment can prevent or halt the mental deterioration associated with Alzheimer's disease. The search for effective drug therapy has focused on preventing the destruction of neurons, with the ultimate goal of preserving cognitive function for as long as possible. One avenue researchers have explored is based on the theory that memory deficits in Alzheimer's are partly the result of a deficiency of the neurotransmitter acetylcholine. Scientists have sought ways to boost the amount of acetylcholine in the brain by administering substances containing it, stimulating the brain to manufacture it in increased quantities, or preventing the breakdown of the limited quantities of acetylcholine that the brain is able to make. Lecithin and choline, two substances that occur naturally in many foods, are used by the body to produce acetylcholine. Supplements of lecithin and choline, available in health food stores, have been given to Alzheimer's patients in the hope of improving their mental function, but results have been disappointing.

Cholinesterase inhibitors. Drugs known as cholinesterase inhibitors were the first to be approved by the U.S. Food and Drug Administration (FDA) for the treatment of Alzheimer's disease. These medications work by slowing the breakdown of acetylcholine. Although they may ease some symptoms associated with Alzheimer's, they do not halt its progression. According to guidelines published by the American Academy of Neurology in 2001, these drugs are consistently better than a placebo, but the average benefit is modest, and the disease continues to progress despite treatments.

Tacrine (Cognex)—the first cholinesterase inhibitor to receive FDA approval—works in only about 20% to 40% of people with Alzheimer's disease. Common side effects are nausea, vomiting, and liver damage. Tacrine is rarely used now that a second generation of cholinesterase inhibitors has been developed.

Second-generation cholinesterase inhibitors are similar to tacrine but produce fewer or less severe side effects. The first one approved by the FDA was donepezil (Aricept). Clinical trials have shown significant improvement in cognitive and overall function in people receiving donepezil (compared with those receiving a placebo), with fewer adverse effects than with tacrine. In one 24-week study, at least 80% of the donepezil patients suffered no cognitive decline, compared with 57% of patients taking a placebo. Improvement was greater with higher dosages of the drug: 54% of the patients taking 10 mg of donepezil improved slightly in one cognitive test compared with 38% of those taking 5 mg and 27% taking the placebo. In a more recent study, patients taking 10 mg of donepezil for one year had half the rate of disease progression of those who received a placebo.

The second of these drugs to be approved was rivastigmine (Exelon). In four placebo-controlled clinical trials, involving a total of 3,900 people, those taking rivastigmine had significantly better scores on standard tests of cognitive function than people taking a placebo. One of these trials included 725 people with Alzheimer's disease and found that 24% of the people in the rivastigmine

NEW RESEARCH

Drug May Halve Progression of Early Alzheimer's

The Alzheimer's drug galantamine (Reminyl) may cut in half the rate of mental decline among people in the earlier stages of the disease, a study suggests.

Among patients with mild to moderate Alzheimer's disease who took galantamine for three years, the rate of mental decline was roughly half of what would be expected without treatment. The drug bought patients an extra 18 months of preserved mental functioning. Galantamine is the newest member of a class of drugs called acetylcholinesterase inhibitors (AChEls) approved for Alzheimer's disease.

The study included 194 patients given galantamine (at least 24 mg per day) for up to three years, about 61% of whom took the drug for the entire study period. For those on continuous treatment, the rate of mental decline on standard tests was about 50% of what would be expected (based on a historical sample of Alzheimer's patients given a placebo); patients who discontinued the drug had shown a similarly delayed decline before stopping treatment.

The findings bolster evidence that AChEls delay Alzheimer's progression and emphasize the importance of early diagnosis and treatment of the disease. However, people who stayed on the medicine for three years were a "self-chosen" subsample. Whether the results can be extrapolated to people more broadly is unknown.

ARCHIVES OF NEUROLOGY
Volume 61, page 252
February 2004

group showed significant improvements in cognitive function over a 26-week period compared with 16% of those taking a placebo.

The newest cholinesterase inhibitor to be approved is galantamine (Reminyl). Its approval was based on data from four placebo-controlled clinical trials involving more than 2,650 people. Patients taking galantamine scored better on measures of cognitive performance and function than people taking a placebo. The most common adverse effects of cholinesterase inhibitors are nausea, vomiting, loss of appetite, diarrhea, and weight loss.

NMDA receptor antagonist. In October 2003, the FDA approved memantine (Namenda) for the treatment of moderate to severe Alzheimer's disease. The drug has been the mainstay of Alzheimer's treatment in Germany for years, and the European Union approved it for Alzheimer's disease in 2002. The medication helps block the activity of the neurotransmitter glutamate by binding to N-methyl-D-aspartate (NMDA) receptors on the surface of brain cells.

Memantine has been on the market in the United States for much less time than the cholinesterase inhibitors, and therefore not as much information is available about its long-term cognitive effects. However, one 28-week study comparing memantine with a placebo found that the drug was associated with significantly decreased cognitive decline during that brief period. Also, about 20% of patients taking memantine showed some improvement in cognition and/or activities of daily living by the study's end. Another study found that patients taking memantine plus donepezil averaged less cognitive decline over 24 weeks than those taking a placebo plus donepezil; about 40% of people taking memantine plus donepezil experienced cognitive improvements, and 30% had improved daily functioning.

Although some patients may experience improvements over the short term, most can expect to see a modest delay in declines of memory and activities of daily living with memantine. The medication may also help extend the time patients can spend at home before requiring assisted living. However, memantine does not reverse or halt the degeneration that occurs in the brains of people with dementia.

Because memantine became available only recently, practice patterns are still developing. However, in Europe, where cholinesterase inhibitors and memantine have been available for longer times, the two drugs are often prescribed together early in the disease, although memantine is only approved for the later stages in the United States.

Medications To Treat Alzheimer's Disease 2005

Generic Name	Brand Name	Average Daily Dosage*	Average Retail Cost†	How They Work	Comments
Cholinesterase Inhibitors					
galantamine	Reminyl	16 to 24 mg	8 mg: $75	Block acetylcholinesterase, an enzyme that destroys the neurotransmitter acetylcholine. This action elevates the level of acetylcholine in the brain, thereby increasing messages between nerve cells.	Produce slight improvements in memory and reasoning ability, and mental decline is less pronounced. Side effects include nausea, vomiting, diarrhea, loss of appetite, dizziness, fatigue, and possible liver damage. Rivastigmine and galantamine are taken twice a day and are available in liquid form for people who cannot swallow tablets. Donepezil is taken once a day.
rivastigmine	Exelon	6 to 12 mg	3 mg: $78		
donepezil	Aricept	5 to 10 mg	10 mg: $132		
NMDA Receptor Antagonist					
memantine	Namenda	5 to 20 mg	10 mg: $68	Selectively inhibits glutamate at NMDA receptors, preventing overstimulation of cells and cellular dysfunction.	Slows memory decline and behavioral deterioration. Increases in dosages should occur at increments of 5 mg for at least one week.

NMDA = N-methyl-D-aspartate.

* These dosages represent an average range for the treatment of Alzheimer's disease. The precise effective dosage varies from patient to patient and depends on many factors. Do not make any changes in your medication without consulting your doctor.

† Average price for 30 tablets or capsules (unless otherwise indicated) of the dosage strength listed. Actual price may vary. If a generic version is available, the cost is listed in parentheses. Sources: drugstore.com, eckerd.com, and walgreens.com.

Vitamin E and selegiline. The antioxidant properties of vitamin E made it the focus of a well-designed study published in *The New England Journal of Medicine* in 1997. People with moderately severe Alzheimer's disease received a daily dose of 2,000 IU of vitamin E, 10 mg a day of selegiline (a medication used to treat Parkinson's disease), both, or a placebo. Taking selegiline or vitamin E slowed the time to institutionalization and increased survival by about seven months. The two agents taken independently also cut by one quarter the number of people who lost the ability to do daily activities, such as handling money or bathing. Combining vitamin E and selegiline did not further improve results, however.

Based on this study, the American Academy of Neurology concluded that good evidence exists for the use of vitamin E in an attempt to slow the progression of Alzheimer's disease. The evidence for selegiline is weaker, and it has more side effects than vitamin E. There is no advantage to using selegiline if vitamin E is already being used.

It is too soon to recommend that people take vitamin E to prevent dementia. But the Memory Impairment Study, a randomized, placebo-controlled trial of vitamin E and the cholinesterase inhibitor donepezil is now under way and will help determine whether vitamin E can prevent Alzheimer's disease in people with mild cognitive impairment.

Although vitamin E is generally safe, large doses have been associated with bleeding in some people who are deficient in vitamin K.

Investigational therapies. For reasons that are not entirely clear, a recent study found that people with Alzheimer's disease who participated in a clinical trial were less likely to be placed in a nursing home over a three-and-a-half-year period than patients who never participated. Of the people in clinical trials, 17% entered nursing homes compared with 37% of eligible nonparticipants and 32% of ineligible people. This delay could have a number of explanations. For example, it may be the result of a direct benefit from the drug being studied or from improved coping skills that caregivers gained from additional contact with medical personnel during the study. It is also possible that people who elect to participate in clinical trials are different from those who do not. In any case, enrollment in a clinical trial may be beneficial—and may be even more worthwhile for people with Alzheimer's than for those with other medical conditions because there is no cure for Alzheimer's.

The following are currently being tested or were once thought to have potential as therapeutic agents. They are still regarded as highly investigational and are by no means established as effective—but some do offer hope for the future.

CX516 (Ampalex). The neurotransmitter glutamate, which memantine targets, binds not only to NMDA receptors in the brain but also to α-amino-3-hydroxy-5-methyl-4-isoxazolepropionic acid (AMPA) receptors. By binding to AMPA receptors, the investigational medication CX516 enhances the function of these receptors and possibly improves memory. An early clinical trial showed that the drug was relatively safe and that it improved learning and memory in healthy people. Current research is examining the safety and effectiveness of the drug in treating cognitive deficits in people with Alzheimer's disease.

Cognishunt. The spaces in and around the brain and spinal cord are filled with a substance called cerebrospinal fluid. Researchers are testing a drainlike device called Cognishunt, which is surgically implanted in the brain in the hope of removing cellular debris such as beta-amyloid and tau from the brain. The device helps drain cerebrospinal fluid from the brain into the abdominal cavity, where the body reabsorbs the fluid. The hope is that this would slow or halt worsening of Alzheimer's symptoms by encouraging beta-amyloid and tau to diffuse from the brain into the cerebrospinal fluid. However, investigators have completed only preliminary research into this approach, and the shunt is associated with a number of potential side effects, such as seizures, nausea, pain, subdural hematoma, and the risks involved with any surgical procedure, including death.

In one small study published in *Neurology* in 2002, people who received Cognishunt experienced a slight decline in mental function after a year, while those who received no treatment experienced a more marked decline. Further, patients with the shunt had lower beta-amyloid and tau levels in their cerebrospinal fluid at the end of the study than they did at the beginning. However, this study was not double-blind and too few people were studied to draw definitive conclusions about the effectiveness and safety of Cognishunt. A larger, controlled trial is now in progress.

Statins. Population studies have found that certain medications used to lower LDL ("bad") cholesterol levels may also reduce the risk of Alzheimer's disease. Now, evidence from small, preliminary studies suggests that high doses of statins might also be helpful in treating mental decline in patients with Alzheimer's disease. It is unclear how statins may help treat Alzheimer's disease. Researchers speculate that decreased cholesterol levels may help lower the production of beta-amyloid or improve blood vessel functioning in the brain. Also, statins may have an anti-inflammatory effect. The manufacturers of atorvastatin (Lipitor) are currently testing this drug in the treatment of Alzheimer's disease in a large clinical trial.

Alzheimer's vaccine. In 2000, researchers began testing a vaccine (called AN-1792) designed to trigger the immune system to eliminate beta-amyloid plaques from the brain. Investigators stopped the study in January 2002 after 15 of the 360 Alzheimer's patients studied developed central nervous system inflammation.

However, two 2003 follow-up studies from the halted trial revealed that the vaccine might have helped clear plaques from the brain and reduced cognitive decline in some people. In the first study, from *Nature Medicine*, a 72-year-old woman who was vaccinated developed brain inflammation. She later died from a cause unrelated to the vaccine. An autopsy revealed that the vaccine appeared to have attacked beta-amyloid deposits in the blood ves-

---

NEW RESEARCH

Drug Combo Beats Traditional Medicine for Alzheimer's

Patients with moderate to severe Alzheimer's disease who take the drug memantine (Namenda) together with donepezil (Aricept) experience better mental functioning and quality of life than those who take only donepezil, according to a recent study. Memantine inhibits actions of the neurotransmitter glutamate (which, in excess, can kill neurons) while donepezil boosts levels of acetylcholine, a neurotransmitter involved in memory.

Researchers randomly assigned 404 patients with moderate to severe Alzheimer's to receive memantine (20 mg daily) or a placebo. All patients had taken 5 to 10 mg of donepezil daily for six months of continued donepezil treatment during the study. Mental function, daily living skills, and behavior were monitored using various tests over the course of the 24-week trial.

By the end of the study, patients who received memantine plus donepezil scored higher on scales that rated cognition, activities of daily living, and behavior than those who took placebo and donepezil. The rate of side effects was similar in both groups. The results suggest that together, these two drugs with different mechanisms of action significantly improve outcomes among Alzheimer's patients better than treatment with cholinesterase inhibitors alone. However, the benefits are modest.

JOURNAL OF THE AMERICAN MEDICAL ASSOCIATION
Volume 291, page 317
January 21, 2004

To Drive or Not To Drive

When is it time for a person with dementia to stop driving?
New research and recent recommendations offer some insights.

After decades of the freedom and independence that driving can bring, many people with dementia are reluctant to stop driving. But the decline in cognition found in people with diseases such as Alzheimer's often makes them unsafe drivers. For example, people with dementia are about three to five times as likely as others their age to be involved in a car crash.

Although experts agree that those with moderate or severe dementia should not drive, the data on people with very mild or mild dementia are not as clear. Evidence shows that people with very mild Alzheimer's are no more likely to cause a car crash than a young person who just obtained a driver's license. And new research is beginning to clarify when patients with dementia are fit to drive and when they should give up the keys.

How Safe Are Drivers With Dementia?

One recent report, a 2003 study from the *Journal of the American Geriatrics Society,* used a road test to evaluate and compare the driving skills of people without dementia with those of people with very mild Alzheimer's disease and mild Alzheimer's over two years. (Very mild Alzheimer's is roughly equivalent to a Mini-Mental State Exam score of 25; patients with mild Alzheimer's tend to have scores

between 20 and 24.) The researchers reached the following conclusions:

- At the start of the study, far more people with mild Alzheimer's disease (41%) were unsafe drivers compared with those with very mild Alzheimer's disease (14%) and people without dementia (3%).
- Of those fit to drive at the study's onset, the driving skills of those with mild Alzheimer's disease declined to an unsafe level the fastest, followed by those with very mild Alzheimer's. People without dementia declined the slowest.
- Most of the people with mild Alzheimer's who were initially fit to drive became unsafe drivers within two years.

Signs and Signals of Problem Driving

Some people with dementia might seem like safe drivers in familiar traffic conditions, but they actually have underlying deficits that prevent them from reacting appropriately to unanticipated events. So what problems can family members look for? According to the *Journal of the American Geriatrics Society* article, the first driving skills to go are judgment, awareness of how one's driving affects other drivers, and speed control. Other behaviors that indicate that someone's driving skills may be deteriorating include

the following:

- braking often or unexpectedly;
- not obeying traffic signs and signals;
- becoming aggressive or angry while driving;
- trouble staying in one's lane; and
- difficulty navigating through familiar locations.

A report from a 2004 issue of *Neuropsychology,* which reviewed the results of 27 studies, found that deficits in visuospatial skills (see the inset box) and, to a lesser extent, attention and concentration were the best predictors of which people with early dementia had problems with driving. Visuospatial deficits in people with early dementia are "red flags" indicating that their driving skills should be evaluated carefully, the researchers conclude.

What the Experts Recommend

Guidelines from the American Academy of Neurology (AAN), published in 2000, say that people with mild or more severe dementia should not drive because of an increased crash risk.

However, while noting that people with very mild Alzheimer's disease have an elevated crash risk compared with age-matched controls, the AAN explains that this elevated risk is no different from that in other acceptably "impaired" drivers: 16- to 21-year-olds and people with a blood alcohol con-

sels of her brain, causing inflammation and possibly leading to poor blood flow. However, large sections of her cerebral cortex were almost entirely clear of beta-amyloid plaques.

In another report, from the journal *Neuron,* researchers analyzed cognitive data from 30 of the 360 people who received the vaccine. After one year, the 20 people who developed antibodies to beta-amyloid had significantly less decline in cognition and daily living skills than the 10 who did not develop antibodies. The results

tent below 0.08%. Therefore, the AAN says that people with very mild Alzheimer's may still be able to drive. The academy recommends that caregivers of people with very mild dementia should consider having the person initially have his or her driving examined by a professional, and a clinician should reassess the person's fitness for driving every six months.

Adding to this information, the authors of the *Journal of the American Geriatrics Society* study say that a small proportion of people with mild dementia retain the ability to drive safely and that fitness to drive should not always be determined by a diagnosis of mild dementia, per se, but through semiannual evaluations of driving performance. Some occupational and physical therapists are able to perform such evaluations, or you can request that someone at your state's department of motor vehicles evaluate the person using a road test.

When and How To Restrict Driving

Although some people with very mild or mild dementia may retain the ability to drive safely, they should restrict their driving to nonchallenging situations, such as driving only in familiar areas, during the daytime, in good weather, for short distances, and in light traffic. They should never drink any amount of alcohol before driving. Also, family members need to ascertain that these drivers maintain skills necessary for driving: a quick reaction

---

What Are Visuospatial Skills?

Visuospatial skills are those abilities that allow a person to relate their visual perception to concrete spatial relationships. In driving, these skills allow people to judge distances, maneuver correctly, and navigate unfamiliar territory. When diagnosing a person with dementia, clinicians typically test visuospatial skills as a subset of overall cognitive testing using tests that include clock drawing (accurately drawing a clock depicting a specific time), block design (assembling real-life blocks to look like a two-dimensional drawing), picture completion (pointing out the missing details of a line drawing), and diagram drawing and copying (having a person draw a picture, such as a flower, from memory or copy a complex line drawing). Family members can ask the patient's clinician for the results of their loved one's visuospatial testing.

---

time; the ability to make decisions appropriately and rapidly; an alertness to what is going on in the environment; and good coordination, vision, and hearing.

Eventually, the time to stop driving will come to every person with dementia. Yet a loved one with dementia may have a strong desire to keep driving and little awareness of his or her deficits. How can you get someone with dementia to stop driving if asking isn't enough? Experts recommend that you ask the person's doctor to tell the person not to drive, or even ask the doctor write a "Do Not Drive" prescription. Health care professionals in some states must report to the motor vehicle division that a person in their care has a medical condition that interferes with driving ability. The state may then revoke the person's driver's license.

If the person still insists on driving,

caregivers can take more drastic measures. These include hiding the car keys, parking the car where the person can't see it, or selling the car. A mechanic may be able to show you how to disable the car temporarily by removing the distributor cap or disconnecting the battery.

The Bottom Line

Determining when a person in the early stages of dementia can no longer drive is not always easy. Enlist the help of doctors, lawyers, therapists, or the department of motor vehicles when difficult questions arise. But above all, patients, caregivers, and family members should let common sense be their guide. A good rule of thumb may be the "grandchild test": If you would not feel safe having the person with dementia drive his or her grandchild in the car, you should talk to the person about not driving.

---

suggest that elimination of beta-amyloid does, in fact, slow mental deterioration.

Alternative forms of the vaccine have been identified, but it will take several years to know if they are effective.

Anti-inflammatory drugs. Because Alzheimer's disease is associated with inflammation in the brain, many researchers had considered nonsteroidal anti-inflammatory drugs (NSAIDs) as a potential treatment for the disease. (NSAIDs are a class of drugs commonly used to treat arthritis.) Disappointingly, however, a 2003 randomized study from the *Journal of the American Medical Association* showed that one year of treatment with two commonly used NSAIDs—naproxen (Aleve and other brands) and rofecoxib (Vioxx)—does not improve cognition or slow cognitive decline any better than a placebo in people with mild to moderate Alzheimer's disease. Also, the NSAIDs exposed patients to side effects like fatigue, dizziness, high blood pressure, strokes, heart attacks, and gastrointestinal bleeding. The authors of this study recommend against using NSAIDs to treat Alzheimer's. A 2004 study of 692 people with Alzheimer's published in *Neurology* confirmed that rofecoxib is ineffective in slowing the progression of the disease. (Rofecoxib was taken off the market in 2004 because it was found to increase the risk of heart attacks and strokes.)

Clioquinol. Another drug being studied for the treatment of Alzheimer's disease is clioquinol, an antibiotic and antifungal medication that was, in the past, available in oral form but is now only prescribed as a topical medication to treat conditions such as eczema and athlete's foot. In a preliminary phase II clinical trial of 36 people with moderately severe Alzheimer's disease, clioquinol (in oral form) slowed mental decline and decreased plasma levels of beta-amyloid compared with a placebo. Clioquinol may work by promoting the elimination of metals—such as zinc and copper—in the brain and may allow beta-amyloid to be removed more easily. However, much more research is needed before this drug can be recommended.

Estrogen. Recent studies show that, in addition to being ineffective in preventing dementia—and possibly promoting it—HRT is also not helpful once Alzheimer's begins. A 12-week study conducted in Taiwan showed that estrogen did not improve cognitive function in 50 women with Alzheimer's disease who were randomized to receive either estrogen or a placebo. A more well-designed study, which lasted one year and included 120 women with Alzheimer's, also found that estrogen replacement had no effect on cognitive function.

However, it is still possible that estrogen alone (that is, without progesterone) will be beneficial in some people. Studies to examine this are ongoing.

Ginkgo biloba. Ginkgo biloba has been hypothesized to have antioxidant and anti-inflammatory effects within the brain. However, the supplement appears to be ineffective for people with Alzheimer's disease. A study published in the *Journal of the American Medical Association* in 2002 shows that the supplement does not improve memory or other cognitive functions in older people who are free of memory impairment, either. It is possible that it may benefit some people with

NEW RESEARCH

Men's Testosterone Levels Tied to Alzheimer's Risk

Low testosterone levels may make men vulnerable to developing Alzheimer's disease, a long-term study suggests.

Researchers found that, in a group of U.S. men followed for decades, those with low blood levels of free testosterone had an elevated risk of developing Alzheimer's. Free testosterone is a form of the hormone that is not bound to a protein in the blood and is therefore available to body tissue.

Whether giving older men testosterone replacement therapy might stave off Alzheimer's is far from clear, but the study authors say their findings should spur research into the possibility. They also urge caution, however, noting that although scientists had hoped hormone replacement therapy would lower the risk of dementia in older women, this has not been borne out in recent clinical trials.

The current study included 574 men, ages 32 to 87, who were free from Alzheimer's and followed for an average of 19 years. The researchers found that for every 10-unit increase in a man's free testosterone, his risk of later developing Alzheimer's dipped 26%, even with factors such as age, education, and smoking considered.

According to the authors, the findings are bolstered by past research in animals and humans suggesting that natural testosterone may protect brain cells and limit the buildup of Alzheimer's-linked beta-amyloid proteins.

NEUROLOGY
Volume 62, page 188
January 27, 2004

unspecified dementia (not Alzheimer's), but the American Academy of Neurology states that the evidence for ginkgo biloba is weak. A large, well-designed trial of ginkgo biloba is now under way.

Because ginkgo biloba is considered a food supplement, it is not regulated by the FDA. People who are considering the use of ginkgo biloba should be aware that taking it with aspirin may lead to an increased risk of bleeding.

Alternative measures. Some of the alternative treatments promoted for memory enhancement include choline, a building block of acetylcholine, which has not proven effective; dimethyl-aminoethanol (DMAE), a nutrient found in seafood; ergoloid mesylates (Gerimal, Hydergine), which is used to treat some mood, behavior, or other problems associated with Alzheimer's disease or vascular dementia; piracetam (Nootropil), which may improve the metabolism of acetylcholine; and vasopressin, a hormone produced by the hypothalamus. One potentially promising agent is huperzine A (hupA), which appears to work in a similar fashion to cholinesterase inhibitors. The results from a Chinese trial comparing hupA with a placebo are encouraging, but further studies are needed to prove effectiveness and safety, especially because it may cause many undesirable side effects.

Because no controlled studies have yet demonstrated that any of these substances improves memory, they cannot be recommended for use in the treatment of Alzheimer's disease or any form of memory impairment.

Standard care for Alzheimer's disease. The amount of care that a patient with Alzheimer's disease requires will change over the course of the disorder. A cholinesterase inhibitor and/or memantine, possibly in conjunction with vitamin E, is recommended for use in the last two stages of Alzheimer's, although the FDA has not approved cholinesterase inhibitors for the last stage of the disease. Other treatments can be instituted with the appearance of specific symptoms or associated disorders, such as depression or agitation.

According to the American Academy of Neurology, antipsychotic medications can be useful for the treatment of agitation and psychosis in dementia. Newer antipsychotic agents, such as risperidone (Risperdal), olanzapine (Zyprexa), and quetiapine (Seroquel), seem to be better tolerated than traditional antipsychotic agents such as haloperidol (Haldol).

Depression and Alzheimer's disease commonly occur together, with about 25% of Alzheimer's patients having depression. The options for the treatment of depression are medication, psy-

NEW RESEARCH

Mental "Rehab" Aids in Mild Alzheimer's Disease

Mental exercises may help people in the earlier stages of Alzheimer's disease improve some aspects of their memory.

Cognitive rehabilitation therapy presents patients with several tasks designed to improve their everyday functioning—including matching names with faces and making change from a $20 bill. That the therapy helped patients in this study supports the notion that people with Alzheimer's "can learn and maintain cognitive and functional gains," the say authors.

The study involved 25 mildly impaired Alzheimer's patients who underwent cognitive rehab twice a week for three to four months, and 19 who received "mental stimulation" sessions that used computer games to try to boost memory and concentration skills. All were on cholinesterase inhibitor medication.

Patients in both groups made gains in their memory skills and showed fewer depressive symptoms. But the families of those who received cognitive rehabilitation reported greater improvements than did families in the other group. Moreover, the benefits were still clear three months after the therapy ended.

The fact that patients in the rehab group improved in everyday skills such as making change suggests that the therapy could improve the quality of life of patients, but the biggest impact may be on their caregivers.

AMERICAN JOURNAL OF GERIATRIC PSYCHIATRY
Volume 12, page 395
July–August 2004

The Sundowning Phenomenon

Some people with Alzheimer's disease experience a worsening of agitation and confusion in the afternoon and early evening— a condition for which a variety of coping strategies exist.

Every day at 4 P.M., Mrs. Haas puts on her jacket and announces to her husband that she's going home. Although he explains that she already is home in the retirement community where they've been living for the past two years, she insists that she needs to leave immediately. Over the next hour she becomes increasingly agitated, screaming that her children are alone in the house and that she has to go get them. Finally, at 6 or 7 P.M., she agrees to sit down and eat dinner with her husband.

Becoming agitated in the late afternoon or early evening is a common phenomenon among people with Alzheimer's disease. In fact, a special word—sundowning—is used to describe this behavior. Sundowning can take the form of behaviors not seen during other times of day, or it may represent a worsening of ongoing daily behaviors.

Exactly what causes sundowning is unclear. Possible explanations include fatigue at the end of the day, being overwhelmed by too much sensory input, lack of stimulation (not enough activities or attention), and becoming confused in dim light. Sleep problems, such as sleep apnea and disturbances in the sleep/wake cycle (circadian rhythm), may also play a role. The behavior seems to be more common among people living in nursing homes than in those living at home. Of course, not everyone with Alzheimer's experiences sundowning, and some individuals have more behavior problems early in the day rather than later.

How To Cope

If you are caring for someone with Alzheimer's disease who experiences sundowning, think about what might be triggering the episodes and take steps to minimize those triggers. For example:

Exhaustion. A confused person may be tired in the evening from a day of trying to make sense of his environment. Plan the person's day so that fewer demands, such as bathing, are placed on him in the evening.

Too much input. Noise, glare, and distractions can contribute to agitation. If sundowning coincides with a busy time in your household (for example, dinner preparation, family members arriving, the television being turned on), try to reduce the number of activities going on, or move the person to a quieter area of the house.

Too little input. Some people with Alzheimer's are used to having constant attention and will become agitated when you turn to other responsibilities, such as returning phone calls. Try giving the person a simple task to do nearby, or enlist another family member to spend time with her.

Inadequate lighting. A person who cannot see clearly because of dim light may become confused and visualize objects that aren't there, so make sure the house is well lit in the evening.

If an episode of sundowning occurs, reassure the person using calm, positive statements, or direct the person's attention to another activity, such as going for a walk. Do not raise your voice or argue with the person.

chotherapy, other therapeutic measures such as electroconvulsive therapy, or any combination of these. Treatment for depression is usually highly effective. The first antidepressant medication tried is successful at relieving depression in up to 70% of people; psychotherapy alone works in about half of people; and up to 70% of people with depression and dementia improve with electroconvulsive therapy.

A 2003 study from Johns Hopkins demonstrated the effectiveness of one antidepressant medication, sertraline (Zoloft), in the treatment of depression in Alzheimer's disease. People with Alzheimer's and depression were randomized to receive sertraline or a placebo.

The Role of Sleep

People with Alzheimer's disease suffer disproportionately from sleep disturbances. Helping the person get a good night's sleep can reduce daytime sleepiness and may reduce disruption of the circadian rhythm, a common problem in elderly people.

Sleep hygiene. Encouraging proper sleep practices—known as sleep hygiene—can promote restful sleep:

- Establish a consistent schedule for the person to go to bed and get up.
- If the person has trouble sleeping at night, limit napping to a short period in the early afternoon.
- Engage the person in exercise during the day that is appropriate to his or her level of functioning. Do not encourage strenuous exercise within three hours of bedtime.
- Discourage the person from watching television if he or she awakens at night.
- Don't allow food or beverages containing caffeine (including chocolate) within six hours of bedtime.
- Restrict the use of nicotine and other stimulants.
- Don't provide heavy meals or alcohol before bedtime.
- Limit fluid intake in the evening and encourage the person to empty his or her bladder before bedtime.

- Address factors that may interrupt sleep, such as household pets in the bedroom or traffic noise from outside.

Medication. Because cholinesterase inhibitors sometimes have a stimulant effect, try giving them in the mornings if the person is not sleeping well. In fact, there is some evidence that their use during the day can help reduce daytime sleepiness. The morning is also the best time to give diuretics ("water pills") because they can cause nighttime urination if given in the evening.

In addition, evaluate whether the person is taking other medications that can interfere with sleep. Such medications include beta-blockers (used in high blood pressure and heart disease), bronchodilators (used in lung disorders), corticosteroids (used in arthritis), H_2 blockers (used in acid reflux), and selegiline (used in Parkinson's disease)

Sleep apnea. More than 70% of people with dementia suffer from sleep apnea—temporary, recurrent breathing interruptions during sleep. The best treatment for sleep apnea is continuous positive airway pressure (CPAP), which involves the delivery of pressurized air through a nasal mask to keep the airways open. Although CPAP is highly effective and, in some cases, may even pro-

duce small improvements in cognitive functioning, coaxing a person with dementia to use it is often difficult or impossible.

Light therapy. Inadequate exposure to light can contribute to sundowning; in fact, there may be a link between seasonal affective disorder (SAD) and the condition. Getting the person outdoors during the day or placing the person's chair next to a sunny window can remedy this problem. Some experts suggest using light boxes in the winter, although it may be difficult to get the person to sit in front of a light box.

Melatonin. Although several small studies have found that melatonin may be effective in reducing insomnia and sundowning in people with Alzheimer's disease, others have not. This approach is not recommended.

Activity. Because inactivity can lead to sundowning, try to schedule an activity the person has always enjoyed—such as going to the store or meeting friends—on most afternoons.

Distraction. Sometimes, distracting the person can help control sundowning. Try engaging the person in a conversation about a topic he or she finds important, such as family, hobbies, or politics.

After 12 weeks, those receiving sertraline had less depression, fewer behavioral problems (such as agitation), and less disability (that is, they had less difficulty with daily functions such as grooming) than the placebo group. Also, the patients' caregivers experienced less distress. The rate of side effects, including dry mouth, upset stomach, decreased appetite, agitation, and tremor, was similar in the sertraline and placebo groups. However, the drug did not affect cognitive functioning.

Other commonly used antidepressants include paroxetine (Paxil), citalopram (Celexa), bupropion (Wellbutrin), and venlafaxine (Effexor). The effectiveness of these drugs and their side effects vary from one individual to another. Some antidepressant drugs can themselves cause side effects that impair memory; therefore, a patient's response to treatment must be monitored carefully. It can take as long as six to eight weeks before depression improves with medication or psychotherapy. Electroconvulsive therapy can work more quickly.

COPING WITH CAREGIVING

More than 7 out of 10 people with Alzheimer's disease live at home, where family and friends provide almost 75% of their care. The daily challenges and frustrations of caring for an individual with dementia can leave family members feeling physically exhausted and emotionally drained. Because they are often faced with overwhelming day-to-day responsibilities, most family caregivers tend to neglect their own physical and mental health. Caregivers must pay attention to their own well-being, however—for the ultimate benefit of both themselves and the person with dementia.

Caregivers are advised to accept the fact that feelings of love for a relative may be tempered with anger, anxiety, frustration, or embarrassment. These reactions are perfectly natural and should not be a source of guilt for the caregiver. Equally important are looking after your own health, joining a caregiver support group, scheduling regular respites, asking for help, setting realistic goals, and considering professional counseling if necessary.

Choosing a Nursing Home

As dementia progresses, the patient's increasing dependency and need for supervision may make it more difficult for the family to provide all necessary care. At this point in the illness, the family may need to move the person with dementia to an assisted living facility, a nursing home, or hospice care. Because caring for someone with dementia often requires the skills of professionally trained people, nursing home placement may be in the best interest of the person with dementia. Half of all nursing home residents suffer from Alzheimer's or a related disorder.

This decision to place the person with dementia in a nursing home can be hard for the family to accept and may be accompanied by feelings of guilt, sadness, and anger. In addition, the bad publicity some nursing homes have received for giving inadequate and sometimes dangerous care can add to the anxiety. You should keep in mind that many nursing homes do provide excellent care;

with some research, you should be able to find a suitable facility.

Before deciding on a nursing home, you may want to explore other residential care programs, such as assisted-living facilities, which provide a combination of housing, personalized assistance, and medical care. Whether such facilities—which vary in size, cost, services, location, and quality—are appropriate for a person with Alzheimer's disease depends on the level of care needed.

If you determine that a nursing home proves the best option after discussions with the doctor and other members of your family, the first step toward finding a good one is to consult as many people as possible. Helpful information may come from the patient's physician, from friends and acquaintances who have resided in or have a family member in a home, and from the nursing home ombudsperson (who is responsible for investigating complaints). Also, the local chapter of the Alzheimer's Association (see page 58) may have a list of recommended homes or personal references. Remember, also, to visit any candidate nursing home several times before making a final decision. Some factors to consider during those visits are outlined below.

Licensing and regulations. Check to make sure that the nursing home meets basic safety requirements. The home and the administrator should have current licenses from the state, and the home should meet state fire regulations, which include sprinkler systems and fire doors.

Care and services. It is important that the staff be familiar with common issues arising from dementia. Therefore, you should ask if the staff is continually trained on dementia-care issues, what kinds of programs are offered to the residents, how individual care plans are developed, and how different levels of function are supported. Give examples of your patient's behaviors or challenges to find out how situations that are difficult might be handled. And be sure the facility provides for the special needs of each patient. Other questions may include the following:

- Does the facility have its own physician? How are other medical, dental, and vision needs met?
- Can the home accommodate any improvements or declines in a resident's condition? Under what circumstances can a home discharge the person, and how much notice is given?
- What is the policy regarding life-sustaining measures? Although a painful subject to deal with at the time of the patient's admission, it is generally important to record in the resident's chart the wishes of the family and patient regarding terminal care.

NEW RESEARCH

Care for Alzheimer's Caregivers May Ease Depression

Counseling and support may lower the long-term risk of depression among people who care for a spouse with Alzheimer's disease, a study suggests.

Among 406 men and women caring for a spouse with the disease, those who received professional counseling and help from a support group had fewer symptoms of depression over three years than caregivers who did not receive counseling. The program consisted of six counseling sessions at the time the illness was diagnosed—some involving other family members as well—plus weekly support group meetings for at least four months and access to a counselor over the course of the spouse's illness.

The researchers had found in an earlier study that the program seemed to combat depression among caregivers in the first year. These latest findings show that the benefit extends into the long term and can be seen even after a caregiver's spouse dies or enters a nursing home.

If such support services were widely available, the authors conclude, it could have a "major impact" on caregivers' well-being as well as health care costs related to depression,

"Since family caregiving affects about 25 million American families," they write, "providing effective interventions for caregivers should become a high priority."

AMERICAN JOURNAL OF PSYCHIATRY
Volume 161, page 850
May 2004

Staff. Talk with the staff members who work directly with residents to see if they are competent, friendly, and content in their jobs. Observe how residents are treated and whether they get help when they ask for it. Also, meet with the administrator and directors of nursing and social services. They will be able to tell you such things as the number of people each aide must take care of and how the facility is staffed on weekends and evenings.

Costs. Because nursing home care is expensive, it is important that all costs be clearly outlined and understood. Before making a decision, address how costs will be met and whether paying for them will create a financial burden for family members. Since the laws regarding payment for nursing home care can be complex and vary among the states, be sure to contact a reliable source for accurate information. The Alzheimer's Association, insurance companies, attorneys who specialize in financial planning, Medicare representatives, and some staff members of in-home care programs may be well informed on payment options. Questions include the following:

- Does the home accept the patient's funding sources (for example, Medicare)?
- Will the resident receive a refund of advance payments if he or she leaves the facility?
- How does the home protect cash and assets that are entrusted to it? How are withdrawals noted in order to keep track of the account?
- What charges are extra (for example, television, telephone, laundry, personal-care supplies, special nursing procedures)?

Cleanliness and safety. Be sure the nursing home is clean and safe (especially the kitchen and bathroom). Note unpleasant odors, such as mold, garbage, or urine. Persistent odors upon return visits may indicate poor patient care or poor housekeeping. Make sure that the bathrooms have handrails and nonskid floors, the furniture is sturdy, the doors to the outside are secure, and the facility protects the safety of people who wander.

Comfort. Spend time observing everyday life and how people are treated in a variety of facilities. Ask residents and visitors about their opinions of the facility and its staff. See if the residents look happy, comfortable, relaxed, and involved in activities. Ask yourself these questions:

- Is the facility relatively quiet, well lit, and pleasant to be in?
- Is there a well-planned indoor or outdoor wandering path?
- Are there familiar elements in the environment, such as

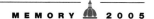

home-like lighting and furnishings, a center of activity, a separate dining room, and areas in the resident's room that can be personalized?

• Does the facility avoid disorienting sensory stimuli, such as overhead speaker systems, loud alarms, and blaring televisions?

Visiting. Be sure the home is close enough so that family members can visit regularly. Also, confirm that the home has long and convenient visiting hours and that the resident can have privacy with visitors.

Meals and activities. Make sure the food is wholesome, appealing, adequate, and suitable for older people. Find out what services and activities are included in the fee. You should ask if participation in activities is required and what is done if a resident does not like the food or the activities. Finally, make sure there are creative and effectively planned social activities in addition to supervised daily exercise. ■

GLOSSARY

acetylcholine—A neurotransmitter crucial to memory and learning.

ADmark Assays—Two clinical tests for Alzheimer's disease. One measures beta-amyloid and tau protein in the spinal fluid; the other tests for the apolipoprotein E ε4 genotype.

age-associated memory impairment—Normal forgetfulness that increases with age.

Alzheimer's disease—A progressive disorder of the brain that is characterized by deterioration of mental faculties resulting from the loss of nerve cells and the connections between them. Also called Alzheimer disease.

amnestic syndrome—Severe memory loss despite maintenance of normal intelligence.

amyloid plaques—Dense deposits of beta-amyloid, pieces of damaged nerve cells, and other proteins. Found in the brains of virtually all people with Alzheimer's disease.

amyloid precursor protein—A protein that is split in two by enzymes to produce beta-amyloid.

aphasia—A partial or complete inability to use or understand language.

apolipoprotein E (APOE)—A gene on chromosome 19. The ε4 version of this gene is associated with an increased risk of Alzheimer's disease.

beta-amyloid—A sticky, starch-like protein that is the main component of amyloid plaques.

bovine spongiform encephalopathy (BSE)—An infectious disease of cows with manifestations similar to Creutzfeldt-Jakob disease in humans. More commonly known as mad cow disease.

carotid endarterectomy—Surgical removal of a blockage of the carotid artery, the main artery leading from the aorta to the brain.

cerebellum—A fist-sized structure, located at the base of the brain beneath the cerebral cortex, that coordinates movement and balance.

cerebral cortex—The convoluted outer layer of gray matter that constitutes the "thinking" portion of the brain.

choline—A substance used by the body to produce acetylcholine. Present in food.

cholinesterase inhibitors—Medications that slow the breakdown of acetylcholine. Used in the treatment of Alzheimer's disease.

colchicine—An anti-inflammatory drug commonly used to treat gout. Currently being tested as a treatment for Alzheimer's disease.

complete blood cell count—Measures cellular elements of blood: red blood cells, white blood cells, and platelets. Helps rule out anemia, infections, and vitamin B_{12} deficiency as causes of dementia or factors that can exacerbate dementia.

computed tomography (CT)—An imaging technique that uses x-rays to create a two-dimensional image of the brain or other parts of the body.

Creutzfeldt-Jakob disease (CJD)—A rare, fatal brain disorder that causes a rapid, progressive dementia. Sometimes mistaken for Alzheimer's disease.

Cushing's disease—A disorder resulting from the overproduction of hormones by the adrenal gland. Also called Cushing disease.

dementia—A significant intellectual decline or impairment that persists over time in several areas of thinking.

dementia with Lewy bodies—A type of dementia characterized by episodes of confusion, falls, and repetitive hallucinations, as well as signs of parkinsonism early in the disease.

frontotemporal dementia—A spectrum of disorders associated with impaired initiation of plans and goal setting, personality changes, language difficulties, and unawareness of any loss of mental function.

gray matter—The area of the brain, gray in appearance, that contains cell bodies (as opposed to white matter, which contains the nerve fibers that extend from the cell bodies).

hippocampus—A small, S-shaped structure in the brain that appears to play a major role in the process of forging memories.

Huntington's disease—A rare, hereditary disorder of the central nervous system characterized by uncontrollable movements and dementia. Also called Huntington disease.

incontinence—An inability to control urination or defecation.

lecithin—A substance used by the body to produce acetylcholine. Occurs naturally in food.

Lewy bodies—Abnormal structures that are found in cells throughout the brain in people with dementia with Lewy bodies.

long-term memory—Holds information that was learned as recently as a few minutes ago and as long ago as early childhood.

magnetic resonance imaging (MRI)—An imaging technique that uses a powerful magnet, rather than x-rays, to create a two-dimensional image of various areas of the body, including the brain.

GLOSSARY—continued

microtubules—An internal transport system in nerve cells. Collapsed microtubules form neurofibrillary tangles.

mild cognitive impairment (MCI)—Forgetfulness that is worse than normal for one's age but is not associated with certain cognitive problems common in dementia, such as disorientation or confusion. Severity falls between age-associated memory impairment and early dementia.

Mini-Mental State Examination—A test of mental status used to check for any basic cognitive impairment.

neurofibrillary tangles—Found in the brains of virtually all people with Alzheimer's disease. Composed mainly of the protein tau. Appear as twisted, hairlike threads and remain after the collapse of the microtubules in the nerve cell.

neuron—Nerve cell.

neurotransmitter—A specialized chemical that relays messages between nerve cells.

nonsteroidal anti-inflammatory drugs (NSAIDs)—A class of drugs, commonly used to treat arthritis, which may be effective in the treatment and prevention of Alzheimer's disease.

normal-pressure hydrocephalus—A condition characterized by excess fluid in the brain that can result in dementia.

palilalia—Compulsive repetition of a word or phrase with increasing rapidity.

Parkinson's disease—A progressive neurological disease characterized by tremors, stooped posture, slow movement, poor balance, and shuffling gait. Also called Parkinson disease.

parkinsonism—The symptoms of Parkinson's disease: tremors; rigid, stooped posture; slowness; and shuffling gait.

Pick's disease—A type of frontotemporal dementia characterized by impaired initiation of plans and goal setting, personality changes, unawareness of any loss of mental function, and language difficulties. Also called Pick disease.

piracetam—An alternative treatment to enhance memory that may improve the metabolism of acetylcholine.

prednisone—A steroid drug with powerful anti-inflammatory effects. Currently being tested as a treatment for Alzheimer's disease.

presenilin-1 (PS-1)—A gene on chromosome 14. May be linked to Alzheimer's disease.

presenilin-2 (PS-2)—A gene on chromosome 1. May be linked to Alzheimer's disease.

prions—Unusual infectious agents that cause Creutzfeldt-Jakob disease.

selegiline—A medication used to treat Parkinson's disease that is currently being tested as a therapy for Alzheimer's disease. It has antioxidant effects similar to vitamin E but is associated with more side effects.

short-term memory—Also known as working memory. Sometimes equated with consciousness.

Short Test of Mental Status—A test of mental status given to check for any basic cognitive impairment.

subdural hematoma—A collection of blood between the skull and the brain that can lead to memory problems and loss of consciousness.

vascular dementia—A disorder, often resulting from a series of tiny strokes in the brain, that can lead to dementia.

vasopressin—A hormone produced by the hypothalamus and used as an alternative treatment to enhance memory.

HEALTH INFORMATION ORGANIZATIONS AND SUPPORT GROUPS

U.S. Administration on Aging
1 Massachusetts Ave., SW
Washington, DC 20201
☎ 202-619-0724
www.aoa.dhhs.gov
A federal agency that works to plan, develop, and fund programs for older Americans through grants to states and nonprofit organizations. Supports regional agencies that provide meals, transportation, and other services for people over age 60. Access to information about local services can be found by contacting the National Eldercare Locator (800-677-1116) or using www.eldercare.gov.

Alzheimer's Association
225 N. Michigan Ave., Ste. 1700
Chicago, IL 60601
☎ 800-272-3900/312-335-8700
www.alz.org
Provides general information about Alzheimer's disease and issues relevant to caregivers. Local chapters have support group resources and information on caregiving.

Alzheimer's Disease Education and Referral (ADEAR) Center
P.O. Box 8250
Silver Spring, MD 20907-8250
☎ 800-438-4380
www.alzheimers.org
Provides information on Alzheimer's disease, including the latest research, new treatments, and referrals, for both health professionals and the general public.

American Stroke Association
7272 Greenville Ave.
Dallas, TX 75231
☎ 888-4-STROKE
    800-553-6321 ("Warmline")
www.strokeassociation.org
A division of the American Heart Association; provides referrals to community stroke groups and information and peer counseling to survivors and caregivers. Call the "Warmline" to subscribe to their magazine, *Stroke Connection*.

American Psychiatric Association
1000 Wilson Blvd., Ste. 1825
Arlington, VA 22209-3901
☎ 703-907-7300
www.psych.org
Medical specialty society that provides clinical patient information about mental illnesses, medication, and psychiatric treatment. Information and brochures are available by contacting the organization's Division of Public Affairs.

National Institute of Mental Health
6001 Executive Blvd.
Rm. 8184, MSC 9663
Bethesda, MD 20892-9663
☎ 866-615-NIMH/301-443-4513
www.nimh.nih.gov
Dedicated to reducing the personal and economic costs of mental illness. Supports ongoing research on behavior and the brain, provides brochures, and sponsors related programs.

National Institute of Neurological Disorders and Stroke
P.O. Box 5801
Bethesda, MD 20824
☎ 800-352-9424
www.ninds.nih.gov
Leading supporter of neurological research in the United States. Provides list of clinical resource centers and voluntary health agencies.

National Mental Health Association
2001 N. Beauregard St., 12th Fl.
Alexandria, VA 22311
☎ 800-969-NMHA/703-684-7722
www.nmha.org
Provides referrals to treatment services and support groups and offers literature on various mental health topics; has branches throughout the country.

LEADING HOSPITALS FOR NEUROLOGY AND NEUROSURGERY

U.S. News & World Report and the National Opinion Research Center, a social-science research group at the University of Chicago, recently conducted their 15th annual nationwide survey of 8,160 board-certified physicians in 17 medical specialties. The doctors nominated the hospitals that they considered to be the best from among 6,012 U.S. medical centers. Below is the current list of the best hospitals for neurology and neurosurgery, as determined by a combination of factors:

doctors' recommendations from 2002, 2003, and 2004; federal death rates; and factual data regarding quality indicators, such as the ratio of registered nurses to patients and use of advanced technology. However, because the results reflect the doctors' opinions to some extent, they are partly subjective. Any institution listed is considered a leading center, and the rankings do not imply that other hospitals cannot or do not deliver excellent care.

1. **Mayo Clinic**
Rochester, MN
☎ 507-284-2511
www.mayoclinic.org

2. **Johns Hopkins Hospital**
Baltimore, MD
☎ 410-955-5000
www.hopkinsmedicine.org

3. **Massachusetts General Hospital**
Boston, MA
☎ 617-726-2000
www.mgh.harvard.edu

4. **New York-Presbyterian Hospital**
New York, NY
☎ 212-305-2500
www.nyp.org

5. **University of California, San Francisco, Medical Center**
San Francisco, CA
☎ 888-689-UCSF/415-476-1000
www.ucsfhealth.org

6. **Cleveland Clinic**
Cleveland, OH
☎ 800-223-2273/216-444-2200
www.clevelandclinic.org

7. **Barnes-Jewish Hospital**
St. Louis, MO
☎ 314-747-3000
www.barnesjewish.org

8. **University of California, Los Angeles, Medical Center**
Los Angeles, CA
☎ 800-825-2631/310-825-9111
www.healthcare.ucla.edu

9. **St. Joseph's Hospital and Medical Center**
Phoenix, AZ
☎ 602-406-3000
www.ichosestjoes.com

10. **Methodist Hospital**
Houston, TX
☎ 713-790-3333
www.methodisthealth.com

Source: *U.S. News & World Report,* July 12, 2004.

THE JOHNS HOPKINS WHITE PAPERS

Selected Medical Journal Article

ALZHEIMER'S DISEASE AND ATHEROSCLEROSIS

Evidence is growing for a link between late-onset Alzheimer's disease—by far the most common type—and atherosclerosis. In the article reprinted here from *The Lancet*, Ivan Casserly, M.D., and Eric Topol, M.D., present their case that the two conditions have independent causes but represent convergent disease processes.

Many researchers speculated that an accumulation of an abnormally folded protein, beta-amyloid, within the brain is a main cause of Alzheimer's disease. Atherosclerosis occurs when fatty plaques build up within the arteries, impairing blood flow, and can lead to heart attack, stroke, and other problems.

The main risk factor for both late-onset Alzheimer's and atherosclerosis is increasing age, and both conditions have long "latency periods," meaning the disease process may advance for many years without producing any clinical signs of illness, the authors note. High cholesterol is a well-known risk factor for atherosclerosis, and cholesterol imbalance may also promote the formation of plaques (accumulations of beta-amyloid) and tangles found in the brain in Alzheimer's disease. Inflammation also appears to play a role in both disease processes, although the event triggering the inflammation is not clear.

Atherosclerosis and Alzheimer's share a number of other risk factors, including high blood pressure, diabetes, cigarette smoking, and obesity. The main genetic risk factor for Alzheimer's disease, known as the apolipoprotein E ε4 allele, also slightly increases atherosclerosis risk. There is also growing evidence that misfolded proteins such as beta-amyloid may play some role in atherosclerosis as well as Alzheimer's disease.

The author's note another piece of evidence for a connection between Alzheimer's and atherosclerosis: Studies suggest that drugs known as statins, which reduce cholesterol levels and may have other heart- and blood-vessel–protecting effects, cut the risk of developing Alzheimer's by 40% to 70%.

The proposal that Alzheimer's and atherosclerosis are convergent disease processes represents a new way of thinking about both illnesses, the authors conclude, and could lead to a better understanding of Alzheimer's and perhaps new strategies for preventing and treating the degenerative brain disease.

Review

Convergence of atherosclerosis and Alzheimer's disease: inflammation, cholesterol, and misfolded proteins

Ivan Casserly, Eric Topol

Late-onset sporadic Alzheimer's disease is a heterogeneous disorder. In elderly patients, increasing evidence suggests a link between this neurodegenerative disease, and vascular risk factors and atherosclerosis. The nature of this link remains speculative. Some investigators have suggested that the disease arises as a secondary event related to atherosclerosis of extracranial or intracranial vessels. A toxic effect of vascular factors on the microvasculature of susceptible brain regions has also been argued. An alternative explanation is that atherosclerosis and Alzheimer's disease are independent but convergent disease processes. This hypothesis is lent support by observations of shared epidemiology, pathophysiological elements, and response to treatment in both disorders. It provides a potential framework for an improved understanding of the pathogenesis of Alzheimer's disease, especially in elderly patients with vascular risk factors, and offers some promise toward the search for preventive and therapeutic treatments.

Introduction

Alzheimer's disease is a progressive neurodegenerative disease that in western society accounts for most cases of dementia.[1] Over the past five decades, there has been a sharp rise in the death rate from Alzheimer's disease in the USA (figure 1).[2,3] By 2050, the number of Americans with Alzheimer's disease is expected to triple (from 4·6 to 16 million).[4] This epidemic has enormous implications for society, in terms of both human suffering and monetary cost.

The prevailing paradigm of Alzheimer's disease pathogenesis contends that the primary pathogenic event is the extraneuronal or intraneuronal, or both, accumulation of the misfolded protein, amyloid β-peptide (Aβ), which initiates a pathogenic cascade resulting in neurotoxicity and ultimately the clinical syndrome of Alzheimer's disease (figure 2).[5] This paradigm has its origins in the autosomal dominant forms of the disease, which account for 1–2% of all cases. These inherited forms are associated with mis-sense mutations of genes that encode the amyloid precursor protein (APP), or proteolytic enzymes that cleave APP (eg, presenilin 1 and 2). Such mutations are associated with an increased production of Aβ (figure 3), and result in early-onset Alzheimer's disease that typically presents in the third or fourth decade of life.

Clinical and basic investigation has revealed that Alzheimer's disease should not be regarded as a single nosological entity.[6] Late-onset disease, which accounts for 90–95% of all cases, differs from early-onset disease. Within the category of late-onset disease, considerable heterogeneity also exists, in terms of risk factor profiles, pathogenesis, and neuropathological findings. In elderly patients, increasing evidence suggests a link between Alzheimer's disease, and both vascular risk factors and atherosclerosis. The nature of this link remains

Lancet 2004; **363**: 1139–46

Department of Cardiovascular Medicine, Cleveland Clinic Foundation, Cleveland, OH, USA (I P Casserly MB BCh, E J Topol MD)

Correspondence to: Eric J Topol, Department of Cardiovascular Medicine, The Cleveland Clinic Foundation, 9500 Euclid Avenue, Cleveland, OH 44195, USA.

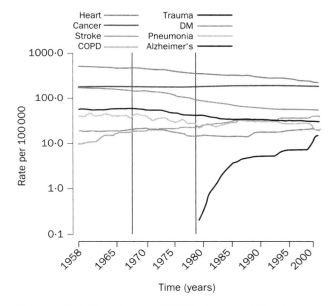

Figure 1: **Mortality rates per 100 000 of the population from leading causes of death over the past five decades**
Reproduced from *National Vital Statistics* 2002; **50**.
COPD=chronic obstructive pulmonary disease. DM=diabetes mellitus.

speculative. Some investigators have suggested that Alzheimer's disease occurs as a secondary event related to atherosclerosis of extracranial[7] or intracranial[8] vessels on

Search strategy

We searched MEDLINE using Ovid Technologies, Version 9.0.0 for 1996–2003 with the keywords atherosclerosis and Alzheimer's disease. This search was supplemented by our knowledge of the primary published work in both the clinical and basic science literature, and from the bibliography of retrieved articles. 468 scientific reports were chosen for in-depth review based on their relevance to this review topic. In addition, we searched the internet using Google, and specifically searched http://www.cdc.gov/nchs/nvss.htm and http://www.alzforum.org/home.asp.

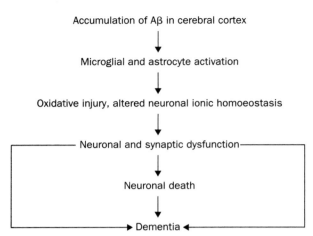

Figure 2: **Hypothetical sequence of events in the pathogenic cascade initiated by Aβ deposition resulting in Alzheimer's disease**

the basis of brain hypoperfusion[9] or discrete brain infarction.[10] A toxic effect of these vascular factors on the microvasculature of susceptible brain regions (ie, medial temporal lobe) has also been argued.[11] An alternative explanation is that atherosclerosis and Alzheimer's disease are independent but convergent disease processes. Based on observations of common epidemiology, pathophysiological elements, and response to therapies in both disorders, we believe this to be a tenable hypothesis.

Epidemiology

Increasing age represents the dominant risk factor for both atherosclerosis and Alzheimer's disease. The disorders are uniquely characterised by lengthy "latency periods" in which subclinical evidence of disease is evident for decades before clinical presentation. Pathological and intravascular ultrasound studies of teenagers and young adults show non-obstructive coronary atheroma.[12] In Alzheimer's disease, histological evidence of senile plaque and neurofibrillary tangle formation can be seen in the temporal lobe up to 40–50 years before the onset of dementia, and might even extend into adolescence[13] (figure 4).

The overlap between additional "vascular" risk factors for both Alzheimer's disease and atherosclerosis is also striking (panel). The association of each of these factors with atherosclerosis is indisputable. Although the importance of some of these factors in Alzheimer's disease pathogenesis is debatable, those studies that were prospectively designed, used a population-based approach, measured the exposures in middle age, and followed patients for long periods (up to 25 years) have suggested the largest effect. Such investigations have the greatest power to suggest a causal association between the exposure and disease. The influence of vascular risk factors in Alzheimer's disease is consistent with the finding that atherosclerosis and Alzheimer's disease seems to be predominant in developed countries,[6] suggesting a strong environmental link; the influence is also consistent with the association between Alzheimer's disease and both cerebrovascular[7,8] and coronary atherosclerosis[8,14] seen from clinical and post-mortem studies.

Common pathophysiological elements

Hypercholesterolaemia and inflammation have emerged as the dominant mechanisms implicated in the development of atherosclerosis, and have important interactions.[15] Superimposed on these basic elements are several factors that seem to affect the disease process largely through effects on cholesterol homoeostasis or the inflammatory response to injury. Inflammation has been implicated in Alzheimer's disease pathogenesis for over a decade, and increasing evidence suggests that abnormalities in cholesterol homeostasis could have an important role. Similarly, many of the contributory factors in atherogenesis have emerged as potential contributors in Alzheimer's disease.

Cholesterol

The causal link between elevated serum cholesterol and atherosclerosis is well established.[16] Prompted largely by results of epidemiological studies,[17] the concept of altered cholesterol homoeostasis as an important factor in the pathogenesis of Alzheimer's disease has emerged. In cell cultures, increased and decreased cholesterol levels promote and inhibit the formation of Aβ from APP, respectively[18,19] (figure 3). Animals fed a high cholesterol

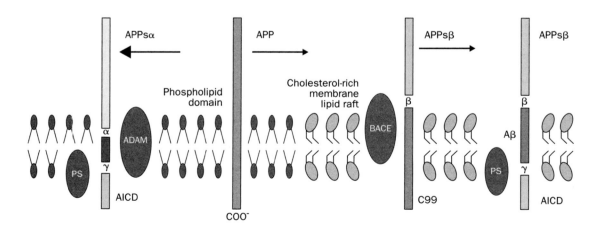

Figure 3: **Alternative cleavage of APP by α or β secretase**

APPsα, the product of cleavage with α secretase has neurotrophic properties. Cleavage with b secretase yields APPsβ molecule and C99. C99 is cleaved by γ secretase (eg, PS1) producing the neurotoxic Aβ peptide (dark green). β and γ secretases can co-localise at sites of increased membrane cholesterol favouring the production of Aβ peptide. ADAM=a disintegrin and metalloproteinase domain. PS=presenilin. AICD=APP intracellular domain. BACE=β site APP-cleaving enzyme. Reproduced with modifications from Wolozin B. *Proc Natl Acad Sci* 2001; **98:** 5371–73.

diet have shown increased intraneuronal Aβ immunoreactivity and occasionally extracellular plaques.[20] Finally, a polymorphism of the *CYP46* gene (*CYP46A1*), which encodes cholesterol 24S-hydroxylase, and is thought to reduce activity of the enzyme and raise concentrations of cholesterol in the brain, has been linked with histological evidence of increased Aβ deposition in the medial temporal lobe, and an increased risk of late-onset Alzheimer's disease.[21]

Increased concentrations of free cholesterol in the neuronal membrane stimulate increased Aβ production through intracellular and membrane effects. In cell cultures, high membrane cholesterol levels induce cellular acyl-coenzyme A: cholesterol acyltrans-ferase (ACAT) to produce cholesterol esters within intracellular granules.[22] Through an unspecified mechanism, this raised ACAT activity seems to modulate Aβ production causing increased synthesis. ACAT has become a target for the treatment of atherosclerosis. Inhibition of ACAT reduces atherosclerosis in apolipopro-tein E-deficient mice,[23] and restricts foam cell formation by enhancing cholesterol efflux from human monocyte macrophage foam cells.[24] Acting at the membrane surface, increased free cholesterol may cause the formation of "lipid rafts", cholesterol-rich areas of membrane, where APP, and β and γ secretases tend to co-localise (figure 3).[25] By favouring the formation of such regions, increased membrane cholesterol levels could result in the preferential processing of APP toward the formation of Aβ.

Inflammation

Over the past 15 years, investigation has shown the importance of inflammation in the pathogenesis of atherosclerosis and Alzheimer's disease.[26,27] As in many human inflammatory diseases, the inciting stimulus in each case remains uncertain, although experimental evidence supports a role for modified low density lipoprotein[28] and Aβ peptide[27] in atherosclerosis and Alzheimer's disease, respectively. Although the initial inflammatory response can be protective (ie, clearance of modified low density lipoprotein or Aβ peptide[29]), failure to adequately clear the inciting stimulus results in a chronic inflammatory response that greatly contributes to the clinical manifestation of the disorder.

The presence of inflammation in brain tissue protected by a blood brain barrier might initially appear incongru-ous. However, the brain is populated by microglia, which are resident brain macrophages, similar to those found in the intima of atherosclerotic lesions.[30] Remarkably, brain microglia are capable of producing almost all of the same cytokines, chemokines, growth factors, enzymes, comple-ment and coagulation factors, and reactive oxygen species, as their peripheral counterparts, and express many of the same surface receptors that mediate peripheral immune interactions.[31]

The supporting cellular cast in Alzheimer's disease is provided by another glial cell, the astrocyte, that secretes a

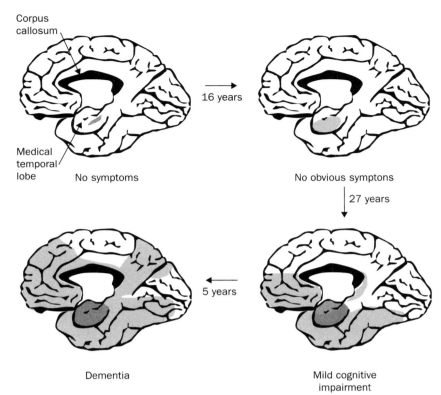

Figure 4: Sagittal view of medial aspect of cerebral cortex showing postulated spatial sequence of spread of pathology in Alzheimer's disease from medial temporal lobe to sensory association cortices.

The postulated temporal sequence is also shown indicating the prolonged incubation period of this disease. The depth of colour is in proportion to the density of pathology. Reproduced with permission from Smith DA, *Proc Natl Acad Sci* 2002; **99:** 4135–37.

more restricted array of pro-inflammatory products and matrix proteins, and by neurons themselves, which produce inflammatory mediators, including C-reactive protein, amyloid P, and complement factors.[32] These cellular elements co-localise at sites of Alzheimer's disease pathology (ie, senile plaque) and occupy a consistent spatial relation at these sites. Their pro-inflammatory and immune mediator products are upregulated and seen in increased concentrations in these regions. Although the precise sequence of events is uncertain, this inflammatory response is believed to contribute significantly to neuronal dysfunction, and ultimately to neuronal death. Results of an in vivo study provided evidence of microglial activation at typical sites of Alzheimer's disease pathology in patients with early disease.[33] Additionally, investigators from the Honolulu-Asia study[34] reported that elevated C-reactive protein in middle age was associated with an increased

Common genetic and environmental risk factors for Alzheimer's disease and atherosclerosis

Epidemiological Factor
ApoEe4 polymorphism[36]
Hypercholesterolaemia[17,98]
Hypertension[98]
Hyperhomocysteinaemia[99]
Diabetes mellitus[100]
Metabolic syndrome[101]
Smoking[102]
Systemic inflammation[34]
Increased fat intake and obesity[103]

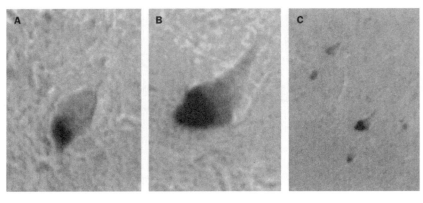

Figure 5: **Immunohistochemical analysis**
(A) Control patient showing normal angiotensin-converting enzyme (ACE) immunoreactivity in a pyramidal neuron. (B) Patient with Alzheimer's disease showing increased ACE immunoreactivity in a pyramidal neuron. (C) Only a subset of pyramidal neurons show immunoreactivity for ACE activity in Alzheimer's disease brain. Reproduced with permission from Savaskan E, Hock C, Olivieri G, et al. *Neurobiol Aging*, 2001; **22:** 541–46.

incidence of Alzheimer's disease in the subsequent 25 years, independent of cardiovascular risk factors.[34] These studies suggest that, as in atherosclerosis, inflammation might play an important part during the earliest phase of Alzheimer's disease pathogenesis.

Other common pathophysiological elements
Apolipoprotein E e4 polymorphism
The e4 allele of the apolipoprotein E gene (*APOE*) represents a modest genetic risk factor for atherosclerosis,[35] and is the most important genetic risk factor for sporadic Alzheimer's disease in the general population.[36] Although this allelic variant seems to function as a disease susceptibility gene (ie, it is neither necessary nor sufficient), its importance is underscored by the prevalence of the carrier status for e4 allele in the general population, estimated at about 25%.[37]

Peripheral apolipoprotein E is synthesised in the liver, and brain apolipoprotein E is synthesised in situ largely by astrocytes.[38] The mechanism by which these compartmentalised pools of apolipoprotein E e4 (product of *APOEe4* allele) contribute to these two diseases is uncertain, however, there are common mechanisms by which apolipoprotein E e4 might affect both processes. In cell cultures, apolipoprotein E e4 is associated with reduced efflux of cholesterol from macrophages,[39] and also neurons and astrocytes.[40] Within macrophages, this association is likely to promote foam cell formation, whereas in neurons, an increase in APP processing toward Aβ production is possible. Evidence also suggests that apolipoprotein E e4 shows less antioxidant effects compared with apolipoprotein E e3.[41] Both atherosclerosis and Alzheimer's disease are associated with the production of reactive oxygen and nitrogen species that oxidise aminoacids and lipids, which contribute to disease pathogenesis. Loss of a protective antioxidant factor may exacerbate any damage due to oxidant stress.

Renin-angiotensin system
Several experimental models and clinical trials support a modulatory role for the renin-angiotensin system in atherosclerosis, independent of its haemodynamic homoeostatic function. In atherosclerotic plaque, angiotensin II can be derived from systemic sources or produced locally in the vascular wall.[42] Angiotensin receptor (AT) 1 activation by angiotensin II produces a series of responses that augment vascular inflammation, which contributes to endothelial

dysfunction and enhances the atherogenic process.[42] Many of the components of the renin-angiotensin system have been described in mammalian brain including angiotensinogen, angiotensin-converting enzyme, angiotensin II, and AT1 and AT2 receptors.[43,44] This has led to the concept of a "self contained" renin-angiotensin system in brain tissue. There is also evidence that over-activation of this system might contribute to the pathogenesis of Alzheimer's disease. In rats, long-term administration of angiotensin-converting-enzyme inhibitors and AT-1 receptor antagonists is associated with improvement in memory function.[45] Compared with controls, immunohistochemical analyses of the brains of patients with Alzheimer's disease show increased staining for membrane-bound angiotensin-converting enzyme, angiotensin II, and AT1, suggesting an increase in activity of the renin-angiotensin system (figure 5).[43] Of interest, the increased staining for these antigens was localised to the pyramidal neurons of the cortex, which are typically the most prominently affected neuronal type in Alzheimer's disease. Activation of the renin-angiotensin system might contribute to Alzheimer's disease pathology by inhibiting the release of acetylcholine from cortical neurons[46] or by promoting the inflammatory response in the brain parenchyma. A contradictory note regarding this hypothesis is the finding that in vitro angiotensin-converting enzyme prevents Aβ aggregation, and that angiotensin-converting enzyme inhibition blocked this effect.[47]

Platelets
The presence of APP in the brain has been most focused on, but it also exists in substantial quantities in non-neural tissues.[48] Platelets contain APP in their α granules and represent the primary source (>90%) of circulating APP and Aβ.[49] Evidence suggests that platelet-derived Aβ might play a part in atherosclerosis. Immunohistochemical analysis of advanced carotid atherosclerotic plaques showed the presence of APP, Aβ, platelets, and activated macrophages surrounding intimal microvessels.[50] In-vitro studies demonstrated that macrophages are capable of platelet phagocytosis, which resulted in macrophage activation and foam cell formation. Macrophage activation seemed to be mediated by the processing of platelet-derived APP to Aβ by secretase enzymes within the macrophage. Other investigators have shown that activation of platelets that enter atherosclerotic plaque through neovessels by collagen, thrombin, or arachidonic acid, results in APP and Aβ release.[51,52] Subsequent uptake of APP by scavenger (class P) receptors on the macrophage surface could lead to similar activation of macrophages as that mediated by platelet phagocytosis.[52] These studies highlight the possible role of misfolded proteins in atherogenesis.[53]

Liver X receptors
Liver X receptors (LXRs) are a subfamily of the nuclear receptor superfamily of transcription factors. These receptors are of interest in both atherosclerosis and Alzheimer's disease, since they regulate the expression of several genes involved in both lipid metabolism and transport, and immune responses.[54] Consistent with this

idea is that LXRs have been identified in macrophages and are broadly expressed in animal brain.[55] Activation of these receptors results in reciprocal upregulation of genes that accelerate cholesterol efflux from cells (eg, Apo E, ABCA1) and inhibition of the expression of inflammatory mediators such as inducible nitric oxide synthase, cyclooxygenase-1, and interleukins 1 and 6.[56] Investigations into LXR-deficient mice have shown an increase in foam cell formation in the arterial wall,[57] and increased aortic atherosclerosis.[58] In atherosclerotic mice, LXR agonists reduced the expression of proinflammatory genes in response to cytokine administration.[56] These findings point to the relevance of this receptor system in atherogenesis. A recent knockout mouse model also provides evidence of an age-dependent neuroprotective effect of this receptor, and an important role in lipid homoeostasis in the brain.[55] The relevance of these findings to Alzheimer's disease merits further study.

RAGE

RAGE (receptor for advanced glycation end-products) is a multi-ligand receptor of the immunoglobulin super-family.[59] The first recognised ligand for this receptor was a heterogeneous group of structures, termed advanced glycation end-products, which are produced as a result of non-enzymatic glycation and oxidation of the free amino groups of proteins. Hyperglycaemia promotes the production of advanced glycation end-products, but they are also produced in the setting of increasing age and renal failure, and at sites of oxidant stress and inflammation in tissues.[60] In diabetic animals, advanced glycation end-products are enriched in the vasculature and activate RAGE receptors on endothelial and smooth muscle cells, and macrophages.[59] In in-vitro and animal studies, interaction between advanced glycation end-products and RAGE is associated with increased vascular permeability and vascular inflammation. These effects are mediated by increased nuclear translocation of NF-κB transcription factor, which leads to the expression of a range of pro-inflammatory molecules.[61] Because interaction between advanced glycation end-products and RAGE leads to increased expression of the receptor rather than down-regulation, a positive feedback loop is initiated which might contribute to chronic inflammation and tissue injury. RAGE can also bind cytokines of the S100/calgranulin family,[61] providing a further link between RAGE activation and inflammation. In-vivo evidence of the role of RAGE in atherosclerosis is provided by animal models, in which blockade of RAGE has been associated with inhibition of both atherosclerotic lesion formation and lesion progression.[59,62]

Within the brain, RAGEs have been seen on the surface of neurons and microglia.[63] Immunoreactivity for advanced glycation end-products is increased three-fold in Alzheimer's disease patients compared to controls, and co-localises with the typical Alzheimer's disease histopathology.[64] It seems likely that increasing age, oxidant stress, and the inflammatory response associated with Alzheimer's disease pathology contributes to the presence of these structures. However, advanced glycation end-products might not be the primary ligand for RAGE in the nervous system. RAGE can act as a signal transduction receptor for Aβ. In cell cultures, RAGE activation by Aβ was associated with oxidant stress in neurons, and cellular activation of microglia.[63] If these in-vitro actions are replicated in vivo, they may contribute directly to neurotoxicity, or indirectly by promoting the inflammatory response.

Angiogenesis

In human atherosclerotic lesions, neovascularisation of the intima is thought to promote plaque progression through the supply of nutrients and oxygen and the accumulation of blood monocytes in the intima.[65] These new vessels arise from the vasa vasorum, which under normal circumstances supply only the adventitia.[66] The stimuli for atherosclerotic neovascularisation include hypoxia and cytokines that function as angiogenic growth factors (eg, VEGF).[67,68] Evidence for these concepts comes from animal models of atherosclerosis, in which VEGF enhanced plaque progression, whereas angiogenesis inhibitors reduced intimal neovascularisation and plaque growth.[69,70]

Vagnucci and colleagues[71] have also hypothesised that angiogenesis may have a role in pathogenesis of Alzheimer's disease. The robust inflammatory response in Alzheimer's disease could serve as the source of angiogenic growth factors, many of which are present in the brain parenchyma of these patients (eg, VEGF, MCP1, TNFα and interleukin 6). Several investigators have noted ultrastructural and functional abnormalities in the microcirculation of brains of people with Alzheimer's disease, and have argued that they promote ischaemia and hypoxia of brain parenchyma, which are further stimuli for angiogenesis.[72,73] Cerebrovascular microvessels in Alzheimer's disease have the potential to contribute to tissue damage. Grammas and colleagues[74] identified a peptide neurotoxic factor secreted by microvessels from patients.[74] Cerebral microvessels in Alzheimer's disease might also produce inflammatory mediators and contribute to the extracellular pool of Aβ through increased expression of APP.[75] Thus, although unlikely to be a sufficient cause of Alzheimer's disease, pathological angiogenesis in the Alzheimer's disease brain might have a contributory role. Further definitive experimental and clinicopathological data are needed.

Response to therapies
Statins

Randomised placebo-controlled trials of statin treatment have shown the beneficial effects of the drugs in primary and secondary prevention of cardiovascular and cerebro-vascular disease events.[76] Through direct effects on LDL cholesterol and triglyceride levels, and cholesterol-independent effects on endothelial function, smooth muscle cell proliferation and migration, platelet reactivity, macrophage activation, and vascular inflammation,[77] statins slow the progression of atherosclerosis and promote plaque stabilisation.

Epidemiological studies with different study designs and patient populations have shown a 40–70% reduction in the risk of Alzheimer's disease associated with statin use.[78-81] Despite the inherent limitations of these data to ascribe a causal link between statin use and a decreased risk of Alzheimer's disease, the magnitude and consistency of the effect observed is remarkable. Two recent randomised placebo-controlled trails have failed to show a benefit of statin therapy on age-associated cognitive decline,[82,83] but some scepticism about the implication of these findings for the role of statins in the prevention of Alzheimer's disease is warranted. The short follow-up of 3·2 years and 5 years in both trials,[82,83] and the elderly population studied in the PROspective Study of Pravastatin in the Elderly at Risk (PROSPER) trial[82] might have undermined the ability of these studies to show an effect. Also, age-associated cognitive decline is at best a poor surrogate for Alzheimer's disease.

As in atherosclerosis, both cholesterol and cholesterol-independent effects could explain the benefit of statins in Alzheimer's disease. In neuronal and peripheral cell lines, statins seem to promote a favourable shift in APP processing toward secretion of the neurotrophic APPsα peptide and away from Aβ production.[25,84] Depletion of membrane cholesterol by statins produces an increase in the activity of enzymes with α secretase activity, and a reciprocal decrease in β-secretase-mediated APP proteolysis. In vivo studies provide additional support for these effects. In guinea pigs given a statin for 3 weeks, reduced levels of Aβ in the CSF, and reduced brain tissue Aβ levels were recorded.[84] In view of the long half-life (about 6 months) of brain cholesterol, any benefit of statins in preventing Alzheimer's disease in humans that is mediated by cholesterol reduction is likely to be very slow and could have particular relevance in clinical studies.

Several previously described pleiotropic effects of statins might also be implicated in any potential benefit in Alzheimer's disease. In animal models of cerebral ischaemia, and in preliminary investigations in human beings, statins favourably alter the expression of adhesion molecules preventing leucocyte-endothelial and leucocyte glial interactions, suppress cytokine production, inhibit astrocyte, microglial, and macrophage inducible nitric oxide synthase production, and have anti-oxidant effects.[85-87] Whereas inflammation in Alzheimer's disease is not thought to be driven by systemic mediators, and the inflammatory response is distinct from that induced by ischaemic injury, the potential benefit of an in-situ anti-inflammatory effect of statins in the brain in the disease seems likely, and is supported by in-vitro studies.[88]

Aspirin and NSAIDs

The argument for the convergence of atherosclerosis and Alzheimer's disease based on a common response to aspirin and non-steroidal anti-inflammatory drugs (NSAIDs) is speculative. Despite the negative results from a randomised study of the effects of a non-selective NSAID and selective COX-2 inhibitor on disease progression,[89] findings from multiple cross-sectional and prospective epidemiological studies support a treatment benefit of low-dose aspirin and NSAIDs in Alzheimer's disease.[90] The magnitude of this benefit seems to be greatest in individuals with long-term use (ie, >2 years), and to be stronger with NSAID compared with aspirin.[90] Although initial attempts to explain the mechanism of this beneficial effect have centered on the anti-inflammatory effect of these agents due to inhibition of COX1 and COX2 (present in microglia[91] and neurons[92]), inflammation-independent effects may be operative in the case of NSAIDs. In cell cultures, a subset of NSAIDs (not including aspirin) greatly reduced the production of Aβ independent of an effect on cyclo-oxygenase activity.[93] In-vivo results seem to confirm this finding (Breteler MM, unpublished data, http://www.alzforum.org).

In patients with coronary or cerebral atherosclerosis, aspirin has proven highly effective in the secondary prevention of ischaemic events in patients with established coronary or cerebrovascular disease.[94] Although the benefit of aspirin in this setting has traditionally been attributed to its anti-platelet effect, clinical[95] and basic[96] findings support an anti-inflammatory effect of aspirin, even at low (ie, anti-platelet) doses, which might improve the progression and evolution of atherosclerotic plaque. Despite the absence of clinical data, experimental evidence also suggests an attenuating effect of NSAIDs in atherogenesis. In LDL-receptor knockout mice, indomethacin suppresses systemic markers of inflam-

mation, and reduces the extent of aortic atherosclerosis by more than 50%.[97] Whether this anti-atherogenic effect results from inhibition of the COX1 or COX2 isoform of the cyclo-oxygenase enzyme is unclear.

Implications

The recognition that atherosclerosis and Alzheimer's disease are independent but convergent disease processes represents a paradigm shift in our thinking about their pathogenesis. We argue that this hypothesis provides a framework for an improved understanding of the pathogenesis of Alzheimer's disease, especially in elderly patients with vascular risk factors, and offers some promise toward the search for preventive and therapeutic treatments for Alzheimer's disease.

Support for this hypothesis could begin with a rigorous quantitative assessment of atherosclerotic burden in various vascular territories and Alzheimer's disease pathology in brain parenchyma in post-mortem cases. The finding of an association between the global burden of atherosclerosis and Alzheimer's disease, which disappears after adjustment for known vascular risk factors, would provide evidence for our hypothesis.

The use of treatments with proven effects on the process of atherosclerosis should be tested systematically in Alzheimer's disease. This should begin with in vitro and animal studies to provide preliminary evidence of efficacy. In view of our hypothesis, agents tested should be capable of achieving therapeutic levels in brain tissue to be effective, since merely treating peripheral atherosclerosis will have little impact on Alzheimer's disease. Cardiovascular medicine has several potential candidate drug groups that might prove useful (table), and more are likely to emerge. Future cardiovascular trials should incorporate pre-specified substudies of cognitive function, and specifically should include mechanisms to allow the diagnosis of incident Alzheimer's disease. Based on our current understanding of the disease and the disappointing results of previous randomised studies, the best chance of proving a benefit of these therapies in the prevention of Alzheimer's disease would seem to need treatment for many years (20–30 years), ideally with life-long follow-up and histological analysis of brain tissue post mortem. The collaboration of cardiologists, neurologists, and histopathologists for these investigations is essential. This proposal represents a major departure from current cardiovascular trial design, and the resources needed are substantial.

Possibly, the pathogenic mechanisms discovered in Alzheimer's disease might advance our understanding of atherosclerosis. Knowledge of the pathogenic role of innate

Drug class	Potential mechanism			
	Cholesterol homoeostasis	Anti-inflammatory	Anti-angiogenic	Aβ effects
ACE inhibitors	–	+	–	?
AII blockers	–	+	–	?
PPARG agonists	–	+	–	?
ACAT inhibitors	+	?	–	?
Statins	+	+	+	+
Aspirin	–	+	+	–
NSAIDs	–	+	+	+
COX2 inhibitors	–	+	+	?
Thienopyridines	–	?	?	?

+ indicates positive; – indicates negative; and ? indicates uncertainty. ACE=angiotensin-converting enzyme. AII=angiotensin II. PPAR=peroxisomal proliferator activating receptor. ACAT=acyl Co-A cholesterol acyl transferase, COX=cyclo-oxygenase.

Cardiovascular drug groups with potential therapeutic benefit in Alzheimer's disease and possible mechanism

immunity in atherosclerosis and the potential pathogenic role of APP and Aβ in carotid atherogenesis represent the first examples of what will hopefully be a fertile symbiosis between investigation into both disease processes. It is reasonable to suggest that our search for the elusive factor initiating atherosclerosis should begin to focus more closely on further species of misfolded proteins.

We thank Jonathan Smith for discussion and review of this manuscript, and S Turner for assistance with graphics.

References

1 Cummings JL, Cole G. Alzheimer disease. *JAMA* 2002; **287:** 2335–38.

2 Minino AM, Arias E, Kochanek KD, Murphy SL, Smith BL. Deaths: final data for 2000. *Natl Vital Stat Rep* 2002; **50:** 1–119.

3 Collen MF. Vicissitudes of preventive medicine and a new challenge. *Methods Inf Med* 2002; **41:** 224–29.

4 Brookmeyer R, Gray S, Kawas C. Projections of Alzheimer's disease in the United States and the public health impact of delaying disease onset. *Am J Public Health* 1998; **88:** 1337–42.

5 Selkoe DJ. Alzheimer's disease: genes, proteins, and therapy. *Physiol Rev* 2001; **81:** 741–66.

6 Ritchie K, Lovestone S. The dementias. *Lancet* 2002; **360:** 1759–66.

7 Hofman A, Ott A, Breteler MM, et al. Atherosclerosis, apolipoprotein E, and prevalence of dementia and Alzheimer's disease in the Rotterdam Study. *Lancet* 1997; **349:** 151–54.

8 Roher AE, Esh C, Kokjohn TA, et al. Circle of willis atherosclerosis is a risk factor for sporadic Alzheimer's disease. *Arterioscler Thromb Vasc Biol* 2003; **23:** 2055–62.

9 de la Torre JC. Alzheimer disease as a vascular disorder: nosological evidence. *Stroke* 2002; **33:** 1152–62.

10 Vermeer SE, Prins ND, den Heijer T, Hofman A, Koudstaal PJ, Breteler MM. Silent brain infarcts and the risk of dementia and cognitive decline. *N Engl J Med* 2003; **348:** 1215–22.

11 Farkas E, Luiten PG. Cerebral microvascular pathology in aging and Alzheimer's disease. *Prog Neurobiol* 2001; **64:** 575–611.

12 Tuzcu EM, Kapadia SR, Tutar E, et al. High prevalence of coronary atherosclerosis in asymptomatic teenagers and young adults: evidence from intravascular ultrasound. *Circulation* 2001; **103:** 2705–10.

13 Ohm TG, Muller H, Braak H, Bohl J. Close-meshed prevalence rates of different stages as a tool to uncover the rate of Alzheimer's disease-related neurofibrillary changes. *Neuroscience* 1995; **64:** 209–17.

14 Sparks DL, Hunsaker JC, Scheff SW, Kryscio RJ, Henson JL, Markesbery WR. Cortical senile plaques in coronary artery disease, aging and Alzheimer's disease. *Neurobiol Aging* 1990; **11:** 601–07.

15 Steinberg D. Atherogenesis in perspective: hypercholesterolemia and inflammation as partners in crime. *Nat Med* 2002; **8:** 1211–17.

16 Steinberg D. The cholesterol controversy is over. Why did it take so long? *Circulation* 1989; **80:** 1070–08.

17 Notkola IL, Sulkava R, Pekkanen J, et al. Serum total cholesterol, apolipoprotein E epsilon 4 allele, and Alzheimer's disease. *Neuroepidemiology* 1998; **17:** 14–20.

18 Frears ER, Stephens DJ, Walters CE, Davies H, Austen BM. The role of cholesterol in the biosynthesis of beta-amyloid. *Neuroreport* 1999; **10:** 1699–705.

19 Simons M, Keller P, De Strooper B, Beyreuther K, Dotti CG, Simons K. Cholesterol depletion inhibits the generation of beta-amyloid in hippocampal neurons. *Proc Natl Acad Sci USA* 1998; **95:** 6460–64.

20 Refolo LM, Malester B, LaFrancois J, et al. Hypercholesterolemia accelerates the Alzheimer's amyloid pathology in a transgenic mouse model. *Neurobiol Dis* 2000; **7:** 321–31.

21 Papassotiropoulos A, Streffer JR, Tsolaki M, et al. Increased brain beta-amyloid load, phosphorylated tau, and risk of Alzheimer disease associated with an intronic CYP46 polymorphism. *Arch Neurol* 2003; **60:** 29–35.

22 Puglielli L, Konopka G, Pack-Chung E, et al. Acyl-coenzyme A: cholesterol acyltransferase modulates the generation of the amyloid beta-peptide. *Nat Cell Biol* 2001; **3:** 905–12.

23 Kusunoki J, Hansoty DK, Aragane K, Fallon JT, Badimon JJ, Fisher EA. Acyl-CoA:cholesterol acyltransferase inhibition reduces atherosclerosis in apolipoprotein E-deficient mice. *Circulation* 2001; **103:** 2604–09.

24 Rodriguez A, Usher DC. Anti-atherogenic effects of the acyl-CoA:cholesterol acyltransferase inhibitor, avasimibe (CI-1011), in cultured primary human macrophages. *Atherosclerosis* 2002; **161:** 45–54.

25 Kojro E, Gimpl G, Lammich S, Marz W, Fahrenholz F. Low cholesterol stimulates the nonamyloidogenic pathway by its effect on the alpha-secretase Alzheimer's disease AM 10. *Proc Natl Acad Sci USA* 2001; **98:** 5815–20.

26 Hansson GK, Libby P, Schonbeck U, Yan ZQ. Innate and adaptive immunity in the pathogenesis of atherosclerosis. *Circ Res* 2002; **91:** 281–91.

27 Akiyama H, Barger S, Barnum S, et al. Inflammation and Alzheimer's disease. *Neurobiol Aging* 2000; **21:** 383–421.

28 Witztum JL, Berliner JA. Oxidized phospholipids and isoprostanes in atherosclerosis. *Curr Opin Lipidol* 1998; **9:** 441–48.

29 Wyss-Coray T, Yan F, Lin AH, et al. Prominent neurodegeneration and increased plaque formation in complement-inhibited Alzheimer's mice. *Proc Natl Acad Sci USA* 2002; **99:** 10837–42.

30 Gehrmann J, Matsumoto Y, Kreutzberg GW. Microglia: intrinsic immuneffector cell of the brain. *Brain Res Brain Res Rev* 1995; **20:** 269–87.

31 McGeer PL, McGeer EG. The inflammatory response system of brain: implications for therapy of Alzheimer and other neurodegenerative diseases. *Brain Res Brain Res Rev* 1995; **21:** 195–218.

32 Yasojima K, Schwab C, McGeer EG, McGeer PL. Human neurons generate C-reactive protein and amyloid P: upregulation in Alzheimer's disease. *Brain Res* 2000; **887:** 80–89.

33 Cagnin A, Brooks DJ, Kennedy AM, et al. In-vivo measurement of activated microglia in dementia. *Lancet* 2001; **358:** 461–67.

34 Schmidt R, Schmidt H, Curb JD, Masaki K, White LR, Launer LJ. Early inflammation and dementia: a 25-year follow-up of the Honolulu-Asia Aging Study. *Ann Neurol* 2002; **52:** 168–74.

35 Wilson PW, Schaefer EJ, Larson MG, Ordovas JM. Apolipoprotein E alleles and risk of coronary disease. A meta-analysis. *Arterioscler Thromb Vasc Biol* 1996; **16:** 1250–55.

36 Farrer LA, Cupples LA, Haines JL, et al. Effects of age, sex, and ethnicity on the association between apolipoprotein E genotype and Alzheimer disease. A meta-analysis. APOE and Alzheimer Disease Meta Analysis Consortium. *JAMA* 1997; **278:** 1349–56.

37 Lehtimaki T, Moilanen T, Viikari J, et al. Apolipoprotein E phenotypes in Finnish youths: a cross-sectional and 6-year follow-up study. *J Lipid Res* 1990; **31:** 487–95.

38 Boyles JK, Pitas RE, Wilson E, Mahley RW, Taylor JM. Apolipoprotein E associated with astrocytic glia of the central nervous system and with nonmyelinating glia of the peripheral nervous system. *J Clin Invest* 1985; **76:** 1501–13.

39 Huang ZH, Mazzone T. ApoE-dependent sterol efflux from macrophages is modulated by scavenger receptor class B type I expression. *J Lipid Res* 2002; **43:** 375–82.

40 Michikawa M, Fan QW, Isobe I, Yanagisawa K. Apolipoprotein E exhibits isoform-specific promotion of lipid efflux from astrocytes and neurons in culture. *J Neurochem* 2000; **74:** 1008–16.

41 Miyata M, Smith JD. Apolipoprotein E allele-specific antioxidant activity and effects on cytotoxicity by oxidative insults and beta-amyloid peptides. *Nat Genet* 1996; **14:** 55–61.

42 Brasier AR, Recinos A, Eledrisi MS. Vascular inflammation and the renin-angiotensin system. *Arterioscler Thromb Vasc Biol* 2002; **22:** 1257–66.

43 Savaskan E, Hock C, Olivieri G, et al. Cortical alterations of angiotensin converting enzyme, angiotensin II and AT1 receptor in Alzheimer's dementia. *Neurobiol Aging* 2001; **22:** 541–46.

44 MacGregor DP, Murone C, Song K, Allen AM, Paxinos G, Mendelsohn FA. Angiotensin II receptor subtypes in the human central nervous system. *Brain Res* 1995; **675:** 231–40.

45 Hirawa N, Uehara Y, Kawabata Y, et al. Long-term inhibition of renin-angiotensin system sustains memory function in aged Dahl rats. *Hypertension* 1999; **34:** 496–502.

46 Barnes JM, Barnes NM, Costall B, et al. Angiotensin II inhibits cortical cholinergic function: implications for cognition. *J Cardiovasc Pharmacol* 1990; **16:** 234–38.

47 Hu J, Igarashi A, Kamata M, Nakagawa H. Angiotensin-converting enzyme degrades Alzheimer amyloid beta-peptide (A beta); retards A beta aggregation, deposition, fibril formation; and inhibits cytotoxicity. *J Biol Chem* 2001; **276:** 47863–68.

48 Haass C, Schlossmacher MG, Hung AY, et al. Amyloid beta-peptide is produced by cultured cells during normal metabolism. *Nature* 1992; **359:** 322–25.

49 Chen M, Inestrosa NC, Ross GS, Fernandez HL. Platelets are the primary source of amyloid beta-peptide in human blood. *Biochem Biophys Res Commun* 1995; **213:** 96–103.

50 De Meyer GR, De Cleen DM, Cooper S, et al. Platelet phagocytosis and processing of beta-amyloid precursor protein as a mechanism of macrophage activation in atherosclerosis. *Circ Res* 2002; **90:** 1197–204.

51 Skovronsky DM, Lee VM, Pratico D. Amyloid precursor protein and amyloid beta peptide in human platelets. Role of cyclooxygenase and protein kinase C. *J Biol Chem* 2001; **276:** 17036–43.

52 Santiago-Garcia J, Mas-Oliva J, Innerarity TL, Pitas RE. Secreted

forms of the amyloid-beta precursor protein are ligands for the class A scavenger receptor. *J Biol Chem* 2001; **276**: 30655–61.

53 Tedgui A, Mallat Z. Platelets in atherosclerosis: a new role for beta-amyloid peptide beyond Alzheimer's disease. *Circ Res* 2002; **90**: 1145–46.

54 Freeman MW, Moore KJ. eLiXiRs for restraining inflammation. *Nat Med* 2003; **9**: 168–69.

55 Wang L, Schuster GU, Hultenby K, Zhang Q, Andersson S, Gustafsson JA. Liver X receptors in the central nervous system: from lipid homeostasis to neuronal degeneration. *Proc Natl Acad Sci USA* 2002; **99**: 13878–83.

56 Joseph SB, Castrillo A, Laffitte BA, Mangelsdorf DJ, Tontonoz P. Reciprocal regulation of inflammation and lipid metabolism by liver X receptors. *Nat Med* 2003; **9**: 213–19.

57 Schuster GU, Parini P, Wang L, et al. Accumulation of foam cells in liver X receptor-deficient mice. *Circulation* 2002; **106**: 1147–53.

58 Tangirala RK, Bischoff ED, Joseph SB, et al. Identification of macrophage liver X receptors as inhibitors of atherosclerosis. *Proc Natl Acad Sci USA* 2002; **99**: 11896–901.

59 Bucciarelli LG, Wendt T, Rong L, et al. RAGE is a multiligand receptor of the immunoglobulin superfamily: implications for homeostasis and chronic disease. *Cell Mol Life Sci* 2002; **59**: 1117–28.

60 Schleicher ED, Wagner E, Nerlich AG. Increased accumulation of the glycoxidation product N(epsilon)-(carboxymethyl)lysine in human tissues in diabetes and aging. *J Clin Invest* 1997; **99**: 457–68.

61 Hofmann MA, Drury S, Fu C, et al. RAGE mediates a novel proinflammatory axis: a central cell surface receptor for S100/calgranulin polypeptides. *Cell* 1999; **97**: 889–901.

62 Park L, Raman KG, Lee KJ, et al. Suppression of accelerated diabetic atherosclerosis by the soluble receptor for advanced glycation endproducts. *Nat Med* 1998; **4**: 1025–31.

63 Yan SD, Chen X, Fu J, et al. RAGE and amyloid-beta peptide neurotoxicity in Alzheimer's disease. *Nature* 1996; **382**: 685–91.

64 Vitek MP, Bhattacharya K, Glendening JM, et al. Advanced glycation end products contribute to amyloidosis in Alzheimer disease. *Proc Natl Acad Sci USA* 1994; **91**: 4766–70.

65 Sueishi K, Yonemitsu Y, Nakagawa K, Kaneda Y, Kumamoto M, Nakashima Y. Atherosclerosis and angiogenesis. Its pathophysiological significance in humans as well as in an animal model induced by the gene transfer of vascular endothelial growth factor. *Ann N Y Acad Sci* 1997; **811**: 311–24.

66 Zhang Y, Cliff WJ, Schoefl GI, Higgins G. Immunohistochemical study of intimal microvessels in coronary atherosclerosis. *Am J Pathol* 1993; **143**: 164–72.

67 Shweiki D, Itin A, Soffer D, Keshet E. Vascular endothelial growth factor induced by hypoxia may mediate hypoxia-initiated angiogenesis. *Nature* 1992; **359**: 843–45.

68 Vasse M, Pourtau J, Trochon V, et al. Oncostatin M induces angiogenesis in vitro and in vivo. *Arterioscler Thromb Vasc Biol* 1999; **19**: 1835–42.

69 Celletti FL, Waugh JM, Amabile PG, Brendolan A, Hilfiker PR, Dake MD. Vascular endothelial growth factor enhances atherosclerotic plaque progression. *Nat Med* 2001; **7**: 425–29.

70 Moulton KS, Heller E, Konerding MA, Flynn E, Palinski W, Folkman J. Angiogenesis inhibitors endostatin or TNP-470 reduce intimal neovascularization and plaque growth in apolipoprotein E-deficient mice. *Circulation* 1999; **99**: 1726–32.

71 Vagnucci AH, Li WW. Alzheimer's disease and angiogenesis. *Lancet* 2003; **361**: 605–08.

72 Kalaria RN. The blood-brain barrier and cerebral microcirculation in Alzheimer disease. *Cerebrovasc Brain Metab Rev* 1992; **4**: 226–60.

73 Farkas E, De Jong GI, de Vos RA, Jansen Steur EN, Luiten PG. Pathological features of cerebral cortical capillaries are doubled in Alzheimer's disease and Parkinson's disease. *Acta Neuropathol (Berl)* 2000; **100**: 395–402.

74 Grammas P, Moore P, Weigel PH. Microvessels from Alzheimer's disease brains kill neurons in vitro. *Am J Pathol* 1999; **154**: 337–42.

75 Rhodin JA, Thomas T. A vascular connection to Alzheimer's disease. *Microcirculation* 2001; **8**: 207–20.

76 Maron DJ, Fazio S, Linton MF. Current perspectives on statins. *Circulation* 2000; **101**: 207–13.

77 Takemoto M, Liao JK. Pleiotropic effects of 3-hydroxy-3-methylglutaryl coenzyme a reductase inhibitors. *Arterioscler Thromb Vasc Biol* 2001; **21**: 1712–19.

78 Wolozin B, Kellman W, Ruosseau P, Celesia GG, Siegel G. Decreased prevalence of Alzheimer disease associated with 3-hydroxy-3-methyglutaryl coenzyme A reductase inhibitors. *Arch Neurol* 2000; **57**: 1439–43.

79 Jick H, Zornberg GL, Jick SS, Seshadri S, Drachman DA. Statins and the risk of dementia. *Lancet* 2000; **356**: 1627–31.

80 Rockwood K, Kirkland S, Hogan DB, et al. Use of lipid-lowering agents, indication bias, and the risk of dementia in community-dwelling elderly people. *Arch Neurol* 2002; **59**: 223–27.

81 Green R, Farrer LA. World Alzheimer Congress 2002, Stockholm.

82 Shepherd J, Blauw GJ, Murphy MB, et al. Pravastatin in elderly individuals at risk of vascular disease (PROSPER): a randomised controlled trial. *Lancet* 2002; **360**: 1623–30.

83 MRC/BHF Heart Protection Study of cholesterol lowering with simvastatin in 20 536 high-risk individuals: a randomised placebo-controlled trial. *Lancet* 2002; **360**: 7–22.

84 Fassbender K, Simons M, Bergmann C, et al. Simvastatin strongly reduces levels of Alzheimer's disease beta -amyloid peptides Abeta 42 and Abeta 40 in vitro and in vivo. *Proc Natl Acad Sci USA* 2001; **98**: 5856–61.

85 Delanty N, Vaughan CJ, Sheehy N. Statins and neuroprotection. *Expert Opin Investig Drugs* 2001; **10**: 1847–53.

86 Vaughan CJ, Delanty N. Neuroprotective properties of statins in cerebral ischemia and stroke. *Stroke* 1999; **30**: 1969–73.

87 Amin-Hanjani S, Stagliano NE, Yamada M, Huang PL, Liao JK, Moskowitz MA. Mevastatin, an HMG-CoA reductase inhibitor, reduces stroke damage and upregulates endothelial nitric oxide synthase in mice. *Stroke* 2001; **32**: 980–86.

88 Pahan K, Sheikh FG, Namboodiri AM, Singh I. Lovastatin and phenylacetate inhibit the induction of nitric oxide synthase and cytokines in rat primary astrocytes, microglia, and macrophage. *J Clin Invest* 1997; **100**: 2671–79.

89 Aisen PS, Schafer KA, Grundman M, et al. Effects of rofecoxib or naproxen vs placebo on Alzheimer disease progression: a randomized controlled trial. *JAMA* 2003; **289**: 2819–26.

90 Etminan M, Gill S, Samii A. Effect of non-steroidal anti-inflammatory drugs on risk of Alzheimer's disease: systematic review and meta-analysis of observational studies. *BMJ* 2003; **327**: 128.

91 Yermakova AV, Rollins J, Callahan LM, Rogers J, O'Banion MK. Cyclooxygenase-1 in human Alzheimer and control brain: quantitative analysis of expression by microglia and CA3 hippocampal neurons. *J Neuropathol Exp Neurol* 1999; **58**: 1135–46.

92 Yasojima K, Schwab C, McGeer EG, McGeer PL. Distribution of cyclooxygenase-1 and cyclooxygenase-2 mRNAs and proteins in human brain and peripheral organs. *Brain Res* 1999; **830**: 226–36.

93 Weggen S, Eriksen JL, Das P, et al. A subset of NSAIDs lower amyloidogenic Abeta42 independently of cyclooxygenase activity. *Nature* 2001; **414**: 212–16.

94 Collaborative overview of randomised trials of antiplatelet therapy—I: Prevention of death, myocardial infarction, and stroke by prolonged antiplatelet therapy in various categories of patients. Antiplatelet Trialists' Collaboration. *BMJ* 1994; **308**: 81–106.

95 Ridker PM, Cushman M, Stampfer MJ, Tracy RP, Hennekens CH. Inflammation, aspirin, and the risk of cardiovascular disease in apparently healthy men. *N Engl J Med* 1997; **336**: 973–79.

96 Cyrus T, Sung S, Zhao L, Funk CD, Tang S, Pratico D. Effect of low-dose aspirin on vascular inflammation, plaque stability, and atherogenesis in low-density lipoprotein receptor-deficient mice. *Circulation* 2002; **106**: 1282–87.

97 Pratico D, Tillmann C, Zhang ZB, Li H, FitzGerald GA. Acceleration of atherogenesis by COX-1-dependent prostanoid formation in low density lipoprotein receptor knockout mice. *Proc Natl Acad Sci USA* 2001; **98**: 3358–63.

98 Kivipelto M, Helkala EL, Laakso MP, et al. Midlife vascular risk factors and Alzheimer's disease in later life: longitudinal, population based study. *BMJ* 2001; **322**: 1447–51.

99 Seshadri S, Beiser A, Selhub J, et al. Plasma homocysteine as a risk factor for dementia and Alzheimer's disease. *N Engl J Med* 2002; **346**: 476–83.

100 Ott A, Stolk RP, van Harskamp F, Pols HA, Hofman A, Breteler MM. Diabetes mellitus and the risk of dementia: The Rotterdam Study. *Neurology* 1999; **53**: 1937–42.

101 Kalmijn S, Foley D, White L, et al. Metabolic cardiovascular syndrome and risk of dementia in Japanese-American elderly men. The Honolulu-Asia aging study. *Arterioscler Thromb Vasc Biol* 2000; **20**: 2255–60.

102 Prince M, Cullen M, Mann A. Risk factors for Alzheimer's disease and dementia: a case-control study based on the MRC elderly hypertension trial. *Neurology* 1994; **44**: 97–104.

103 Gustafson D, Rothenberg E, Blennow K, Steen B, Skoog I. An 18-year follow-up of overweight and risk of Alzheimer disease. *Arch Intern Med* 2003; **163**: 1524–28.

NOTES

NOTES

NOTES

NOTES

NOTES

NOTES

ISBN 1-933087-10-2
ISSN 1542-1708
Ninth Printing
Printed in the United States of America

The questionnaire on page 39 reprinted by permission from "A functional dementia scale." *Journal of Family Practice* 16(3): 499–503, 1983.

The chart on page 7 is reprinted with permission from *Diagnosis, Management and Treatment of Dementia: A Practical Guide for Primary Care Physicians*, p. 4, American Medical Association ©1999.

The graph on page 17 is reprinted with permission from Lopez, O.L. et al. "Risk factors for mild cognitive impairment in the Cardiovascular Health Study Cognition Study: Part 2." *Archives of Neurology* Vol. 60, No. 10 (October 2003): 1397.

Casserly, I. and Topol E. "Convergence of atherosclerosis and Alzheimer's disease: Inflammation, cholesterol, and misfolded proteins." Reprinted with permission from *The Lancet* Vol. 363, No. 9415 (April 2004): 1139–1146. Copyright © 2004 The Lancet Publishing Group.

The Johns Hopkins White Papers are published yearly by Medletter Associates, Inc.

Visit our Web site for information on Johns Hopkins Health After 50 publications, which include White Papers on specific disorders, home medical encyclopedias, consumer reference guides to drugs and medical tests, and our monthly newsletter
The Johns Hopkins Medical Letter: Health After 50.
www.HopkinsAfter50.com

The Johns Hopkins White Papers

Paul Candon
Managing Editor

Catherine Richter
Senior Editor

Devon Schuyler
Consulting Editor

Kimberly Flynn
Writer/Researcher

Leslie Maltese-McGill
Copy Editor

Tim Jeffs
Art Director

Vincent Mejia
Graphic Designer

Betsy Meredith Rigo
Editorial Assistant

Robert Duckwall
Medical Illustrator

Kate Brackney
Intern

Johns Hopkins Health After 50 Publications

Rodney Friedman
Editor and Publisher

Thomas Dickey
Editorial Director

Tom Damrauer, M.L.S.
Chief of Information Resources

Jerry Loo
Product Manager

Darren Leiser
Promotions Coordinator

Joan Mullally
Head of Business Development

NUTRITION AND WEIGHT CONTROL FOR LONGEVITY

Lora Brown Wilder, Sc.D., M.S., R.D.,

Lawrence J. Cheskin, M.D.,

and

Simeon Margolis, M.D., Ph.D.

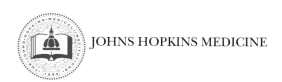

Dear Readers:

Low-carb, low-fat, low-calorie … what's the best eating plan for leading a long, healthy life? This White Paper gives you answers based on the latest research. It provides you with up-to-date recommendations on how to start an exercise program, lose unwanted pounds, and reduce your risk of heart disease, cancer, high blood pressure, diabetes, and osteoporosis. You'll find out which fad diets are dangerous, and which ones are less risky. So grab an apple and read on—and when you're done, consider going for a walk.

Here are some of this year's highlights:

- Understanding the latest changes in **food labels**. (page 4)
- Balancing the benefits and risks of **eating fish**. (page 12)
- The good news about **dairy intake** and your risk of colorectal cancer. (page 27)
- The latest recommendations on **antioxidant vitamin supplements**. (page 31)
- **Genetic engineering**: Is it safe to tweak a food's genes? (page 44)
- Which is better for weight loss: **High-intensity or moderate-intensity** exercise? (page 51)
- Johns Hopkins weighs in on the **South Beach diet**. (page 64)
- Why reducing abdominal fat with **liposuction** doesn't improve your health. (page 76)

We hope that this White Paper will serve as a blueprint for a lifetime of healthy eating and weight control.

Sincerely,

Lora Brown Wilder, Sc.D., M.S., R.D.
Assistant Professor
Johns Hopkins School of Medicine

Lawrence J. Cheskin, M.D.
Director
Johns Hopkins Weight Management Center

P. S. Don't forget to visit HopkinsWhitePapers.com for the latest health information that will complement your Johns Hopkins White Paper.

THE AUTHORS

Lora Brown Wilder, Sc.D., M.S., R.D., a registered dietitian, received her M.S. in nutrition from the University of Maryland and her Sc.D. in public health from Johns Hopkins University. She is currently an assistant professor at the Johns Hopkins University School of Medicine and is also affiliated with the United States Department of Agriculture and the University of Maryland's Department of Nutrition and Food Science. Dr. Wilder has served on various advisory committees related to nutrition, including committees at the American Heart Association and the National Institutes of Health, and helped set up the first Johns Hopkins Preventive Cardiology Program. In her research, Dr. Wilder has studied the effects of coffee on fatty acids and investigated behavioral strategies to reduce coronary risk factors. Her current research is in the area of dietary assessment methodology. She contributed to *Nutritional Management: The Johns Hopkins Handbook*, and her research has been published in *Circulation, The American Journal of Medicine*, and the *Journal of the American Medical Association*.

■ ■ ■

Lawrence J. Cheskin, M.D., graduated from Dartmouth Medical School and completed a fellowship in gastroenterology at Yale-New Haven Hospital. Currently, he is an associate professor of international health and human nutrition at the Johns Hopkins Bloomberg School of Public Health and an associate professor of medicine at the Johns Hopkins University School of Medicine. Dr. Cheskin is also the director of the Johns Hopkins Weight Management Center. In his research, Dr. Cheskin has studied the effects of medications on body weight, the gastrointestinal effects of olestra, how cigarette smoking relates to dieting and body weight, and the effectiveness of lifestyle changes in weight loss and weight maintenance. He is also the author of four books: *Losing Weight for Good, New Hope for People with Weight Problems, Better Homes and Gardens' 3 Steps to Weight Loss*, and *Healing Heartburn*. Dr. Cheskin has appeared on television news programs and lectured both professional and lay audiences on the topics of weight loss and management.

■ ■ ■

Simeon Margolis, M.D., Ph.D., received his M.D. and Ph.D. from the Johns Hopkins University School of Medicine and performed his internship and residency at Johns Hopkins Hospital. He is currently a professor of medicine and biological chemistry at the Johns Hopkins University School of Medicine and medical editor of *The Johns Hopkins Medical Letter: Health After 50*. He has served on various committees for the Department of Health, Education and Welfare, including the National Diabetes Advisory Board and the Arteriosclerosis Specialized Centers of Research Review Committees. In addition, he has been a member of the Endocrinology and Metabolism Panel of the United States Food and Drug Administration.

CONTENTS

Nutrition

The Basics of Nutrition . . . . .p. 1

Fat . . . . .p. 3

Fiber . . . . .p. 14

Vitamins and Minerals . . . . .p. 18

B Vitamins: Folic Acid, Vitamin B_6, and Vitamin B_{12} . . . . .p. 19

Calcium and Vitamin D . . . . .p. 23

Sodium and Potassium . . . . .p. 26

Antioxidants . . . . .p. 31

Phytochemicals . . . . .p. 36

Alcohol . . . . .p. 40

Enhanced Foods . . . . .p. 42

Organic Foods . . . . .p. 43

Food Safety . . . . .p. 45

Chart: Vitamins: Sources, Actions, and Benefits . . . . .p. 20

Chart: Minerals: Sources, Actions, and Benefits . . . . .p. 24

Weight Control

Metabolism . . . . .p. 47

Factors That Affect Body Weight . . . . .p. 48

Medical Consequences of Obesity . . . . .p. 52

Medical Evaluation of Weight . . . . .p. 52

Lifestyle Treatments for Weight Loss . . . . .p. 56

Medical and Surgical Treatments for Obesity . . . . .p. 67

Chart: Weight Loss Drugs 2005 . . . . .p. 74

Glossary . . . . .p. 78

Health Information Organizations and Support Groups . . . . .p. 81

Leading Centers for Weight Control . . . . .p. 81

Selected Medical Journal Article . . . . .p. 82

NUTRITION AND WEIGHT CONTROL
FOR LONGEVITY

Eating right will help you maintain a healthy weight and may protect you against a variety of chronic diseases, including coronary heart disease (CHD), certain types of cancer, diabetes, and osteoporosis. Most people recognize the importance of a healthy diet, and yet they do not always follow one. A recent report issued by the Congressional General Accounting Office notes that only 23% of Americans get their recommended servings of fruit and only 41% get their recommended servings of vegetables.

People cite a multitude of obstacles to practicing good nutrition: time constraints, the ready availability of packaged and processed foods, the perception that they will have to give up their favorite foods, and confusion over conflicting information on nutrition and weight loss. And many people harbor the misguided belief that dietary changes made late in life are of little consequence. In fact, changing dietary habits and losing weight in middle or even old age can significantly influence health. This White Paper addresses these concerns and counters them with simple, effective strategies for achieving good nutrition and, in particular, keeping your weight under control.

Nutrition

This section of the White Paper gives an overview of nutrition principles and specific recommendations—based on research studies—for the intake of various nutrients.

THE BASICS OF NUTRITION

Food provides not only the energy we need to function but also the nutrients required to build all tissues (such as bone, muscle, fat, and blood) and to produce substances used for the chemical processes that take place in our bodies millions of times a day. There are two broad categories of nutrients: macronutrients (carbohydrates, protein, and fats), which supply energy and are needed in large amounts to maintain and repair body structures; and micronutrients, the vitamins and minerals required in small amounts to help regulate chemical processes and build strong bones. Fiber, technically not a nutrient, also is part of a healthy diet.

Calories (technically called kilocalories) measure the amount of energy in a food. One calorie represents the amount of heat needed to raise the temperature of 1 L of water by 1° C. Carbohydrates and protein contain four calories per gram; fat contains nine calories per gram; alcohol contains seven calories per gram. All calories consumed in excess of need—whether in the form of carbohydrate, protein, or fat—get stored as fat.

Carbohydrates are starches and sugars obtained from plants. Sugars are known as simple carbohydrates and starches as complex carbohydrates. All carbohydrates are broken down in the intestine and converted in the liver into glucose, a sugar that is carried through the bloodstream to the cells, where it is used for energy. Some glucose is converted into glycogen, which is stored in limited amounts in the liver and muscles for future use. Carbohydrates are converted into fat when intake exceeds immediate needs and glycogen storage capabilities.

Proteins are nitrogen-containing substances that make up muscles, bones, cartilage, skin, antibodies, some hormones, and all enzymes. The proteins in foods are broken down in the intestine into amino acids, the building blocks for body proteins. The body can manufacture 13 of the 22 amino acids present in proteins; these 13 are called nonessential amino acids because they need not be obtained from the diet. The other nine are known as essential amino acids because they must be supplied by food.

Fats belong to a group of substances called lipids and are made up of chains of carbon, hydrogen, and oxygen that vary in length and in the number of hydrogen atoms attached to the carbon atoms. All fats are combinations of saturated and unsaturated fatty acids. The degree to which a fatty acid is loaded with hydrogen determines its "saturation" and impact on health. Along with protein and carbohydrates, fat is one of the three nutrients that supply calories to the body. Fat is vital for the proper functioning of the body. For example, fats are used to store energy in the body, insulate body tissues, and transport fat-soluble vitamins through the blood.

Cholesterol is a waxy, fat-like substance that is produced mainly in the liver but can also be made by any cell in the body except red blood cells. The liver produces all the cholesterol the body needs, but cholesterol is also found in any animal product you eat, such as meats, poultry, fish, eggs, butter, cheese, and milk. (Plant foods contain no cholesterol.) For transport in the blood, cholesterol associates with certain proteins to form lipoproteins. Cholesterol is present in the membranes of all cells, acts as insulation around nerve fibers, and serves as a building block for some hormones.

Vitamins are organic substances (meaning that they contain carbon) needed to regulate metabolic functions within cells. Vitamins do not supply energy, but one of their functions is to aid in the conversion of macronutrients into energy. Fat-soluble vitamins (A, D, K, and E) are stored in the body for long periods, whereas water-soluble vitamins (the B vitamins and vitamin C) can only be stored for a short time (although vitamin B_{12} is stored for longer periods). See the chart on pages 20–21 for the functions of the individual vitamins.

Minerals are inorganic substances that serve many functions, including helping to build certain tissues and maintain water content and acid–base balance (pH) in the body. Macrominerals (calcium, phosphorus, chloride, sodium, magnesium, potassium, and sulfur) are present in the body in large amounts. Microminerals, though no less important, are present in smaller amounts. The most important minerals and their functions are listed in the chart on pages 24–25.

Fiber is present in fruits, vegetables, grains, and legumes. Supplying no nutrients or calories, fiber is not digestible, but it is valuable in speeding foods through the digestive system and (possibly) binding toxins and diluting their concentration in the intestine. Some types of fiber also help to control blood sugar and blood cholesterol levels.

Water is an essential nutrient because it is involved in all body processes. Since an individual's water needs vary with diet, physical activity, environmental temperature, and other factors, it is difficult to pin down an exact water requirement. The general recommendation to drink at least six to eight 8-oz. glasses of water daily was recently revisited in a 2004 report by the Institute of Medicine (IOM). In the report, the IOM established general fluid recommendations at 91 oz. a day for women and 125 oz. a day for men, but concluded that most people can meet their hydration needs by letting their thirst guide them. Fluid requirements can be met, they said, by drinking water as well as other fluids (milk and fruit juice), including caffeinated beverages, and eating foods that contain a large percentage of water (fruits, vegetables, and soups).

FAT

By now, almost everyone is aware that reducing dietary fat can lessen the risk of several chronic diseases. While a high fat intake contributes to obesity, CHD, and some forms of cancer, not all types

NEW RESEARCH

Combination of Lifestyle Measures Prolongs Life in Old Age

Adhering to a Mediterranean diet and following other healthful lifestyle measures are associated with a significant decrease in the risk of death in elderly people, a new study finds.

A study team analyzed data on 2,300 older men and women from the Healthy Ageing: a Longitudinal study in Europe (HALE) population. Participants between 70 and 90 years old were followed for 10 years.

Study results indicated that after adjusting for such factors as age, sex, years of education, and body mass index, the risk of death was reduced by 33% in those who followed a Mediterranean diet—a diet rich in plant foods and low in saturated fat from animal foods—22% in those who drank alcohol moderately, 37% in those who got regular physical activity, and 35% in nonsmokers. Those who exhibited all four protective behaviors had a 65% reduction in the risk of death. These lifestyle factors were also associated with reductions in death from coronary heart disease, cardiovascular disease, and cancer.

Although this observational study cannot prove a cause-and-effect relationship between a low-risk lifestyle and risk of death, it suggests that a healthy lifestyle continues to provide benefits into old age. Previous studies have examined these four lifestyle factors, but not in combination.

JOURNAL OF THE AMERICAN MEDICAL ASSOCIATION
Volume 292, page 1433
September 22/29, 2004

How To Read a Food Label

Reading the Nutrition Facts panel on your groceries can help you make better food choices.

You've seen them in the supermarket—people who read the label on every package they buy. Although reading labels can be time consuming (and sometimes aisle clogging), comparing the nutritional content of products can help you make healthier food choices and plan a balanced diet. For example, a box of cereal that lists whole grains or bran first is going to be healthier that one composed primarily of regular (not whole) wheat flour, sugar, or corn syrup. To get more in-depth information, however, you'll need to look at the Nutrition Facts panel.

The U.S. Food and Drug Administration (FDA) devised the Nutrition Facts panel in 1994 as part of the Nutrition Labeling and Education Act. This standardized food label appears on nearly all packaged food sold in the United States and must list calories, total fat, saturated fat, cholesterol, sodium, vitamin A, vitamin C, calcium, and iron. Other nutrients may be listed voluntarily. Here's how to understand the label.

Decoding Daily Values

The percentages on the Nutrition Facts panel are based on Daily Val-

Nutrition Facts

Serving Size 1 cup (228g)
Servings Per Container 2

Amount Per Serving

Calories 260   Calories from Fat 120

	% Daily Value*
Total Fat 13g	20%
Saturated Fat 5g	25%
Trans Fat 2g	
Cholesterol 30mg	10%
Sodium 660mg	28%
Total Carbohydrates 31g	10%
Dietary Fiber 0g	0%
Sugars 5g	
Protein 5g	

Vitamin A 4%	•	Vitamin C 2%
Calcium 15%	•	Iron 4%

* Percent Daily Values are based on a 2,000 calorie diet. Your Daily Values may be higher or lower depending on your calorie needs.

		Calories	2,000	2,500
Total Fat	Less than		65g	80g
Sat Fat	Less than		20g	25g
Cholesterol	Less than		300mg	300mg
Sodium	Less Than		2,400mg	2,400mg
Total Carbohydrates			300g	375g
Dietary Fiber			25g	30g

Calories per gram:
Fat 9   Carbohydrate 4   Protein 4

ues, which encompass Daily Reference Values and Reference Daily Intakes. Daily Values for vitamins and minerals are the amounts you should aim for, whereas Daily Values for total fat, saturated fat, cholesterol, and sodium are the upper limits that are considered acceptable.

The label presents nutritional information as grams and milligrams and as percentages of Daily Values. Percent Daily Value is the amount one serving of the food contributes toward your daily goal, based on consuming 2,000 calories a day. In the example shown opposite, one serving provides 15% of the suggested daily amount of calcium. No Percent Daily Value is listed for trans fat, sugars, and protein because a Daily Value has not been established for these nutrients.

Getting Started With Serving Size

The top portion of the Nutrition Facts panel lists the serving size and the servings per container, which are based on the amount of that particular product that most people eat. Each product type (such as bread) has a standardized serving size (one slice for bread), which makes it easier to compare labels for similar products.

The remainder of the information listed below the serving size—including the calories, total fat, and vitamins and minerals—is based on one serving of the product. On the sample food label, one serving equals 1 cup, which provides 260

of fat have the same effects on health.

Triglycerides are the most abundant fats in foods and are the body's main source of stored energy in the body's fat cells. Triglycerides are manufactured in the liver and fat cells as well as obtained from food. It takes about eight hours for all of the triglycerides ingested during a meal to be removed from the blood where, like cholesterol, they are transported on lipoproteins called chylomicrons.

Triglycerides can be any combination of three types of fatty acids—saturated, monounsaturated, and polyunsaturated—which

calories and 13 g of fat. If you eat more than the listed serving, you will need to adjust all the other figures accordingly.

Fat and Cholesterol
Total fat represents the sum of all fatty acids (saturated, monounsaturated, and polyunsaturated, plus the glycerol backbone to which the fatty acids are attached) in one serving of the food. Food manufacturers are also required to separately list the amount of saturated fat and cholesterol on the Nutrition Facts panel. Because trans fats are now recognized as unhealthy, the FDA will also require manufacturers to list the amount of trans fat on the label beginning in January 2006.

Total Carbohydrate
The total carbohydrate is the sum of all of the starches, fiber, and sugars in the product. Dietary fiber and sugars are also broken down separately beneath the total carbohydrate.

It is important to note that the value for sugar includes both added sugars and sugars that occur naturally, such as lactose in dairy products and fructose in fruit juice.

Food Label Terms
The FDA also regulates descriptive terms on food labels. Some common terms and their definitions are listed below.

• **Excellent source, good source:** A product is said to be an "excellent source" ("rich in" or "high source" may also be used) of a nutrient—for instance, fiber or calcium—if it provides at least 20% of the Daily Value for that nutrient in a single serving. A product that contains 10% to 19% of the Daily Value of a nutrient is considered a "good source."

• **Lean, extra-lean:** These terms are often used to describe meat, poultry, and seafood. "Lean" implies that the product has less than 10 g of fat, 4.5 g of saturated fat, and 95 mg of cholesterol per 100-g serving. "Extra-lean" foods contain less than 5 g of fat, 2 g of saturated fat, and 95 mg of cholesterol per 100-g serving.

• **Low, free:** "Low-fat" foods have less than 3 g of fat per serving; "low-sodium" foods contain 140 mg or less of sodium per serving, and "low-cholesterol" foods provide 20 mg or less of cholesterol per serving and 2 g or less of saturated fat. "Free" means that a serving contains none or a trivial amount of the nutrient. Foods can be labeled "fat-free" if a serving contains less than 0.5 g of fat. A "sodium-free" or "salt-free" food has less than 5 mg of sodium per serving and "cholesterol-free" food contains less than 2 mg of cholesterol per serving.

• **Reduced:** This is a comparison claim. Foods labeled "reduced" contain at least 25% less fat, saturated fat, cholesterol, or sodium than the traditional counterpart.

Though manufacturers use the terms "low-carbohydrate," "carbohydrate-free," and "reduced carbohydrate" to market foods, those terms have no standard definition. However, the FDA is planning to set definitions for these.

differ in their chemical structures. As a result, no food contains just one type of fatty acid. Instead, the fat in a particular food is classified as saturated or unsaturated based on the type of fatty acid that predominates. For example, olive oil is typically thought of as a monounsaturated fat, but it also contains some polyunsaturated and saturated fat.

Fatty acids serve crucial functions in the body: They are required for the membranes of cells, keep skin and hair healthy, and form triglycerides that provide a layer of insulation under the skin. Since the body cannot manufacture them, certain fatty acids must be obtained from foods and are therefore called essential fatty acids. They are required components of cell membranes and can be converted to important hormone-like substances. In addition, dietary fat is needed to help the intestine absorb the fat-soluble vitamins A, D, and E.

Saturated fatty acids carry all the hydrogen atoms that their carbon chains can hold. Saturated fats are solid at room temperature and are found in abundance in animal products, such as meats, cheese, milk, and butter. Tropical oils—palm, palm kernel, and coconut—are also saturated. Saturated fats raise blood cholesterol levels and possibly contribute to certain forms of cancer.

Monounsaturated fatty acids are missing one pair of hydrogen atoms. As a result, two neighboring carbon atoms form what is known chemically as a double bond. The "mono" in monounsaturated indicates that these fatty acids have just one double bond. Liquid at room temperature, they predominate in foods such as olive oil, canola oil, almonds, and avocados. Cholesterol levels drop when monounsaturated fats replace saturated fats in the diet.

Researchers discovered the value of monounsaturated oil in part by studying the Mediterranean diet, which is associated with low rates of CHD and, possibly, cancer, despite a relatively high total fat intake. Olive oil is the main source of fat in that diet. The Mediterranean diet is also high in fruit, vegetables, and grains. The relatively low intake of animal foods may also account for the diet's heart-healthy effects.

Polyunsaturated fatty acids have two or more ("poly," meaning many) double bonds. Also liquid at room temperature, polyunsaturated fats make up the majority of the fatty acids in safflower, sunflower, and corn oils; fish; and some nuts, such as walnuts. Most of the polyunsaturated fats in plants are called omega-6 fatty acids, because the first of the double bonds is located at the sixth carbon atom in the fatty acid chain.

Fish contains both omega-6 fatty acids and another type of fatty acid called omega-3 (so named because the first double bond is located at the third carbon). Researchers believe that two specific omega-3 fatty acids, eicosapentaenoic acid (EPA) and docosahexaenoic acid (DHA)—found primarily in seafood—may help reduce blood pressure and prevent cardiac arrhythmias (abnormal heart rhythms). Small amounts of omega-3 fatty acids are also found in vegetable sources such as walnuts, and soy, canola, and flaxseed oils. While they appear to have some of the benefits of omega-3 fatty acids in fish, more research is required to determine their benefits.

Like monounsaturated fats, all polyunsaturated fats lower blood cholesterol levels when substituted for saturated fats in the diet.

Trans fatty acids (TFAs) are formed when food manufacturers add hydrogen atoms to unsaturated fats to make them more saturated and therefore more solid and shelf stable. The American Heart Association recommends cutting down on trans fats, which are used in many packaged cookies, crackers, and other baked goods; commercially prepared fried foods; and most margarines. A report recently issued by the Institute of Medicine (IOM) concludes that there are no safe levels of trans fats. The IOM recommends reducing TFA consumption to as little as possible to decrease risk of heart disease, cancer, and gastrointestinal disorders.

Dietary Fat and Coronary Heart Disease

A diet high in saturated fats increases CHD risk by raising blood cholesterol levels. Body cells use fat as an energy source and need cholesterol as a component of their membranes. Because fat is not soluble in the watery environment of the bloodstream, the liver wraps the cholesterol and triglycerides in a layer of proteins to transport them through the blood. There are three main types of these protein-wrapped packages called lipoproteins:

Very–low-density lipoprotein (VLDL) carries triglycerides from the liver to other cells. As the triglycerides are removed from VLDL, they are converted into smaller, cholesterol-rich particles, called low-density lipoproteins (LDL). The cholesterol in LDL is often referred to as "bad" cholesterol. LDL is first oxidized before it is taken up by cells in the arterial walls, where it initiates a series of changes that result in the formation of atherosclerotic plaques. These plaques can eventually hinder blood flow in arteries throughout the body. The formation of a blood clot on the plaques can halt blood flow altogether: Blockage of an artery supplying the heart causes a heart attack, while a blockage in an artery leading to the brain leads to a stroke.

The third type of lipoprotein is called high-density lipoprotein (HDL). As it travels through the bloodstream, HDL helps reduce the buildup of arterial plaque by removing cholesterol from arterial walls and returning it to the liver for disposal. For this reason, HDL cholesterol is often called "good" cholesterol.

Measures to prevent the formation of plaques include reducing blood levels of triglycerides and LDL cholesterol while raising HDL cholesterol. The different types of fatty acids in foods have varying

NEW RESEARCH

Mediterranean Diet Reduces Inflammation and Coagulation

A Mediterranean diet is known to protect against coronary heart disease (CHD), but researchers don't understand exactly how it offers protection. To learn more about the cardioprotective effects of this diet, scientists recently investigated the relationship between this diet and blood markers of inflammation and coagulation that are associated with CHD.

The research team evaluated the diets of over 3,000 Greek men and women. They found that people whose diets adhered most closely to the traditional Mediterranean model—rich in fruits, vegetables, legumes, whole grains, fish, nuts, and low-fat dairy products with olive oil being the main added fat and wine in moderation—had significantly lower markers of inflammation and coagulation than those whose diets adhered least closely. Adherence to the diet improved blood levels of C-reactive protein (CRP), interleukin-6, homocysteine, and fibrinogen as well as white blood cell count.

The researchers conclude that adhering to a traditional Mediterranean diet reduces measures of inflammation and coagulation that are believed to play a role in the development of CHD.

JOURNAL OF THE AMERICAN COLLEGE OF CARDIOLOGY
Volume 44, page 152
July 7, 2004

effects on the levels of LDL and HDL cholesterol. Saturated fatty acids increase levels of LDL cholesterol, while diets low in saturated fats reduce LDL levels. Although not everyone responds to the same degree, on average, every 1% reduction in saturated fat calories reduces total blood cholesterol levels by about 2 mg/dL, mostly from a decrease in LDL cholesterol. Saturated fats raise LDL levels by reducing LDL's removal from the blood by the liver.

Blood cholesterol levels are also raised by dietary cholesterol, but not as much as by saturated fat. A few foods—egg yolks, lobster, and shrimp—are especially high in dietary cholesterol.

Studies suggest that trans fats are even more harmful to health than saturated fats because trans fats not only raise LDL cholesterol, but also lower HDL cholesterol levels more than saturated fats. Elevated levels of blood triglycerides, which are especially common in people with diabetes, may also increase CHD risk.

Eating fish is associated with a reduced risk of CHD. This benefit may be due to special effects of the omega-3 fatty acids found in fish or may simply reflect the fact that many people who eat fish tend to eat less red meat. A growing body of research shows that omega-3 fatty acids may protect against sudden cardiac arrest and irregular heart rhythms. Omega-3 fatty acids are believed to make blood platelets less sticky and thus less likely to form blood clots that can cause heart attacks. Furthermore, omega-3 fatty acids can help lower triglyceride levels and decrease blood pressure slightly in people with hypertension. It should be noted, however, that fish oils in capsule form do not lower blood cholesterol levels, although these supplements can reduce triglycerides in people with very high triglyceride levels.

In addition, consuming foods that contain naturally occurring plant compounds called plant sterols (also known as phytosterols) can help lower cholesterol levels and may reduce the risk of CHD. Plant sterols are chemically similar to cholesterol. When they are ingested, the body mistakes them for cholesterol and tries to absorb them without success. As a result, the absorption of cholesterol is partially blocked.

Plant sterols are present in all plant foods but are particularly concentrated in vegetable oils, including corn and sunflower oil. Chemically modified phytosterols are added to certain margarines and orange juice. When used properly, these products, such as the butter substitutes Benecol and Take Control, can help lower LDL cholesterol levels.

Just Released: New Dietary Guidelines

What should you eat to stay healthy and maintain an appropriate weight? This question is addressed in the newly released 2005 *Dietary Guidelines for Americans,* a joint publication by the Department of Health and Human Services (HHS) and the United States Department of Agriculture (USDA). Last issued in 2000, the guidelines are revamped every five years to include the latest scientific information on nutrition and health.

Past guidelines have been geared toward healthy people age two and older, but the latest report includes recommendations for the elderly and for people with chronic health conditions, such as obesity, high blood pressure, and abnormal blood lipids. As in previous versions, these guidelines give advice on how to eat to promote health and a desirable weight.

Below are the nine major messages from the 2005 *Dietary Guidelines,* along with some information to help you interpret the recommendations and tips to help you meet them.

1. Consume a variety of foods within and among the basic food groups while staying within energy needs. People should meet their nutrient needs by choosing a variety of foods. To avoid weight gain, limit intake of items that are rich in calories but poor in nutrients, such as alcoholic beverages and foods with added sugars or fats. People over age 50 benefit from extra vitamin B_{12} from supplements or foods fortified with B_{12}, and certain people, such as the elderly, may need extra vitamin D from vitamin D–fortified foods or supplements.

2. Control calorie intake to manage body weight. Many people gain a small amount of weight each year, but reducing your daily calorie intake by just 50 to 100 calories can help prevent such weight gain.

3. Be physically active every day. The report recommends a minimum of 30 minutes of moderate activity daily to reduce the risk of chronic diseases. To prevent weight gain, it may be necessary to participate in 60 to 90 minutes of moderate to vigorous activity on most days of the week. Avoiding regain of lost weight may require up to 90 minutes per day of moderate activity.

4. Increase daily intake of fruits and vegetables, whole grains, and nonfat or low-fat milk and milk products. The range of fruits and vegetables advised is 5 to 13 servings—the equivalent of 2^1/2 to 6^1/2 cups daily. (This is another departure from the 2000 *Guidelines,* which suggested eating two fruits and three vegetables daily.) Aim for at least three servings each of whole grains and three servings of nonfat or low-fat dairy products per day.

5. Choose fats wisely for good health. Keep total fat intake between 20% and 35% of total calories, and limit intake of saturated fat and trans fat. Choose mono- and polyunsaturated fats instead.

6. Choose carbohydrates wisely for good health. Fruits, vegetables, grains, and milk products are all sources of carbohydrates. Choose fiber-rich carbohydrates, such as whole fruits over juices and whole-wheat grains rather than refined grains.

7. Choose and prepare foods with little salt. Reduce sodium intake to less than 2,300 mg daily. Some people, such as the elderly and those with hypertension, should try to lower sodium intake even further.

8. If you drink alcoholic beverages, do so in moderation. Drinking in moderation (two drinks a day for men and one drink a day for women) reduces the risk of coronary heart disease. However, people should abstain from drinking if they are taking medications that interact with alcohol, will be driving, or have trouble controlling their alcohol intake.

9. Keep food safe to eat. People can substantially reduce the risk of foodborne illness by washing their hands and all surfaces that come into contact with raw meat and poultry before preparing meals, thoroughly washing all fruits and vegetables, cooking foods to a safe temperature, and storing foods at the proper temperature.

Dietary Fat and Weight

Fat is a concentrated source of calories—it has nine calories per gram, compared with four calories per gram in protein and carbohydrates. Small amounts of fatty foods, therefore, pack a lot of calories. Reducing fat intake, however, does not guarantee weight loss. Weight is ultimately determined by the total number of calories consumed—whether from fat, carbohydrates, or protein—and the total number expended by metabolism, daily activity, and exercise. Overeating even fat-free foods can result in weight gain if they are also high in calories.

A low-fat diet that is also low calorie and is combined with regular exercise will help people maintain an appropriate weight, or lose weight if necessary. Weight loss is the most effective way to lower elevated triglyceride levels. It also helps to raise HDL cholesterol levels. Weight loss is also the first line of treatment for type 2 diabetes. In addition, a weight loss of as little as 5 to 10 lbs. may lower blood pressure enough to make antihypertensive drugs unnecessary. The many factors that affect weight control—and healthy strategies for losing weight—are discussed in detail in the section beginning on page 46.

Dietary Fat and Cancer

As with CHD, the hypothesis that a high-fat diet promotes the development of certain cancers first came from observational studies of different populations. In cultures where fat consumption is low, such as Japan and China, rates of breast, colon, ovarian, and prostate cancer are also low. In countries where people eat high-fat diets—the United States and Finland, for example—the incidence of these cancers is high. Furthermore, as people emigrate from a country where a low-fat diet is the norm to one where a high-fat diet predominates, and they adopt the dietary habits of their new homeland, their rates of these cancers increase. Thus, some researchers believe that the fat content of the diet, rather than differences in the genetic makeup of people from different countries, is responsible for the increased cancer risk.

Animal studies supported the link between dietary fat and cancer, but human studies have produced conflicting results. While some studies have shown that total fat intake is directly related to cancer risk, others have suggested that a high calorie intake, a diet rich in red meat, or a high intake of saturated fats may be the causative factor. Still other research shows that even if total fat intake is not involved in the development of cancer, it can accelerate progression of the disease.

Research into the role of dietary fat in breast cancer is a good example of the conflicting data on fat and cancer risk. Several studies have linked fat intake to breast cancer development, while others have found no connection. One possible explanation is that dietary fat itself does not raise breast cancer risk but does so indirectly by promoting weight gain. Several studies have shown that weight gain in adulthood is associated with an increased risk of developing breast cancer.

Alternatively, the fat content of the diet in childhood or early adulthood may determine cancer risk, so changes made in mid- to late life may not appreciably decrease risk.

One difficulty with connecting a high-fat diet to cancer is that no measurable factor in the body can be used to determine the increased risk, as with blood cholesterol levels and CHD, for example. It may be that cancer risk is not reduced until fat intake is very low. Because of the relatively high fat content of typical Western diets, modest reductions in fat intake by participants in U.S. studies may be too small to affect cancer risk.

The way that food is cooked also may play a role in the development of cancer. For example, studies suggest carcinogens, called polycyclic aromatic hydrocarbons, form when the fat from animal foods drips onto hot coals or stones during grilling. The resulting smoke from flare-ups can then transfer these cancer-causing compounds to food.

In addition, studies indicate that the type of fat in the diet may also be significant. In Mediterranean countries, for example, where monounsaturated fats (in the form of olive oil) make up a large part of the diet, women have a lower risk of breast cancer than women in the United States, even though their average total fat intake is about 42% of calories, compared with 35% in the United States. Fats derived from some fish and plant sources (such as avocados, nuts, and seeds) also may reduce the risk of cancer. In countries like Japan where the consumption of fatty fish (tuna, mackerel, and salmon) is high, cancer rates (particularly for breast and prostate cancer) tend to be low. It has been suggested that the omega-3 fatty acids found in fish (and in flaxseeds) may stunt tumor growth by "crowding out" harmful fats that seem to spur cancer growth in the cells.

Recommendations for Fat Intake

1. Above all, keep saturated and trans fat intake to 10% of calories or less. People with CHD, diabetes, or elevated LDL cholesterol levels should get less than 7% of their calories from saturated and trans fat. Meats, poultry skin, and whole-milk dairy products contain the most saturated fat and thus should be limited in the diet. Also, limit your trans fat intake. Although trans fats are not required to be listed on the food label until 2006, the tip-off in the ingredient list is the word "hydrogenated."

2. With few exceptions, limit total fat intake to less than 35% of calories. For those whose fat intakes have exceeded the recom-

Eating Fish: What's Safe, What Isn't

Seafood has been making headlines lately, for not only the health benefits but also the pollutants found in many species of fish.

Fish is an excellent part of a healthy diet, particularly for people who have or are at risk for coronary heart disease (CHD). In fact, the American Heart Association (AHA) recommends eating at least two servings a week of fish—especially oily fish—because of evidence that the omega-3 fatty acids in fish can lower triglyceride levels, decrease the rate of atherosclerotic plaque growth, and lower the chance of arrhythmias (abnormal heart rhythms). However, consumers need to be aware of pollutants found in fish and how to minimize exposure to them in their efforts to reap the benefits of eating fish.

Polychlorinated Biphenyls

Polychlorinated biphenyls (PCBs) are man-made chemicals used mainly in plastics, rubbers, and certain types of equipment, such as electrical and hydraulic equipment. Production was banned in 1977 owing to concerns about the potential risks of PCBs, for example, liver and kidney disease, developmental abnormalities, and cancer. Despite this ban, PCBs still exist in older electrical equipment and when the chemicals vaporize, they are either absorbed by the soil or carried by wind and water erosion to lakes, rivers, and oceans.

Fish farming practices have made certain types of fish less expensive and more widely available. Unfortunately, farmed fish tend to have higher concentrations of PCBs than wild fish because they feed on contaminated fish meal. Of particular concern is salmon, which is often farmed.

A study published in a 2004 issue of *Science* examined the PCB concentration of 700 salmon worldwide and found that farmed salmon had significantly higher levels of PCBs than wild salmon. PCB levels depended on where the salmon was raised. Salmon produced in North and South America had significantly lower levels of PCBs then salmon produced in Europe.

Another study, presented by the Environmental Working Group (a nonprofit organization) in 2003, analyzed PCB levels in 10 samples of salmon purchased at grocery stores throughout the United States. The researchers found that the farmed salmon contained 16 times more PCBs than the wild salmon.

Though authors of each study cautioned consumers to limit farmed salmon consumption to no more than once a month, the take-home message isn't quite so clear. PCB levels in farmed salmon are way below levels deemed acceptable by the U.S. Food and Drug Administration (FDA), though they are higher than levels tolerated by the Environmental Protection Agency (EPA), another government organization. Part of this discrepancy stems from the fact that the FDA's limits apply to commercially sold fish, whereas the EPA's limits apply to recreationally caught fish. The EPA levels are lower because people who catch their own fish are presumably eating more fish from one source, which might be heavily contaminated.

Moreover, nearly all of the farmed salmon consumed in the United States comes from North and South America—areas where salmon had lower levels of PCBs in the *Science* study. In addition, PCB levels were reported in raw fish; cooking the fish could reduce the contaminants by about 30%.

Mercury

Mercury is another environmental contaminant present in fish. Like PCBs, mercury can accumulate in people who frequently consume fat-

mended amount, fat calories should be replaced with ones from complex carbohydrates, with an emphasis on whole grains, vegetables, fruits, and legumes (beans and peas). As much as possible, avoid calories from products that contain a lot of refined carbohydrates, such as sugar and white flour.

While modifying fat intake is desirable, most people should not reduce fat intake to less than 15% of total calories. According to the American Heart Association, short-term studies reveal that lowering fat intake below this amount does not reduce LDL cholesterol levels much further than a standard low-fat diet. In addition, very–low-fat diets decrease HDL cholesterol and increase triglyceride levels.

ty fish. However, unlike PCBs, mercury is found in the fish muscle and therefore can't be reduced during preparation or cooking. The highest concentrations of mercury are found in larger, longer-lived fish, such as swordfish, shark, king mackerel, and tilefish. Fresh tuna and canned albacore tuna are also relatively high in mercury.

Bottom Line

Like all things, it is important to weigh the risks and benefits of eating fish. Certain individuals, such as young children and pregnant and nursing women, are especially susceptible to health problems stemming from fish contamination, particularly mercury. Therefore, the FDA and EPA recently issued guidelines regarding fish consumption for this high-risk population. The guidelines specify avoiding shark, swordfish, king mackerel, and tilefish (because of high mercury levels) and limiting overall fish consumption to 12 oz. per week. Also advised is limiting albacore tuna consumption to 6 oz. per week.

On the other hand, according to the AHA guidelines, the benefits of eating fish "far outweigh the risks" for middle-aged and older men, and women after menopause. To minimize exposure to pollutants, eat different types of fish from numerous sources and limit consumption of large, long-lived species. To reduce PCB contamination, trim the skin and visible fat before you cook the fish, and try baking, broiling, or grilling instead of frying, which cooks the fish in its own fat. Alternate consumption of farmed salmon with wild salmon (which is low in contaminants but also more expensive than farmed salmon). Canned salmon (which comes from wild salmon) is an excellent, lower-cost choice.

Broiled Tuna Burgers

Although tuna burgers are often made by combining tuna with breadcrumbs, try using heart-healthy oats instead. Sun-dried tomato "bits" can be found in many supermarkets. If all you can find are whole sun-dried tomato halves, choose soft, tender tomatoes and cut them into bits with a pair of scissors or a knife.

2	cans (6 oz. each) water-packed albacore tuna, drained
1/4	cup plain fat-free yogurt
2	tablespoons light mayonnaise
1/4	cup sun-dried tomato bits (not oil-packed)
3	scallions, thinly sliced
3	tablespoons quick-cooking oats

1. In a large bowl, combine the tuna, yogurt, mayonnaise, sun-dried tomatoes, scallions, and oats. Stir until well combined.
2. Preheat the broiler. Spray a broiler pan with nonstick cooking spray. Shape the tuna mixture into four patties. Broil 4 to 6 inches from the heat for three to four minutes per side or until crusty and heated through.
3. Serve the tuna burgers on toasted sourdough English muffins. On the side, serve finely shredded carrots and scallions tossed with fat-free ranch dressing. Makes four servings.

Broiled Salmon Burgers. Broiling salmon allows the fat to drip out, which reduces PCB contamination. Substitute one can (14 3/4 oz.) pink salmon, drained, for the tuna. Increase the yogurt to 1/3 cup and reduce the mayonnaise to 1 tablespoon.

---

3. Get half your total fat intake from monounsaturated fats. Monounsaturated fats are the major fats in the diet and are found in many foods. They are particularly plentiful in olive oil, canola oil, almonds, walnuts, and avocados. Because these sources are also concentrated sources of total fat, they must be eaten in moderation to maintain a diet containing no more than 35% of calories from fat.

4. Get less than 300 mg of dietary cholesterol per day, and less than 200 mg if you have elevated LDL levels. Although saturated fat raises blood cholesterol levels more than cholesterol from foods, experts still recommend limiting dietary cholesterol.

5. Eat fatty fish at least twice a week. The omega-3 fatty acids in fatty fish appear to have some protective effect, and fish are a good source of protein and are low in saturated fat. Salmon, sardines, and albacore tuna are all good choices. Omega-3 fatty acids are also found in soybeans, walnuts, flaxseed canola seeds, and products made from these foods (such as tofu and various oils).

6. Minimize cancer risk while grilling. The American Institute for Cancer Research advises simple measures, such as selecting lean cuts of meat, trimming fat, marinating, precooking, and minimizing fire flare-ups and smoke.

7. Remember that these recommendations need not be followed for each meal. It is more important to even out fat intake over the course of a week. If you eat a high-fat lunch, for example, you can compensate by eating a low-fat dinner or a little less fat than usual over the next several meals.

FIBER

For many years, fiber (the indigestible component of plant foods) was thought to be useful only for adding bulk to the diet to prevent constipation. But the shift in the diets of Western societies from ones based on whole grains, vegetables, fruits, and legumes to diets based on meats, refined grains, and processed foods has been associated with an increase in the incidence of CHD and type 2 diabetes; several studies point to a lack of dietary fiber as a primary cause. Some debate has ensued over whether fiber has a protective effect or is simply a marker for a healthy diet. But in recent studies, fiber has emerged as an independent factor for the prevention of disease.

Both types of fiber—soluble (sometimes called viscous) fiber, which dissolves in water and forms a gel-like substance, and insoluble fiber, which does not dissolve in water—are important for disease prevention. Most plant foods contain some of each type, but often one or the other predominates. Soluble fiber is found in legumes, barley, oats, and most fruits, while wheat and other whole grains and some vegetables contain insoluble fiber.

The two types of fiber exert different effects in the intestine. Soluble fiber binds bile acids and removes them in the stools. By absorbing many times its weight in water, insoluble fiber increases stool bulk and helps wastes pass more easily and rapidly through the digestive tract.

Fiber and Heart Disease
The connection between fiber and heart disease has focused on the

effect of soluble fiber on blood cholesterol levels. In the liver, cholesterol is used to make bile acids. Soluble fiber binds with bile acids in the intestines and removes them in the stool. The liver responds by converting more cholesterol into bile acids. The resulting fall in cholesterol in liver cells leads them to take up more LDL from the blood.

Studies suggest that an increase of 5 to 10 g per day in soluble fiber intake—two to four extra servings of fruits and vegetables—reduces cholesterol levels by about 5%. Other studies have shown that fiber intake directly affects the risk of fatal and nonfatal heart attacks. Other research indicates that soluble fiber is more strongly associated with a reduced risk of heart attack and CHD death than insoluble fiber. However, the effect of soluble fiber on blood cholesterol levels does not fully account for the protective effect of dietary fiber. This finding opens the possibility that fiber may work in additional ways—by affecting the body's use of glucose and insulin, for example, or by reducing triglyceride levels.

Fiber and Diabetes

People with type 2 diabetes, which accounts for 95% of all diabetes, are resistant to the actions of insulin, a hormone that controls the removal of glucose from the blood. To compensate, the pancreas must secrete more insulin to allow glucose in the blood to enter muscle cells, where it is used for energy. Diabetes develops if the pancreas cannot keep up with the continual demand for large amounts of insulin. Dietary fiber is thought to help prevent diabetes—as well as make it easier for people with diabetes to maintain good control of blood glucose levels—because it slows the absorption of sugars from the intestine and diminishes the rise in blood glucose following the ingestion of carbohydrates.

Fiber and Cancer

After skin cancer, colon cancer is the second most common cancer in the United States, where diets tend to be high in fat and low in fiber. Rates are much lower in countries where inhabitants consume a high-fiber, low-fat diet. The relationship between colon cancer and fiber was questioned by a 1999 study that tracked approximately 88,000 female nurses over a 16-year period. Surprisingly, the women who ate the most fiber—nearly 25 g a day—were just as likely to develop colon cancer and adenomas as those who ate the least fiber (about 10 g per day). Because the study had limitations in its design and because its findings contradict those of several previous studies, the results cannot be considered definitive.

NEW RESEARCH

Low-fat Diet Aids Weight Loss In Type 2 Diabetes

One concern with low-fat diets for people with type 2 diabetes is that they might increase triglycerides and worsen blood glucose control. But a new study finds that a low-fat diet has the same effect on triglycerides and blood glucose levels as a diet rich in monounsaturated fat—with the added benefit of weight loss.

Researchers randomly assigned 11 people with type 2 diabetes to either a low-fat diet that provided 20% of calories from fat or a high–monounsaturated-fat diet that provided 40% of calories from fat. Carbohydrates accounted for 65% of calories in the low-fat diet and 45% in the high–monounsaturated-fat diet. The participants ate as much as they wanted on either diet.

After six weeks, low-density lipoprotein (LDL) and total cholesterol levels improved the same amount in both groups. High-density lipoprotein (HDL) cholesterol levels decreased slightly on both diets. Triglycerides and glycemic control were similar for both diets. However, participants following the low-fat diet lost weight, whereas those following the high–monounsaturated-fat diet did not.

Though longer studies with more people are needed to determine the long-term effects of a low-fat, high-carbohydrate, high-fiber diet, it is encouraging to see that, at least in the short term, such a diet did not worsen control of blood glucose and triglyceride levels.

AMERICAN JOURNAL OF CLINICAL NUTRITION
Volume 80, page 668
September 2004

Tips for Eating Alone

Living by yourself doesn't mean you can't enjoy nutritious, varied meals.

Nearly a third of older people who don't live in an institution live by themselves, and living alone usually means eating alone. For someone who's not used to cooking for one, such as a widow or widower, being alone can interfere with proper nutrition.

Indeed, several studies over the past decade have determined that the loss of a spouse has a detrimental effect on the body weight and eating behaviors of the remaining spouse. One study of 58 recent widows and widowers found that widowed participants ate more meals alone, ate more commercial meals per week, and ate fewer snacks and homemade meals than their married counterparts. Moreover, widows and widowers reported that they derived less enjoyment from eating than the married participants. Other studies have shown that widows and widowers experience unintentional weight loss, which can signal malnutrition among older adults.

Yet good nutrition remains important in the later years of life. In fact, a healthy diet has impressive benefits, even for those with chronic conditions, such as diabetes, coronary heart disease, and hypertension. While dietary measures can't cure these disorders, they can help patients maintain their independence, improve their health and quality of life, and possibly reduce their need for costly prescription medication. In contrast, poor nutrition contributes to many chronic conditions, makes it harder to recover from illnesses, and increases the likelihood of institutionalization. Therefore, taking the time to shop for healthy foods and prepare nutritious meals is worth the effort.

Shopping For One

Buying healthy foods is the first step toward improving your diet. Below are some strategies to help you get started.

- Prepare a shopping list in advance. This will keep you on track once you get to the grocery store. It also helps to plan your menus ahead of time and to ensure that you purchase the right ingredients for your meals.
- Save money by clipping coupons (many stores will even double coupon savings on particular days) and reading store circulars for sales.
- Check the expiration or "sell by" dates on all perishable foods. Though most items are cheaper when bought in bulk, buying a smaller amount may save you money in the long run because you'll waste less.
- Buy frozen vegetables, particularly the bagged types, which are as nutritious as their fresh counterparts but allow you to make enough for a single meal while preserving the rest for another time. Keeping several types of frozen vegetables on hand (for instance, broccoli, spinach, and corn) will help add variety to your diet.
- Ask someone in the meat department to repackage fresh meat and poultry in smaller portions so that you can prepare a small amount and freeze the rest for another meal. You can safely freeze properly wrapped

---

While debate continues as to whether a high fiber intake can help prevent breast cancer, some research has shown that dietary fiber may lower blood levels of estrogen, thereby possibly reducing breast cancer risk.

Fiber and Weight Control

A diet rich in fiber helps people control their weight. Studies have found that those who consume fiber-rich diets feel less hungry between meals, get fuller more quickly at mealtime, and tend to consume fewer calories throughout the day.

Fiber-rich foods help to promote feelings of fullness and reduce caloric intake in a variety of ways. Foods high in fiber require more time and effort to chew, so they may reduce the amount of food consumed at a meal. The extra time required to chew high-fiber

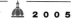

ground meat for up to 4 months, steak for 6 to 12 months, and turkey and chicken breast for up to 9 months.

- Maintain a small supply of nonperishable foods, such as boxed milk, hot cereals, dried fruit, peanut butter, pasta, tuna fish, and canned beans, in the event that you can't make it to the grocery store one week.

Preparing Meals

Though cooking for one person can seem like a chore, there are many ways to make nutritious meals that don't need a lot of preparation time. Here are some suggestions.

- Whole-grain cereal—either hot or cold—prepared with low-fat milk and fruit makes a nutritious meal any time of day.
- Make an omelet using low-fat cheese and frozen vegetables. Serve with a slice of whole-wheat toast and fruit to round out the meal.
- Heat up a can of soup, such as black bean or lentil, when you don't feel like cooking or cleaning up. (Most canned soups are high in sodium and may not be appropriate for some people, such as those with high blood pressure.).

- Make a simple stir-fry with low-sodium soy sauce, frozen vegetables, and chunks of beef, chicken, shrimp, or tofu.
- A variety of toppings can turn a baked potato into a healthy meal. A few to try: low-fat cheddar cheese and black beans; cottage cheese and cooked frozen spinach; cooked frozen chopped broccoli and low-fat cheddar cheese; and salsa and black beans. Experiment with your own favorite foods.
- Make a bowl of pasta with jarred sauce. Add frozen vegetables, such as broccoli or peas, to the boiling pasta water for a quick, one-dish meal.
- Prepare double portions of food and refrigerate half for the following day.

Eating Alone

Recent studies indicate that dining alone has a big impact on enjoyment of food. When possible, try dining with friends or family, or visit a local senior center for a free or low-cost meal and meal-time company. Of course, there will still be occasions when you will need to eat alone. Here are some strategies to liven up lonely mealtimes.

- Set the table with your nice china and silverware. Turn on the music for added ambiance.
- Enjoy your favorite television show while eating a meal.
- Sometimes, just a change in setting can make a meal seem more pleasurable. Try dining on your deck or in the living room by a window.

Assistance

If you or someone you know or care for isn't able to shop for or prepare meals, special services are available for older adults. Some programs, like Meals on Wheels, provide food to homebound people while other programs offer group meals where older adults can socialize with one another. Some communities even have services that deliver groceries to older adults. Though these programs tend to target low-income seniors, they are often available to everyone. To learn more about resources available in your area, contact the Eldercare Locator, a hotline established by the U.S. Department of Health and Human Services that will direct you to local agencies and programs, at 1-800-677-1116 or www.eldercare.gov.

foods produces more saliva, which, along with the extra water that fiber absorbs, is believed to distend the stomach and create a feeling of fullness. Furthermore, dietary fiber is thought to block the absorption of some fat and protein in the intestinal tract, thus reducing the calories derived from these nutrients.

Both soluble and insoluble fiber contribute to weight control in specific ways: Soluble fiber (found in oats, barley, legumes, and dried and fresh fruit) forms a gel around food particles, which slows the passage of food through the stomach and delays hunger signals sent to the brain. Insoluble fiber (found in broccoli, potatoes with their skins, apples, beans, and whole-grain breads and cereals) supplies bulk by absorbing water in the digestive tract, which, in turn, contributes to a feeling of fullness and thereby helps to discourage overeating. Consuming the recommended servings of fruits, vegetables, and whole grains each day makes it unnecessary to count grams of fiber or to keep track of how much you are eating of each type of fiber.

Recommendations for Fiber Intake

1. Consume the recommended daily intake of fiber, which is set at 38 g per day for men up to age 50 and 25 g per day for women up to age 50. Men and women over age 50 should aim for 30 and 21 g of fiber daily, respectively.

2. Eat whole grains and vegetables for insoluble fiber. Refined, grain products—white bread, white flour, white rice, and pasta—are not good sources of fiber. To get insoluble fiber, you must consume the bran (the outer coating of the grain) that is removed in the processing of many grains, especially wheat milled for flour. Good sources of insoluble fiber include whole-grain cereals, whole-wheat bread, whole-wheat crackers, bulgur, and wheat berries. Vegetables such as broccoli and potatoes with their skins also are good sources of insoluble fiber.

3. Eat oats, barley, legumes, and fruits for soluble fiber.

4. Increase fiber intake gradually over several weeks. A sudden increase of fiber in the diet may cause uncomfortable gas pains.

5. Drink enough fluids. Insoluble fiber needs fluid to be effective.

6. Do not go overboard on fiber. A very high intake can interfere with the absorption of some vitamins and minerals.

VITAMINS AND MINERALS

Vitamins and minerals are essential for virtually all of the biochemical processes necessary for life. They are needed to produce energy, fight disease, and repair injured tissue. One of their most important functions is the activation of enzymes to initiate and control chemical reactions in the body.

The 13 essential vitamins are divided into two major groups: water soluble (vitamin C and the B vitamins) and fat soluble (vitamins A, D, E, and K). With the exception of vitamin B_{12}, water-soluble vitamins cannot be stored in the body and need to be replaced frequently. Fat-soluble vitamins can be stored and require less frequent replacement. Especially important minerals include calcium, magnesium, sodium, potassium, and iron.

While true vitamin and mineral deficiencies are rare in developed countries, less-than-optimal intake of certain nutrients is common among Americans. A diminished intake of vitamins and minerals may raise the risk of chronic disease, including cardiovascular disease, colon and breast cancer, bone fractures, as well as pregnancies resulting in neural tube defects.

Multivitamins

Because studies suggest that the diets of most American adults fall short in ideal amounts of vitamins and minerals, a 2002 report in the *Journal of the American Medical Association* advises all adults to consume a daily multivitamin supplement. The recommendation is based on accumulated evidence from more than 100 research studies. Taking a multivitamin supplement can help to fill nutritional gaps in the typical American diet, although the practice is no substitute for eating a balanced diet rich in unprocessed whole foods, which are naturally full of thousands of potentially bioactive substances.

Most multivitamin supplements contain the RDA of all the essential vitamins, except biotin and vitamin K, which are easy to obtain from foods. The supplements also contain a smattering of key minerals. Most men and nonmenstruating women are advised to select a multivitamin supplement that contains little or no iron. Products formulated especially for seniors, however, typically contain less iron and vitamin A, and more calcium, vitamin B_{12}, and vitamin B_6.

While optimal multivitamin doses are beneficial for everyone, high doses of some nutrients, particularly fat-soluble vitamins, are dangerous. (For more on supplements, see the feature on pages 32–33.)

Everyone is advised to consume a multivitamin with food because nutrients are absorbed best together. In addition, to avoid the expense of name-brand vitamins, experts recommend buying inexpensive, generic-brand multivitamins sold at pharmacies or discount shops.

B VITAMINS: FOLIC ACID, VITAMIN B_6, AND VITAMIN B_{12}

B vitamins are vital for the breakdown and utilization of carbohydrates, fats, and proteins, and they also help to ensure the proper functioning of the nervous system and the synthesis of red blood cells and genetic material. Folic acid is essential during the early months of pregnancy to prevent birth defects, such as spina bifida and cleft palate.

Older adults may have greater requirements for certain B vita-

Vitamins: Sources, Actions, and Benefits

This chart describes and provides sources for the 13 vitamins. In addition, it enumerates the adult Recommended Dietary Allowance (RDA) established by the National Academy of Sciences. For some vitamins, not enough is known to recommend a specific amount; in these cases, the Academy has recommended a range called the Estimated Safe and Adequate Daily Dietary Intake (ESADDI).

Vitamin/Food Sources	What It Does/Potential Benefits	Recommended Intake
Vitamin A. Liver, eggs, fortified milk, fish, fruits and vegetables that contain beta-carotene, such as carrots, sweet potatoes, cantaloupe, leafy greens, tomatoes, apricots, winter squash, red bell peppers, broccoli, and mangoes.	Essential for night vision; helps form and maintain healthy skin and mucous membranes. Beta-carotene is converted in the body to vitamin A; beta-carotene (and other carotenoids) from foods may protect against some cancers and increase resistance to infection in children.	*700 mcg for women; 900 mcg for men* Vitamin A may be toxic in high doses (over 3,000 mcg), so supplements are not recommended. Beta-carotene supplements may increase lung cancer risk in smokers. In contrast to vitamin A, beta-carotene in food is never toxic.
Vitamin C (ascorbic acid). Citrus fruits and juices, strawberries, peppers, broccoli, potatoes, kale, cauliflower, cantaloupe.	Promotes healthy gums and teeth; aids in iron absorption; maintains normal connective tissue; helps in wound healing. As an antioxidant, it combats adverse effects of free radicals. May reduce the risk of certain cancers.	*75 mg for women; 90 mg for men* For supplementation, smokers should add 35 mg a day. Tissue levels are not increased further when supplements exceed 250 mg.
Vitamin D. Milk, fish oil, fortified margarine; also produced by the body in response to sunlight.	Promotes strong bones and teeth by aiding absorption of calcium. Helps maintain blood levels of calcium and phosphorus. May reduce the risk of osteoporosis.	*200 IU for adults age 19 to 50; 400 IU for adults age 51 to 70; 600 IU for adults age 70+* The limited amount of vitamin D in food often makes it necessary to take a supplement.
Vitamin E. Nuts, vegetable oils, margarine, wheat germ, leafy greens, seeds, almonds, olives, whole grains.	As an antioxidant, it combats adverse effects of free radicals. Consult your doctor before using vitamin E supplements if you are taking aspirin or warfarin.	*15 mg*
Vitamin K. Cauliflower, broccoli, leafy greens, cabbage, milk, soybeans, eggs. Bacteria in the intestine produce most of the vitamin K needed each day.	Essential for normal blood clotting.	*90 mcg for women; 120 mcg for men* No supplementation necessary or recommended.
Thiamin (B$_1$). Whole grains, dried beans, lean meats, liver, wheat germ, nuts, brewer's yeast.	Required for the conversion of carbohydrates into energy; necessary for normal function of the brain, nerves, and heart.	*1.1 mg for women; 1.2 mg for men* No supplementation necessary or recommended.

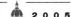

Vitamin/Food Sources	What It Does/Potential Benefits	Recommended Intake
Riboflavin (B$_2$). Dairy products, liver, meat, chicken, fish, leafy greens, beans, nuts, eggs.	Helps cells convert carbohydrates into energy; essential for growth, production of red blood cells, and health of skin and eyes.	*1.1 mg for women; 1.3 mg for men* No supplementation necessary or recommended.
Niacin (B$_3$). Nuts, grains, meat, fish, chicken, liver, dairy products.	Aids in release of energy from foods; helps maintain healthy skin, nerves, and digestive system. Large doses may be prescribed by a doctor to lower low-density lipoprotein (LDL) cholesterol and triglyceride levels and raise high-density lipoprotein (HDL) cholesterol levels.	*14 mg for women; 16 mg for men* When used in large doses to lower cholesterol, may cause flushing, nausea, gout, liver damage, and increased blood glucose levels. Do not exceed 35 mg/day unless prescribed by a doctor.
Vitamin B$_6$ (pyridoxine). Whole grains, bananas, meat, beans, nuts, wheat germ, chicken, fish, liver.	Important in chemical reactions of proteins and amino acids; helps maintain brain function and form red blood cells. May boost immunity in the elderly. May lower homocysteine levels, high levels of which may increase risk of coronary heart disease (CHD).	*1.5 mg for women age 51+; 1.7 mg for men age 51+* Megadoses can cause numbness and other neurological disorders.
Folate (B$_9$) (folic acid, folacin). Leafy greens, wheat germ, liver, beans, whole and fortified grains, broccoli, citrus fruit.	Important in the synthesis of DNA, in normal growth, and in protein metabolism. Adequate intake reduces risk of certain birth defects. May protect against CHD by lowering homocysteine levels.	*400 mcg* Can be derived from both fortified foods and supplements. Doses should not exceed 1,000 mcg/day.
Vitamin B$_{12}$ (cobalamin). Liver, beef, pork, poultry, eggs, dairy products, seafood, fortified cereals.	Necessary for production of red blood cells; maintains normal functioning of nervous system.	*2.4 mcg* Strict vegetarians may need supplements. Despite claims, no benefits from megadoses.
Pantothenic acid. Whole grains, dried beans, eggs, milk, liver.	Vital for metabolism of food and production of essential body chemicals.	*5 mg* No supplementation necessary or recommended.
Biotin. Eggs, milk, liver, brewer's yeast, mushrooms, bananas, grains.	Important in metabolism of protein, carbohydrates, and fats.	*30 mcg* No supplementation necessary or recommended.

mins, particularly vitamins B_6 and B_{12}. A lack of vitamin B_{12} can cause a form of dementia in older people that may be mistaken for Alzheimer's disease, which is noteworthy because the absorption of vitamin B_{12} diminishes with age. Some experts estimate that 10% to 30% of older adults are unable to absorb vitamin B_{12} efficiently from food, owing to alterations in the cells lining the digestive tract or diminished secretion of a substance called intrinsic factor that is needed to absorb vitamin B_{12}. An insufficient intake of vitamin B_6 may impair immune function in older adults. Experts believe that most older adults can benefit from taking a daily B_{12} supplement in addition to a multivitamin to ensure adequate intake of B vitamins.

B Vitamins and Heart Disease

Vitamin B_6, vitamin B_{12}, and especially folic acid may be important for the prevention of cardiovascular disease. They affect blood levels of the amino acid homocysteine by regulating its formation and conversion to other amino acids. It has been known for 30 years that people with a condition called homocystinuria—an inherited metabolic defect that results in extremely high blood levels of homocysteine—develop premature atherosclerosis and often suffer a heart attack or stroke before age 30. Now, researchers have found that people with far more moderate homocysteine elevations are at increased risk for cardiovascular disease.

Just how excess homocysteine contributes to arterial disease is not known. Some animal studies suggest that homocysteine damages the cells lining blood vessels and paves the way for the buildup of plaque. Other research suggests that homocysteine increases the formation of blood clots, which can obstruct an artery and cause a heart attack or stroke.

There is no doubt that folic acid and homocysteine levels in the blood are inversely related—that is, when folic acid levels are higher, homocysteine levels are lower. Many studies have clearly shown that folic acid supplements lower homocysteine levels. It is not yet clear whether increasing folic acid intake, alone or in combination with vitamin B_6, can lower the risk of arterial disease, but much of the evidence points in that direction.

Recommendations for Intake of B Vitamins

1. Get plenty of folic acid every day. The Recommended Dietary Allowance (RDA) for this vitamin is 400 mcg. Good sources include enriched breads and cereals, dried peas and beans, oranges, orange juice, green vegetables, and whole grains.

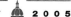

2. Eat foods rich in vitamin B$_6$. Meeting the RDA of 1.3 mg (for women) to 1.7 mg (for men) is all that is necessary. Good sources of vitamin B$_6$ include fish, meats, poultry, avocados, and bananas.

3. Maintain an adequate vitamin B$_{12}$ intake. The RDA for people over 50 is 2.4 mcg per day. People age 50 and older can meet the RDA mainly by consuming foods fortified with B$_{12}$ or with a supplement containing B$_{12}$. On the other hand, vegetarians who eat no animal products (B$_{12}$ is found only in meat, poultry, shellfish, fish, eggs, and dairy products) need to take a vitamin B$_{12}$ supplement. Vitamin B$_6$ and iron enhance vitamin B$_{12}$ absorption. People taking supplements of folic acid should also add 1 mcg of vitamin B$_{12}$ daily.

4. Take a multivitamin. Most multivitamins contain the amounts recommended above.

CALCIUM AND VITAMIN D

Most people are aware that calcium is essential for the formation and strength of bones, but few people realize that it fulfills other important functions. For example, calcium in the bloodstream is involved in blood clotting, blood pressure control, enzyme activation, contraction and relaxation of muscles (including the heart), nerve transmission, and membrane permeability (controlling the passage of fluids and other substances in and out of cells).

Along with calcium, you also need vitamin D to maintain the body's calcium stores. Without vitamin D, ingested calcium is poorly absorbed from the intestines. In addition, vitamin D strengthens the immune system. Although vitamin D is found naturally in only a few foods, the body can usually produce enough in response to sunlight.

Calcium, Vitamin D, and Osteoporosis

An adequate intake of calcium protects against the development of osteoporosis, which causes bones to become porous, brittle, and susceptible to fractures. While postmenopausal women are at highest risk, men also are susceptible to osteoporosis, particularly when they reach age 65.

When blood levels of calcium are too low, calcium can be released from bones, which contain 99% of body calcium. Bones are constantly broken down and rebuilt throughout life. This bone turnover becomes a problem only when calcium use outpaces calcium intake, because the body will then sacrifice bone in order to maintain blood calcium levels needed for these other crucial functions. Over time, a deficit in dietary calcium can result in osteoporo-

Minerals: Sources, Actions, and Benefits

As with vitamins, the National Academy of Sciences has established a Recommended Dietary Allowance (RDA) or Estimated Safe and Adequate Daily Dietary Intake (ESADDI) for minerals. The chart below gives a description of each mineral as well as the Academy's recommendation for intake.

Mineral/Food Sources	What It Does	Recommended Intake
Calcium. Milk and milk products, canned salmon and sardines eaten with bones, dark green leafy vegetables, shellfish, some fortified cereals.	Major component of bones and teeth; helps prevent or minimize osteoporosis; helps regulate heartbeat, blood clotting, muscle contraction, and nerve conduction. May help prevent hypertension.	*1,000 mg for adults age 19 to 50; 1,200 mg for adults age 51+*
Chloride. Table salt, fish.	Helps maintain fluid and acid–base balance; component of gastric juice.	*No RDA*
Chromium. Meat, cheese, whole grains, brewer's yeast.	Important in metabolism of carbohydrates and fats. Deficiency may impair the action of insulin.	*25 mcg for women age 19 to 50; 20 mcg for women age 51+; 35 mcg for men age 19 to 50; 30 mcg for men age 51+*
Copper. Shellfish, nuts, beans, seeds, organ meats, whole grains, potatoes.	Formation of red blood cells; helps keep bones, nerves, and immune system healthy.	*900 mcg*
Fluoride. Fluoridated water and foods grown or cooked in it, marine fish (with bones), tea.	Contributes to solid bone and tooth formation. Reduces dental cavities.	*3 mg for women; 4 mg for men*
Iodine. Primarily from iodized salt, but also seafood, seaweed food products, vegetables grown in iodine-rich areas. Widely dispersed in the food supply.	Necessary for the formation of thyroid hormone and thus for normal cell metabolism; prevents goiter (enlargement of the thyroid).	*150 mcg*
Iron. Liver, kidneys, red meats, eggs, peas, beans, nuts, dried fruits, green leafy vegetables, enriched grain products, fortified cereals. Cooking in iron pots adds iron, especially to acidic foods.	Essential component of hemoglobin (which carries oxygen in red blood cells) and myoglobin (in muscle); part of several enzymes and proteins in the body. Heme iron, found in animal products, is better absorbed by the body than non-heme iron, found in plants.	*18 mg for women age 19 to 50; 8 mg for women age 51+; 8 mg for men* There may be a danger from iron supplements for people who do not know they have hemachromatosis.

Mineral/Food Sources	What It Does	Recommended Intake
Magnesium. Wheat bran, whole grains, raw leafy green vegetables, nuts, soybeans, bananas.	Aids in bone growth; aids function of nerves and muscles, including regulation of normal heart rhythm.	*310 mg for women age 19 to 30; 320 mg for women age 31+; 400 mg for men age 19 to 30; 420 mg for men age 31+.*
Manganese. Nuts, whole grains, vegetables, fruits, instant coffee, tea, cocoa powder, beans.	Needed for energy production and reproduction. May also be essential for building bones. Excess may interfere with iron absorption.	*1.8 mg for women; 2.3 mg for men.*
Molybdenum. Peas, beans, cereal grains, organ meats, some dark green vegetables.	Aids in bone growth and strengthening of teeth; important in energy metabolism.	*45 mcg.*
Phosphorus. Meats, poultry, fish, dairy products, eggs, dried peas and beans, soft drinks, nuts; present in almost all foods.	Major component of bones and teeth; present in cell membranes and genetic material. Vital for energy metabolism.	*700 mg.*
Potassium. Most foods, especially oranges and orange juice, bananas, tomatoes, potatoes, greens, dried beans, brussels sprouts, dried fruits, yogurt, meat, poultry, milk.	Vital for muscle contraction, nerve impulses, and function of heart and kidneys. Helps regulate blood pressure and water balance in cells.	*1,600 to 2,000 mg minimum.*
Selenium. Fish, shellfish, red meat, nuts, grains, eggs, chicken, garlic, organ meats; amount in vegetables depends on soil.	Part of enzymes that act as antioxidants to prevent cell damage. Needed for proper immune response.	*55 mcg.* Large doses can be toxic.
Sodium. Table salt, salt added to prepared foods (such as cheese, smoked meats, and fast foods), baking soda.	Helps regulate blood pressure and water balance in the body.	*2,400 mg maximum.*
Zinc. Oysters, crabmeat, liver, eggs, poultry, brewer's yeast, wheat germ, milk, beans.	Important in activity of enzymes for cell division, growth, and repair (wound healing), as well as proper functioning of immune system. Maintains taste and smell acuity.	*8 mg for women; 11 mg for men.*

sis. (For more on dietary strategies to build bone, see the feature on pages 28–29.)

Calcium, Vitamin D, and Other Disorders

Calcium may offer a small reduction of blood pressure in people with high blood pressure, and vitamin D may help people with osteoarthritis. Both calcium and vitamin D appear to have a modest protective effect against colon cancer.

Recommendations for Calcium and Vitamin D Intake

If you are between the ages of 19 and 50, try to get 1,000 mg of calcium a day. This level of calcium intake helps to maintain calcium stores in bones. At age 51, increase calcium intake to 1,200 mg per day. To build peak bone mass and prevent osteoporosis, however, men and postmenopausal women over age 65 require 1,500 mg of calcium daily as well as an intake of vitamin D ranging from 400 to 600 IU a day.

SODIUM AND POTASSIUM

Sodium, found outside cells, and potassium, found mainly inside cells, are minerals that work together to maintain fluid balance in the body. In addition, they are involved in the regulation of muscle contraction and nerve transmission and play an important role in controlling blood pressure.

Although sodium occurs naturally in foods, the average person consumes most dietary sodium from salt added to foods in processing, in cooking, or at the table, and from other compounds—for example, sodium bicarbonate (baking soda) or monosodium glutamate (MSG).

Keep in mind when reading the information in this section that sodium and salt are not the same thing. Only 40% of table salt (sodium chloride) is sodium. All of the values in the following section refer to amounts of sodium, not salt.

Sodium, Potassium, and Hypertension

Overall, Americans tend to get too much sodium—about 3,900 mg per day, which is nearly twice the recommended amount—and too little potassium. This imbalance may contribute to high blood pressure. Experts continue to debate whether everyone needs to lower sodium intake to prevent or control high blood pressure. While many experts maintain that everyone should cut back on sodium intake, some hold that sodium reduction is worthwhile only when blood pressure is borderline or too high or in those who have a family history of high blood pressure.

Part of the debate results from an incomplete understanding of how sodium increases blood pressure. Researchers know that higher sodium levels promote water retention, which in turn increases blood volume and may ultimately lead to higher blood pressure. Excess sodium is usually excreted in the urine, but 30% to 50% of people with hypertension cannot efficiently get rid of excess sodium. Sodium can also constrict small blood vessels, which causes greater resistance to blood flow. How sodium produces blood vessel constriction remains unknown.

High blood pressure is defined as having a systolic blood pressure (the upper number) of 140 mm Hg or higher and/or a diastolic blood pressure (the lower number) of 90 mm Hg or higher. Studies estimate that if everyone stopped adding salt to food (which accounts for about a third of the sodium in most diets), the number of people who need antihypertensive medication would be cut in half.

In 1997, the results from the DASH (Dietary Approaches to Stop Hypertension) trial proved that diet could reduce blood pressure. The diet used in the eight-week study consisted of 8 to 10 servings of fruits and vegetables and 2 to 3 servings of low-fat dairy products each day. The diet also promoted plant sources of protein at least once or twice a week. By the end of the trial, the DASH diet had reduced blood pressure by an average of 5.5/3 mm Hg compared with the control diet. While the DASH diet is highly effective for prevention of hypertension, some of the most impressive results were in people who already had hypertension. These individuals, who had blood pressures of 140/90 mm Hg or greater, lowered their levels by 11/5.5 mm Hg, which is as low as (or lower than) the results produced by a single antihypertensive medication.

Results from a subsequent study, the DASH-Sodium trial, published in *The New England Journal of Medicine* in 2001, indicate that combining the DASH diet with a reduced sodium intake can lower blood pressure more than either measure alone. In the trial, participants followed a diet that combined the DASH diet with one of three levels of sodium intake (3,300 mg, 2,400 mg, or 1,500 mg per day). Those participants with hypertension who consumed the DASH diet with the least sodium had a systolic blood pressure that was almost 12 mm Hg lower than that of people who ate the typical American diet with a high sodium level.

NEW RESEARCH

Milk and Calcium May Decrease Risk of Colorectal Cancer

Drinking milk may offer protection against cancer of the distal colon and rectum, according to findings from a recent international study.

Researchers pooled data from 10 observational studies with over 534,000 men and women, 4,992 of whom developed colorectal cancer during 6 to 16 years of follow-up. Those who drank the most milk—at least a cup a day—had about a 15% lower risk of colorectal cancer than those who drank the least milk. Other dairy products studied, such as cheese, yogurt, and ice cream, were not clearly linked to a decreased risk of colorectal cancer.

A high overall intake of calcium—from diet and supplements—was also related to a decreased risk of colorectal cancer, although amounts beyond 1,000 mg a day produced little or no additional benefit. It is unclear whether this effect was related to intake of milk, which is an important source of dietary calcium, or to the effects of calcium alone.

Calcium and dairy food are hypothesized to reduce the risk of colorectal cancer by slowing the proliferation of cells in the colon, and some animal research supports this theory. Because this study is observational (rather than a clinical trial), it cannot prove a cause-and-effect relationship. However, it does add support to recommendations to obtain calcium in the diet.

JOURNAL OF THE NATIONAL CANCER INSTITUTE
Volume 96, page 1015
July 7, 2004

The Right Diet for Building Bone

Osteoporosis affects millions of Americans, but eating well and taking supplements if needed can help prevent this common problem.

About 10 million Americans have osteoporosis, and another 18 million have low bone density, according to the National Osteoporosis Foundation. Women are especially susceptible: They account for 80% of cases of osteoporosis, and nearly half of all American women past menopause have thinning bones but do not realize it, according to a major study published in the *Journal of the American Medical Association* in 2004.

Although osteoporosis predominantly affects women, men are susceptible, too. Once they reach age 65 or 70, men start to lose bone mass at the same rate as women, and about one third of all hip fractures each year occur in men.

In addition to age, risk factors for osteoporosis include low body weight (less than 127 lbs.), cigarette smoking, a personal or family history of fractures, Caucasian or Asian heritage, prolonged low calcium intake, and lack of exercise.

Calcium and Vitamin D
Though some risk factors for osteoporosis are unavoidable, getting enough calcium and vitamin D can help build strong bones and maintain bone strength for a lifetime.

Consume plenty of calcium. About 99% of calcium in the body is stored in the bones and teeth; the rest is in the blood, other body fluids, and cells where it is needed for vital body functions, including contractions of the heart and other muscles. If low calcium intake or poor calcium absorption lowers blood calcium levels, parathyroid hormone promotes the removal of calcium from bones to raise blood calcium levels and maintain these vital functions. A lifetime of inadequate calcium intake can result in low bone density because more calcium is taken from the bones than is deposited in them.

The Dietary Reference Intake (DRI) for calcium is 1,200 mg per day for men and women over age 50. (The DRI is 1,000 mg daily for men and women age 19 to 50.) Some experts advise a daily calcium intake of up to 1,500 mg for older adults. Despite these recommendations, and the fact that calcium is the single most important nutrient for building peak bone mass and preventing osteoporosis, only 50% to 60% of the population meets their calcium requirements.

Try to get as much calcium as possible through your diet. The best sources of calcium are low-fat milk and other dairy products, which contain as much calcium as their full-fat counterparts but contain less saturated fat. To boost the calcium content of your diet, consider adding low-fat milk to hot cereal or canned soup in lieu of water, sprinkle low-fat cheese on salads or other vegetables, or try snacking on pudding, low-fat yogurt, or a fruit smoothie made with low-fat yogurt. You can also add nonfat powdered dry milk to baked goods, soups, and casseroles.

While dairy products are the principal and most absorbable source of dietary calcium, calcium-fortified juice, canned salmon and sardines with the bones (the bones are soft and edible), and firm tofu (make sure the label says the tofu has been processed with calcium) are good nondairy choices.

Use supplements to make up for calcium shortfalls. A variety of calcium supplements are available to help you meet your calcium requirements. Calcium carbonate and calcium citrate contain the highest percentage of elemental calcium in each tablet, but calcium citrate is more readily absorbed from the intestine. Calcium carbonate pills should be taken with meals because gastric calcium improves calcium absorption from such tablets.

Calcium—whether from supplements or dietary sources—is best absorbed when consumed several times a day in amounts of 500 mg or

A large part of the success of the DASH-Sodium diet may be its high potassium content of about 4,400 mg daily (roughly the amount in 11 bananas). Research indicates that potassium lowers blood pressure by relaxing arteries. But the interplay of all essential nutrients in the diet, as well as fiber, is probably just as important as any single vitamin or mineral.

The DASH diet may also help to improve cholesterol levels. According to a study in the *American Journal of Clinical Nutrition*, the diet reduces total cholesterol an average of 13.7 mg/dL and LDL

less. Also, calcium supplements should not be taken within 30 minutes of bisphosphonates, such as alendronate (Fosamax) or risedronate (Actonel), which are prescribed to prevent osteoporosis.

Get enough vitamin D. Vitamin D enhances calcium absorption from the intestines. The recommended intake for vitamin D is 400 IU per day for men and women age 51 to 70, and 600 IU for those over 70. Most vitamin D is synthesized by the skin in response to sunlight. Therefore, you should spend 10 to 15 minutes outside prior to applying sunscreen. Older people may need slightly longer exposure to compensate for the decreased ability of their skin to synthesize vitamin D in response to sunlight.

Vitamin D is not found naturally in a wide variety of foods; the best sources include fortified dairy products and ready-to-eat cereals that have been fortified with vitamin D (check the label). Therefore, if you live in a northern climate, are homebound, or live in a nursing home, you may benefit from supplemental vitamin D. Furthermore, if you currently have osteoporosis or low bone mineral density, you should take a vitamin D supplement. Many calcium supplements contain vitamin D (again, check the label). Consult your physician as to which supplement is appropriate for you.

Other Nutrients

Though calcium and vitamin D are the key nutrients involved in developing bone mass, other nutrients play supporting roles. Fortunately, following a well-balanced diet—like the one recommended in this White Paper—will provide sufficient amounts of these nutrients.

Potassium. This mineral helps bones retain calcium. It is plentiful in fruits and vegetables, including bananas, potatoes, and orange juice.

Phosphorous. This mineral binds with calcium to form hydroxyapatite, a compound that makes bones strong and rigid. Phosphorous is abundant in the diet, particularly in protein-rich foods like meat, poultry, fish, and milk.

Magnesium. Magnesium, another important component of bone, is found in many foods, including fruits, vegetables, and grains.

Vitamin C. Vitamin C is involved in the formation of collagen, part of the matrix that holds bones together. Along with citrus and other fruits, vitamin C is found in vegetables like green peppers, broccoli, and tomatoes.

Vitamin K. Sufficient vitamin K intake is necessary for the bone matrix protein osteocalcin to function properly. Several studies have linked low vitamin K intake with low bone mineral density and increased risk of fractures. Vitamin K is predominantly found in leafy green vegetables, which include spinach, collard greens, broccoli, and kale.

Vitamin A. New research published in *The American Journal of Medicine* found an increased risk of hip fracture among women with low vitamin A intake. But research also suggests that a high intake of vitamin A from retinol (also called preformed vitamin A) might increase the risk of fractures, so make sure that any supplements you take contain at least 20% of their vitamin A in the form of beta-carotene (a precursor of vitamin A that does not contribute to fractures). Vitamin A is found in fortified milk and other animal products, like eggs and meat. Beta-carotene is primarily found in orange-colored fruits and vegetables, like carrots, pumpkin, and cantaloupe.

Folate and other B vitamins. A 2004 study published in *The New England Journal of Medicine* found that people with high homocysteine levels had an increased prevalence of osteoporosis. Though this early research does not show whether high homocysteine levels cause low bone density or whether it is a marker for some other cause of low bone density, high homocysteine levels are easily corrected with sufficient intake of folate and vitamin B_6. In addition to fortified grains, folate is found in leafy green vegetables. Sources of vitamin B_6 include whole grains, beans, nuts, and legumes.

cholesterol an average of 10.7 mg/dL.

Sodium and Other Disorders

There are several other reasons to reduce sodium in your diet. A high-sodium diet can increase the loss of calcium in the urine, which in turn triggers removal of calcium from bones. A very high intake of sodium (3,000 mg or more daily) can also raise the risk of stomach cancer because sodium irritates the lining of the stomach, especially in people who have had ulcers. Finally, excess sodium contributes to kidney disease as an extension of its effect on hypertension. Chronic high blood pressure damages organs by injuring the blood vessels that supply them, and the kidneys are particularly vulnerable to such damage.

Recommendations for Sodium and Potassium Intake

1. Don't add salt to foods. One teaspoon of salt contains 2,130 mg of sodium. At first, a low-sodium diet may make food taste bland, but within six to eight weeks your palate will adjust.

2. If you have hypertension, do not consume more than 2,000 mg of sodium daily. Those individuals who have a particular sensitivity to sodium should consume even less.

3. Flavor foods with herbs, spices, and citrus juices. These seasonings can help perk up foods and compensate for the flavor lost from the reduction in salt.

4. Read food labels carefully for sodium content. Packaged and processed foods supply about two thirds of the sodium in the average diet. Minimize your use of high-sodium products, such as luncheon meats, sausages, smoked meats and fish, hot dogs, canned shellfish, canned soups, frozen dinners, condiments (relish, mustard, ketchup, soy sauce, and pickles), cheese, and processed snack foods.

5. Remember that sodium comes in many forms, not just salt. Baking soda, monosodium glutamate (MSG), onion salt, soy sauce, and some other flavorings also are sources of sodium.

6. Try salt alternatives. Salt alternatives—such as Cardia and Morton's Lite Salt, which contain about half the sodium of table salt—can be an option for some people. However, people with kidney problems and those taking potassium-sparing diuretics for hypertension or heart failure should not use these products because they replace some sodium with potassium. Speak with your doctor first before using these salt alternatives.

7. Look for reduced-sodium packaged foods. Sodium claims made on labels must meet certain standards: Low-sodium foods have 140 mg or less per serving, very low sodium means 35 mg or less, and sodium free has 5 mg or less. Unsalted or no-salt-added foods generally contain only naturally occurring sodium.

8. Get about 2,000 mg of potassium a day. Eat more fruits, vegetables, legumes, and grains. Bananas, kidney beans, lentils, oranges, orange juice, yogurt, cantaloupe, prunes, and potatoes are just a few of the foods that are both high in potassium and low in sodium.

ANTIOXIDANTS

Antioxidants are substances that help to counteract cell damage resulting from the formation of free radicals during normal metabolism. Free radicals are molecules that are highly reactive because they are missing one or more electrons. They seek to combine with other molecules and can set off a chain reaction that rapidly passes electrons from molecule to molecule. At times, this process can be beneficial: For example, free radicals help the body fight bacteria and viruses. However, the rapid exchange of electrons can also damage cell membranes and DNA. Excess free radical production is now thought to contribute to many diseases, including CHD, cancer, and cataracts.

A variety of antioxidants can either neutralize free radicals or repair the damage caused by them. Health problems can arise, however, when the body's production of free radicals overwhelms its natural antioxidant defenses. Foods that contain antioxidants—which include vitamins C and E, the mineral selenium, and a collection of plant pigments known as carotenoids (which includes beta-carotene)—can add to the body's supply of antioxidants. Other plant substances, known collectively as phytochemicals (see pages 36–40), may also act as antioxidants. Each antioxidant has a different mode of action, and many of them appear to work together. For example, vitamin C helps to regenerate vitamin E once it has become oxidized. Therefore, it is important that your diet supply adequate amounts of all of the antioxidants to achieve this synergy.

Antioxidants and CHD

Numerous studies have shown that people who eat a lot of fruits and vegetables are less likely to develop CHD. Some researchers attribute this benefit to the antioxidants in these foods, especially vitamin C, vitamin E, beta-carotene, and other carotenoids. In studies that measured blood levels of these nutrients, high levels were associated with a reduced risk of CHD.

However, three large trials have shown that vitamin E supplements provided no benefits in patients with known CHD. A major report recently issued by the Food and Nutrition Board of the National Academy of Sciences—the main authority in the United States for nutritional recommendations—also concluded that vitamin E in supplement form serves no purpose in helping to reduce CHD. And a study in *The New England Journal of Medicine* found that taking antioxidant supplements containing vitamins E and C, beta-carotene, and selenium did not reduce heart attacks in patients with

NEW RESEARCH

Antioxidant Supplements Not Found To Reduce Cardiovascular Disease

In a recent advisory, the American Heart Association (AHA) did not recommend the use of antioxidant vitamin supplements to prevent or treat cardiovascular disease (CVD).

Some observational studies have found that people who take antioxidant supplements are less likely to develop CVD than those who don't, but such findings may simply reflect healthier lifestyles among people who take vitamins. Only randomized clinical trials are able to establish cause-and-effect relationships.

The review showed that "clinical trials have failed to demonstrate a beneficial effect of antioxidant supplements on CVD morbidity and mortality." In fact, several studies found increased rates of death and coronary heart disease in people given vitamin supplements. AHA reviewers support additional research to resolve the discrepancy between observational studies and clinical trials.

Instead of taking supplements, the AHA advises people to obtain antioxidants by eating a diet rich in fruits, vegetables, whole grains, and nuts—a measure proven to reduce the risk of CVD.

The AHA consultants reviewed 20 randomized clinical trials that examined the effects of vitamins C and E, beta-carotene, and antioxidant supplements containing more than one antioxidant on the risk of CVD. Most of the study participants had already had a heart attack or were at elevated risk for CVD.

CIRCULATION
Volume 110, page 637
August 2004

Supplements: Unsafe at Certain Doses

Between supplements and fortified foods, it's not difficult to overdose on vitamins and minerals.

About half of American adults take vitamin or mineral supplements in an effort to ward off chronic conditions or offset a possible deficiency, a strategy that may benefit certain individuals. For example, the elderly are advised to take supplements of calcium and vitamin D to help prevent bone loss because the aging body manufactures less vitamin D, as well as a vitamin B_{12} supplement. Women of childbearing age are advised to consume an additional supplement of 400 micrograms (mcg) of folic acid per day.

However, while a daily multivitamin pill can help fill any nutritional gaps in your diet, certain vitamins and minerals may be hazardous when taken over time in high doses. Not only can high doses of individual supplements or doubling up on multivitamins prove dangerous, but foods that are fortified with vitamins and minerals—such as cereals, breads, and some snack products—can be harmful when eaten in large amounts, especially if you are already taking a supplement. For example, iron is often added to cereals and grains. This can pose a problem for individuals who are at risk for hemochromatosis (see the opposite page). So before taking a supplement, check with your physician about the proper dosage and be sure to inform him or her about other supplements or medication you are taking. Fortunately, it's difficult, if not impossible, to consume unsafe levels of vitamins and minerals through unfortified foods.

To make sure you're taking supplements that have been tested by the U.S. Pharmacopeia for strength and purity, look for "USP" on the label.

Defining Safety Limits

The Food and Nutrition Board of the National Academies of Science developed the Dietary Reference Intakes (DRIs) in 1995 to reflect evolving scientific knowledge about vitamins and minerals. DRIs encompass three values for nutrients: the Estimated Average Requirement (EAR), the Recommended Dietary Allowance (RDA), and the Tolerable Upper Intake Level (UL).

The EAR specifies the value that meets the needs of half the people in a specified group, while the RDA is designed to meet the needs of nearly everyone in a group. Both of these are below the level at which toxicity may occur, whereas the UL represents the maximum amount designated to be safe for most people.

Taking vitamins and minerals in excess of ULs can cause adverse effects ranging from the relatively benign, such as diarrhea with high vitamin C intake, to serious, such as liver damage with high vitamin A intake. Excessive intake usually must continue for several months at high levels before such reactions are apparent, but it is important not to consistently exceed the UL.

Below are some nutrients that can have serious health consequences when taken in high doses.

Vitamin A

Too much vitamin A may interfere with bone formation and increase the risk of fracture. A study of 72,000 postmenopausal women published in the *Journal of the American Medical Association* in 2002 found that those with a high intake of vitamin A from retinol were at increased risk for hip fractures; vitamin A from beta-carotene did not affect fracture risk. More recently, a study of more than 2,000 older men published in *The New England Journal of Medicine* in 2003 linked high blood levels of vitamin A with fractures. High levels of vitamin A are also associated with birth defects and liver problems.

Men should aim for 900 mcg (3,000 IU) of vitamin A per day and women

established heart disease, normal LDL cholesterol levels, and low HDL cholesterol levels. Drug therapy with simvastatin (Zocor) and niacin produced marked improvements in HDL cholesterol levels, arterial narrowing, and heart attack risk. But combining the drug therapy with antioxidants lessened these benefits.

Moreover, antioxidant supplementation may blunt the benefits of cholesterol-lowering drugs, suggests a study in *Arteriosclerosis, Thrombosis, and Vascular Biology*. Researchers treated 153 coronary artery disease patients with drug therapy (a statin with niacin) alone, drug therapy with antioxidants (vitamins E and C, beta-

700 mcg (2,333 IU) a day. Nobody should consume more than the upper limit of 3,000 mcg (10,000 IU) daily, the highest level likely not to produce adverse effects. Few Americans need vitamin A supplements, but if you take multivitamins that contain vitamin A, at least 20% should be in the form of beta-carotene.

Folate

The concern with too much folate, which is found in fortified breads and cereals as well as in leafy green vegetables, is how it interacts with vitamin B_{12}. High levels of folate can mask symptoms of pernicious anemia, a blood abnormality caused by a B_{12} deficiency, and make it more difficult to diagnose the disorder. B_{12} deficiency surfaces frequently after middle age.

People with insufficient levels of vitamin B_{12} may experience generalized symptoms of anemia, such as fatigue, pallor, headaches, and shortness of breath during physical exertion, in addition to symptoms more specific to B_{12} deficiency, including alternating bouts of constipation and diarrhea, weight loss, numbness and tingling in the hands and feet, burning of the tongue, poor balance, confusion, depression, and dementia. Undetected, advanced vitamin B_{12} deficiency may result in permanent nerve damage.

Adults should aim for 400 mcg of folate daily. Although the UL is 1,000 mg, people should be aware that getting more than 400 mcg could mask pernicious anemia in individuals with B_{12} deficiency. To avoid the risk of pernicious anemia, people who take multivitamins should also take a daily supplement containing 1,000 mcg (1 mg) of B_{12}.

Vitamin D

Unlike other vitamins and minerals, the body can manufacture vitamin D in response to small amounts of sunlight. Other sources of vitamin D include fortified dairy products and oily fish, such as mackerel, salmon, and sardines. Amounts of vitamin D in excess of the UL can cause nausea and vomiting, poor appetite, constipation, and weight loss. Megadoses of vitamin D can also lead to high blood calcium levels, which can cause mental changes and nausea and increase the risk of kidney stones.

Moreover, a 2004 study published in the *International Journal of Cancer* examined the rates of prostate cancer among nearly 200,000 Scandinavian, middle-aged men. Researchers found that men with both the lowest and the highest blood levels of vitamin D had an increased risk of prostate cancer. Previously, it had been thought that only low serum levels of vitamin D posed a risk, leading some scientists to believe vitamin D supplementation would reduce the risk of prostate can-

cer. In this study, however, researchers speculated that taking vitamin D supplements for a long period of time might increase the risk of prostate cancer. This conflicting information highlights the fact that doctors and researchers don't yet know all of the potential adverse effects of vitamin and mineral supplementation.

Vitamin D deficiency is common in adults; those 50 and older should get 400 IU of vitamin D through food and/or supplements while those 70 and older require 600 IU. The UL for vitamin D is set at 2,000 IU.

Iron

Most men and postmenopausal women have adequate iron stores and do not need supplemental iron. But excess iron—from iron-enriched breads and cereals, supplements, or foods high in iron, such as liver and red meat—is a potential problem for people with hemochromatosis, an often undiagnosed genetic disorder that affects one of every 200 to 300 people. Hemochromatosis may lead to diabetes, liver disease, heart failure, and impotence.

Adults over 50 should aim to consume 8 mg of iron daily. As with all nutrients, the upper limit for iron is set at the amount that would likely pose no risk for most people (45 mg). However, even this amount is likely too much for people at risk for hemochromatosis.

carotene, and selenium), antioxidants alone, or placebo. Cholesterol levels improved more in patients on drug therapy alone. The improvement produced by drug therapy with antioxidants was similar to that of placebo. Make sure to check with your doctor before taking extra vitamin E if you are taking daily blood-thinning medications such as warfarin (Coumadin) or aspirin, because vitamin E also reduces the ability of the blood to clot.

Antioxidants and Cancer

Adequate intakes of beta-carotene and vitamin C have been linked to a reduced risk of cancers of the esophagus, stomach, pancreas, lung, colon, rectum, prostate, breast, ovaries, and cervix. Several studies found that people with low intakes or blood levels of antioxidants have a higher risk of these cancers.

In the studies that showed protective effects, fruits and vegetables—not supplements—were the key sources of these nutrients. In fact, clinical studies with supplements have proven how difficult it is to distinguish between the effect of a food and the effect of one of its many specific components. At best, such studies have produced disappointing results, and a few have even raised the possibility that high doses of a single antioxidant may be harmful. For example, the Physicians' Health Study found that beta-carotene supplements provided no protection against cancer, and two other studies found that beta-carotene supplements increase the incidence of lung cancer in smokers. In none of the three studies did beta-carotene supplements protect against CHD.

Some researchers hypothesize that the large amounts of beta-carotene in the supplements increased lung cancer incidence in these studies because the beta-carotene blocked the absorption of other carotenoids that are protective. This possibility underscores the potential dangers of overloading with one particular nutrient by taking large doses of supplements. Such studies should not stop people from eating foods that supply beta-carotene, which is only one of hundreds of carotenoids in foods. It is virtually impossible to get too much of any particular nutrient from foods alone.

Other carotenoids are also emerging as possibly protective against cancer and other disorders. For example, studies have suggested that tomatoes and tomato-based products (such as tomato sauce, tomato juice, and ketchup) are linked to a reduced risk of cancer, particularly prostate cancer. Tomatoes are a leading source of lycopene, the carotenoid that gives tomatoes their red color.

More studies are needed to firmly establish whether lycopene, alone or in combination with other dietary components, actually reduces prostate cancer risk. In the meantime, it is reasonable for men to consume tomato-based products and other foods with lycopene on a regular basis. The greatest protective effect of tomatoes appears to come from cooked tomato products, such as sauce, since cooking concentrates the lycopene content and increases its absorption. Watermelon is another good source of lycopene.

Selenium is a mineral that has been associated with a reduced risk of developing various cancers. Selenium acts indirectly as an antioxidant; it is an essential component of certain enzymes that inactivate free radicals. Research indicates that people with a high intake of this mineral, and those who live in areas where the selenium content of the soil is high, have a lower risk of lung, colon, and other cancers. Selenium is found in Brazil nuts, sunflower seeds, fish, turkey, wheat germ and other grains, fruits, and vegetables. The amount of selenium in plant foods depends on the amount of the mineral in the soil where the food is grown. Preliminary studies suggest that selenium supplements may help reduce cancer incidence, but further research is necessary.

Antioxidants and Other Disorders

A diet rich in carotenoids, especially lutein and zeaxanthin, has been linked to a reduced risk of developing macular degeneration, an age-related visual disorder that reduces central vision. The retina (the light-sensitive portion of the eye that receives and transmits visual impulses to the brain via the optic nerve) is rich in lutein and zeaxanthin, and studies suggest that these carotenoids protect the macula—the most sensitive portion of the retina—from damaging ultraviolet rays.

In October 2001, researchers from the Age-Related Eye Disease Study (AREDS) reported in the *Archives of Ophthalmology* that taking a combination of antioxidant vitamins and zinc reduced the rate of progression of age-related macular degeneration (AMD) in some people. The AREDS researchers studied 3,640 people, age 55 to 80, who had no AMD, early AMD in one or both eyes, intermediate AMD in one or both eyes, or advanced AMD in one eye. Neither antioxidants nor zinc, alone or in combination, reduced the risk of developing AMD in people without the disease or slowed its progression in those with early AMD. However, people with intermediate AMD or advanced AMD in one eye who took both antioxidants and zinc reduced their risk of progression to more advanced AMD by about 25%; in addition, these individuals lowered their risk of vision loss from AMD by 19%.

Because the supplements that were used in the AREDS study contain larger dosages of vitamins and minerals than those present in a normal diet or a typical vitamin tablet, you should check with your primary care physician before starting to take any supplements. This caution applies especially to people receiving treatment for diabetes, heart disease, or cancer. In addition, the AREDS supplements may interfere with over-the-counter or prescription medications or interact with other dietary supplements or herbal preparations.

Finally, vitamin E may help to improve the immune system and

memory in older people. One study found that extremely high doses of vitamin E—2,000 IU per day—slowed the progression of
Alzheimer's disease (although no improvement in symptoms was
noted in the patients). These possible effects are promising, but
more research is needed. Make sure to check with your doctor
before taking extra vitamin E if you are taking daily blood-thinning
medications such as warfarin (Coumadin) or aspirin, because vitamin E, too, reduces the ability of the blood to clot.

Recommendations for Antioxidant Intake
**1. Get most of your antioxidants from fruits and vegetables, not
supplements.** A diet containing five to nine servings of fruits and
vegetables per day can easily provide an adequate amount of vitamin
C, beta-carotene, other carotenoids, dietary fiber, and phytochemicals, as well as other vitamins and minerals. It's possible that the beneficial effect of antioxidants only occurs when they are consumed in
combination with each other or with other substances, known and
not known, in plant foods. Furthermore, the long-term effects of
high-dose antioxidants are unknown and may include increased
lung cancer risk in smokers; high-dose zinc can interfere with some
medications and may produce gastrointestinal side effects.

**2. Focus on dark green vegetables and orange, red, and yellow
fruits and vegetables.** Fruits and vegetables of these colors are the
most nutritious. They provide substantial amounts of antioxidants
and vitamin C, as well as other beneficial nutrients.

**3. Be sure to get the RDA for vitamin C: 75 mg for women and
90 mg for men.** These amounts are easily obtained through diet.
The vitamin chart on pages 20–21 lists some common dietary
sources.

4. Don't take selenium supplements. The difference between an
adequate and a toxic dose of selenium is quite small. People concerned that they are not getting enough selenium might consider a
multivitamin-mineral supplement that contains no more than the
RDA for selenium (55 mcg).

PHYTOCHEMICALS

Fruits, vegetables, and other plant foods may protect against disease.
From anthocyanins (the red pigment in strawberries and cherries)
to allylic sulfides (which are responsible for the pungent flavor of
garlic and onions), plant foods contain a plethora of chemical compounds that give them color and flavor and even protect them from

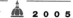

insects. These compounds, termed phytochemicals, may be responsible for part of the disease-preventing effect of fruits and vegetables.

Phytochemicals have no traditional nutritive value—that is, they are not vitamins or minerals—but they may have positive effects on the body over the long term. These effects include inhibiting tumor formation, producing an anticoagulant effect, blocking the cancer-promoting effect of certain hormones, and lowering cholesterol levels.

As noted in the antioxidant section (see pages 31–36), studies exploring the effects of supplements (other than possibly vitamin E) have failed to show that a high intake of isolated nutrients reduces the risk of disease. These observations leave open the possibility that other substances in plant foods, namely phytochemicals, may be important in disease prevention, either on their own or in combination with the antioxidants. A 2003 report in the *American Journal of Clinical Nutrition* lends support to this theory. The researchers provided several examples showing that fruits and vegetables offer superior health benefits over dietary supplements. For instance, 128 of 156 studies found that people who eat a diet rich in fruits and vegetables had half the risk of most types of cancer as people who ate a diet low in fruits and vegetables. By contrast, supplements of the single phytochemical beta-carotene (present in green and yellow fruits and vegetables) did not protect against cancer in several studies. The researchers concluded that phytochemicals and other bioactive substances present in fruits and vegetables work together to protect against cancer and other diseases.

Phytochemicals are found in a wide variety of plant foods, and indeed many different phytochemicals are often present in a single food—for example, more than 170 have been identified in oranges. The vast number of compounds in fruits, vegetables, grains, and legumes makes it nearly impossible for supplements to substitute for a healthy diet. While the beneficial effects, if any, of phytochemicals have yet to be proven, the following show some promise for disease prevention.

Allylic sulfides. Found in onions and garlic, these substances may enhance immune function, help the body to excrete cancer-causing compounds, and interfere with the development of tumors.

Flavonoids. These compounds function as antioxidants. They may be involved in several actions, including extending the life of vitamin C, inhibiting tumor development, preventing the oxidation of LDL cholesterol, and controlling inflammation. Various flavonoids are found in a host of fruits and vegetables, as well as in red wine, red and purple grape juice, and green and black tea.

Pumping Iron

Just about everyone over 50 can benefit from lifting weights.

Regular strength training is an important part of an exercise program. Unlike aerobic exercise, which raises the heart and breathing rate and improves cardiovascular fitness, the goal of strength training (also called resistance training and muscle conditioning) is to build muscle mass.

Evidence of the health benefits of strength training is so overwhelming that the American College of Sports Medicine (ACSM) recommends strength training for virtually everyone over 50.

Strength Training and Body Composition
Muscle mass declines dramatically after middle age—by approximately 15% per decade beginning at age 60 and even more rapidly after age 80. This decline in muscle mass, known as sarcopenia, leads to a corresponding reduction in strength. Reduced strength can make it difficult to carry out daily tasks like lifting groceries or

climbing stairs. Fortunately, strength training can help prevent or reverse age-related muscle loss, helping people maintain their independence as they get older.

Because muscle burns more calories than fat, even at rest, loss of muscle mass can also lead to weight gain unless you compensate by exercising more or eating less. The remedy is to increase muscle mass, which will speed up your metabolism. In fact, every pound of muscle you add burns up to 50 more calories a day, even when you are not exercising. That's why strength training is an important part of a weight loss program. In addition, because dieting is typically associated with a decline in muscle mass, strength training can help dieters preserve muscle and ensure that pounds they shed are fat.

Additional Benefits
In addition to aiding in weight loss, numerous studies have demonstrated

the advantages strength training offers people with obesity-related diseases, such as diabetes, coronary heart disease, and osteoarthritis.

Diabetes. Studies show that adults with type 2 diabetes who participate in strength training improve their glucose tolerance, insulin sensitivity, and glycemic control. Part of this improvement is caused by an increase in muscle mass because muscle tissue is the primary site for glucose disposal.

In fact, one recent study of middle-aged men and women with type 2 diabetes and poor glycemic control found that strength-training sessions three times a week increased muscle mass, improved glycemic control, and reduced systolic blood pressure (the higher number in a blood pressure reading) among participants. Moreover, study subjects who participated in strength training had reduced abdominal fat, increased muscle strength, and less need for

Indoles, isothiocyanates, and sulforaphane. In 1992, researchers at Johns Hopkins found that broccoli, kale, brussels sprouts, and other members of the cabbage family (also known as cruciferous vegetables) contain a potent substance—sulforaphane—that stimulates cells to produce cancer-fighting enzymes. Since then, indoles and isothiocyanates, also present in cruciferous vegetables, have been found to act in a similar manner.

Phenolic acids. Ellagic acid, ferulic acid, and other phenolic acids may prevent damage to DNA. They are found in strawberries, raspberries, tomatoes, citrus fruits, whole grains, and nuts.

Phytoestrogens. Phytoestrogens are plant substances that are converted to estrogen-like compounds by bacteria in the intestine. They are present in many common foods, especially soybeans and soy products such as tofu and soy milk. Lignans and isoflavones are examples of phytoestrogens. Researchers believe that these compounds may protect against hormone-dependent cancers of the breast, uterus, and prostate by blocking the actions of certain hor-

their diabetes medications compared with a control group that did not participate in strength training. The exercise group also became more active outside of their exercise sessions compared with the control group.

Coronary heart disease. A strength-training program is also recommended for the prevention of cardiovascular disease and as part of a cardiac rehabilitation program because building muscle mass can modify a number of risk factors for coronary heart disease. For example, evidence suggests that strength training is as effective as aerobic exercise in increasing high-density lipoprotein (HDL) cholesterol and lowering low-density lipoprotein (LDL) cholesterol and diastolic blood pressure (the lower number in a blood pressure reading) levels in healthy adults and low-risk men with heart disease. Though more research is needed on women, there is every reason to believe that they would also benefit from a strength-training program.

Osteoarthritis. Strength training is also often recommended for people with osteoarthritis. Although working out with weights can't reverse arthritic changes, the practice can help alleviate pain by improving range of motion and strengthening the muscles that surround arthritic joints.

Recommendations

Most experts agree that twice weekly sessions of 8 to 10 exercises will benefit nearly all adults, including the elderly. Usually, exercises are performed using free weights or machines, though the ACSM prefers machines for beginners. Exercise machines stabilize your body so they don't require as much balance as lifting free weights. Machines also assist you through the proper range of motion for each exercise so there is less chance that you will perform an exercise incorrectly.

Aim to work out each of the following muscle groups at each session: the chest, shoulders, arms,

back, abdomen, and legs. Another option is to exercise certain muscle groups one day and other muscle groups on another day. Do not exercise the same muscle groups two days in a row because your muscles need time, preferably 48 hours, to rest.

Choose weights that are sufficiently heavy so that you can perform the exercise at least 8 times, but no more than 15 times. And as your strength improves, continue choosing heavier weights that will help build your muscle strength.

Of course, always check with your doctor before you begin a strength-training program (weight lifting may not be safe for certain people, such as those with high blood pressure). You may also want to enlist the help of a trainer (preferably someone certified by the American College of Sports Medicine or the American Council on Exercise) for at least a few sessions. The trainer can develop an appropriate series of exercises and help orient you to the equipment.

mones that stimulate tumor growth. However, one 2004 study published in the *American Journal of Clinical Nutrition* did not lend support to this theory. The study involved over 15,0000 Dutch women between 49 and 70 years old. After evaluating the isoflavone content in their diets, researchers determined that those with the highest daily isoflavone levels did not have a significant difference in breast cancer risk compared to those with the lowest daily isoflavone levels.

Some reports also suggest that women who eat a lot of soy products have fewer hot flashes associated with menopause.

Soy products may also lower blood cholesterol levels. In a meta-analysis of 38 studies where soy protein replaced animal protein in people's diets, eating an average of 47 g of soy protein per day lowered levels of total cholesterol by about 9%, LDL cholesterol by 13%, and triglycerides by 11%. Evidence of the cholesterol-lowering effects of soy products is so convincing that the U.S. Food and Drug Administration permits food manufacturers to tout the heart-healthy benefits of soy on products that contain at least 6.25 g of soy protein.

According to the FDA, four daily servings of such products can lower levels of LDL cholesterol by up to 10%. It is not known whether soy products lower cholesterol levels simply by replacing saturated fats with unsaturated fats (soybeans derive 38% of their calories from fat, mostly unsaturated) or from the isoflavones in soybeans.

Saponins. These sugar-like compounds have an antibacterial effect. Saponins may strengthen the immune system, prevent microbial and fungal infections, and fight viruses. They are found in potatoes, tomatoes, legumes, oats, and spinach.

Recommendations for Phytochemical Intake

1. Follow a plant-based diet. Eat five to nine servings of fruits and vegetables and at least six servings of grain products each day, and consume legumes several times a week. Vary the choices to get a wide range of phytochemicals, but focus on dark green vegetables, red and orange fruits and vegetables, and whole grains.

2. Season foods with herbs and spices. Such seasonings also contain phytochemicals. Try using garlic, shallots, ginger, basil, oregano, parsley, rosemary, cumin, curry powder, cayenne pepper, red chili pepper, and cinnamon, to name a few.

3. Incorporate soy products. Tofu, soy protein, soy milk, soy flour, soy butter, and edamame (edible green soybeans) are all examples. Tofu and other soy products are mild tasting and pick up the flavor of the foods they are cooked with. Tofu can be stir-fried with vegetables or added to soups. Soy flour can substitute for up to one quarter of the total flour in baking recipes, and soy butter can be spread on bread in place of peanut butter.

ALCOHOL

The role of alcohol in a healthy diet is confusing. While moderate alcohol consumption has some undeniable health benefits, alcohol also adds extra calories, interferes with the action of many medications and, when consumed in excess over a long period of time, can cause some types of heart disease and raise blood pressure. Fatty liver and cirrhosis are major consequences of alcohol abuse. In addition, alcohol is a leading cause of car accidents.

Studies in both men and women have shown that having one to two alcoholic drinks per day is associated with a 30% to 60% reduction in the risk of developing CHD and also helps protect against ischemic stroke (the type caused by a blood clot in an atherosclerotic carotid or cerebral artery). Just how alcohol prevents CHD and strokes is a subject of much scientific debate, but it is generally accepted that about half of the risk reduction comes from an increase in HDL cholesterol levels. The rest of the protection may be due to alcohol's ability to reduce clot formation in the coronary and cerebral arteries.

For women, however, there is a downside to moderate drinking. Daily consumption of even small amounts of alcohol appears to increase the chances of breast cancer. Studies have shown a 30% to 60% rise in breast cancer risk for women who have one or two alcoholic drinks per day. The risk increases steeply—some studies show it more than doubles—as alcohol consumption rises to three or more drinks per day. Recent alcohol consumption appears to have a greater impact on risk than alcohol consumption early in life.

A report from the Iowa Women's Health Study, involving over 41,000 women, found that the effect of alcohol on breast cancer risk was limited to women taking estrogen replacement therapy (ERT). This result was not confirmed by other studies; however, one study found that in postmenopausal women on ERT, drinking alcohol tripled blood levels of estradiol, a form of estrogen, and estrogen has been shown to promote breast cancer. The researchers who conducted this study speculated that the combination of ERT and alcohol may increase the risk of breast cancer more than either one alone.

Recommendations for Alcohol Consumption

1. If you don't currently drink alcohol, don't start. Experts do not recommend that teetotalers begin drinking alcohol, but instead should take other steps to reduce their risk of CHD.

2. Men who drink should limit themselves to one to two alcoholic drinks per day. This amount of alcohol is enough to reduce CHD risk. However, it may impact the ability to drive and operate other machinery. (A drink is defined as 12 oz. of beer, 5 oz. of wine, or 1.5 oz. of 80-proof spirits.)

3. Women who drink but have no CHD risk factors should limit alcohol to fewer than seven drinks per week. Having a few drinks per week probably does not increase the odds of getting breast cancer, but it is not known whether this amount of alcohol can prevent CHD.

4. Women who drink and have CHD (or an increased risk of CHD) should have no more than one drink per day. For a woman at risk for CHD, the benefits of moderate alcohol consumption may outweigh the risks. However, keep in mind that there are many ways to reduce CHD risk but few known ways to reduce the risk of breast cancer.

5. The type of alcoholic drink does not matter. Some studies have emphasized the protective effect of red wine in reducing CHD risk, but most experts agree that wine (red or white), beer, or spirits all have the same effect.

6. Remember that heavy alcohol consumption is a health risk. Heavy drinking (more than two alcoholic drinks per day) can cause a variety of life-threatening diseases, including hypertension, stroke, cardiomyopathy (an enlargement of the heart), and cirrhosis.

7. Certain people should avoid alcohol altogether. They include people with hypertriglyceridemia, pancreatitis, liver disease, porphyria, uncontrolled hypertension, and heart failure. Anyone with a past or current problem with alcohol should not drink. And of course, anyone who will be driving should abstain from alcohol.

ENHANCED FOODS

As part of an effort to ensure that people eat well, and to help with disease prevention, several areas of food research are devoted to improving the types of foods we eat. These foods include ones that have been enriched or fortified with the addition of healthy components, as well as foods that have been genetically modified to provide certain nutrients. The concept of using food as a way to prevent disease is not new. Beginning in the 1920s, iodine was added to salt to prevent goiters; later, milk was fortified with vitamin D to prevent rickets.

Enriched food. An enriched food contains nutrients that are added to increase the amount originally present or to replace nutrients lost during processing. An example is white rice that is enriched with B vitamins and iron that were lost during processing.

Fortified food. Foods that have been fortified have had vitamins and/or minerals added to them; they are marketed to promote health and prevent disease. The added nutrients were not present in the original food or were present in lower amounts. Such foods include folic acid-fortified wheat products, orange juice fortified with calcium, and vitamin D–fortified milk.

Functional food. Although the U.S. Food and Drug Administration (FDA) has made no legal definition of functional foods (see www.cfsan.fda.gov/label.html), many groups use this term to refer to foods with specific health benefits that go beyond traditional nutritional effects. Because there is no uniform definition, the term can be applied in different ways. It is sometimes used to refer only to enhanced foods, such as enriched and fortified foods, and sometimes the term refers to natural foods with probable benefits. An example is the tomato as a source of lycopene.

Nutraceuticals. Pharmaceutical companies have also started to manufacture functional foods that are intended to have drug-like effects. Broadly known as nutraceuticals, these functional foods rack up billions of dollars in sales. Fruit juice and iced tea with added herbs like ginkgo biloba are examples of nutraceuticals. Experts predict that nutraceuticals could be one of the biggest growth areas in food production. The incredible increase in the number of nutraceuticals on the market in the past few years does not indicate that their health claims have been substantiated. There is little evidence that these products are beneficial, and many of the ingredients used in nutraceuticals have not been tested in clinical trials.

Genetically modified food. Genetic modification of food is another food science initiative, which introduces new genes into crops to improve their health benefits or make them hardier. However, genetic modification of food crops has been the subject of a great deal of controversy; critics argue that the unpredictable consequences of genetic modifications may have a serious impact on the ecosystem. (For more on genetic modification of food, see the feature on pages 44–45.)

ORGANIC FOODS

More Americans are turning to organic foods out of a concern for the environment as well as a desire to minimize their exposure to certain chemicals in their food. As a result, the market for organic foods is thriving. Over the past decade, consumer demand for organic foods has increased 20% or more each year in the United States. The Food Marketing Institute estimates that approximately 40% of all U.S. shoppers have purchased at least one organic product. A diverse array of organic goods—from produce to frozen foods—is readily available to consumers, and the popularity of organic foods is expected to continue.

A national definition of the term "organic" was established in 2002 by the federal government. This definition encompasses a set of standards that governs the production, labeling, and marketing of organic foods. In order to be called organic, a food must be produced without the use of bioengineered foods, herbicides, irradiation, pesticides, synthetic fertilizers, or sewage sludge. Organic livestock must be raised on 100% organic feed, and antibiotics and growth hormones are prohibited. To find out if a food is organic,

Tweaking a Food's Genes

Genetic science can produce less-expensive, better-tasting, more nutritious crops—but are there downsides?

Traditional plant breeding has led to hardier varieties of apples, uniformly hued corn, and hybrid foods such as the nectarine (a cross between a peach and a plum). But now there's a new way to alter a plant's genetic makeup: genetic engineering.

Also referred to as bioengineering or transgenic technology, genetic engineering involves isolating a desirable gene, such as one for drought tolerance, and inserting it into a plant. Usually the gene is taken from a plant, but nonplant sources can also be used. The goal is to immediately and predictably produce a desired characteristic or weed out an undesirable one.

The U.S. Food and Drug Administration (FDA) has approved more than 50 genetically engineered foods. The most prevalent genetically engineered crops in the United States are soybeans, corn, and cotton, all of which can be altered to resist common herbicides used to kill weeds. Although few genetically engineered whole fruits and vegetables are available in the produce aisle of your local supermarket, an estimated 75% of processed foods contain at least some genetically engineered ingredients.

Potential Benefits
Helping crops cope with environmental stressors is a major benefit of genetic engineering. Traditionally, insects and weather (for example, early frosts or droughts) can have a huge impact on crop yield. But genetically engineered crops are altered to be pest resistant or otherwise better able to cope with environmental damage. These crops use fewer pesticides and may require fewer environmental resources, like water and fertilizer.

Some genetically engineered food may have nutritional advantages over conventional foods. For instance, food companies are manufacturing soybean oil with a higher heart-healthy omega-3 content and potatoes that absorb less fat during frying. In addition, scientists are working to produce less allergenic versions of foods that many people can't eat, such as peanuts and wheat.

Food is also being altered to make it more stable for transport or give it a longer shelf-life. A genetically altered tomato made its debut to the public in 1994; this vine-ripened tomato does not rot as rapidly as its traditional counterpart, resulting in a better-quality product after shipping.

Other areas under investigation include edible vaccines and plants that have disease-fighting properties.

Safety Concerns
One major concern regarding genetically engineered food is the potential to release new allergens into the food supply. For example, a life-threatening allergen might be transferred into foods that an allergic person has always been able to eat safely.

Another possible risk to human health involves the use of antibiotic resistance marker genes in genetically engineered foods. Scientists use these marker genes to help determine whether modification of the desired

check the label for a "USDA Certified Organic" seal. (USDA stands for U.S. Department of Agriculture.)

While all organic foods carry the basic seal of approval, labels identifying foods as organic differ according to the quantity of organic ingredients the food contains:

- "100% organic" means the food contains only organically produced raw or processed ingredients, with the exception of water and salt.
- "Organic" indicates that 95% of the ingredients are organically produced and the remaining 5% are from the USDA–approved national list.
- "Made with organic ingredients" denotes that at least 70% of the ingredients in the product are organic. For more information on organic food labels and regulations, visit the USDA's

characteristic was successful. However, some researchers worry that human consumption of foods using this technology could contribute to the growing problem of antibiotic-resistant strains of bacteria.

There are also several environmental concerns regarding the use of genetically engineered food. For example, a common insecticide derived from the bacterium *Bacillus thuringiensis* (Bt) is widely used in creating transgenic crops. Some scientists believe there is the potential for insects to overcome pesticides in resistant crops and that the widespread use of Bt in transgenic crops will render the spray form less useful on traditional crops.

There is also the potential threat to other nontarget organisms that feed on pest-resistant crops. One landmark study found that Monarch butterflies that fed on Bt corn pollen had high mortality rates. However, many experts dismissed these findings since Monarch butterflies don't typically feed on corn pollen. Though additional research is needed, most studies have not found a harmful effect on nontarget organisms.

Another environmental concern is the possibility of generating hardier weeds that are resistant to herbicides, though this risk also needs further investigation.

Finally, opponents of genetic engineering fear that herbicide- and pest-resistant crops may have an impact further down the food chain. For instance, a reduction in weeds or pests may affect the population of organisms that feed on them. Therefore, long-term studies are needed to determine the effect of such crops on the ecosystem.

Regulation of Genetically Engineered Foods

Bioengineered food has been studied and tested for safety worldwide. In the United States, three government agencies regulate genetically engineered foods: the FDA, the Environmental Protection Agency (EPA), and the United States Department of Agriculture (USDA). These three agencies help ensure that genetically engineered foods are safe for human consumption, animal consumption, and the environment. Internationally, Codex Alimentarius Commission, a branch of the World Health Organization and the Food and Agriculture

> ### Produce Codes Decoded
> Have you ever wondered about the stickers on your fruits and vegetables? It turns out that not only does the sticker help the cashier figure out how much to charge you, it also lets you know how the item was grown. A four-digit code means that the item was conventionally grown, a five-digit code starting with the number nine means that the food was organically grown, and a five-digit code starting with the number eight means that the food was genetically engineered.

Organization of the United Nations, oversees safety guidelines of bioengineered foods.

Along with these agencies, the National Academy of Sciences (NAS), the Government Accounting Office, and the Organization of Economic Cooperation and Development agree that to date, there is no evidence that genetically engineered foods are unsafe for humans or animals to eat.

National Organic Program Web site at www.ams.usda.gov/nop.

Currently, there is no scientific evidence that organic foods are safer, better in quality, or more nutritious than conventional foods. In addition, although many consumers perceive organic foods as healthier than conventional foods, a USDA Certified Organic seal does not signify freshness, enhanced taste, or superior quality or nutritional content. Nor does organic guarantee a food is pesticide free: Up to 5% pesticide residues are permitted in organic foods.

FOOD SAFETY

U.S. consumers have one of the safest supplies of food in the world, but the increasing global exchange of food has recently highlighted the risk of foodborne diseases and suggests the need for an international agreement on standards for food production. In any case, research continues on ways to prevent food contamination.

The National Animal and Disease Center is developing several faster and more advanced tests to identify foodborne pathogens, and the USDA and FDA are supporting a "farm-to-table" approach to eliminate and control foodborne toxins at all steps along the chain of food production and consumption. One recent advance uses antibodies that bind to toxins produced by bacteria and fungi (molds) to measure the content of the organisms in foods. Referred to as ELISA (enzyme-linked immunosorbent assay), these highly sensitive tests can identify trace amounts of a toxin and take less time than traditional disease-detection strategies. ELISA test kits to detect bacterial toxins in food are currently in development for use by farmers.

Other strategies to fight foodborne bacteria are evolving from developments in genetic therapy and molecular biology. For example, scientists found that inactivating a gene called DAM can disarm the ability of a strain of Salmonella to cause disease. These approaches to detection and prevention, combined with proper food preparation and refrigeration techniques, should help to further improve the safety of our food supply.

Weight Control

In addition to adopting good overall nutritional habits, one of the most important ways to preserve good health is to control your weight. Rates of overweight and obesity are higher than ever, according to the Centers for Disease Control and Prevention, which estimates that more than 6 in 10 American adults are overweight or obese. By shedding pounds, overweight people can reduce their risk of type 2 diabetes, high blood pressure, and coronary heart disease (CHD). Losing weight may lower levels of low-density lipoprotein (LDL) cholesterol, which is often referred to as "bad" cholesterol. Losing weight can also lower levels of triglycerides and even increase high-density lipoprotein (HDL) cholesterol, referred to as "good" cholesterol. In addition, weight loss can help reduce the risk of osteoarthritis and gallstones.

In theory, weight control is a simple matter of balancing energy intake (the calories supplied by food) with energy output (the calories expended by physical activity and metabolism). To lose weight, you need to expend more energy than you take in. In practice, how-

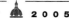

ever, the task is clearly not that simple. Obesity—the medical term for excessive amounts of body fat—is a chronic condition, like hypertension or diabetes. While the basic principle of energy balance remains true, several mechanisms—genetic, metabolic, and environmental—control how much you eat and how your body uses and stores energy.

Even if some of the components involved in weight regulation are beyond your control, environmental factors have a significant impact. By manipulating these factors to your advantage, you can successfully lose weight and keep it off.

METABOLISM

A certain amount of calories are needed to supply the energy required for metabolism and everyday activities. When more calories are consumed than are needed, these extra calories are stored primarily as fat—whether the calories come from fat, carbohydrates, or proteins, though dietary fat is converted into body fat most efficiently.

During digestion, enzymes in the small intestine break down carbohydrates into simple sugars like glucose, proteins into amino acids, and triglycerides (dietary fat) into fatty acids and glycerol. Simple sugars and amino acids are rapidly absorbed from the small intestine into the bloodstream. The liver converts other sugars, like fructose and lactose, into glucose, which is used as a source of energy. Amino acids can be used as an energy source but serve mainly as building blocks for body proteins. Fatty acids combine with bile salts to form tiny droplets that promote their entry into cells in the intestinal wall, where they are again formed into triglycerides. The triglycerides are packaged into transport lipoproteins called chylomicrons, which carry the triglycerides to the adipose tissue (fat) for storage of any triglycerides not immediately used to provide energy.

Any excess carbohydrates and protein not immediately used for energy are converted to glycogen and triglycerides in the liver. These triglycerides are transported from the liver on another lipoprotein (very–low-density lipoprotein) for storage in various parts of the body in individual adipose tissue cells, located just beneath the skin or around the intestines.

To store more fat, the body either creates more fat cells (a process called hyperplasia, which generally occurs only in childhood-onset obesity, during pregnancy, or with rapid weight gain in adults) or enlarges existing fat cells (hypertrophy, the primary way that adults increase their adipose tissue). If faced with a shortage of

NEW RESEARCH

Increasing Portion Sizes May Contribute to Obesity

Portion sizes have increased in the United States over the last few decades, at the same time that obesity rates have risen. What role might larger portion sizes of common foods play in the obesity epidemic?

To address this question, scientists served 75 young adults varying portion sizes of a deli-style sandwich to see whether subjects would consume more food when offered larger portion sizes. Each person was given a different-sized sandwich (6, 8, 10, and 12 inches long) for lunch once a week for four weeks. Most subjects indicated they were still hungry after eating the 6-inch sandwich, so a comparison was made between hunger levels after being served the 8- and 12-inch sandwiches.

Researchers found that women consumed 12% more calories and men consumed 23% more calories when served the 12-inch sandwich compared with the 8-inch sandwich. However, there was no significant difference between ratings of hunger and fullness after each of these test meals.

The authors conclude that these findings "indicate that consumers respond to increases in portion size by eating more." They note that over time, consuming extra calories by eating larger portion sizes could contribute to obesity.

JOURNAL OF THE AMERICAN DIETETIC ASSOCIATION
Volume 104, page 367
March 2004

calories—as when a person diets—the body uses the fat stored in these cells as a source of energy. Unfortunately, once fat cells are formed they can shrink, but they are not eliminated.

FACTORS THAT AFFECT BODY WEIGHT

Controllable factors—such as a high-calorie diet, inappropriate psychological responses to food, and a lack of exercise—play a critical role in the development of obesity. But research has confirmed that more is involved than just a lack of willpower or a sedentary lifestyle.

Risk Factors That Cannot Be Changed

Although these factors are beyond your control, their impact on weight can be modified by changes in diet and physical activity.

Heredity. Studies show that 80% of children born to two obese parents will themselves become obese, compared with 14% of children born to normal-weight parents. Research on identical twins shows similarly high rates of inheritance. However, studies comparing the weights of adoptees with the weights of their biological and adopted parents indicate that genetic factors are responsible for only about one third of the variance in weight, a figure experts believe is more accurate. Heredity seems to influence the number of fat cells in the body, how much and where fat is stored, and the resting metabolic rate. About 80% of obese children become obese adults, though only 20% of obese adults were obese as children.

A number of genes appear to be responsible for the regulation of body weight. A major advance occurred in 1994 when researchers at Rockefeller University discovered that mutations in a gene—termed the obesity (ob) gene—in one strain of mice prevented them from producing leptin, a hormone normally manufactured by adipose tissue cells and released into the bloodstream to inform the brain about the body's level of fat stores. When this communication system works correctly, the hypothalamic area of the brain responds to leptin by reducing appetite and speeding up metabolism to maintain a normal level of body fat. Because mice with the mutated ob gene did not produce leptin, their brains continued to prompt the storage of fat and they became obese. When leptin was injected into these obese mice, they quickly lost weight through a combination of decreased food intake and increased activity.

Mice who had no mutation but had simply been overfed lost some weight with leptin injections, but they lost much less weight than the leptin-lacking mice. A second strain of obese mice (db)

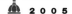

Poor Diet: A Top Cause of Preventable Death

A supersized diet of French fries, soft drinks, and other high-calorie, nutrient-poor foods—combined with a lack of physical activity—is taking its toll on Americans. In fact, poor diet and physical inactivity may soon overtake tobacco as the leading cause of death in the United States.

Researchers from the Centers for Disease Control and Prevention (CDC) analyzed data from between 1990 and 2000 to determine how certain risk factors (such as tobacco, alcohol use, poor diet, and physical inactivity) have become the nation's leading killers. The researchers termed these risk factors "actual" causes of death because they underlie the leading causes of mortality in the United States, such as heart disease, cancer, and stroke.

According to the study results, published in the *Journal of the American Medical Association* in 2004, poor diet and physical inactivity were responsible for approximately 400,000 deaths in 2000, topped only by tobacco use. Poor diet and physical inactivity also represented the most significant increase in actual cause of deaths from 1990 to 2000.

Actual Causes of Death in the United States in 1990 and 2000

Actual Cause	No (%) in 1990	No (%) in 2000
Tobacco	400,000 (19)	435,000 (18.1)
Poor diet and physical inactivity	300,000 (14)	400,000 (16.6)
Alcohol consumption	100,000 (5)	85,000 (3.5)
Microbial agents	90,000 (4)	75,000 (3.1)
Toxic agents	60,000 (3)	55,000 (2.3)
Motor vehicle	25,000 (1)	43,000 (1.8)
Firearms	35,000 (2)	29,000 (1.2)
Sexual behavior	30,000 (1)	20,000 (0.8)
Illicit drug use	20,000 (<1)	17,000 (0.7)
Total	**1,060,000 (50)**	**1,159,000 (48.2)**

Source: *Journal of the American Medical Association,* March 10, 2004, p. 1240.

The CDC researchers note that most deaths from poor eating habits and lack of exercise are related to being overweight or obese, though a small percentage of deaths are due to poor nutritional status and inactivity among normal-weight people. Because rates of overweight and obesity in the United States continue to climb, CDC researchers speculate that poor diet and physical inactivity will soon become the number-one actual cause of death.

An accompanying editorial states that because the leading causes of death are largely preventable, better public policy initiatives are necessary to promote lifestyle changes.

had high leptin levels but did not respond to leptin because of a mutation in the gene for the leptin receptor in the hypothalamus (the site in the brain that normally receives the leptin message). Unraveling the links between leptin and weight may lead to the development of more effective drugs for weight loss.

Metabolism. This is the process that extracts and utilizes energy (measured in calories) from food. Even at rest, energy is needed for many functions, such as respiration, heart contractions, and cell repair and growth. The amount of energy used for these basic functions while a person is awake and at rest is known as the resting metabolic rate (RMR), which accounts for about 70% of energy utilization each day (although this percentage is lower in physically active individuals). RMR is affected by weight, age, and the ratio of lean tissue (muscle) to adipose tissue (fat), since muscle is metabolically more active than fat—that is, muscle utilizes more energy even at rest. RMR is also in part genetically determined.

Food intake itself generates energy expenditure because energy is needed to digest food, absorb nutrients, and store excess calories as body fat. This process—called the thermic effect of food, or thermogenesis—accounts for 10% to 15% of the body's total daily energy expenditure. Some research suggests that obese people require slightly less energy for thermogenesis, and so more of the calories they eat are stored as body fat rather than used to process food.

Whether or not obese people have an abnormally slow metabolism is a matter of controversy. Because it takes more energy to maintain a greater body mass, a person who weighs 200 lbs. has a higher RMR than one who weighs 150 lbs. In addition, a heavier person expends more calories than a leaner one for any given physical activity. But even when people of the same height, weight, age, sex, and lean body mass are compared, RMR may vary by 20% or more. Consequently, someone who would be predicted to use 1,200 calories through RMR may actually use anywhere from 1,080 to 1,320 calories. This variability could explain why two people who weigh the same may require different amounts of calories to maintain, lose, or gain weight.

Set point theory. According to this theory, each person has a predetermined level of body fat. How the body controls its fat stores is unknown, but the regulatory mechanism, sometimes called the adipostat, is probably located in the hypothalamus. (Other regions of the brain may also play a role.) The adipostat monitors body fat stores, possibly through the actions of leptin on its hypothalamic receptor, and works to maintain the prescribed level of fat, or set point, by adjusting appetite, physical activity, and RMR to conserve or expend energy. Thus, actions perceived to be voluntary, such as eating and physical activity, may be subtly controlled by the set point mechanism.

Factors That Can Be Changed
The following known factors are amenable to individual control.

Dietary intake. Eating more calories than you expend is an important cause of obesity. In fact, regardless of genetic predisposition or any other factors, you cannot gain weight without consuming more calories than you burn. Even small excesses in calorie intake—too small to measure accurately in the most rigorous study—can contribute to obesity over the long term. For example, a person who overeats by just 25 calories a day will consume 9,125 excess calories over the course of a year and so will gain 2.5 lbs. (a pound of body fat is equivalent to 3,500 calories). A woman weighing 125 lbs. who starts this pattern at age 20 would weigh 175 lbs. by the time she is 40.

To point to overeating as the cause of obesity is overly simplistic, however. It does not explain why one 125-lb. woman needs 1,800 calories a day to meet her body's energy needs and avoid losing weight, while another 125-lb. woman struggles to avoid gaining weight on 1,200 calories a day.

Numerous other factors contribute to weight gain, including RMR and physical activity. Nevertheless, obese people must be consuming more calories than required by their individual make-ups and activity levels; otherwise they would not store excess body fat. A reduction in calorie intake is essential for weight loss.

Physical activity. Variations in physical activity can have a tremendous impact on total daily energy expenditure. A sedentary person may burn just a few hundred calories above RMR while going about daily activities (performing household chores or walking to the mailbox, for example), whereas an athlete can burn an additional 3,000 calories each day through vigorous exercise. Regular exercise not only burns calories, but also builds lean muscle mass and raises RMR because muscle requires more energy for maintenance. A low level of activity may be the most important factor responsible for the high and rising rate of obesity in the United States.

Behavioral and psychological issues. Several psychological factors affect weight control. The message to eat often comes from external cues rather than hunger—noon means it's time for lunch, for example. Food and emotions are closely linked; many people use food for comfort or to release tension. Obese people often eat quickly, and eating too fast can lead to taking in more calories than are needed to satisfy hunger. The amount of exercise a person engages in is also shaped by habit and attitudes toward physical activity. Some studies suggest that lean people may expend more energy than obese people in ordinary activities, as well as during formal exercise. For example, lean people may walk around (rather than sit) while on the phone, or may take the stairs rather than an elevator or escalator.

Hormonal (endocrine) abnormalities. An underactive thyroid (hypothyroidism) is often a layperson's explanation for obesity, but even when present, hypothyroidism is rarely a primary cause. Other conditions that may affect weight include polycystic ovary disease; tumors of the pituitary or adrenal glands; an insufficient production of sex hormones; and insulin-producing tumors of the pan-

NEW RESEARCH

Modest Exercise Helps Prevents Weight Gain

Getting a modest amount of exercise—the equivalent of walking 30 minutes a day—prevents weight gain and promotes positive changes in body composition, according to results of a new study. The finding supports existing recommendations from the Centers for Disease Control and Prevention that adults get 30 minutes or more of moderate-intensity physical activity on most, preferably all, days of the week.

Researchers randomized 120 sedentary, middle-aged, overweight people to one of four groups: high amount/vigorous intensity exercise, low amount/vigorous intensity exercise, low amount/moderate intensity exercise, and no change (the control group). None of the study subjects changed their diets, so the outcomes on weight and body composition were related solely to exercise.

People in all three exercise groups lost weight and body fat and saw their waist size go down during the eight-month study period. By contrast, those in the control group gained weight. The high-amount exercisers experienced greater improvements than the low-amount exercisers, but the effect of exercise intensity (vigorous or moderate) was less clear.

The study authors conclude that "a modest amount of exercise can prevent weight gain with no changes in diet, and more exercise may lead to important weight loss in initially overweight individuals."

ARCHIVES OF INTERNAL MEDICINE
Volume 164, page 31
January 12, 2004

creas. Although they are uncommon, these disorders need to be ruled out by a thorough medical evaluation before determining the best course of action to achieve weight loss.

MEDICAL CONSEQUENCES OF OBESITY

Overweight and obesity are linked with an increased risk of life-threatening conditions, such as type 2 diabetes, stroke, CHD, and cancer. Studies show that mortality rates are substantially higher in obese adults, especially in those whose excess fat is stored in the abdomen rather than in the hips. In fact, abdominal obesity is particularly dangerous because it leads to resistance to the actions of insulin, the hormone that regulates blood glucose. Insulin resistance results in elevated blood levels of insulin, which is associated with high triglycerides, low HDL cholesterol, high blood pressure, and increased CHD risk, a constellation of conditions called metabolic syndrome. Almost one in four American adults has metabolic syndrome, which increases the risk of diabetes, coronary heart disease, and strokes.

A recent report in the *Journal of the American College of Cardiology* further clarified the link between obesity and insulin resistance. Researchers measured insulin sensitivity in 314 individuals free from diabetes and hypertension and determined that the likelihood of insulin resistance rose in tandem with a rising body mass index (BMI). However, the BMI alone did not predict insulin resistance: About 20% of those with the syndrome had a normal weight (BMI less than 25), and some obese individuals (a BMI over 30) were not insulin resistant, indicating that other factors also play a role. For any given level of obesity, however, insulin-resistant individuals are at significantly greater risk for developing coronary artery disease than those with normal insulin sensitivity. The study also found that the risk factors most strongly associated with insulin resistance were elevated triglyceride levels and low levels of HDL cholesterol.

Excess weight also increases the risk of gallbladder disease and places greater stress on the back, hips, and knees, which may aggravate arthritis. In addition, obesity can lead to mental anguish due to poor body image, social isolation, and social discrimination.

MEDICAL EVALUATION OF WEIGHT

Anyone who is over age 40 or has health problems should have a thorough medical evaluation prior to beginning a weight loss program. In addition, your physician may refer you to a nutritionist for an assessment of eating habits.

Medical History

The medical history will include the following:

Weight history. Your physician will determine how long you have been overweight, because obesity present since childhood may reflect a genetic predisposition and is often more difficult to treat than adult-onset obesity. Other questions may address dieting history: Have you tried a variety of diets? Is there a pattern of weight loss and gain (called weight cycling or "yo-yo" dieting)?

Medical history. Do you have any symptoms or history of obesity-related disorders (such as CHD, stroke, hypertension, cancer, or diabetes)? Are there any symptoms suggesting an endocrine cause of obesity, such as hypothyroidism?

Family history. Is obesity prevalent in your family? Is there a family history of any obesity-related disorders?

Medications. Drugs that can cause weight gain, increase appetite, or hinder weight loss include corticosteroids, progestins, tricyclic antidepressants, phenothiazines, lithium, sulfonylureas, thiazolidinediones, and insulin.

Depressive symptoms. Depression affects many overweight people, especially those who are severely obese. A thorough evaluation includes questions about mood to determine whether depression needs to be treated along with obesity.

Physical Examination

Blood pressure, height, weight, and waist circumference are measured. The physician will look for evidence of cardiovascular disease (diseases of the heart and blood vessels), osteoarthritis, and hypothyroidism or other hormonal conditions.

Obesity is often defined as weighing 20% or more above ideal body weight (which varies with height, age, and gender). This definition is somewhat misleading, however, since it is not the amount of excess weight, but the amount of excess adipose tissue—or body fat—that determines the threat to health. It is possible to be overweight without being obese, as in the case of a weight lifter who has built up muscle mass. Moreover, the distribution of body fat is an important predictor of health risk—fat stored in the abdominal area is more harmful than fat stored in the hips, thighs, and buttocks. The degree of obesity is also important; a mildly obese person is at less risk for developing obesity-related conditions than some-

NEW RESEARCH

Waist Circumference Valuable In Predicting Health Risk

Waist circumference may be more useful than body mass index (BMI) at predicting obesity-related health risk, according to the results of a recent study.

Researchers analyzed data from nearly 15,000 participants in the third National Health and Nutrition Examination Survey to determine the relationship among BMI, waist circumference, and the risk of health conditions such as high blood pressure, elevated blood cholesterol, and metabolic syndrome.

They classified individuals as either normal weight, overweight, or obese based on BMI, and looked at people's waist circumferences. They categorized waist circumferences as either normal or high; the cutoff was 40 inches for men and 35 inches for women.

BMI coupled with waist circumference category was a better indicator of health risk than BMI alone. However, when BMI was added to waist circumference values on a continuous scale the BMI did not contribute to the health risk. The authors conclude that waist circumference, not BMI, determines the health risk of obesity.

However, the author of an accompanying editorial cautions against replacing BMI with waist circumference because BMI is a well-established indicator of health status.

AMERICAN JOURNAL OF CLINICAL NUTRITION
Volume 79, pages 347 and 379
March 2004

one who is morbidly obese (a BMI of 40 or more).

In addition to height, age, and gender, a person's ideal weight depends on many factors, including body composition (the proportion of fat and muscle), body shape (where fat is deposited), and general health. The most accurate way to assess the degree of obesity is to measure the amount of body fat. Since this task is not easy to perform, doctors generally rely on surrogate measures, such as body mass index and waist circumference, or use height/weight tables.

The National Heart, Lung, and Blood Institute and the National Institute of Diabetes and Digestive and Kidney Diseases have issued guidelines on the identification, evaluation, and treatment of overweight and obesity. Body mass index and waist circumference were found to be most useful for determining the need for weight loss. The pros and cons of most methods of weight assessment are discussed below.

Height/weight tables. Height/weight tables are the most straightforward way to assess your weight, but there are drawbacks to relying solely on this method. The tables are not based on scientific calculations of ideal weight but instead are derived from height, weight, and mortality data of people seeking life insurance. Moreover, they do not take into account body composition.

Body mass index (BMI). As the result of the difficulty in directly measuring the amount of body fat and the drawbacks of using height/weight tables alone, researchers have turned to a measurement called body mass index to define obesity and its severity. BMI is a measurement of your weight as it relates to your height. BMI correlates strongly with the amount of body fat, though it does not measure it directly. Federal guidelines define overweight as a BMI from 25 to 29.9 and obesity as a BMI of 30 or greater. Morbid obesity is a BMI of 40 or greater. To calculate your BMI, multiply your weight (in pounds) by 703; divide the result by the square of your height (in inches).

Waist circumference. While BMI is a general assessment of body weight and disease risk, waist circumference provides an added and more specific measure of health risk because waist circumference indicates harmful abdominal fat. Research shows that the mortality rates and incidence of certain chronic diseases, such as diabetes and high blood pressure, are substantially higher in those with a disproportionate amount of body fat stored in the abdomen.

Fortunately, abdominal fat is often the first to go with weight loss. Typically, men are prone to fat deposition in the abdomen—developing what is commonly called a pot belly, beer belly, or apple shape—

Shopping for Home Exercise Equipment

Treadmills and other types of home exercise machines can be expensive investments. Make sure you get your money's worth.

Each year, Americans buy more than $5 billion worth of home exercise equipment, including treadmills, stationary bicycles, home gyms, free weights, and elliptical machines. It's no wonder, because home equipment can overcome almost every excuse for not working out. You can exercise at night or in bad weather, avoid long lines at the health club, squeeze in a session before you leave for work, and avoid boredom by reading, switching on the television, or listening to the radio.

Nonetheless, a large proportion of people who purchase home exercise machines stop using them. After all, like any type of exercise, establishing a regular home workout regimen requires planning, goal setting, and self-discipline. Therefore, investing in a home exercise machine calls for careful thought and research. Before buying any equipment, follow the steps below.

Check for quality. A good exercise machine feels sturdy (not wobbly) and provides continuous, smooth movement. In general, those made with lightweight sheet metal or with many plastic parts are not likely to be long-lasting. (One strategy for ensuring durability: Check the floor models at the store and see how they've stood up to wear.) Always be skeptical of advertising claims, and stick with reliable manufacturers. Both

Consumer Reports and *Consumers Digest* magazines publish periodic ratings of home exercise equipment, including brand names and prices.

Take time to try it out. Before deciding what type of machine to get, consider buying a temporary pass to a local health club. Try the various options and decide which you like best. Then, wear workout gear to the store, and test the various models for a few minutes each. Make sure the machine you choose feels comfortable and easy to use and that it's adjustable if more than one person will be using it. (Even if you're buying from a catalog, you should still try out your selected model at a store or health club.) It's crucial that very tall, short, or heavy individuals test machines before making a purchase, since they may not fit on some models.

Shop around. Prices vary from store to store, so it's best to call a number of places to find the best deal. Always stick to reputable sporting goods stores, catalogs, or Web sites. The salespeople should be knowledgeable and able to answer any questions you have on delivery, installation, and how to use the machines—even after the equipment is at home.

Find out the length and terms of the warranty. Select a machine

with at least a 90-day warranty. Some warranties guarantee only parts and not services; if possible, choose a model with a warranty that covers both, and make sure that service facilities are located nearby.

Consider price. Prices for home exercise equipment range from $40 for a set of free weights to over $3,000 for a treadmill. When it comes to electronic equipment, the cheapest versions may be flimsy, hard to use, and easily breakable, but the most expensive machines are not necessarily the best. You can often trim hundreds of dollars off your purchase by forgoing such high-tech options as heart rate monitors and video displays. In most cases, the best values are in the mid-price range. However, if used and maintained properly, exercise equipment is an investment that can last at least a decade. While discount stores are generally not a good idea, you might consider checking stores that specialize in used exercise equipment from reliable manufacturers.

Measure the machine's size. Before you purchase any type of exercise machine, measure its dimensions and make sure it will fit through your front door and sit comfortably in its allotted floor space.

whereas women tend to accumulate fat around the hips, buttocks, and thighs, a distribution called a pear shape. Some researchers believe that women are naturally programmed to store fat in the lower body for use as an energy reserve during pregnancy and breast feeding. However, women are not immune to accumulating abdominal fat, and weight tends to be stored in a pattern typical to a particular individual (in other words, once a pear, always a pear).

Even in people of normal weight, an increased waist circumference may be linked to an elevated health risk. (A normal waist circumference is less than 40 inches in men and less than 35 inches in women.) And in men and women who are overweight or obese, a large waist circumference increases the already elevated risk of disease. But people with a BMI of 35 or higher have a high risk of disease, regardless of their waist circumference.

Techniques for measuring body fat. Obesity is defined as fat stores exceeding 25% of total body weight for men or 30% for women. Direct measurement of the amount of body fat is the most accurate way to determine obesity-related health risk. A variety of methods can be used to estimate body fat, including underwater weighing (hydrodensitometry), dual-energy x-ray absorptiometry (DEXA), and bioelectrical impedance analysis (in which a small current of electricity is sent through the body). These techniques have the advantage of providing a more direct assessment of the proportion of total body weight that is fat. However, none of them is exact, some are expensive and not widely available, and all require trained personnel to administer them. Thus, they are not practical for general use.

Laboratory tests. Blood will be drawn to measure total and HDL cholesterol, triglycerides, liver function, and blood glucose to screen for some of the complications of obesity. If a thyroid abnormality is suspected, thyroid stimulating hormone (TSH) is often measured.

LIFESTYLE TREATMENTS FOR WEIGHT LOSS

Successful weight loss requires a three-pronged approach: changing behavior patterns, making dietary adjustments, and increasing physical activity. Culled from medical research, the following guidelines incorporate strategies employed by people who have lost weight and kept it off. Use them to construct a weight loss program on your own or as an adjunct to medical or surgical treatments.

Behavioral Modification
An ability to alter lifelong attitudes toward diet and exercise may ultimately be the key to successful weight management: You must be motivated enough to change habits not for a few weeks or months, but for a lifetime. The importance of this resolve cannot be underestimated.

The desire to lose weight must come from within. A person who wants to shed 20 lbs. to please a spouse is not likely to be as motivated, or as successful, as someone whose goal is to improve health or

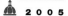
increase self-esteem. Choosing the right time to start a weight-loss program is also important. People under stress or pressure may not be able to devote the considerable attention and effort required to make lifestyle changes.

If you are motivated and ready to lose weight, the following guidelines will help.

1. Set realistic goals. Remember that weight tables give estimates of ideal weights; you can probably be healthy at weights above "ideal" if you have a nutritious diet and exercise. Instead of attempting to lose a specific number of pounds, make it your goal to adopt healthier eating and exercise habits. If you are obese and feel compelled to set a weight goal, losing 10% to 15% of your current body weight is a realistic objective. The good news is that evidence shows that weight loss of as little as 5% to 10% of body weight can significantly improve heart disease risk factors such as blood pressure and blood glucose. The safest rate of weight loss is 1/2 to 2 lbs. a week.

2. Seek support from family and friends. People who receive social support are more successful in changing their behaviors. Ask family and friends for help, whether this means keeping high-fat foods out of the house or relieving you of some chore so that you have time to exercise. It will be easier to stick to your new eating plan if everyone in the household eats the same types of foods. (A low-fat diet that includes plenty of fruits, vegetables, and grains will benefit your family's health even if they do not need to lose weight.) You may be more motivated to exercise if you work out with a friend or family member.

3. Make changes gradually. Trying to make many changes quickly can leave you feeling overwhelmed and frustrated. Instead, ease into exercise; do not overdo it. Incorporate low-fat eating in stages. For example, if you typically drink whole milk, switch to reduced-fat (2%) milk, then to low-fat (1%), and then to fat-free milk.

4. Eat slowly. Many people consume more calories than needed to satisfy their hunger because they eat too quickly. Since it takes about 20 minutes for the brain to recognize that the stomach is full, slowing down helps you feel satisfied on less food. Moreover, eating slowly allows you to better appreciate the flavors and textures of your food.

5. Eat three meals a day, plus snacks. Skipping meals is counterproductive, as is severely reducing food intake, since such strict changes are impossible to maintain and are ultimately unhealthy. In addition, eating the bulk of your calories at one sitting may impair metabolism. You will be more successful in the long run if you allow

NEW RESEARCH

**Boosting Fruit Consumption
May Prevent Weight Gain**

Eating more fruit and less fat may help reduce weight gain that often occurs over time, according to a recent Canadian study.

Nearly 250 adults filled out a food questionnaire and had their body weight recorded, once at baseline and again six years later. Although participants gained an average of 7 lbs. over the follow-up period, those who reduced their consumption of fat and boosted their intake of skim milk and fruit during that time gained less weight. The association between increased fruit intake and weight control was especially strong.

Interestingly, no association was found between weight control and increased vegetable consumption. Although an increase in vegetable consumption should help moderate calorie intake, it is possible that people add extra fat and calories (butter, oil, and cheese, for instance) to vegetable dishes, whereas fruit is usually eaten plain.

This study supports evidence that eating a low-fat diet can help control weight gain that commonly occurs over time, thereby helping to prevent or reduce obesity. Moreover, the authors suggest that dietary recommendations should focus on food groups, such as low-fat dairy and fruit, instead of nutrients, such as fat and carbohydrates.

AMERICAN JOURNAL OF
CLINICAL NUTRITION
Volume 80, page 29
July 2004

yourself to eat when you are hungry, eat enough nutritious low-fat food to satisfy that hunger, and spread your calorie intake over the course of the day.

6. Plan for exercise. Choose activities that are convenient and enjoyable for you to do on a regular basis, and then treat exercise like any other appointment—set a time and jot it down in your date book. Many people find it easier to exercise first thing in the morning, before the demands of the day interfere, but others find lunchtime or right after work more convenient.

7. Record your progress. Start a food diary and exercise log to keep track of your accomplishments. Keeping such detailed diaries may seem cumbersome, but they can help you stay motivated, and reviewing the entries can reveal any problem areas. In addition, the information can help facilitate treatment by your nutritionist or doctor.

8. Evaluate your relationship to food. Behavioral and emotional cues frequently trigger an inappropriate desire to eat. The most common cues are habit, stress, boredom, sadness, anxiety, loneliness, and the use of food as a reward. Many people also relate food to love or care and derive comfort from it. Although eating may appear to soothe uncomfortable feelings, its effect is temporary at best and ultimately does not solve any problems. In fact, it may distract you from focusing on the real issues.

9. Recall your accomplishments. Over your lifetime you have probably been successful in tackling many difficult tasks—quitting smoking, learning a new skill, or advancing in the workplace, for example. Reminding yourself of past achievements can help you feel more confident about making the changes that will lead to weight loss.

10. Don't try to be perfect. While losing weight requires significant changes in eating and exercise habits, not every high-calorie food must be banished forever, and you need not exercise vigorously every day.

Diet

To determine how many calories you should eat per day, first calculate the number of calories needed to maintain your current weight—roughly 15 calories per pound of body weight in a moderately active person (someone who gets at least 30 minutes of moderate to intense physical activity every day). A completely sedentary person may require just 12 calories per pound to maintain weight.

A pound of body fat contains 3,500 calories. To lose one to two pounds per week—a gradual and safe rate of weight loss—you must eat 500 to 1,000 fewer calories per day than what is needed to maintain your weight. (The calorie cutback need not be so severe if you also begin to exercise regularly.) Calorie intake should not drop below 1,200 per day in women or 1,500 per day in men (unless the diet is medically supervised and you are taking a vitamin/mineral supplement), since it would be difficult to get all the nutrients you need.

While reducing calorie intake is essential for losing weight, focusing on calories per se may leave people feeling hungry and frustrated unless the overall composition of the diet is also considered. Replacing dietary fat with complex carbohydrates automatically lowers calorie intake, while allowing a satisfying volume of food. For any given number of calories, you can eat a much larger amount of food on a low-fat diet than on a high-fat diet. The reason for this is simple: Gram for gram, fat contains more than twice as many calories as carbohydrates or protein: nine versus four calories. Fatty foods also contain less water and fiber—substances that help make a food more filling—than foods high in complex carbohydrates. But, all too often, people reduce their intake of fat and instead consume an equal or greater amount of calories in the form of simple carbohydrates.

There are other reasons to reduce the fat content of your diet. Some evidence suggests that a prolonged high-fat diet may trigger an upward adjustment in the body's set point. In addition, fewer calories are burned when dietary fat is converted into body fat than when carbohydrates or protein are converted into fat. Moreover, a low-fat diet can help to lower blood cholesterol levels and may reduce the risk of colon and prostate cancer.

Once you decide on an appropriate calorie intake, you need to determine the amount of total fat you should eat. Most experts now recommend that a diet should derive no more than 35% of its calories from fat (even when substituting monounsaturated for saturated fats). Most people should not reduce fat intake to less than 20% of calories, and the American Heart Association (AHA) cautions against cutting fat below 15% for certain groups of people (older adults, for example) owing to concerns over malnutrition and a possible negative effect on blood lipids. The following guidelines will help you adopt a low-fat, high-complex-carbohydrate diet.

1. **Eat mostly fruits, vegetables, legumes, and grains.** These foods are naturally low in fat and high in fiber. (Fiber provides bulk, which helps to fill you up without adding calories.)

2. **Do not add fat during cooking.** Avoid sautéing foods in butter

NEW RESEARCH

Big Portions of Calorie-dense Foods Boost Overall Calorie Intake

Eating large portions of high-calorie foods boosts calorie intake without making people feel extra full, according to a new study. Previous studies have focused on portion size or calorie density, but not both together.

The study involved serving breakfast, lunch, and dinner once a week for six weeks to 39 women. Breakfasts and dinners were standardized, but lunches varied in portion size and calorie density.

When the women were served the largest portion of the study lunch, they ate 20% more calories than when they were served the smallest portion. When they were given the calorie-dense lunch, they consumed 26% more calories than when they were given the less–calorie-dense version. And when they were served a lunch that combined large portion size and high calorie density, they consumed 56% more calories than when they were served a lunch that combined small portion size and low calorie density. Participants did not compensate for the additional calories consumed at lunch by eating fewer calories at dinner, and did not feel more or less full when they ate the different lunches.

The researchers concluded that "large portions of foods with a high energy density may facilitate the overconsumption of energy."

AMERICAN JOURNAL OF CLINICAL NUTRITION
Volume 79, page 962
June 2004

or oil. Use nonstick pans; coat them lightly with cooking spray if necessary, or try using broth, wine, fruit juice or even water for sautéing. Bake, broil, steam, or roast foods instead of frying them.

3. Choose lean cuts of meat and poultry. Meat and poultry are rich in nutrients and good sources of high-quality protein, but they can also contain a lot of fat. Top round, eye of round, and round are the leanest cuts of beef; tenderloin, top loin, and lean ham are the leanest pork cuts; and light-meat chicken and turkey are leaner than dark meat. Completely trim all external fat from meat before cooking. Do not eat poultry skin—it contains a lot of fat. But you can leave it on during roasting or baking to help keep the meat moist and tender; just be sure you do not cook the poultry with other ingredients, such as potatoes, that could absorb the fat released from the skin as it cooks. Limit portion sizes to 3 oz.—about the size of the palm of your hand or a deck of cards—and round out the meal with plenty of grains and vegetables.

4. Switch to low-fat or fat-free dairy products. Whole milk and cheeses can contain more fat than meat. For example, 1 oz. of cheddar has the same amount of fat as a 6-oz. chicken breast or a 3.5-oz. sirloin. But do not eliminate dairy products: They are an important source of calcium and protein. Moreover, a recent study published in the *Journal of Obesity Research* found that overweight adults on a reduced-calorie diet that included three to four daily servings of dairy products lost significantly more weight—notably in the abdominal region—than participants who just cut calories or reduced calories and took calcium supplements. Researchers suggest that the combination of nutrients in dairy products may speed up metabolism and improve the body's ability to burn fat.

5. Read food labels. The nutrition labels that are required on all packaged foods provide important information about their calorie and fat content, which makes it easy to compare brands. (For more on reading food labels, see the feature on pages 4–5.)

6. Experiment with reduced-fat, low-fat, and fat-free versions of foods. From fat-free milk to reduced-fat salad dressing and cream cheese, these foods can help you cut fat from your diet. Just because a food is low in fat does not mean you can eat unlimited quantities, however, since it can still provide a lot of calories. For example, some fat-free cakes and cookies contain as many—or more—calories than the regular versions because manufacturers add extra sugar to compensate for flavor lost when fat is removed.

7. Use fat substitutes judiciously. While fat substitutes definitely reduce the number of calories consumed from fat and saturated fat,

Exploring Diet Plans

Making sense of the claims of various diet programs and books can prove quite confusing at times. To help you sort through them, this chart examines some of the most common diet plans. Ones that offer quick results may work initially, but remember that the only proven way to maintain weight loss over the long run is to make permanent changes in dietary and exercise habits. Only follow a diet that can provide solid evidence of its benefits.

Diet Plan	Claims	Comments
Commercial weight loss companies (Weight Watchers; LA Weight Loss)	A high-carbohydrate, low-fat diet is best for weight loss. These plans provide advice on making healthy food choices and reducing calorie intake. They stress moderate weight loss (1 to 2 lbs. per week). Group or individual counseling sessions provide support and behavior modification techniques.	This approach is safe and effective. Because these programs emphasize gradual, healthy weight loss, they can be followed for a long time and lead to the permanent adoption of healthy diet and exercise modifications. As a result, weight loss should be maintained.
Fasting	Periodic fasting will help keep calorie intake low and aid in weight loss. Fasting also has the advantage of cleansing the body of toxins that can contribute to weight gain.	Starvation diets are rarely recommended, even for the severely obese. One-day fasts are unlikely to contribute to weight loss, and longer fasts deprive the body of nutrients. There's no evidence that fasting removes toxins from the body.
Fat-burning diets (Cabbage soup diet; grapefruit diet)	Certain foods can accelerate the body's ability to burn fat stores. Eating large quantities of these foods results in fast weight loss.	No food burns fat. If these diets work, it's usually because they are low in calories. In addition, the focus on one food makes these diets boring and nutritionally unbalanced.
Food-combining diets (Beverly Hills Diet; Suzanne Somers' Eat Great, Lose Weight)	Certain foods should not be eaten together (e.g., carbohydrates and protein; foods of varying textures; fruit at any time of day but morning) because they do not digest well, slow down metabolism, and produce toxins that prevent the elimination of waste.	There's no evidence to support food combining. All foods, even when eaten individually, are a combination of protein, fats, and carbohydrates. The food texture theory has no scientific basis. Fruit is nutritious at any time of day.
Insulin-resistance diets (The South Beach Diet; The Zone)	Consuming unrefined or low glycemic index carbohydrates or eating foods in proper protein-to-carbohydrate ratios will combat insulin resistance (a poor response to the actions of insulin that leads to overproduction of insulin), which otherwise prompts fat storage and makes weight loss difficult.	These diets combine the rationales of high-protein diets and food-combining diets, and are ineffective for the same reasons. There's no evidence that a diet high in complex carbohydrates increases appetite or causes the body to store more fat. Obese people are often insulin resistant, but obesity is the cause, rather than the result, of this condition.
Low-carbohydrate/ high-protein diet (Atkins diet; Protein Power)	Glucose (a primary source of body fuel) is usually derived from carbohydrates but can be formed from protein. This conversion requires extra energy that speeds fat breakdown and produces substances called ketones that suppress appetite.	High-protein diets are low-calorie diets. An initial rapid weight loss is mostly water, not fat. Even the small amount of carbohydrate in these diets is enough to prevent ketosis. A high-protein diet usually cannot be continued indefinitely; when eating returns to normal, weight may be regained. The high-fat content of high-protein diets may increase the risk of heart disease.
Meal-replacement drinks (Dyna-Trim; Slim-Fast)	A liquid shake (either prepackaged or made from powdered mix and milk) or candy-type bar replaces one or two meals a day, thus helping to cut calories. Shakes contain sugar, protein, fiber, vitamins, and minerals and about 200 calories each.	Hunger may not be satisfied by the shakes, and some individuals may add these drinks to their food intake rather than replace food. If the shake is used for two meals a day, calorie intake may be too low. Weight is usually regained when the product is no longer used.
Prepackaged meal plans (Jenny Craig; Nutri/System)	This approach teaches portion control by supplying the food. Counselors help set weight goals and provide information on exercise and behavioral techniques. In-house doctors may prescribe appetite suppressant drugs or supplements.	People lose weight because calorie intake is strictly controlled. Weight loss maintenance depends on how successful you are at making the transition from prepackaged meals to regular food. These plans are expensive to join, and the food and drugs must be purchased separately.

their impact on total caloric intake and body weight, as well as general health in the long term, is uncertain. And one fat substitute, olestra—used in some chips and crackers—inhibits the absorption of fat-soluble nutrients. Vitamins A, D, E, and K are added to products to offset this effect.

8. Watch out for hidden fats. It is easy to overlook the fat and calories contributed by toppings such as margarine, cream sauce, mayonnaise, salad dressings, peanut butter, sour cream, and cheese. Limit the amounts of these items; choose low-fat versions (such as nonfat sour cream or mayonnaise); or find substitutes (for example, tomato sauce instead of cream sauce on pasta).

9. Consider the calories in beverages. Although regular soda, fruit juices, and alcoholic beverages are fat free, they contain a significant number of calories. And, with the exception of citrus juices, these beverages are not a good source of vitamins and minerals. Choose calorie-free beverages—water or seltzer, and moderate amounts of coffee and tea—most of the time.

10. Control portion sizes. While fat consumption has dropped in the past 20 years in the United States, serving sizes and total calorie consumption have increased. Americans tend to eat large portions of food, especially meat, and what many people think of as a serving is usually more than the amount that is listed in nutrition tables and on food labels. And according to recent research, almost all foods and beverages currently sold in the United States are excessive in size and dramatically increased from their original sizes. Hamburgers, french fries, and sodas are two to five times larger than they used to be in the 1970s. In addition, the average American eats about four restaurant meals a week; and studies show that most restaurant meals are not only larger in size than home-cooked meals, but they are also higher in calories, saturated fat, and sodium while being lower in fiber and calcium. Experts estimate that the dramatic increase in portion sizes could add 15 lbs. a year to the average person. And although the public has been educated about the fat in their diets, they may not realize that consuming the extra calories in super-sized portions can lead to weight gain.

To get an accurate picture of the amount of food you normally eat, serve yourself a typical portion, then use a measuring cup, measuring spoons, or a food scale to measure or weigh the food. Next, try serving yourself a smaller portion. You can dispense with weighing and measuring food once you become accustomed to estimating smaller portion sizes.

Fad Diets

Popular "fad" diets have been around for decades and are appealing because they often result in rapid, seemingly effortless weight loss, at least initially, owing to loss of body water. Recently, there has been an enormous resurgence in the popularity of low-carbohydrate (high-protein) diets. Such diets promote the same basic idea that was put forth in the 1960s: Eat high-protein foods (such as meat and eggs) and restrict carbohydrate-rich foods (such as potatoes, pasta, fruits, and certain vegetables).

Once relegated to the realm of quackery, these diets are being advocated because carbohydrates are thought to promote weight gain by increasing the body's production of insulin, which speeds up the conversion of food to body fat. Proponents of low-carbohydrate diets also claim that carbohydrates are less filling than other foods, causing people to consume more calories in an effort to satisfy their hunger. Furthermore, in some people, a low-fat, high-carbohydrate diet has been shown to raise triglyceride levels and lower HDL cholesterol levels—two components of metabolic syndrome, which can lead to heart disease and type 2 diabetes.

High-protein diets are being taken seriously by some researchers who recognize that people can lose weight on them. In two recent studies, overweight and obese people who were placed on a very-low-carbohydrate diet program lost more weight over a 6 month period than subjects who followed a low-fat, reduced-calorie diet. However, in both studies, there was no significant difference between the two groups in the amount of weight lost after a year of following the diets. These findings indicate that a low-carbohydrate diet produces more weight loss initially, but that dieters following a low-fat diet continue to lose weight over time. More research is needed to determine whether dieters following a low-carbohydrate diet can maintain weight loss or continue to lose weight over a longer period of time.

Furthermore, the long-term effects of a low-carbohydrate diet, which is typically heavy on meat and saturated fat, on coronary heart disease are currently unknown. In the aforementioned studies, subjects following the low-carbohydrate diet experienced a reduction in triglyceride levels and an increase in HDL levels, however these lipid changes are typical following weight loss. Future studies need to evaluate lipid changes on a long-term basis.

Moreover, the long-term effects of a diet devoid of antioxidants and phytochemicals from fruits, vegetables, and whole grains, which are very restricted on a low-carbohydrate meal plan, are unknown.

NEW RESEARCH

Study Ties Sugary Soft Drinks to Weight Gain, Diabetes

High consumption of sugar-sweetened beverages leads to weight gain and increases the risk of developing type 2 diabetes, according to a large new study.

The study included more than 90,000 women in the Nurses Health Study who filled out questionnaires on health and diet every two years from 1991 to 1999. Those who reported increasing their intake of sugar-sweetened soft drinks or fruit punch over a four-year period from one drink or less each week to one drink or more a day gained the most weight. The women who reduced their consumption gained the least weight. On average, women who boosted their soft-drink intake increased their overall energy intake by 358 calories per day; those who cut soft drink consumption consumed 319 fewer calories daily.

After adjusting for other diabetes risk factors, the researchers found women who drank one or more sugar-sweetened soft drinks a day were nearly twice as likely to develop diabetes as those who had less than one soft drink each month.

Sugar-sweetened drinks promote weight gain because they are less likely to make one feel full than solid foods, the researchers say, adding that soft drinks may also promote the development of diabetes because they contain large amounts of quickly absorbed carbohydrates.

JOURNAL OF THE AMERICAN MEDICAL ASSOCIATION
Volume 292, page 927
August 25, 2004

Weighing in on the South Beach Diet

Should you try the diet of the moment? Here's what you need to know.

You don't have to live in the tony Miami neighborhood of South Beach to have heard about—and possibly even tried—*The South Beach Diet*. At press time, it had been on the *New York Times* list of hardcover advice books for over a year and was among the top 10 books sold at amazon.com. But will this diet plan work for you?

The Plan
In a nutshell, the South Beach Diet is a reduced-carbohydrate meal plan that is set up in three phases. Phase one, the most restrictive part of the plan, lasts two weeks and is designed to initiate rapid weight loss by eliminating most carbohydrates. Dieters are advised to go back on phase one of the plan if they experience any setbacks to weight loss, such as overindulging on vacation. Phase two allows dieters to resume eating more carbohydrates, including whole-grain breads and cereals, sweet potatoes, and most fruits, but limits the portion sizes of these foods. Phase three is the maintenance part of the meal plan and is supposed to be more flexible than the other two phases.

The premise behind the book is that overindulging in highly processed carbohydrates raises blood glucose levels, leading to surges in insulin that cause sugar cravings and weight gain. By limiting such carbohydrates, the South Beach Diet suggests that you can virtually eliminate cravings for carbohydrates and sugary sweets and lose weight—all without counting calories or measuring portion sizes.

Moreover, *The South Beach Diet* author, Dr. Agatston, claims that avoiding so-called "bad" carbohydrates such as white bread and sweets in favor of "good" ones like whole grains, fruits, and vegetables will cure insulin resistance and decrease your risk of coronary heart disease.

A Day in South Beach
Despite Dr. Agatston's claims that the South Beach Diet "is distinguished by the absence of calorie counts; percentage counts of fats, carbs, and proteins; or even rules about portion size," the meal plans involve recipes that state portion sizes, and portions are given for most items on the menus. Therefore, the diet ultimately restricts calories. In fact, a calorie analysis of day one on phases one and two reveals that a dieter who strictly follows the meal plan would consume about 1,500 calories a day; day one on phase three—the maintenance part of the plan—contains about 2,000 calories. Certainly, many people could lose weight on 1,500 calories a day and maintain their weight consuming 2,000 calories daily.

Weight and Insulin Resistance
The South Beach Diet suggests that overeating highly processed carbohydrates contributes to weight gain, which leads to insulin resistance. Though it's true that overeating causes weight gain, the source of the calo-

Also, several specific health concerns are associated with a diet that places such a heavy emphasis on the consumption of protein and the restriction of carbohydrate. Consuming too much protein places extra stress on the liver and kidneys because they have to metabolize and excrete more than normal amounts of waste products. Kidney stones can be caused or aggravated by the high uric acid levels created by high-protein foods. And for those who have diabetes or kidney disease, high-protein diets may speed the progression of kidney disease, even if the diet is followed for a short time. Furthermore, some studies suggest that eating too much protein causes excessive calcium loss, which can contribute to osteoporosis.

Restricting carbohydrate intake is unhealthy as well. Drastically reducing carbohydrate consumption increases the metabolism of fatty acids and causes ketosis. This condition results when excessive amounts of acidic substances known as ketone bodies are released

ries doesn't affect weight. In addition, the book oversimplifies the cause of insulin resistance. Although obesity is the more common cause of insulin resistance, genetic factors, diet, physical inactivity, cigarette smoking, and older age contribute to it as well.

The Glycemic Index

The meal plan in the South Beach Diet is built upon the glycemic index, which assigns each food a number based on the rise in blood glucose it produces during the first two hours after eating it compared with the rise triggered by eating an equivalent amount of carbohydrate in a standard food like white bread.

The South Beach Diet, particularly in phase one, calls for choosing foods that are low on the glycemic index in order to avoid surges in blood glucose. Moreover, the book suggests that consuming low-glycemic foods will curb your appetite and minimize your cravings. Again, this message is oversimplified.

According to the American Diabetes Association, the amount of carbohydrate consumed each day is more important in determining the body's glucose response than the glycemic index of each individual carbohydrate.

Another problem with the index is that it is not practical. The index rates only single foods eaten individually, which is not the way people eat. Finally, the effect of a food on blood glucose levels can vary depending on whether a particular food is cooked or eaten in combination with other foods, and what the blood glucose level is before eating.

Furthermore, many nutritious foods, such as corn, carrots, and raisins, are high on the glycemic index, but that doesn't mean they need to be eliminated in order to stay healthy or lose weight.

The Bottom Line

Despite some of the problems mentioned above, the South Beach Diet does make some good points, particularly about choosing whole-grain foods, fruits, and vegetables over processed carbohydrates. As Agatston points out, these foods contain fiber, which helps fill you up, but are naturally low in fat and calories. Furthermore, unlike Atkins—who revolu-tionized low-carbohydrate eating—Agatston focuses on lean meats, low-fat dairy products, and healthy sources of fats, like nuts and fish.

Though phase one severely limits carbohydrates, several clinical trials over the last few years have shown that dieters lose weight on these types of meal plans—at least in the short term. It's possible that the initial weight loss will motivate people to remain on the diet. Phase two calls for filling up on lots of fruits and vegetables, along with lean meats and reduced fat cheeses, which is a reasonable way to lose weight. Finally, phase three allows for more carbohydrates from fruits and whole grains, which is a sensible plan for maintenance. Though South Beach does allow low-fat dairy products, most adults could benefit from additional servings to meet their calcium needs.

Of course, in addition to reducing calories, exercise is a critical component of a weight loss program. Though Dr. Agatston claims the South Beach Diet doesn't depend on exercise in order to work, studies have shown that people who exercise are more likely to maintain their weight loss.

into the bloodstream. Ketosis can be dangerous for people with known or unrecognized heart disease, diabetes, or kidney problems. In addition, restricting carbohydrates can lead to vitamin and mineral deficiencies. Healthful, carbohydrate-rich foods, such as whole grains, fruits, and vegetables, provide essential nutrients as well as fiber and phytochemicals that work together to help prevent disease and promote good health. In fact, one of the basic underlying problems with most high-protein diets is their failure to promote a balanced diet and to teach long-term healthful eating habits.

High-protein, low-carbohydrate diets are best used selectively on a short-term basis, if at all, and under medical supervision. The many limitations and risks associated with high-protein diets raise important questions about their long-term safety and effectiveness. In fact, a 2003 advisory by the American College of Preventive Medicine (ACPM) states that there is currently little evidence to support the safety and effectiveness of popular diets that promote unlimited consumption of protein or fat.

Exercise

Exercise is a valuable element in a weight loss program, but exercise alone results in only modest weight loss, and at a slower rate than calorie restriction. Although combining exercise with diet results in greater loss of weight and body fat than dieting alone, exercising is especially important for maintaining weight loss. And adding exercise to calorie restriction makes the dietary changes easier because they need not be as drastic. It is easy to see why this is so. To lose one pound per week requires a deficit of about 500 calories a day. By adding a half hour of moderate to vigorous exercise per day (enough to burn 250 calories), you reduce the dietary restriction to a more manageable 250 calories per day.

Engage in activities that involve stretching, balance, aerobic exercise, and strength training. These types of exercises are generally recommended for older adults because they are low impact and help maintain overall strength, lower blood pressure, and strengthen bones. Exercise—especially strength training—helps to maintain muscle mass. Because muscle weighs more than fat, a person who does strength training exercises and cuts calories may lose less weight than one who only cuts calories, but the exerciser will lose more body fat.

The effect of exercise is cumulative. For example, while it takes about nine hours of walking at a normal pace for a 175-lb. person to burn 3,500 calories, the walking does not have to be completed all at once. You can achieve the same calorie deficit if you walk for half an hour each day for 18 days, or 45 minutes for 12 days, or an hour for 9 days. Even if you alternate days or work out only three times a week, you can still burn the same number of calories. You can even break up an exercise session into segments: For example, a 10-minute walk in the morning, 10 minutes at lunch, and 10 minutes in the evening still burn the same number of calories as a single 30-minute walk.

If you choose to use a personal trainer (either at home or at a gym), seek out a trainer who is properly qualified. A qualified trainer will have a bachelor's degree in exercise science or physical education or will be certified by the American College of Sports Medicine or the National Strength and Conditioning Association.

Start an exercise program gradually. Trying to do too much, too soon may lead to muscle strain and soreness, or even injury, which

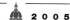

may lead to the desire to quit. Instead, increase your exercise level in the stages described below. It is also important to make sure your exercise plan suits your lifestyle. For example, if you are a morning person, select that time to exercise.

And remember that sedentary people over the age of 50 should consult their doctor before starting any vigorous exercise program.

1. Increase your amount of everyday physical activity. Look for ways to add physical activity into your lifestyle: For example, walk rather than drive, or take the stairs rather than an elevator or escalator. When doing errands or shopping, park some distance from your destination and walk the rest of the way.

2. Add a formal walking program. Walking is appealing because it can be done anywhere, requires no special equipment (other than a supportive pair of shoes), and almost anyone can do it. Set your own pace: You expend approximately the same number of calories during an hour of slow walking as in half an hour of brisk walking. Start by walking for half an hour, three times a week. Once you become comfortable with this level of activity, walk for the same length of time five days a week. Next, gradually increase the duration of your walking to 40 minutes, then 50 minutes, and ultimately 1 hour. As you become more physically fit, you will be able to walk faster and go farther—and thus burn more calories in a given period of time.

3. Vary your activities. If you enjoy walking, make it the foundation of your exercise program. To prevent boredom, and also to work different muscle groups, choose other activities to substitute for walking on some days. Good choices include aerobic dance classes, bicycling, line dancing, or swimming. The most important rule, however, is to engage in activities that are enjoyable and convenient to do regularly.

4. Start a weight-training program. Working a muscle against resistance increases muscle size and strength. Because muscle takes up about 20% less space than fat, building muscle results in a leaner physique. In addition, having more muscle increases your metabolism, because it requires more energy to maintain muscle than fat tissue. (For more on strength training, see the feature on pages 38–39.)

MEDICAL AND SURGICAL TREATMENTS FOR OBESITY

Because the following treatments can be demanding for the patient and carry the risk of adverse side effects, they are appropriate only for people who are severely obese—especially those with, or at

NEW RESEARCH

Large, Low-Calorie Salads Can Aid in Weight Loss

Eating a large salad before a main course can decrease the overall amount of calories a person consumes, a new study finds, but only if the salad is low in calories.

The study included 42 healthy women between the ages of 19 and 45 who ate one study lunch a week. The lunch was served with no salad or started with a salad that was low, medium, or high in calorie density, depending on the type of salad dressing and cheese used. Small and large versions of each were tested, and participants were required to eat the entire salad. The main course of pasta was always the same, but participants weren't required to finish their serving.

Compared with no salad, eating a low-calorie salad decreased overall calorie intake at the meal—by 7% for the small version of this salad and 12% for the large. Eating a calorie-dense salad increased energy intake—by 8% for the small salad and 17% for the large.

The study authors conclude that eating less is not always the best strategy when it comes to weight loss.

They recommend that when dieters prepare salad as a first course, they use plenty of vegetables and keep the overall calorie count to about 100.

JOURNAL OF THE AMERICAN
DIETETIC ASSOCIATION
Volume 104, page 1570
October 2004

high risk for, medical conditions that may be improved with weight loss.

Very–Low-Calorie and Low-Calorie Diets

The term very–low-calorie diet (VLCD) is used to describe diets supplying fewer than 800 calories a day. Typically, patients must replace food with a powdered supplement that is combined with a noncaloric liquid (water or diet soda). To prevent deficiencies, the supplement is primarily made of high-quality protein derived from milk, eggs, or soy, along with a small amount of carbohydrates, minimal fat, and added vitamins and minerals. The high protein content of these diets is essential to help preserve muscle mass when calorie intake is so low. Recently, many centers modified their VLCD formulas to contain more calories. Studies have shown that weight loss is about as good on 800 as on 400 to 500 calories a day, and there are probably fewer risks. The term low-calorie diet (LCD) is used to describe diets that supply from at least 800 calories per day to slightly below the person's daily caloric expenditure. So for a person needing 2,000 calories per day, a VLCD is up to 799 calories and an LCD is 800 to 1,999 calories. (Although a program may be referred to as a low-calorie diet, or LCD, we will use VLCD to describe both types, except where the protocols differ.)

Typically lasting 12 to 16 weeks, VLCDs require close medical supervision and are usually administered by weight loss clinics or hospitals. Programs should include regular medical monitoring; behavioral counseling to help you adjust to the diet; and instruction for changing eating patterns once food is reintroduced. Programs may also provide classes and support groups; many place a great emphasis on exercise. Once the VLCD phase is completed, food is slowly reintroduced over 2 to 10 weeks. The cost of participation is around $2,000 to $3,000. Few insurance companies cover this cost. If they do, it is usually covered only if the program is used to help treat a complication of severe obesity.

VLCDs are appropriate for people with a BMI of 35 or higher who have been unable to lose weight with conventional diet and exercise. LCDs are appropriate for individuals with a BMI between 30 and 34.9, especially for those who have coexisting conditions, such as type 2 diabetes, hypertension, high triglycerides, low HDL cholesterol, sleep apnea, or osteoarthritis.

Contraindications to VLCDs include a recent heart attack or stroke, heart rhythm abnormalities (arrhythmias), angina, liver or kidney disease, or type 1 diabetes. However, insulin-treated, obese patients with type 2 diabetes can benefit from VLCDs. For people who can stay on them, VLCDs produce dramatic reductions in weight. On average, participants lose 2.5 to 4 lbs. per week, at a rate that tends to slow as the duration of the VLCD increases to months.

Adding exercise to the program may enhance weight loss. Within three weeks, VLCDs often help lower blood pressure and cholesterol and triglyceride levels. In addition, glycemic control also improves.

Despite the dramatic success possible with VLCDs, they are not a panacea. About 25% of people who start a VLCD cannot adhere to the strict regimen and drop out of the program. Most of those who do complete treatment regain large amounts of weight within a year or two, typically reaching pretreatment weight within five years. In this way, VLCDs are no different from other diets. Most people can stick with dietary restrictions for a limited period of time. VLCDs may be even easier to follow than low-calorie diets that contain real food, because predetermined meals and controlled portion sizes help you to resist temptations.

However, you must learn to overcome the eating and behavioral patterns that contributed to your obesity in the first place—and you ultimately must make daily food choices on your own. As a result, VLCD programs are worthless without detailed attention to long-term maintenance. In one study, patients participated in a VLCD program with intensive behavioral training that included instructions on self-monitoring of eating behavior, guidelines for increasing physical activity, and techniques for counteracting relapse. The behavioral training continued even after the VLCD was finished and the patients returned to eating food. In six months, the patients lost an average of 45 lbs. One year later, they had regained only an average of 5 lbs.

In general, VLCDs are safe when medically supervised. Early side effects of hunger, fatigue, and light-headedness usually subside within two weeks. People who cannot tolerate milk products may react to a dairy-based formula. Later on, dieters may note constipation and intolerance to cold, and the risk of gallstones is increased.

Medications

Whether the treatment of obesity requires medication is a decision that must be made on a case-by-case basis. Drug therapy was never intended to be anything but a last-choice option when no other treatment had worked. And today, the use of medications to help suppress appetite or otherwise alter the body's energy balance

NEW RESEARCH

Drugs Help Diabetics Lose Modest Amount of Weight

Three drugs prescribed for weight loss all seem to help diabetics shed some pounds, but whether the modest change on the scale makes a difference in long-term health is unclear, according to a recent review of 14 clinical trials. The review also leaves open the question of whether the drugs—weight-loss medications sibutramine (Meridia) and orlistat (Xenical), and the antidepressant fluoxetine (Prozac)—are safe in the long run.

Overall, the studies found that patients with type 2 diabetes lost an average of 6 to 13 lbs. after 6 to 12 months on one of the drugs. All three medications were deemed effective, but the weight loss was "modest," and the long-term effects on diabetics' weight and general health remain unclear. However, research suggests that dropping even a small amount of weight carries health benefits for the general public.

In addition to questions about effectiveness, the drugs' long-range safety is still uncertain, according to the researchers. Sibutramine caused heart palpitations, orlistat caused gastrointestinal upset, and fluoxetine caused tremor, sleepiness, and sweating in many of the studies. The authors say that further research is needed to see whether lifestyle changes add to the effectiveness of medication, and to monitor the rate of drug side effects.

ARCHIVES OF INTERNAL MEDICINE
Volume 164, page 1395
July 12, 2004

Understanding Over-the-counter Diet Aids

The vast array of weight loss products sold over the counter includes diet pills, diuretics, minerals, and herbal supplements and teas. Although diet pills are regulated by the U.S. Food and Drug Administration (FDA), diet supplements are not, leaving manufacturers free to determine doses and, possibly, make misleading claims regarding their effectiveness and how they work. Despite such claims, carefully controlled scientific studies in humans are rare and do no support the efficacy of supplements for reducing body weight. Moreover, the safety of these products is questionable because many of the diet aids contain numerous ingre-

Weight Loss Aid*	Claims
Chromium picolinate	Builds muscle mass and reduces body fat by enhancing the body's use of the hormone insulin.
Garcinia camogia (Hydroxycut)	Promotes weight loss by naturally suppressing appetite.
Conjugated Linoleic Acid (CLA)	Helps burn fat and build muscle.
Diuretics (Aqua-ban; Diurex)	Weight loss occurs because of increased urinary output, which removes water from the body.
Fiber supplements (Chitosan; glucomannan; guar gum; psyllium)	Fiber lessens appetite by enhancing feelings of fullness. Chitosan binds with fat to remove it from the intestine before it's absorbed.
Herbal weight loss teas (with ingredients such as guarana, kola nut, catechins, and senna)	The mix of natural herbs aids digestion, increases energy, and improves metabolism.
L-carnitine	A nutrient that burns fat, increases energy, and improves athletic performance.
Ephedrine/Ma huang	Suppresses appetite and accelerates burning of fat by increasing metabolism.

* Just a few of the many products containing these ingredients are named here. Read product labels carefully for mention of these ingredients.

remains a controversial area in obesity management. Drugs should be used only in people whose BMI exceeds 30, or exceeds 27 when accompanied by serious medical conditions that could be improved by weight loss. Anorectics—drugs that reduce appetite—do not magically melt away pounds: While they may make it easier to adhere to lifestyle changes, they do not eliminate the need to alter behavior permanently.

dients, and no one knows the long-term effects of a single ingredient—much less a combination of herbs. The benefits and possible dangers of these products will only be understood after more long-term, controlled studies are completed. In the meantime, the chart below should help you sort through the maze of some of the most common over-the-counter diet aids. Look for scientific proof of benefits before using any products. Bear in mind, however, that the best approach to weight loss is a commitment to a sensible diet and exercise program.

Comments

Although chromium—obtained from food—is needed in trace amounts for carbohydrate and fat metabolism and for protein synthesis, there are no data showing a meaningful benefit from supplement use..

Results of studies using *Garcinia cambogia* or its active ingredient, hydroxycitric acid, for weight loss have been mixed. Authors of a 2004 review on dietary supplements for weight loss published in the *American Journal of Clinical Nutrition* concluded that "the evidence for *G. cambogia* is not compelling."

Though small amounts of CLA, a fatty acid, are found naturally in dairy products and beef, studies involving CLA have used supplements that contain more CLA than people typically consume in their diet. Moreover, the few existing studies that have investigated CLA in humans have been short term and results have been contradictory. The long-term effects of CLA—both benefits and risks—are unknown.

Any weight lost from using diuretics is temporary and in the form of water, not body fat. Overuse of diuretics can cause dehydration and electrolyte imbalances that can promote abnormalities in cardiac rhythm.

Although high-fiber foods are filling and generally low in calories, fiber supplements do not have the same effect. They contain only small amounts of fiber—five pills of one brand supply about 2.5 g of fiber, the same amount as in an apple—and provide none of the satiety properties of high-fiber foods. There is no evidence to back up the claims about chitosan.

If these teas seem to increase energy, it's probably because they contain caffeine in the form of kola nut or guarana. There's no evidence that they enhance weight loss. Teas or supplements containing catechins such as epigallocatechin gallate (ECGC) do not produce meaningful weight loss. Teas with senna are powerful laxatives that can cause diarrhea, which may lead to dehydration and mineral imbalances.

There is currently no evidence to support the claim that L-carnitine enhances fat metabolism or improves athletic performance.

In 2004, the FDA prohibited the sale of dietary supplements containing ephedrine because recent studies confirmed that ephedrine raises blood pressure and is linked to heart attack and stroke. Consumers should carefully read labels of all over-the-counter weight loss products and avoid or discontinue using those that contain ephedrine.

For good results, drug therapy must be combined with extensive dietary, exercise, and behavior modifications. Anorectics are not effective for everyone. For example, people whose excessive eating is triggered by habits, stress, or emotions may benefit less from drugs that reduce appetite than those who eat because of hunger. If no weight is lost in the first week or two of use, the drug is unlikely to help and should be discontinued (consult your doctor first). Following are the types of drugs currently in use. The prescription drugs, together with side effects and contraindications, are discussed in the chart on pages 74–75.

Antidepressants. Although the FDA has not approved antidepressants for the treatment of obesity, patients taking the selective serotonin reuptake inhibitors (SSRIs) fluoxetine (Prozac) or sertraline (Zoloft) for depression often experience weight loss. Typically, doctors prescribe these drugs for weight loss if the patient is also depressed. SSRIs increase brain levels of serotonin, which produces feelings of fullness. Thus, some patients taking SSRIs feel less hungry, are less concerned with food, and are better able to control their appetites, though the effect may not last long.

Lipase inhibitor. Orlistat (Xenical) blocks the intestinal absorption of about 30% of dietary fat. Side effects—such as cramping, oily anal leakage, and explosive diarrhea—tend to be worse when patients eat greater quantities of fatty foods. These adverse effects discourage the consumption of such foods and contribute to the effectiveness of the drug. Because fat malabsorption associated with orlistat can lead to a loss of fat-soluble vitamins A, D, E and K in the stools, a multivitamin must be taken with this medication.

Noradrenergics. These drugs increase levels of norepinephrine (noradrenaline) in the brain. Norepinephrine reduces appetite by stimulating the central nervous system. On average, people taking a noradrenergic lose about 1/2 lb. more per week than those taking a placebo. A noradrenergic agent called phenylpropanolamine (PPA), present in several medicines and over-the-counter appetite suppressants such as Dexatrim, was recalled by the FDA in November 2000.

Serotonin/norepinephrine reuptake inhibitor. The drug sibutramine (Meridia) enhances both serotonin and norepinephrine levels in the brain. This action promotes feelings of fullness and thus reduces appetite. Studies show that patients who took sibutramine while on a reduced-calorie diet showed significant weight loss during the first six months of treatment. In addition, significant weight loss was maintained for one year. Because of the potential for adverse effects, such as increased blood pressure, sibutramine has come under increased scrutiny. Additional research is currently under way to evaluate the safety of this drug.

Dietary Supplements and Herbal Preparations

A wide variety of dietary supplements and herbal preparations has been heavily promoted for weight loss. A recent critical review of these products found no credible evidence for their safety or effec-

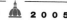

tiveness, with the possible exception of pills containing caffeine and ephedrine. National Institutes of Health guidelines do not recommend herbal preparations for weight loss. The botanical source of the ephedra in herbal weight-loss preparations is the Chinese herb Ma-huang, and its use has been associated with severe cardiovascular and neurological complications. Therefore, in 2004, the FDA banned all supplements containing ephedrine. (See the feature on pages 70–71 for more on dietary supplements for weight loss.)

The past decade has seen a dramatic increase in the marketing of dietary supplements purported to aid in weight loss. Despite the enormous popularity of these supplements, there is surprisingly little reliable information about their safety and effectiveness. While some weight-loss supplements may have components that could potentially promote weight loss, no well-designed studies in humans have proven the supplements effective. As for the safety of weight-loss supplements, there is limited information available, particularly regarding long-term use. In addition, little is known about the interactions of weight-loss supplements with prescription and other over-the-counter drugs.

The FDA requires product labels to be accurate, but this requirement is difficult to enforce because dietary supplements are exempt from the rigorous testing that is required for drugs and food additives. As a result, the amount of an active ingredient in a supplement often does not conform to the quantity listed on the label. Ingredients may be mislabeled or a supplement may contain harmful substances that are not listed on the label. A dietary supplement, however, can be investigated by the FDA if it appears to pose "a significant or unreasonable health risk" to the public.

Exaggerated and false claims are rampant in the advertisements for weight-loss products. They commonly promise that weight loss will require little sacrifice and will be fast, effortless, and safe. At the same time, the advertisements frequently contradict proven methods of successful weight loss—exercise and cutting calories. Rapid weight loss is unlikely and can be unsafe when using these products.

Bariatric Surgery

Each year, approximately 100,000 Americans undergo bariatric surgery for the treatment of severe obesity. Bariatric surgery is considered for morbidly obese people or for obese people with significant complications of obesity. Specifically, it is intended for people who either have a BMI of 40 or greater or are 100 pounds overweight

NEW RESEARCH

Long-Term Benefits of Weight-Loss Drug Unclear

A recent review concludes that sibutramine (Meridia) effectively promotes weight loss in obese adults. However, it is unclear whether the drug prevents or reduces risk factors for cardiovascular disease and diabetes— including elevated blood pressure, blood cholesterol, and blood glucose levels.

The report analyzed 29 trials lasting from 8 to 54 weeks that compared sibutramine with a placebo. Sibutramine produced significantly greater weight loss than a placebo among overweight and obese adults (average of 10 lbs. after one year) along with small improvements in triglyceride and HDL cholesterol levels. In addition, sibutramine improved blood glucose control somewhat in people with diabetes. However, sibutramine was also associated with a modest increase in both systolic and diastolic blood pressure and heart rate.

The researchers conclude that weight loss with sibutramine is associated with both positive and negative changes in risk factors for cardiovascular disease and diabetes. They write that these changes could potentially have "important long-term effects on cardiovascular disease risk that enhance, diminish, or reverse the health benefits that result from modest weight loss." Therefore, future studies need to evaluate the long-term risks and benefits of sibutramine.

ARCHIVES OF INTERNAL MEDICINE
Volume 164, page 994
May 10, 2004

Weight Loss Drugs 2005

Drug Type	Generic Name	Brand Name	Average Daily Dosage*	Average Retail Cost†
Noradrenergics	benzphetamine	Didrex	50 mg	50 mg: $40
	diethylpropion	Tenuate	75 mg	25 mg: $18 ($6)
	phendimetrazine	Bontril	35 mg	35 mg: $13 ($9)
	phentermine	Adipex-P	15 to 37.5 mg	37.5 mg: $54 ($38)
		Ionamin	15 to 30 mg	30 mg: $79
		Pro-Fast	15 to 37.5 mg	37.5 mg: $31
Serotonin/ norepinephrine reuptake inhibitor	sibutramine	Meridia	10 to 15 mg	10 mg: $90
Antidepressants	fluoxetine	Prozac	20 mg	10 mg: $117 ($36)
	sertraline	Zoloft	50 mg	25 mg: $77
	bupropion	Wellbutrin	150 to 200 mg	100 mg: $47 ($22)
Miscellaneous off-label uses of approved drugs	topiramate	Topamax	50 to 400 mg	100 mg: $122
	metformin	Glucophage	500 mg	500 mg: $25 ($13)
Lipase inhibitor	orlistat	Xenical	120 to 360 mg	120 mg: $48

* These dosages represent an average range for the treatment of obesity. The precise effective dosage varies from patient to patient and depends on many factors. Do not make any changes to your medication without consulting your doctor.

† Average price for 30 tablets or capsules (unless otherwise indicated) of the dosage strength listed. Actual price may vary. If a generic version is available, the cost is listed in parentheses. Sources: drugstore.com, eckerd.com, and walgreens.com.

and have been unable to lose weight through nonsurgical means. It may also be appropriate for people with a BMI between 35 and 40 who have serious obesity-related complications.

Bariatric surgery does not remove fat tissue by suction or excision; rather it usually involves reducing the size of the stomach. The three commonly used types of bariatric procedures are vertical banded gastroplasty, laparoscopic adjustable gastric banding, and gastric bypass. Most bariatric operations can be performed using

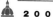
How They Work	Comments
Stimulate the central nervous system and suppress appetite by increasing norepinephrine (noradrenaline) levels in the brain.	Tolerance may develop after a few weeks, slowing the rate of weight loss, but abrupt cessation could cause fatigue and depression. Possible side effects include nervousness, restlessness, difficulty sleeping, irritability, diarrhea, dry mouth, rapid heartbeat, and hypertension. Noradrenergics should be taken with caution by those with mild hypertension and diabetes and not at all by those with arteriosclerosis, moderate to severe hypertension, glaucoma, overactive thyroid, anxiety, a history of drug abuse, or those taking MAO inhibitors. Alcohol should be avoided while taking noradrenergics.
Creates a feeling of fullness by blocking the reabsorption of serotonin and norepinephrine in the brain. May also increase metabolism.	Appears to cause about 5% weight loss over six months. May raise pulse and blood pressure, which should be monitored regularly. Patients with coronary heart disease or uncontrolled hypertension and those who have survived a stroke should not use this drug. Other possible side effects include dry mouth, insomnia, and constipation.
Fluoxetine and sertraline create a feeling of fullness by raising levels of serotonin in the brain. Bupropion raises levels of norepinephrine, serotonin, and dopamine.	Though approved by the U.S. Food and Drug Administration for depression, these drugs may (as a side effect) cause weight loss. Sometimes prescribed for obese people with depression. Possible side effects include insomnia and fatigue.
An antiseizure medicine that produces weight loss as a side effect. Mechanism unknown.	May cause central nervous system side effects, kidney stones, and acidosis.
Improves insulin sensitivity.	May cause bloating, diarrhea, flatulence, or nausea. Lactic acidosis may occur in patients with heart failure or kidney, liver, or lung disease.
Blocks the action of intestinal and pancreatic lipases (which digest dietary fats). As a result, the undigested dietary fat passes through the intestines and out of the body without being absorbed, carrying with it fat-soluble vitamins that otherwise would have been absorbed in the intestines.	Reduces fat absorption by about 30% and promotes significant weight loss when used with a reduced-calorie diet. May raise blood pressure in some individuals. Other possible side effects include abdominal cramping and diarrhea. Patients must take a daily multivitamin to prevent vitamin deficiency.

laparoscopy, a type of surgery in which surgical instruments are inserted through a small incision in the abdominal wall. With improved surgical techniques, as well as an increasingly overweight population, bariatric procedures are expected to become more prevalent in the future.

Vertical Banded Gastroplasty. This surgery, also called gastric partitioning, is a gastric restriction procedure that divides the stomach into two sections. A stapling instrument is used to section off a golf ball-sized pouch at the top of the stomach, and an inflexible ring (or band) is put in place to encircle the small opening between the pouch and the rest of the stomach. This procedure allows small amounts of food to pass from the pouch to the remaining portion of the stomach. The likelihood of overeating is reduced because a small quantity of food creates a feeling of fullness. Several studies have shown that vertical banded gastroplasty may result in significant weight loss and improvement in weight-related medical conditions, although there are some side effects and risk, which include deterioration of the band or staple line. More commonly, people who undergo this procedure experience vomiting from overstretching the stomach. The risk of infection or death from complications of vertical banded gastroplasty is less than 1%.

Laparoscopic Adjustable Gastric Banding. Approved for use by the FDA in June 2001, this gastric restriction procedure cuts off a portion of the stomach to reduce gastric volume without stapling. Using laparoscopic techniques, an adjustable, hollow, silicone band ("Lap-Band") is wrapped around the upper part of the stomach to create a small pouch. Attached to the band is a flexible tube connected to a miniature access port, which is implanted just beneath the skin of the abdomen. Using this reservoir system, a physician can remove or add saline solution to the band to adjust its fit around the stomach and change the size of the narrow passage that connects the pouch to the lower stomach. Laparoscopic gastric banding is considered relatively safe and, unlike some other gastric surgeries, is reversible.

Gastric Bypass. This procedure is done in combination with gastric restriction. The volume of the stomach is first reduced by using a stapling tool to create a small upper gastric pouch that is completely separated from the rest of the stomach. The small pouch decreases the quantity of food an individual can comfortably consume. A segment of the small intestine is then surgically rerouted to connect directly to the gastric pouch. This procedure allows ingested food to bypass the majority of the stomach as well as part of the small intestine. Since nutrient absorption takes place in the small intestine, the number of calories available to the body is reduced by limiting both the amount of time food spends there and the amount of small intestine exposed to food and thus available to absorb it. The risks associated with gastric bypass are similar to those of vertical banded gastroplasty. However, approximately 30% of bypass patients also develop nutritional deficiencies because many nutrients are normally absorbed in the upper part of the jejunum.

NEW RESEARCH

Liposuction Doesn't Provide Health Benefits of Standard Weight Loss

Although liposuction results in weight loss and a slimmer appearance, it does not offer the same health benefits as conventional weight loss through diet and exercise, according to findings from a recent study.

Researchers investigated the effects of large-volume liposuction—removal of about 20 lbs. of fat—on 15 obese women, including 8 with type 2 diabetes. After a 10- to 12-week recovery period, the women were an average of 9 to 11 lbs. lighter than before the surgery and had reductions in body mass index and waist circumference.

Despite these findings, no improvements were seen in insulin sensitivity, blood pressure, blood glucose, insulin, lipid concentrations, and blood markers of inflammation and insulin resistance. A similar degree of weight loss by conventional means typically improves all of these values.

A possible explanation for these findings is that a negative calorie balance—as opposed to just a decrease in fat mass—is necessary to achieve the health benefits seen with conventional weight loss. An alternate explanation is that conventional weight loss reduces harmful deposits of fat around the internal organs, whereas liposuction removes only fat located directly beneath the skin's surface.

THE NEW ENGLAND
JOURNAL OF MEDICINE
Volume 350, page 2549
June 17, 2004

According to clinical studies, gastric bypass is effective for initiating and sustaining weight loss.

Liposuction

While the surgical removal of fat may seem like an ideal method of weight reduction, liposuction is, at best, a questionable solution. Unlike diet and exercise, fat reduction via liposuction has no proven health benefits. And the procedure cannot help those who are diffusely overweight. Instead, liposuction is appropriate only for people of normal or near-normal weight who have stubborn fat deposits that do not respond to diet and exercise. Candidates should also be in good general health and have skin that is elastic enough to shrink evenly after the surgery—which rules out many people over 50. Finally, liposuction comes with no cosmetic guarantees: While the extracted fat cells will not return, weight can still be gained at other sites in the body.

Common sites of liposuction include the abdomen, hips, buttocks, thighs, legs, upper arms, face, and neck; sometimes several areas are treated at once. Patients must wear a special pressure dressing (such as a girdle or body stocking) over the treated area for several weeks afterward to help the skin shrink to fit the new contour and to minimize bruising and swelling (which may persist for months). While the overall risk associated with liposuction is low, the more fat that is removed, the greater the risk of complications such as infection or blood clots. Patients interested in liposuction should consult their doctor for an assessment and, possibly, a referral to an experienced plastic surgeon. ■

GLOSSARY

abdominal obesity—Excessive fat in the abdomen indicated by a waist circumference greater than 40 inches in men and 35 inches in women.

amino acids—Building blocks of protein. Certain amino acids, termed essential or indispensable, must be obtained from the diet because the body does not produce them.

antioxidants—Substances that help the body neutralize free radicals. Beta-carotene, vitamin E, and vitamin C are some examples of the hundreds of naturally occurring antioxidants.

atherosclerosis—An accumulation of deposits of fat and fibrous tissue, called plaques, within the walls of arteries that can narrow the arteries and reduce the flow of blood through them.

bariatric surgery— An operation designed to cause weight loss, often by reducing the size of the stomach. This type of surgery is also called gastric restriction surgery.

bioavailability—A measure of how much and how well a nutrient is absorbed by the body.

body mass index (BMI)—A measurement of weight in relation to height. It is generally considered to be a good indicator of body fat. Calculated by multiplying weight in pounds by 703 and dividing the result by the square of height in inches. Overweight is defined as a BMI between 25 and 29.9 and obesity as a BMI of 30 and over.

calorie—A unit that signifies the quantity of energy in a food. Carbohydrates and protein contain four calories per gram; fat contains nine calories per gram; alcohol contains seven calories per gram. Technically known as a kilocalorie.

carbohydrates—Foods made up of starches and/or sugars. Sugars are simple carbohydrates while complex carbohydrates are starches that may also contain fiber, vitamins, and minerals. Carbohydrates provide four calories per gram.

cardiovascular disease—Disease affecting the heart or arterial vascular system of the body.

carotenoids—A collection of plant pigments that are found in yellow, orange, red, and dark green fruits and vegetables and may lower the risk of heart disease and certain cancers. Certain carotenoids, particularly beta-carotene, can be converted into vitamin A in the body. Lycopene, lutein, and zeaxanthin are other carotenoids.

cholesterol—A soft, waxy substance present in cells throughout the body. Deposition of blood cholesterol in blood vessels initiates the formation of atherosclerotic plaques. Cholesterol and triglycerides, both fatty substances (or lipids), are transported in the blood in combi-

nation with proteins to form three lipoproteins: high-density lipoprotein (HDL), low-density lipoprotein (LDL), and very–low-density lipoprotein (VLDL), which carries mainly triglycerides. Because HDL protects against coronary heart disease, it is often called "good" cholesterol. The plaque-forming cholesterol, or LDL, is referred to as "bad" cholesterol. See also dietary cholesterol.

DASH diet—An eating plan that can help control blood pressure and may also improve cholesterol. Rich in vegetables and fruits, the diet includes low-fat dairy products and is low in saturated fat, total fat, and cholesterol.

diabetes—A disorder characterized by abnormally high levels of glucose (sugar) in the blood.

dietary cholesterol—The cholesterol present in and obtained from animal foods—meats, poultry, fish, shellfish, eggs, and dairy products. Plant foods contain no cholesterol.

dietary supplement—A product (in pill, liquid, or powder form) that is taken in addition to one's regular diet. The supplement can contain a single substance—such as ginkgo biloba, ginseng, or St. John's wort—or a combination of substances.

dysphagia—Difficulty in swallowing food or liquids.

enriched food—A food to which a nutrient or nutrients have been added. Often, the added nutrients were present in the original food but were lost during processing, such as in enriched bread. Sometimes called fortified food.

enzyme—A protein that accelerates chemical reactions in the body.

essential amino acids— Amino acids that the body cannot synthesize and thus must be consumed in the diet. Lysine is an example. Also known as indispensable amino acids.

essential fatty acids—Fatty acids that are not made by the body and must be obtained from food. Essential fatty acids are necessary for cell structure and are converted into certain hormones that assist in the control of blood pressure, blood clotting, inflammation, and other body functions. Polyunsaturated fatty acids, such as linoleic acid, linolenic acid, and arachidonic acid, are essential fatty acids.

fiber—An indigestible component of fruits, vegetables, grains, and legumes that has numerous health benefits. There are two principal types of fiber: Insoluble fiber does not dissolve in water and helps prevent constipation. Soluble fiber (sometimes called viscous fiber) dissolves in water and helps to regulate blood levels of sugar and cholesterol.

fortified food—Food to which a nutrient or nutrients have been added to promote health and prevent disease. The nutrients added to fortified foods are not present in the original food or were present in smaller amounts. Example: vitamin D–fortified milk. Sometimes called enhanced food.

free radicals—Chemical compounds that can damage cells and oxidize LDL cholesterol so that it is more likely to be deposited in the walls of arteries.

functional foods—Foods that provide a health benefit beyond the traditional nutrients they contain.

gastric bypass—A type of gastric restriction surgery that reduces the amount of food that can be eaten and absorbed by the body. Gastric bypass involves sealing off a portion of the stomach and bypassing part of the intestine.

genetically modified food— Food that has been genetically altered. A piece of DNA from one plant or animal species is inserted into the DNA of another species in order to increase food production, decrease the need for pesticides, improve food quality, and/or help prevent diseases in people.

height/weight tables—Tables that display ranges of weights, according to different heights. The information is derived from mortality data of people seeking or obtaining life insurance.

high-density lipoprotein (HDL)—A particle in the blood that can protect against coronary heart disease by removing cholesterol from arterial walls. See also cholesterol.

homocysteine—An amino acid that arises from the breakdown of methionine, another amino acid found in animal-derived foods. High blood levels of homocysteine may promote atherosclerosis.

insulin—A hormone that controls the manufacture of glucose by the liver and permits muscle and fat cells to remove glucose from the blood. Also a medication taken by people with diabetes whose pancreas does not make enough insulin.

ketosis—A state in which the blood contains high levels of appetite-suppressing substances called ketones. When carbohydrate consumption is limited and not available for energy, an increased breakdown of fat results in elevated blood levels of ketones. Both poorly controlled diabetes and low-carbohydrate, high-protein diets can lead to ketosis. Side effects of ketosis can include dehydration, dizziness, weakness, headaches, and confusion.

lactose intolerance—A reduced ability to digest the milk sugar lactose that results in abdominal discomfort within 30 minutes to two hours of consuming milk or milk-based foods.

laparoscopic adjustable gastric banding—A minimally invasive, reversible form of gastric restriction surgery that places an adjustable silicone band around the top of the stomach in order to reduce its size and decrease food intake.

leptin—A protein secreted by human fat cells that informs the brain about the body's level of fat stores. Obese people have higher leptin levels than normal-weight individuals.

low-density lipoprotein (LDL)—A particle that transports cholesterol in the bloodstream. Its deposition in artery walls initiates plaque formation. A major contributor to coronary heart disease. See also cholesterol.

metabolic syndrome—Also called syndrome X or insulin resistance syndrome. The presence of at least three of five risk factors (abdominal obesity, elevated triglycerides levels, low HDL cholesterol levels, elevated blood pressure, elevated blood sugar) increases the risk of diabetes and coronary heart disease.

metabolism—The chemical process by which the body converts food into energy and various functions. Such activities include food digestion, nutrient absorption, waste elimination, respiration, circulation, and temperature regulation.

minerals—Naturally occurring inorganic substances required for growth and the maintenance of body functions.

monounsaturated fat—A fat with only one double bond that is capable of absorbing more hydrogen. Monounsaturated fatty acids are widely found in foods; concentrated sources include avocados, almonds, and olive and canola oils. Can lower LDL cholesterol levels when substituted for saturated fat in the diet.

norepinephrine—A stress hormone that promotes satiety (fullness) by stimulating the central nervous system and affecting levels of blood glucose (sugar). Certain weight loss drugs are designed to enhance levels of norepinephrine in the brain. Also called noradrenaline.

obesity—Conventionally defined as a body weight that is 20% or more than what is ideal for a person's height and body type. Obesity is also defined more precisely as a body mass index (BMI) of 30 or higher.

omega-3 fatty acids—Forms of polyunsaturated fat found primarily in fatty fish (such as mackerel, salmon, and tuna) and in small amounts in canola, soybean and walnut oils, walnuts, soybeans, and purslane.

organic food—A product that is grown and produced without the use of petroleum-based fertilizers, sewage

GLOSSARY—continued

sludge-based fertilizers, most conventional pesticides, genetic modification, ionizing radiation, antibiotics, or growth hormones.

osteoporosis—A disorder characterized by fragile, weak bones that result from a loss of bone mass. Increases the risk of bone fracture.

overweight—An excess of body weight that is defined as a body mass index (BMI) of 25 to 29.9.

oxidation—A reaction of any substance with oxygen—an interaction that may generate harmful free radicals, which contribute to the onset of disease. The oxidation of LDL, for example, contributes to its deposition in arterial plaque.

phytochemicals—Compounds from plant foods that may help lower the risk of disease. Flavonoids and soy isoflavones are examples.

plaques—Deposits of fat and fibrous tissue in arteries that can lead to heart disease and stroke.

polyunsaturated fat—A type of fat found in safflower, sunflower, and corn oils. Can help to lower LDL cholesterol when substituted for saturated fat in the diet.

protein—Compounds made up of varying sequences of amino acids. Dietary protein provides four calories per gram.

Recommended Dietary Allowances (RDA)—The average intake of nutrients required to meet the daily nutritional needs of nearly all healthy people.

resting metabolic rate (RMR)—The amount of energy that is spent on basic functions, such as breathing, digestion, heartbeat, and brain activity, while a person is at rest.

saturated fat—A fat found in most animal foods and in tropical oils, such as palm and coconut oils. A major dietary factor in raising blood cholesterol.

serotonin—A chemical in the brain, called a neurotransmitter, that is synthesized from the amino acid tryptophan. Serotonin affects mood and suppresses appetite.

set point theory—A theory that the body maintains a certain weight and body fat level by regulating its own internal controls.

stroke—A sudden reduction in or loss of brain function that occurs when an artery supplying blood to a portion of the brain becomes blocked or ruptures. Nerve cells, or neurons, in the affected area are destroyed by the lack of oxygen and nutrients normally provided by the blood.

thermogenesis—The release of heat energy that occurs when the body breaks down fat and other fuels for energy.

trans fatty acids—Fats formed when food manufacturers add hydrogen atoms to unsaturated fats to make them more saturated and therefore more solid and shelf stable. Found in margarines, deep-fried fast foods, and store-bought baked goods. Trans fatty acids raise blood cholesterol and lower HDL cholesterol.

triglyceride—A lipid (fat) formed in adipose tissue that serves as the body's major store of energy. Triglycerides released in the liver are carried on lipoproteins, especially very–low-density lipoprotein. Elevated blood triglyceride levels are associated with an increased risk of coronary heart disease.

vertical banded gastroplasty—A type of bariatric surgery that partitions off a portion of the stomach, leaving room for only about 1 oz. of food.

vitamins—Organic substances that are required for many metabolic functions including converting food into energy and aiding in the development of bones and tissues. Vitamins themselves do not provide energy. While vitamins are vital to life, they are needed only in minute amounts.

waist circumference—An indicator of abdominal fat. A healthy waist circumference is 40 inches or less for men and 35 inches or less for women. An increased waist circumference confers a health risk.

HEALTH INFORMATION ORGANIZATIONS AND SUPPORT GROUPS

American Council on Exercise
San Diego, CA
☎ 800-825-3636/858-279-8227
www.acefitness.org

**American Council on Science
and Health (ACSH)**
New York, NY
☎ 212-362-7044
www.acsh.org

American Dietetic Association
Chicago, IL
☎ 800-366-1655/312-899-0040
www.eatright.org

American Heart Association
Dallas, TX
☎ 800-242-8721
www.americanheart.org

**American Institute for
Cancer Research (AICR)**
Washington, DC
☎ 800-843-8114
www.aicr.org

American Running Association
Bethesda, MD
☎ 800-776-2732/301-913-9517
www.americanrunning.org

**Center for Science in the
Public Interest**
Washington, DC
☎ 202-332-9110
www.cspinet.org

**Food and Nutrition
Information Center**
Beltsville, MD
☎ 301-504-5719
www.nal.usda.gov/fnic

The Food and Drug Administration
Rockville, MD
☎ 888-463-6332
www.fda.gov

**International Food Information
Council Foundation (IFIC)**
Washington, DC
☎ 202-296-6540
www.ific.org

**National Institute of Diabetes
& Digestive & Kidney Disease,
Weight-Control Information**
Bethesda, MD
☎ 202-828-1025
www.niddk.nih.gov/health/
    nutrit/win.htm

USDA Meat and Poultry Hotline
Washington, DC
☎ 800-535-4555
www.fsis.usda.gov/OA/
    programs/mphotline.htm

LEADING CENTERS FOR WEIGHT CONTROL

The following list of weight control and eating disorders centers was compiled by Lawrence J. Cheskin, M.D., director of the Johns Hopkins Weight Management Center and coauthor of this White Paper. Listed alphabetically, all of the centers are affiliated with hospitals or universities involved in obesity research. Any institution listed is considered a leading center, and the rankings do not imply that other hospitals cannot or do not deliver excellent care.

**Duke University
Diet and Fitness Center**
Durham, NC
☎ 800-235-3853
www.dukedietcenter.org

**Johns Hopkins Weight
Management Center**
Lutherville, MD
☎ 410-847-3744
www.jhbmc.jhu.edu/weight

**New York Obesity Research Center
St. Luke's-Roosevelt Hospital
Center**
New York, NY
☎ 212-523-4196
www.nyorc.org

**Weight and Eating
Disorders Program
University of Pennsylvania**
Philadelphia, PA
☎ 215-898-7314
www.uphs.upenn.edu/weight

**Comprehensive Weight Control
Program**
New York, NY
☎ 212-583-1000
www.weightscience.com

**Yale Center for Eating and
Weight Disorders**
New Haven, CT
☎ 203-432-4610
www.yale.edu/ycewd

HIGH-FRUCTOSE CORN SYRUP AND OBESITY

A massive increase in the consumption of high-fructose corn syrup—particularly in sweetened beverages—may be a key contributor to the obesity epidemic hitting the United States, according to the report reprinted here from the *American Journal of Clinical Nutrition.*

High-fructose corn syrup (HFCS) was introduced as a sweetener for foods and beverages in the late 1960s, and its use rapidly expanded beginning in the 1980s, George A. Bray, M.D., of the Louisiana State University in Baton Rouge, and colleagues note. HFCS now accounts for 40% of all calorie-containing added sweeteners used in the United States, and about two thirds is consumed in beverages.

The body responds differently to fructose than to glucose, the researchers point out. Glucose stimulates the secretion of insulin and leptin, both of which play a role in appetite regulation. But fructose triggers less secretion of insulin and leptin; as a result of this and other factors, fructose may be more likely to be converted directly into fat and less likely to signal the brain that fullness has occurred. The researchers add that several studies have suggested a link between consumption of sweetened beverages and weight gain, so HFCS–sweetened sodas and fruit drinks may be particularly likely to contribute to obesity.

From 1970 to 1990, consumption of HFCS increased by more than 1000%. An increase in obesity that "mirrored" the rise in HFCS consumption was seen between the 1976–1980 and the 1988–1994 National Center for Health Statistics Surveys.

"We believe that an argument can now be made that the use of HFCS in beverages should be reduced and that HFCS should be replaced with alternative noncaloric sweeteners," the researchers propose. (People who drink diet sodas may not lose weight, but they are less likely to gain as much weight as people who drink beverages with HFCS.) They also suggest removing soda machines from schools and reducing portion sizes of soda.

Consumption of high-fructose corn syrup in beverages may play a role in the epidemic of obesity[1,2]

George A Bray, Samara Joy Nielsen, and Barry M Popkin

ABSTRACT

Obesity is a major epidemic, but its causes are still unclear. In this article, we investigate the relation between the intake of high-fructose corn syrup (HFCS) and the development of obesity. We analyzed food consumption patterns by using US Department of Agriculture food consumption tables from 1967 to 2000. The consumption of HFCS increased > 1000% between 1970 and 1990, far exceeding the changes in intake of any other food or food group. HFCS now represents > 40% of caloric sweeteners added to foods and beverages and is the sole caloric sweetener in soft drinks in the United States. Our most conservative estimate of the consumption of HFCS indicates a daily average of 132 kcal for all Americans aged ≥ 2 y, and the top 20% of consumers of caloric sweeteners ingest 316 kcal from HFCS/d. The increased use of HFCS in the United States mirrors the rapid increase in obesity. The digestion, absorption, and metabolism of fructose differ from those of glucose. Hepatic metabolism of fructose favors de novo lipogenesis. In addition, unlike glucose, fructose does not stimulate insulin secretion or enhance leptin production. Because insulin and leptin act as key afferent signals in the regulation of food intake and body weight, this suggests that dietary fructose may contribute to increased energy intake and weight gain. Furthermore, calorically sweetened beverages may enhance caloric overconsumption. Thus, the increase in consumption of HFCS has a temporal relation to the epidemic of obesity, and the overconsumption of HFCS in calorically sweetened beverages may play a role in the epidemic of obesity.   Am J Clin Nutr 2004;79:537 43.

KEY WORDS   Epidemiology, food intake, obesity, artificial sweeteners, fructose

INTRODUCTION

As obesity has escalated to epidemic proportions around the world, many causes, including dietary components, have been suggested. Excessive caloric intake has been related to high-fat foods, increased portion sizes, and diets high both in simple sugars such as sucrose and in high-fructose corn syrup (HFCS) as a source of fructose (13). In this article, we discuss the evidence that a marked increase in the use of HFCS, and therefore in total fructose consumption, preceded the obesity epidemic and may be an important contributor to this epidemic in the United States.

To provide a common frame of reference for the terms used in this paper, the following definitions should be understood. Sugar is any free monosaccharide or disaccharide present in a food. Sugars includes at least one sugar; composite sugars refers to the aggregate of all forms of sugars in a food and is thus distinguishable from specific types of sugar, such as fructose, glucose, or sucrose. Added sugar is sugar added to a food and includes sweeteners such as sucrose, HFCS, honey, molasses, and other syrups. Naturally occurring sugar is sugar occurring in food and not added in processing, preparation, or at the table. Total sugars represents the total amount of sugars present in a food and includes both naturally occurring and added sugars. Free fructose is fructose that exists in food as the monosaccharide. Fructose refers to both the free and bound forms of fructose (4).

Added sweeteners are important components of our diet, representing 318 kcal of dietary intake for the average American aged ≥ 2 y, or 16% of all caloric intake as measured by a nationally representative survey in 1994 1996 (5). Sweet corn-based syrups were developed during the past 3 decades and now represent close to one-half of the caloric sweeteners consumed by Americans (6, 7). HFCS made by enzymatic isomerization of glucose to fructose was introduced as HFCS-42 (42% fructose) and HFCS-55 (55% fructose) in 1967 and 1977, respectively, and opened a new frontier for the sweetener and soft drink industries. Using a glucose isomerase, the starch in corn can be efficiently converted to glucose and then to various amounts of fructose. The hydrolysis of sucrose produces a 50:50 molar mixture of fructose and glucose. The development of these inexpensive, sweet corn-based syrups made it profitable to replace sucrose (sugar) and simple sugars with HFCS in our diet, and they now represent 40% of all added caloric sweeteners (8). Fructose is sweeter than sucrose. In comparative studies of sweetness, in which the sweetness of sucrose was set at 100, fructose had a sweetness of 173 and glucose had a sweetness of 74 (9). If the values noted above are applied, HFCS-42 would be 1.16 times as sweet as sucrose, and HFCS-55 would be 1.28 times as sweet as sucrose. This contrasts with the estimates reported by Hanover and White (10). In their study, the sweetness of sucrose was set at 100 as in reference 8. Fructose, however, had a sweetness of only 117, whereas a 50:50 mixture of fructose and sucrose had a sweetness of 128. It is difficult to see why fructose and sucrose combined would be sweeter than either one alone and as sweet as HFCS-55. On the basis of data in Agriculture Handbook no. 8 from the US Department of Agriculture (USDA) (11), a cola beverage in 1963

[1] From the Pennington Biomedical Research Center, Louisiana State University, Baton Rouge, LA (GAB), and the Department of Nutrition, University of North Carolina, Chapel Hill (SJN and BMP).

[2] Reprints not available. Address correspondence to GA Bray, Pennington Biomedical Research Center, 6400 Perkins Road, Baton Rouge, LA 70808.

Received October 3, 2003.
Accepted for publication December 15, 2003.

had 39 kcal/100 g, whereas a cola beverage in 2003 had 41 kcal/100 g. Because the number of calories per 100 g has not changed substantially over the past 40 y, current beverages are probably sweeter, depending on the temperature at which they are served.

HFCS has become a favorite substitute for sucrose in carbonated beverages, baked goods, canned fruits, jams and jellies, and dairy products (10). The major user of HFCS in the world is the United States; however, HFCS is now manufactured and used in many countries throughout the world (7). In the United States, HFCS is the major source of caloric sweeteners in soft drinks and many other sweetened beverages and is also included in numerous other foods; therefore, HFCS constitutes a major source of dietary fructose. Few data are available on foods containing HFCS in countries other than the United States (7).

THE BIOLOGY

Absorption of fructose

The digestive and absorptive processes for glucose and fructose are different. When disaccharides such as sucrose or maltose enter the intestine, they are cleaved by disaccharidases. A sodium-glucose cotransporter absorbs the glucose that is formed from cleavage of sucrose. Fructose, in contrast, is absorbed further down in the duodenum and jejunum by a non-sodium-dependent process. After absorption, glucose and fructose enter the portal circulation and either are transported to the liver, where the fructose can be taken up and converted to glucose, or pass into the general circulation. The addition of small, catalytic amounts of fructose to orally ingested glucose increases hepatic glycogen synthesis in human subjects and reduces glycemic responses in subjects with type 2 diabetes mellitus (12), which suggests the importance of fructose in modulating metabolism in the liver. However, when large amounts of fructose are ingested, they provide a relatively unregulated source of carbon precursors for hepatic lipogenesis.

Fructose and insulin release

Along with 2 peptides, glucose-dependent insulinotropic polypeptide and glucagon-like peptide-1 released from the gastrointestinal tract, circulating glucose increases insulin release from the pancreas (13, 14). Fructose does not stimulate insulin secretion in vitro, probably because the β cells of the pancreas lack the fructose transporter Glut-5 (15, 16). Thus, when fructose is given in vivo as part of a mixed meal, the increase in glucose and insulin is much smaller than when a similar amount of glucose is given. However, fructose produces a much larger increase in lactate and a small (1.7%) increase in diet-induced thermogenesis (17), which again suggests that glucose and fructose have different metabolic effects.

Insulin and leptin

Insulin release can modulate food intake by at least 2 mechanisms. First, Schwartz et al (18) have argued that insulin concentrations in the central nervous system have a direct inhibitory effect on food intake. In addition, insulin may modify food intake by its effect on leptin secretion, which is mainly regulated by insulin-induced changes in glucose metabolism in fat cells (19, 20). Insulin increases leptin release (21) with a time delay of several hours. Thus, a low insulin concentration after ingestion of fructose would be associated with lower average leptin concentrations than would be seen after ingestion of glucose. Because leptin inhibits food intake, the lower leptin concentrations induced by fructose would tend to enhance food intake. This is most dramatically illustrated in humans who lack leptin (22, 23). Persons lacking leptin (homozygotes) are massively obese (22), and heterozygotes with low but detectable serum leptin concentrations have increased adiposity (23), which indicates that low leptin concentrations are associated with increased hunger and gains in body fat. Administration of leptin to persons who lack it produces a dramatic decrease in food intake, as expected. Leptin also increases energy expenditure, and during reduced calorie intake, leptin attenuates the decreases in thyroid hormones and 24-h energy expenditure (24). To the extent that fructose increases in the diet, one might expect less insulin secretion and thus less leptin release and a reduction in the inhibitory effect of leptin on food intake, ie, an increase in food intake. This was found in the preliminary studies reported by Teff et al (25). Consumption of high-fructose meals reduced 24-h plasma insulin and leptin concentrations and increased postprandial fasting triacylglycerol concentrations in women but did not suppress circulating ghrelin concentrations.

Fructose and metabolism

The metabolism of fructose differs from that of glucose in several other ways as well (3). Glucose enters cells by a transport mechanism (Glut-4) that is insulin dependent in most tissues. Insulin activates the insulin receptor, which in turn increases the density of glucose transporters on the cell surface and thus facilitates the entry of glucose. Once inside the cell, glucose is phosphorylated by glucokinase to become glucose-6-phosphate, from which the intracellular metabolism of glucose begins. Intracellular enzymes can tightly control conversion of glucose-6-phosphate to the glycerol backbone of triacylglycerols through modulation by phosphofructokinase. In contrast with glucose, fructose enters cells via a Glut-5 transporter that does not depend on insulin. This transporter is absent from pancreatic β cells and the brain, which indicates limited entry of fructose into these tissues. Glucose provides satiety signals to the brain that fructose cannot provide because it is not transported into the brain. Once inside the cell, fructose is phosphorylated to form fructose-1-phosphate (26). In this configuration, fructose is readily cleaved by aldolase to form trioses that are the backbone for phospholipid and triacyglycerol synthesis. Fructose also provides carbon atoms for synthesis of long-chain fatty acids, although in humans, the quantity of these carbon atoms is small. Thus, fructose facilitates the biochemical formation of triacylglycerols more efficiently than does glucose (3). For example, when a diet containing 17% fructose was provided to healthy men and women, the men, but not the women, showed a highly significant increase of 32% in plasma triacylglycerol concentrations (27).

Overconsumption of sweetened beverages

One model for producing obesity in rodents is to provide sweetened (sucrose, maltose, etc) beverages for them to drink (28). In this setting, the desire for the calorically sweetened solution reduces the intake of solid food, but not by enough to prevent a positive caloric balance and the slow development of obesity. Adding the same amount of sucrose or maltose as of a solid in the diet does not produce the same response. Thus, in experimental animals, sweetened beverages appear to enhance caloric consumption.

Fructose and soft drinks

A similar argument about the role of overconsumption of calorically sweetened beverages may apply to humans (29 32).

TABLE 1
Availability of high-fructose corn syrup (HFCS) in the US caloric sweetener supply[1]

Year	HFCS	Total caloric sweeteners	HFCS as percentage of total caloric sweeteners	Percentage of HFCS from HFCS-42	Percentage of HFCS from HFCS-55
	$g \cdot person^{-1} \cdot d^{-1}$	$g \cdot person^{-1} \cdot d^{-1}$	%	%	%
1966	0.0	165.9	0.0		
1970	0.8	175.1	0.4	100.0	0.0
1975	7.1	168.8	4.2	100.0	0.0
1980	27.3	176.0	15.5	71.2	28.8
1985	64.7	184.4	35.1	34.3	65.7
1990	71.0	195.7	36.3	41.0	59.0
1995	82.3	211.7	38.9	39.9	60.1
2000	91.6	218.0	42.0	38.8	61.2

[1] Data from reference 8. HFCS-42 and HFCS-55, HFCS containing 42% and 55% fructose, respectively.

Mattes (29) reported that when humans ingest energy-containing beverages, energy compensation is less precise than when solid foods are ingested. In another study in humans, DiMeglio and Mattes (30) found that when 15 healthy men and women were given a carbohydrate load of 1880 kJ/d (450 kcal/d) as a calorically sweetened soda for 4 wk, they gained significantly more weight than when the same carbohydrate load was given in a solid form as jelly beans. Additional support for our hypothesis that calorically sweetened beverages may contribute to the epidemic of obesity comes from a longitudinal study in adolescents. Ludwig et al (31) showed that in adolescents participating in the Planet Health project, the quantity of sugar-sweetened beverages ingested predicted initial body mass index (BMI; in kg/m^2) and gain in BMI during the follow-up period. Raben et al (32) designed a randomized, double-blind study to compare the effect of calorically sweetened beverages with that of diet drinks on weight gain in moderately overweight men and women. This European study found that drinking calorically sweetened beverages resulted in greater weight gain over the 10-wk study than did drinking diet drinks. Compared with the subjects who consumed diet drinks, those who consumed calorically sweetened beverages did not compensate for this consumption by reducing the intake of other beverages and foods and thus gained weight. The beverages in this study were sweetened with sucrose, whereas in the United States almost all calorically sweetened beverages are sweetened with HFCS. Thus, we need a second randomized controlled study that compares sucrose- and HFCS-sweetened beverages. This could establish whether the form of the caloric sweetener played a role in the weight gain observed in the study by Raben et al (32).

The results of the studies by Raben et al (32) and Ludwig et al (31) suggest that the rapid increase in the intake of calorically sweetened soft drinks could be a contributing factor to the epidemic of weight gain. Between 1970, when HFCS was introduced into the marketplace, and 2000, the per capita consumption of HFCS in the United States increased from 0.292 kg $person^{-1}$ y^{-1} (0.6 lb $person^{-1}$ y^{-1}) to 33.4 kg $person^{-1}$ y^{-1} (73.5 lb $person^{-1}$ y^{-1}), an increase of > 100-fold (8) (**Table 1**). The total consumption of fructose increased nearly 30%. The consumption of free fructose showed a greater increase, which reflected the increasing use of HFCS (**Figure 1**). During the same interval, the consumption of sucrose decreased nearly 50%, and

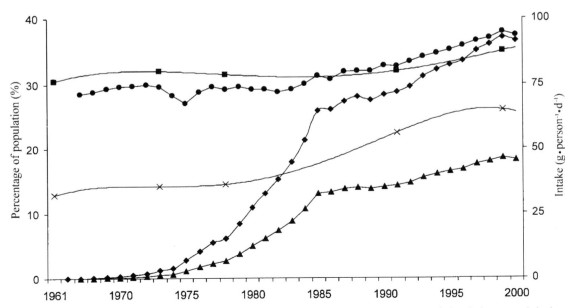

FIGURE 1. Estimated intakes of total fructose (●), free fructose (▲), and high-fructose corn syrup (HFCS, ◆) in relation to trends in the prevalence of overweight ( ) and obesity (x) in the United States. Data from references 7 and 35.

the intakes of sucrose and HFCS are now nearly identical. Although this shift has clearly led to a major increase in free-fructose consumption, it is unclear how much of the increase in consumption of calorically sweetened soft drinks is a result of the shift to beverages in which one-half of the fructose is free rather than bound with glucose as in sucrose. A recent review described many facets of this issue (3).

HFCS USE AND INTAKE

Availability of HFCS in the food supply

In 1970 HFCS represented < 1% of all caloric sweeteners available for consumption in the United States, but the HFCS portion of the caloric sweetener market jumped rapidly in the 1980s and by 2000 represented 42.0% of all caloric sweeteners (Table 1) (8). HFCS-42 was initially the only HFCS component, but by the early 1980s, HFCS-55 had become the major source and constituted 61.2% of all HFCS in 2000. These data are based on per capita food disappearance data. In the absence of direct measures of HFCS intake, these data provide the best indirect measure of the HFCS available for consumption in the United States. The data are useful for studying trends but probably overestimate intake patterns. Although it is useful to understand that HFCS intake represents more than two-fifths of the total intake of caloric sweeteners in the United States, it is also important to recognize that the proportion of HFCS in some foods is much higher than that in other foods.

Foods containing HFCS

In the United States, HFCS is found in almost all foods containing caloric sweeteners. These include most soft drinks and fruit drinks, candied fruits and canned fruits, dairy desserts and flavored yogurts, most baked goods, many cereals, and jellies. Over 60% of the calories in apple juice, which is used as the base for many of the fruit drinks, come from fructose, and thus apple juice is another source of fructose in the diet. Lists of HFCS-containing foods can be obtained from organizations concerned with HFCS-related allergies (33). It is clear that almost all caloric sweeteners used by manufacturers of soft drinks and fruit drinks are HFCS (4, 34). In fact, about two-thirds of all HFCS consumed in the United States are in beverages. Aside from beverages, there is no definitive literature on the proportion of caloric sweeteners that is HFCS in other processed foods. HFCS is found in most processed foods; however, the exact compositions are not available from either the manufacturer or any publicly available food-composition table.

Trends in obesity and HFCS availability

There are important similarities between the trend in HFCS availability and the trends in the prevalence of obesity in the United States (Figure 1). Using age-standardized, nationally representative measures of obesity at 5 time points from 1960 to 1999 (35) and data on the availability of HFCS collected annually over this same period, we graphed both patterns. The data on obesity are from the National Center for Health Statistics for the following periods: 1960 1962 (National Health Examination Survey I), 1971 1975 [National Health and Nutrition Examination Survey (NHANES)], 1976 1980 (NHANES II), 1988 1994 (NHANES III), and 1999 (NHANES 1999 2000) (35). The HFCS data are those from Table 1. The prevalence of overweight (BMI of 25 29.9)

and the prevalence of obesity (BMI > 30) were fit with fourth-order polynomial curves so that the limited number of data points could be fitted into a curve to capture the US trends. We also included estimates of free-fructose intake and total fructose intake. Total fructose is the sum of free fructose and fructose that is part of the disaccharide sucrose. Free fructose is the monosaccharide in HFCS and is also obtained in small amounts from other sources. Free-fructose intake closely follows the intake of HFCS. Total fructose intake increased nearly 30% between 1970 and 2000.

Estimated HFCS consumption

The intake of caloric sweeteners in the United States has increased rapidly, and nationally representative data from 1994 to 1998 from the USDA allow us to estimate an intake of 318 kcal/d for the average US resident aged ≥ 2 y. This value is one-sixth of the intake of all calories and close to one-third of the intake of all carbohydrates and represents a significant increase over the past 2 decades (**Table 2**). As the intake of caloric sweeteners increased, so did the fructose load, which increased from 158.5 to 228 kcal • person^{-1} • d^{-1} between 1977 1978 (36) and 1994 1998 (38, 39).

Furthermore, as shown in Table 2, the major increase in the intake of caloric sweeteners from 1977 to 1998 came from the intake of soft drinks and fruit drinks, and these intake values were 105 and 31 kcal person^{-1} d^{-1}, respectively, of the total added sugar intake of 318 kcal person^{-1} d^{-1} in 1994 1998. Moreover, more than one-half of the increased caloric sweetener intake during this time period came from the intake of these beverages. The intakes of these 2 types of beverages and of desserts total about two-thirds of all caloric sweetener intake in the United States today (Table 2).

We have no way to directly measure total HFCS use. However, one Food and Drug Administration study used very conservative methods to estimate HFCS use for the nationally representative dietary intake sample from 1977 to 1978 from the USDA (35). Using measures of the proportion of HFCS in each food, Glinsmann et al (40) created food categorywide estimates of the proportion of caloric sweeteners that is HFCS. We applied those same proportions to a set of food groups to estimate the use of caloric sweeteners not only during 19771978 but also during later periods. Using our conversion technique applied to the initial 19771978 Nationwide Food Consumption Survey data, we obtained results that were only 4 kcal higher than the estimates of Glinsmann et al (39). This approach is based on HFCS composition in the early 1980s. With the use of the USDA value of 4.2 g HFCS/tsp (0.84 g/mL), the availability of HFCS in the food supply in the early 1980s was only one-half of the current availability on a gram per capita basis (as shown in Table 1). Thus, we feel confident that we can use this approach to provide a conservative lower limit of HFCS intake.

In Table 2, the 2 columns at the right contain our estimates of HFCS intake and total fructose intake. On the basis of the trend in intakes, our estimate of HFCS intake for the most recent period of measurement from 1994 1998 is 132 kcal person^{-1} d^{-1} (37). This represents a shift between 19771978 and 1994 1998 from 4.5% of total calories to 6.7% of total calories, or from 10.1% of carbohydrates to 13.1% of carbohydrates (41). The estimate of total fructose intake, which was obtained from the intakes of sucrose and HFCS, would be somewhat higher if we knew the fructose content of the fruit drinks.

TABLE 2
Trends in intakes of added sugar (sucrose) and high-fructose corn syrup (HFCS) by Americans aged ≥ 2 y[1]

	Soft drinks	Fruit drinks	Desserts	Total added sugar	Estimated HFCS intake[2]	Estimated total fructose intake[3]
Intake (kcal · person^{-1} · d^{-1})						
1977 1978	52	18	54	235	80	158.5
1989 1991	74 [4]	19	47[4]	242	95	170
1994 1998	105 [4,5]	31[4,5]	60[4,5]	318[4,5]	132	228
Percentage of total energy (%)						
1977 1978	2.9	1.0	3.0	13.1	4.5	8.8
1989 1991	4.1 [4]	1.1	2.6[4]	13.5	5.3	9.4
1994 1998	5.3 [4,5]	1.6[4,5]	3.0[4,5]	16.0[4,5]	6.7	11.5
Percentage of total carbohydrates (%)						
1977 1978	6.5	2.3	6.8	29.5	10.1	19.8
1989 1991	8.5 [4]	2.2	5.4[4]	27.8	10.9	19.5
1994 1998	10.4 [4,5]	3.1[4,5]	5.9[4,5]	31.5[4,5]	13.1	22.8

[1] Data from references 36 39.
[2] Coefficients derived from Glinsmann et al (40) were used to estimate HFCS intake.
[3] Estimated as 50% of sucrose + fructose in HFCS.
[4] Significantly different from 1977 1978, P ≤ 0.01 (t test).
[5] Significantly different from 1989 1991, P ≤ 0.01 (t test).

Distribution of HFCS intake matters!

We also explored the distribution of HFCS consumption by examining quintiles of caloric sweetener intake among Americans aged ≥ 2 y (**Table 3**). Most of the increase in caloric sweetener intake from the middle quintile to the upper quintile came from increases in the intake of calorically sweetened beverages, particularly soft drinks. Consumers in the top quintile, which represents 20% of all Americans, consume > 11% of their calories from HFCS. Again, remember that this is a very conservative estimate. This same group obtains almost one-half of its carbohydrates from caloric sweeteners and one-fifth of its carbohydrates from HFCS.

DISCUSSION

Genetic factors play an important role in the development of obesity (42). However, the rapidity with which the current epidemic of obesity has descended on the United States (35) and

TABLE 3
Distribution of consumption of added caloric sweeteners and high-fructose corn syrup (HFCS) by quintile (Q) of added sugar intake in persons aged ≥ 2 y (1994 1996, 1998)[1]

	Q1 (n = 3907)	Q2 (n = 4259)	Q3 (n = 4228)	Q4 (n = 3645)	Q5 (n = 2988)	Total (n = 19 027)	P for trend
Added caloric sweeteners							
Intake (kcal · person^{-1} · d^{-1})							
Soft drinks	6	31	69	129	290	105	0.022
Fruit drinks	4	14	26	43	69	31	0.003
Total	69	169	263	388	703	318	0.001
Percentage of total energy in kcal (%)							
Soft drinks	0.4	1.9	3.7	6.0	10.2	5.3	0.004
Fruit drinks	0.3	0.8	1.4	2.0	2.4	1.6	0.0001
Total	4.9	10.2	14.0	18.1	24.7	16.0	0.0004
Percentage of carbohydrates (%)							
Soft drinks	0.9	3.8	7.3	11.6	18.8	10.4	0.003
Fruit drinks	0.6	1.7	2.8	3.9	4.5	3.1	0.0004
Total	10.5	20.8	27.9	35.0	45.6	31.4	0.0002
HFCS							
Intake (kcal · person^{-1} · d^{-1})							
Soft drinks	4	22	49	91	205	74	0.022
Fruit drinks	3	10	18	30	49	22	0.004
Total	21	58	103	166	316	132	0.012
Percentage of total energy in kcal (%)							
Soft drinks	0.3	1.3	2.6	4.2	7.2	3.7	0.005
Fruit drinks	0.2	0.6	1.0	1.4	1.7	1.1	<0.0001
Total	1.5	3.5	5.5	7.7	11.1	6.7	0.0007
Percentage of carbohydrates (%)							
Soft drinks	0.6	2.7	5.2	8.2	13.3	7.3	0.003
Fruit drinks	0.4	1.2	1.9	2.7	3.2	2.2	0.0002
Total	3.2	7.2	10.9	14.9	20.5	13.1	0.0002

[1] Data from references 38 and 39 (weighted to be nationally representative).

many other countries (43) makes environmental factors the more likely explanation. From a public health perspective, the key question is whether there are modifiable environmental agents that could have triggered this epidemic and that might be altered. Several environmental agents, including reduced levels of physical activity (44), a decrease in smoking, increased portion size (2), eating outside the home and at fast-food restaurants, and changes in the types of food that are ingested (45), have been suggested. In this article, we propose that the introduction of HFCS and the increased intakes of soft drinks and other sweetened beverages have led to increases in total caloric and fructose consumption that are important contributors to the current epidemic of obesity.

In this article, we address an important potential hypothesis by which HFCS may have an environmental link with the epidemic of obesity. When total calorie intake is fixed, ie, if a person eats the same amount of fructose, glucose, or sucrose in a metabolically controlled setting, the response should be the same, and this was shown by McDevitt et al (46). This situation is not one in which differences in taste and portion size are allowed to operate. However, many biological factors that we noted in this article suggest that calorically sweetened beverages are associated with overconsumption when the sweetener is in a liquid form (29 32). The collective data suggest that overconsumption of beverages sweetened with HFCS and containing > 50% free fructose and the increased intake of total fructose may play a role in the epidemic of obesity. Whether HFCS used in solid food produces the same overconsumption as it does in beverages is unknown, but we suspect that if the HFCS was entirely in the solid form, it would not pose the same problem (30). Total fructose, both free fructose and fructose combined in sucrose, in both beverages and solid food may be viewed as a precursor to fat because of the ease with which the carbon skeleton of fructose can form the backbone for triacylglycerols and be used for the synthesis of long-chain fatty acids (25). Additional clinical trials are clearly needed to buttress the conclusions of Raben et al (32) that beverages containing sugar caused more weight gain over 10 wk than did diet beverages.

There is a distinct likelihood that the increased consumption of HFCS in beverages may be linked to the increase in obesity. One US study showed that beverages sweetened with HFCS are linked with increased energy intake and weight gain (31). Furthermore, we showed that the increase in the use of HFCS was concurrent with the increase in obesity rates in the United States. HFCS was introduced into the food supply just before 1970 and increased rapidly to constitute > 40% of the sweeteners used by 2000 (8). The increase in HFCS consumption just preceded the rapid increase in the prevalence of obesity that occurred between the National Center for Health Statistics survey in 1976 1980 and the next survey in 1988 1994 (35) (Figure 1).

HFCS is used in soft drinks, and HFCS and apple juice, which has 65% fructose, are used as the principal sweeteners for fruit drinks. The increasing consumption of calorically sweetened soft drinks has been associated with a decrease in the intake of milk (5, 8, 47, 48). This relation adds another mechanism by which HFCS consumption in beverages may be related to the epidemic of obesity. Per capita calcium intake decreased from 890 to 860 mg/d between 1970 and 1981 but has increased slowly since then (8). This was a mean 3% decrease that probably reflected a much larger decrease in calcium intake at the upper ends of the skewed distribution for intake. In US teenagers, total calcium

intake decreased by > 50 mg/d (> 10%) between 1977 and 1996 (49). A convincing set of epidemiologic and clinical studies suggests that dairy products may have a favorable effect on body weight and insulin resistance in both children and adults (50 52). During the interval from 1970 to 1990, the intake of whole milk decreased 58%. However, the intake of cheese, which is high in fat, increased and partially offset the decrease in calcium intake from milk (8). Because milk is a major source of dietary calcium for most humans, this decrease in milk intake may play an important role in the decrease in calcium in the diet.

One possible public health option is to address the sweet taste preference of humans by reducing HFCS and, if sweetness is needed, relying on artificial sweeteners to make up any difference in sweetness. It is becoming increasingly clear that soft drink consumption may be an important contributor to the epidemic of obesity, in part through the larger portion sizes of these beverages and through the increased intake of fructose from HFCS and sucrose (53). If HFCS acts as an agent in the disease, then reducing exposure to this agent may help to reduce the epidemic (54).

Some will question our measures of HFCS intake and availability. Our very conservative estimate of HFCS use and the Food and Drug Administration data showed high HFCS intakes for a large segment of the US population (39).

In conclusion, we believe that an argument can now be made that the use of HFCS in beverages should be reduced and that HFCS should be replaced with alternative noncaloric sweeteners. Sweetness is a preferred taste as well as an acquired one that may be enhanced by exposure to sweet foods. The hypothesis that providing sodas and juice drinks in which caloric sweeteners are partially or completely replaced with noncaloric sweeteners will help reduce the prevalence of obesity is worth testing. If the intake of calorically sweetened beverages is contributing to the current epidemic, then reducing the availability of these beverages by removing soda machines from schools would be a strategy worth considering, as would reducing the portion sizes of sodas that are commercially available (55).

We thank Dan Blanchette for programming assistance, Tom Swasey for graphics support, and Frances Dancy for support in administrative matters. We also thank Linda Adair for thoughtful comments on an early version of this article.

REFERENCES

1. Bray GA, Popkin BM. Dietary fat intake does affect obesity! Am J Clin Nutr 1998;68:115773.
2. Young LR, Nestle M. The contribution of expanding portion sizes to the US obesity epidemic. Am J Public Health 2002;92:2469.
3. Elliott SS, Keim NL, Stern JS, Teff K, Havel PJ. Fructose, weight gain, and the insulin resistance syndrome. Am J Clin Nutr 2002;76:91122.
4. Smith SM. High fructose corn syrup replaces sugar in processed food. Environ Nutr 1998;11:78.
5. Nielsen SJ, Siega-Riz AM, Popkin BM. Trends in energy intake in U.S. between 1977 and 1996: similar shifts seen across age groups. Obes Res 2002;10:370 8.
6. Higley NA, White JS. Trends in fructose availability and consumption in the United States. Food Technol 1991;45:118 22.
7. Vuilleumier S. Worldwide production of high-fructose syrup and crystalline fructose. Am J Clin Nutr 1993;58(suppl):733S 6S.
8. Putnam JJ, Allshouse JE. Food consumption, prices and expenditures, 197097. US Department of Agriculture Economic Research Service statistical bulletin no. 965, April 1999. Washington, DC: US Government Printing Office, 1999.
9. Krause MV, Mahan LK. Food, nutrition and diet therapy. 7th ed. Philadelphia: WB Saunders Company, 1984.

10. Hanover LM, White JS. Manufacturing, composition, and applications of fructose. Am J Clin Nutr 1993;58(suppl):724S32S.
11. Watt BK, Merrill AL. Composition of foods: raw, processed, prepared. Agriculture handbook no. 8. Washington, DC: US Government Printing Office, 1963.
12. Petersen KF, Laurent D, Yu C, Cline GW, Shulman GI. Stimulating effects of low-dose fructose on insulin-stimulated hepatic glycogen synthesis in humans. Diabetes 2001;50:1263 8.
13. Edwards DM, Todd JF, Mahmoudi M, et al. Glucagon-like peptide 1 has a physiological role in the control of postprandial glucose in humans: studies with the antagonist exendin 9 39. Diabetes 1999;48:86 93.
14. Vilsboll T, Krarup T, Madsbad S, Holst JJ. Both GLP-1 and GIP are insulinotropic at basal and postprandial glucose levels and contribute nearly equally to the incretin effect of a meal in healthy subjects. Regul Pept 2003;114:115 21.
15. Curry DL. Effects of mannose and fructose on the synthesis and secretion of insulin. Pancreas 1989;4:29.
16. Sato Y, Ito T, Udaka U, et al. Immunohistochemical localization of facilitated-diffusion glucose transporters in rat pancreatic islets. Tissue Cell 1996;28:637 43.
17. Schwarz J-M, Schutz Y, Froidevaux F, et al. Thermogenesis in men and women induced by fructose vs glucose added to a meal. Am J Clin Nutr 1989;49:667 74.
18. Schwartz MW, Woods SC, Porte D Jr, Seeley RJ, Baskin DG. Central nervous system control of food intake. Nature 2000;404:661 71.
19. Muller WM, Gregoire FM, Stanhope KL, et al. Evidence that glucose metabolism regulated leptin secretion from cultured rat adipocytes. Endocrinology 1998;39:551 8.
20. Havel PJ. Control of energy homeostasis and insulin action by adipocyte hormones: leptin, acylation stimulating protein, and adiponectin. Curr Opin Lipidol 2002;13:519.
21. Saad MF, Khan A, Sharma A, et al. Physiological insulinemia acutely modulated plasma leptin. Diabetes 1998;47:544 9.
22. Farooqi IS, Matarese G, Lord GM, et al. Beneficial effects of leptin on obesity, T cell hyporesponsiveness, and neuroendocrine/metabolic dysfunction of human congenital leptin deficiency. J Clin Invest 2002;110:1093 1103.
23. Farooqi IS, Keogh JM, Kamath S, et al. Partial leptin deficiency and human adiposity. Nature 2001;414:34 5.
24. Rosenbaum M, Murphy EM, Heymsfield SB, Matthews DE, Leibel RL. Low dose leptin administration reverses effects of sustained weight-reduction on energy expenditure and circulating concentrations of thyroid hormones. J Clin Endocrinol Metab 2002;87:2391 4.
25. Teff K, Elliot S, Tschoep MR, et al. Consuming high fructose meals reduces 24 hour plasma insulin and leptin concentrations, does not suppress circulating ghrelin, and increases postprandial and fasting triglycerides in women. Diabetes 2002;52(suppl):A408(abstr).
26. Mayes PA. Intermediary metabolism of fructose. Am J Clin Nutr 1993;58(suppl):754S 65S.
27. Bantle JP, Raatz SK, Thomas W, Georgopoulos A. Effects of dietary fructose on plasma lipids in healthy subjects. Am J Clin Nutr 2000;72:1128 34.
28. Sclafani A. Starch and sugar tastes in rodents: an update. Brain Res Bull 1991;27:383 6.
29. Mattes RD. Dietary compensation by humans for supplemental energy provided as ethanol or carbohydrate in fluids. Physiol Behav 1996;59:179 87.
30. DiMeglio DP, Mattes RD. Liquid versus solid carbohydrate: effects on food intake and body weight. Int J Obes Relat Metab Disord 2000;24:794 800.
31. Ludwig DS, Peterson KE, Gortmaker SL. Relation between consumption of sugar-sweetened drinks and childhood obesity: a prospective, observational analysis. Lancet 2001;357:505 8.
32. Raben A, Vasilaras TH, Moller AC, Astrup A. Sucrose compared with artifical sweeteners: different effects on ad libitum food intake and body weight after 10 wk of supplementation in overweight subjects. Am J Clin Nutr 2002;76:721 9.
33. Hurt-Jones M. The allergy self-help cookbook: over 350 natural food recipes, free of all common food allergens. Emmaus, PA: Rodale Press, 2002.
34. Park YK, Yetley E. Intakes and food sources of fructose in the United States. Am J Clin Nutr 1993;58(suppl):737S 47S.
35. Flegal KM, Carroll MD, Ogden CL, Johnson CL. Prevalence and trends in obesity among US adults, 1999 2000. JAMA 2002;288:1723 7.
36. Rizek RL. The 1977 78 Nationwide Food Consumption Survey. Fam Econ Rev 1978;2001;4:37.
37. Tippett KS, Mickle SJ, Goldman JD, Sykes KE, Cook DA, Sebastian RS. Food and nutrient intakes by individuals in the United States, 1 day, 1989 91. Continuing Survey of Food Intakes by Individuals 1989 91, Nationwide Food Surveys report no. 91-2. Beltsville, MD: US Department of Agriculture, Agriculture Research Service, 1995.
38. Tippett KS, Cypel YS. Design and operation: the Continuing Survey of Food Intakes by Individuals and the Diet and Health Knowledge Survey 1994 96. Continuing Survey of Food Intakes by Individuals 1994 96, Nationwide Food Surveys report no. 96-1. Beltsville, MD: US Department of Agriculture, Agriculture Research Service, 1998.
39. United States Department of Agriculture, Agricultural Research Service. Design and operation: the Continuing Survey of Food Intakes by Individuals and the Diet and Health Knowledge Survey, 1994 96 and 1998. Beltsville, MD: US Department of Agriculture, Agricultural Research Service, 2000.
40. Glinsmann WH, Irausquin H, Park YK. Evaluation of health aspects of sugars contained in carbohydrate sweeteners. Report of Sugars Task Force, 1986. J Nutr 1986;116:S12 16.
41. Popkin BM, Nielsen SJ. The sweetening of the worlds diet. Obes Res 2003;11:1325 32.
42. Rankinen T, Perusse L, Weisnagel SJ, Snyder EE, Chagnon YC, Bouchard C. The human obesity gene map: the 2001 update. Obes Res 2002;10:196 243.
43. World Health Organization. Obesity: preventing and managing the global epidemic. Report of a WHO consultation. World Health Organ Tech Rep Ser 2000;894:ixii, 1 253.
44. Prentice AM, Jebb SA. Obesity in Britain: gluttony or sloth? Br Med J 1995;311:437 9.
45. Troiano RP, Flegal KM. Overweight children and adolescents: description, epidemiology, and demographics. Pediatrics 1998;101:497 504.
46. McDevitt RM, Poppitt SD, Murgatroyd PR, Prentice AM. Macronutrient disposal during controlled overfeeding with glucose, fructose, sucrose, or fat in lean and obese women. Am J Clin Nutr 2000;72:369 77.
47. Cavadini C, Siega-Riz AM, Popkin BM. US adolescent food intake trends from 1965 to 1996. Arch Dis Child 2000;83:18 24.
48. Harnack L, Stang J, Story M. Soft drink consumption among US children and adolescents: nutritional consequences. J Am Diet Assoc 1999;99:436 41.
49. Carruth BR, Skinner JD. The role of dietary calcium and other nutrients in moderating body fat in preschool children. Int J Obes Relat Metab Disord 2001;25:559 66.
50. Davies KM, Heaney RP, Recker RR, et al. Calcium intake and body weight. J Clin Endocrinol Metab 2000;85:4635 8.
51. Pereira MA, Jacobs DR Jr, Van Horn L, et al. Dairy consumption, obesity, and the insulin resistance syndrome in young adults: the CARDIA study. JAMA 2002;287:2081 9.
52. Zemel MB, Shi H, Greer B, Dirienzo D, Zemel PC. Regulation of adiposity by dietary calcium. FASEB J 2000;14:1132 8.
53. Barr SI, McCarron DA, Heaney RP, et al. Effects of increased consumption of fluid milk on energy and nutrient intake, body weight, and cardiovascular risk factors in healthy older adults. J Am Diet Assoc 2000;100:810 7.
54. Nielsen SJ, Popkin BM. Patterns and trends in portion sizes, 1977 1998. JAMA 2003;289:450 3.
55. Bray GA. The fluoride hypothesis and diobesity. How to prevent diabetes by preventing obesity. In: Mederios-Neto G, Halpern A, Bouchard C, eds. Progress in obesity research: 9. Proceedings of the 9th International Congress on Obesity. Surrey, United Kingdom: John Libbey Eurotext, 2003:26 8.

ISBN 1-933087-11-0
ISSN 1542-1899
Fourth Printing
Printed in the United States of America

The chart on page 49 was adapted with permission from Mokdad, A.H. "Actual causes of death in the United States." *Journal of the American Medical Association* Vol. 291, No. 10 (March 10, 2004): 1240.

Bray, G.A. et al. "Consumption of high-fructose corn syrup in beverages may play a role in the epidemic of obesity." Reprinted with permission from the *American Journal of Clinical Nutrition* Vol. 79, No. 4 (April 2004): 537–543.
Copyright © 2004, The American Society for Clinical Nutrition, Inc.

The Johns Hopkins White Papers are published yearly by Medletter Associates, Inc.

Visit our Web site for information on Johns Hopkins Health After 50 publications, which include White Papers on specific disorders, home medical encyclopedias, consumer reference guides to drugs and medical tests, and our monthly newsletter The Johns Hopkins Medical Letter: Health After 50.
www.HopkinsAfter50.com

The Johns Hopkins White Papers

Paul Candon
Managing Editor

Catherine Richter
Senior Editor

Samantha B. Cassetty, M.S., R.D.
Senior Writer

Devon Schuyler
Consulting Editor

Kimberly Flynn
Writer/Researcher

Leslie Maltese-McGill
Copy Editor

Tim Jeffs
Art Director

Vincent Mejia
Graphic Designer

Betsy Meredith Rigo
Editorial Assistant

Robert Duckwall
Medical Illustrator

Kate Brackney
Intern

Johns Hopkins Health After 50 Publications

Rodney Friedman
Editor and Publisher

Thomas Dickey
Editorial Director

Tom Damrauer, M.L.S.
Chief of Information Resources

Jerry Loo
Product Manager

Darren Leiser
Promotions Coordinator

Joan Mullally
Head of Business Development

PROSTATE DISORDERS

H. Ballentine Carter, M.D.

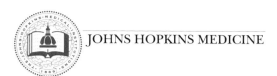
JOHNS HOPKINS MEDICINE

Dear Readers:

The prevalence of prostate disorders has led to a variety of treatment options—but often no clear consensus from the medical community on the best choice for a given situation. This year, a study even called into question the definition of a "normal" prostate specific antigen (PSA) level. To help men make objective decisions, this year's White Paper reviews the latest knowledge and advances in the diagnosis, management, and treatment of prostate disorders.

Here are some of this year's highlights:

- The most recent data on **finasteride** for men with benign prostatic hyperplasia (BPH). (page 13)
- Choosing the best treatment for **BPH**. (page 20)
- New research on the role of **selenium** in prostate cancer. (page 26)
- The role of **PSA velocity** in determining who should have prostate cancer surgery. (page 30)
- The implications of finding **prostatic intraepithelial neoplasia (PIN)** on biopsy. (page 31)
- A practical guide to **getting a second (or third or fourth) opinion**. (page 38)
- Evaluating the newest drugs for **erectile dysfunction**. (page 61)
- The impact of **postejaculatory pain** in men with chronic prostatitis. (page 63)

I hope that this information will be helpful in educating and guiding patients who are interested in prostate disease.

Sincerely,

H. Ballentine Carter, M.D.
Professor
Department of Urology and Oncology
Johns Hopkins University School of Medicine

P.S. Don't forget to visit HopkinsWhitePapers.com for the latest news on prostate disorders and other information that will complement your Johns Hopkins White Paper.

THE AUTHOR

H. Ballentine Carter, M.D., graduated from the Medical University of South Carolina and completed his residency training at New York Hospital-Cornell Medical Center in New York City. Currently, he is a professor of urology and oncology and the director of Adult Urology at the Johns Hopkins University School of Medicine.

Dr. Carter has written extensively on the diagnosis and staging of prostate cancer. In particular, he has researched prostate specific antigen (PSA) levels: how they change as men age, their variability in men with prostate cancer, and their use in staging, predicting, and managing prostate cancer. At this time, he is working closely with the Baltimore Longitudinal Study of Aging to evaluate the development of prostate disease with age. Dr. Carter has had research articles published in *The Journal of Urology, Urology, Cancer Research,* the *Journal of the American Medical Association,* and the *Journal of the National Cancer Institute.*

CONTENTS

Structure of the Prostate . . . . .p. 1

Benign Prostatic Hyperplasia (BPH)
Causes of BPH . . . . .p. 2
Symptoms of BPH . . . . .p. 4
Diagnosis of BPH . . . . .p. 5
   Medical History, Physical Examination, Laboratory Tests, Special Diagnostic Tests
When is BPH Treatment Necessary? . . . . .p. 9
Treatment Options for BPH . . . . .p. 9
   Watchful Waiting, Phytotherapy, Medication, Surgery, Minimally Invasive Therapy,
   Stents

Prostate Cancer
Causes of Prostate Cancer . . . . .p. 24
Prevention of Prostate Cancer . . . . .p. 28
Symptoms of Prostate Cancer . . . . .p. 28
Diagnosis of Prostate Cancer . . . . .p. 28
   Digital Rectal Examination, Prostate Specific Antigen (PSA) Test, Transrectal
   Ultrasound, Prostate Biopsy, Other Diagnostic Tests, Determining the Extent of Cancer
Choosing a Prostate Cancer Treatment . . . . .p. 36
Treatment Options for Prostate Cancer . . . . .p. 37
   Watchful Waiting, Radical Prostatectomy, External Beam Radiation Therapy,
   Brachytherapy, Cryotherapy, Hormone Therapy
Managing Side Effects of Treatment . . . . .p. 56
   Urinary Incontinence, Erectile Dysfunction

Prostatitis
Causes of Prostatitis . . . . .p. 62
Diagnosis of Prostatitis . . . . .p. 63
Treatment of Prostatitis . . . . .p. 63

Chart: Medications Used in the Treatment of Benign Prostatic Hyperplasia . . . . . . .p. 14
Chart: Medications Used in Hormone Treatment of Prostate Cancer . . . . .p. 50

Glossary . . . . p. 65
Health Information Organizations and Support Groups . . . . .p. 68
Leading Hospitals for Urology . . . . .p. 69
Selected Medical Journal Article . . . . .p. 70

PROSTATE DISORDERS

The prostate is a gland that sits below a man's bladder and in front of his rectum. This gland is the size and shape of a crab apple and surrounds the urethra, the tube that carries urine away from the bladder.

The prostate gland has several functions. First, it produces prostatic fluid, which is a component of semen. Second, it serves as a valve to keep both urine and semen flowing in the proper direction. Finally, it pumps semen into the urethra during orgasm. (For more information about how the prostate works, see the feature on page 3.)

When a man reaches his mid-40s and beyond, the inner portion of the prostate begins to enlarge and may put pressure on the urethra, a condition called benign prostatic hyperplasia (BPH). BPH affects about 50% of men age 51 to 60 and about 90% of men older than age 80. Although it can cause a variety of symptoms, BPH is not life-threatening.

Prostate cancer is a much more serious health problem. After skin cancer, it is the second most common cancer in men and is second only to lung cancer as a cause of cancer deaths. In 2004, about 230,000 men were diagnosed with prostate cancer, and about 30,000 died of the disease. The good news is that reliable diagnostic tests and numerous treatment options are available for prostate cancer, and death rates from prostate cancer are on the decline.

BPH and prostate cancer may have similar symptoms, but the two conditions are unrelated. Having BPH neither increases nor decreases an individual's risk of prostate cancer, although a man may have both conditions at the same time.

A third condition that can affect the prostate is prostatitis, an inflammation of the prostate that may cause pain in the lower back and in the area between the scrotum and rectum. Prostatitis may also cause chills, fever, and a general feeling of malaise. Nearly half of all men will develop prostatitis in their lifetime.

STRUCTURE OF THE PROSTATE

The prostate is made up of two kinds of cells: glandular (epithelial) cells and smooth muscle cells. The glandular cells produce part of the fluid portion of semen. The smooth muscles contract to push prostatic fluid into the urethra during ejaculation. These muscles are involuntary (not under the control of the individual), like those of the intestines and blood vessels.

The prostate can be divided into three main regions, or zones. Immediately surrounding the urethra is a thin layer called the transition zone; it is surrounded by the central zone, which is followed by the largest and outermost portion, the peripheral zone. BPH typically develops in the transition zone, while prostate cancer usually occurs in the peripheral zone.

Benign Prostatic Hyperplasia (BPH)

BPH is the most common benign (noncancerous) tumor in men. As is true for prostate cancer, BPH occurs more often in Western than in Eastern countries, such as Japan and China, and may be more common among blacks than among whites. Not long ago, a study also found a possible genetic link for BPH in men younger than age 65 who have a very enlarged prostate: Their male relatives were four times more likely than other men to need BPH surgery at some point in their lives, and their brothers had a sixfold increase in risk.

Symptoms related to BPH are present in about one in four men by age 55 and in half of men by age 75. However, treatment is necessary only if symptoms become bothersome. By age 80, between 20% and 30% of men experience BPH symptoms severe enough to require treatment. The main treatment options are: medications that either shrink the prostate or relax the prostate muscle tissue that constricts the urethra; surgery to remove excess prostate tissue; or heat therapy to vaporize excess prostate tissue.

CAUSES OF BPH

In BPH, the enlargement of glandular tissue and the tightening of smooth muscles may obstruct the urethra. Although the cause of BPH is not understood, testosterone (a male sex hormone) and aging are essential for the development of the condition. Animal studies suggest that the female sex hormone estrogen also may play a role in BPH.

The word *hyperplasia* refers to any abnormal accumulation of cells that causes enlargement of a body part or organ. BPH occurs when an increase in the number of prostate cells produces discrete nodules in the prostate. The increase is due to a slowing of the normal rate of death of these cells, rather than to a heightened production.

How BPH and Prostate Cancer Affect the Urinary System

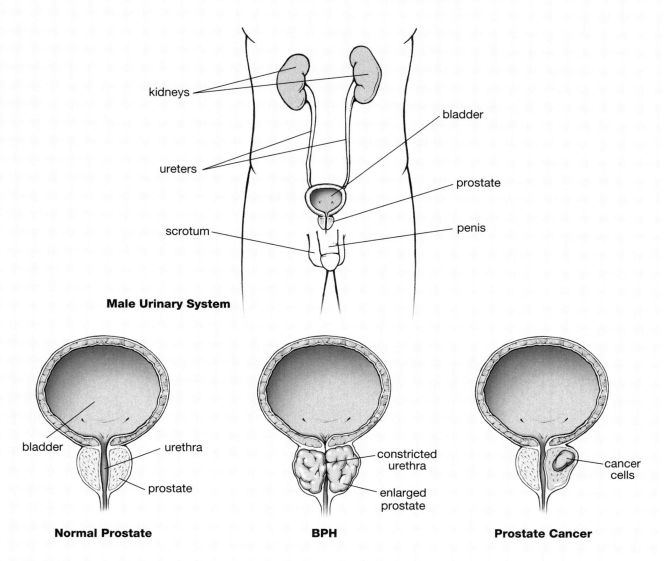

Male Urinary System

kidneys

bladder

ureters

prostate

scrotum

penis

bladder

urethra

prostate

Normal Prostate

constricted
urethra

enlarged
prostate

BPH

cancer
cells

Prostate Cancer

The prostate is a reproductive organ that is situated just below the bladder. It completely surrounds the top portion of the urethra—the channel through which both urine and seminal fluid (including sperm) pass from the body.

The prostate's major function is to produce part of the fluid portion of semen that transports sperm. Glandular tissue within the prostate forms tiny chambers that steadily secrete the prostatic fluid. During ejaculation, smooth muscle in the prostate contracts, pushing the prostatic fluid through ducts or conduits into the urethra, where it mixes with other fluids from the seminal vesicles to carry sperm out of the body. (Sperm is produced in the testes and passes into the urethra via a tube called the vas deferens.)

Although the prostate plays no known direct role in the urinary system, prostate disorders often cause urinary problems owing to the gland's close proximity to the bladder and urethra. The urinary tract begins with the kidneys—located at either side of the base of the rib cage—which filter excess water, salts, and impurities from the bloodstream to form urine. Urine then passes through two long tubes, called ureters, and is stored in the bladder until it is released through the urethra during urination. Enlargement of the prostate due to benign prostatic hyperplasia or cancer, for example, can constrict the urethra, causing a variety of urinary symptoms (such as frequent or difficult voiding) and may eventually damage the bladder itself. Prostate infections can cause painful or burning urination.

The nodules are surrounded by a capsule that contains smooth muscle cells, which also can increase in number.

Whether or not prostate enlargement puts pressure on the urethra and increases resistance to the flow of urine depends on the location of the nodules. Although the transition zone accounts for only about 5% of the prostate mass, the nodules in men with BPH occur primarily in this region. Because the transition zone envelops the urethra, the excess tissue may obstruct urine flow. In addition, the smooth muscle cells surrounding the nodules may contract and obstruct the urethra. Consequently, some men with a very enlarged prostate may have no urethral obstruction, while others with mild enlargement may have marked symptoms because a nodule is located where it compresses the urethra, or because the smooth muscles become too tight.

To compensate for the obstruction of the urethra, the muscular wall of the bladder contracts more strongly to expel urine. These stronger contractions lead to a thickened bladder wall, which decreases the bladder's capacity to store urine. Over time, the bladder holds smaller and smaller amounts of urine, resulting in a need to urinate more frequently. As the urethral obstruction worsens, the contractions can no longer empty the bladder completely. Urine retained in the bladder (residual urine) may then become infected or lead to the formation of bladder stones (calculi). Less often, the kidneys become damaged, either as a result of increased pressure on them from the overworked bladder or because an infection has spread from the bladder to the kidneys.

SYMPTOMS OF BPH

BPH can produce lower urinary tract symptoms. These symptoms include difficulty in starting to urinate, a weak urinary stream, a sudden, strong desire to urinate (urinary urgency), an increased frequency of urination, and a sensation that the bladder is not empty after urinating. In fact, BPH can prevent the bladder from emptying completely (urinary retention), and as the bladder becomes more sensitive to retained urine, a man may become unable to control the bladder (incontinent) because he is unable to respond quickly enough to urinary urgency. A bladder infection or stone can cause burning or pain during urination. Blood in the urine (hematuria) may be a sign of BPH, but most men with BPH do not experience it.

At times, men with BPH may suddenly become unable to urinate at all, even though their condition is responding to treatment. This problem, called acute urinary retention, requires immediate medical attention in a hospital emergency room. It is easily treated with catheterization—passing a tube through the urethra into the bladder to allow urine to drain from the bladder. Acute urinary retention may be triggered by an extended delay in urination, urinary tract infection, alcohol intake, and use of certain drugs such as antidepressants, decongestants, and tranquilizers. Acute urinary retention often occurs unexpectedly, and it is impossible to predict whether a man with only modest lower urinary tract symptoms will develop this condition. Some men who experience acute urinary retention need to undergo surgery to remove excess prostate tissue.

DIAGNOSIS OF BPH

The International Prostate Symptom Score questionnaire, also called the American Urological Association Symptom Index, is used to assess the severity of lower urinary tract symptoms (see page 7 for the questionnaire). It can also help doctors and patients decide on treatment. However, it cannot be used alone for diagnosis for two main reasons. First, other diseases can cause lower urinary tract symptoms similar to those of BPH. Second, as men (and women) age, the bladder naturally becomes less efficient at storing urine and symptoms of urinary frequency and urgency become more common.

Therefore, a careful medical history, physical examination, and laboratory tests are required to exclude such conditions as urethral stricture (narrowing of the urethra) and bladder disease. In fact, some reports indicate that as many as 30% of men who undergo surgery for BPH show no evidence of urethral obstruction (meaning their symptoms were due to another cause).

Medical History

A medical history helps doctors identify the presence of conditions that can mimic BPH, such as urethral stricture, bladder cancer, bladder stones, bladder infection, or neurogenic bladder (problems with holding or emptying urine due to a neurological disorder). Strictures can result from urethral damage caused by trauma, catheter insertion, or an infection such as gonorrhea. Bladder cancer is suspected when a man has a history of blood in the urine. Pain in the penis or bladder area may indicate bladder stones or infection. A neurogenic bladder is suggested when an individual has diabetes or a neurological disease such as multiple sclerosis or Parkinson's disease, or has

NEW RESEARCH

Alfuzosin Improves Recovery After Acute Urinary Retention

Alfuzosin (UroXatral) can help restore normal urination after a bout of acute urinary retention (AUR), researchers report. This should help reduce the need for emergency surgery for benign prostatic hyperplasia (BPH).

In AUR, a complication that occurs in 1% to 2% of older men with BPH, voluntary urination suddenly becomes impossible. Treatment requires immediate medical attention, catheter insertion and, often, surgery. Some men can avoid emergency surgery, but only if they are able to void on their own when the catheter is removed—a procedure called trial without catheter. In the current study, alfuzosin improved the odds of successful trial without catheter.

Men received 10 mg per day of the drug or placebo over three days while a catheter was in place for AUR treatment. Among the 236 men given the drug, 62% returned to normal urination after trial without catheter, while 48% of the 121 men on placebo did. Men over 65 and those who had retained 1,000 mL or more of urine were more likely to fail trial without catheter, but the drug nearly doubled chances of success among these men.

The researchers conclude that alfuzosin can help men avoid emergency surgery for BPH, which is riskier than planned surgery.

THE JOURNAL OF UROLOGY
Volume 171, page 2316
June 2004

experienced a recent deterioration in sexual function.

A thorough medical history also includes questions about previous urinary tract infections or prostatitis, and any worsening of urinary symptoms when taking cold or sinus medications. The physician will also ask whether any medications (over the counter and prescription), nutritional supplements, or herbal remedies are being taken, because some of them can worsen or improve symptoms of BPH.

Physical Examination
The physical examination usually begins with the doctor observing the patient as he urinates to completion to detect any urinary irregularities. The doctor will manually examine the lower abdomen to check for the presence of a mass, which may indicate an enlarged bladder due to retained urine. In addition, a digital rectal exam—to assess the size, shape, and consistency of the prostate—is performed. This important examination, which involves the insertion of a gloved, lubricated finger into the rectum, is mildly uncomfortable. The detection of hard or firm areas in the prostate raises the suspicion of prostate cancer. (For more information on the digital rectal exam, see the feature on page 27.)

If the medical history suggests possible neurological disease, the physical examination may also look for abnormalities such as a loss of sensation or weakness in the lower body, which indicates that the urinary symptoms are likely the result of a neurogenic bladder.

Laboratory Tests
Urinalysis—examination of a urine sample under a microscope—is performed in all patients with lower urinary tract symptoms. It is often the only laboratory test required when symptoms are mild (International Prostate Symptom Score of 1 to 7) and no other abnormalities are suspected from the medical history and physical examination. A urine culture is done when a urinary infection is suspected. In the presence of more severe or chronic symptoms of BPH, blood creatinine or blood urea nitrogen and hemoglobin levels are measured to rule out kidney damage and anemia, respectively.

Measuring blood levels of prostate specific antigen (PSA; see pages 29–32) is generally recommended. PSA values alone are not helpful in determining whether symptoms are due to BPH or prostate cancer because both conditions can elevate PSA levels. However, knowing a man's PSA level may help predict how rapidly his prostate will increase in size over time and whether problems such as urinary retention are more likely to occur.

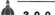

Do You Need Treatment for BPH?

The International Prostate Symptom Score questionnaire (see below) was developed to help men evaluate the severity of their symptoms from benign prostatic hyperplasia (BPH). This self-administered test can help determine which treatment is needed, if any. Symptoms are classified as mild (1 to 7), moderate (8 to 19), or severe (20 to 35). Generally, no treatment is needed if symptoms are mild; moderate symptoms usually call for some form of treatment; and severe symptoms indicate that surgery is most likely to be effective.

Circle one number on each line.

	Not at all	Less than 1 time in 5	Less than half the time	About half the time	More than half the time	Almost always
1. Over the past month, how often have you had the sensation of not emptying your bladder completely after you finished urinating?	0	1	2	3	4	5
2. Over the past month, how often have you had to urinate again less than two hours after you finished urinating?	0	1	2	3	4	5
3. Over the past month, how often have you found you stopped and started again several times when you urinated?	0	1	2	3	4	5
4. Over the past month, how often have you found it difficult to postpone urination?	0	1	2	3	4	5
5. Over the past month, how often have you had a weak urinary stream?	0	1	2	3	4	5
6. Over the past month, how often have you had to push or strain to begin urination?	0	1	2	3	4	5
	None	**1 time**	**2 times**	**3 times**	**4 times**	**5x or more**
7. Over the past month, how many times did you most typically get up to urinate from the time you went to bed at night until the time you got up in the morning?	0	1	2	3	4	5

Total Score: _____

Source: American Urological Association.

Special Diagnostic Tests

Men with moderate to severe symptoms (International Prostate Symptom Score of 8 or higher) may benefit from one or more of the following tests: uroflowmetry, pressure-flow urodynamic studies, imaging studies, filling cystometry, or cystoscopy.

Uroflowmetry. This noninvasive test uses an electronic device to measure the speed of urine flow. If the flow rate is slow, obstruction of the urethra may be present; if the flow rate is high, obstruction is unlikely and therapy for BPH will not be effective in most cases. Normally, urine flow rate is 15 mL per second or greater.

Pressure-flow urodynamic studies. These studies measure bladder pressure during urination by placing a recording device into the bladder and, often, into the rectum as well. The difference between the pressures in the bladder and the rectum indicates the pressure generated when the bladder muscle contracts. A high pressure accompanied by a low urine flow rate indicates obstruction of the urethra. A low pressure with a low urine flow rate signals an abnormality in the bladder itself, for example, due to a neurological disorder.

Imaging studies. In general, imaging studies are performed only in patients with blood in the urine, urinary tract infection, abnormal kidney function, previous surgery on the urinary tract, or a history of urinary tract stones.

Ultrasound is the most commonly used imaging study in men with lower urinary tract symptoms. The test involves pressing a microphone-like device onto the skin covering the urinary system. The device emits sound waves that reflect off internal organs; the reflections are used to create an image of these organs. Ultrasound can be used to search for structural abnormalities in the kidneys or bladder, to determine the amount of residual urine in the bladder after urination, to detect the presence of stones in the bladder, and to estimate the size of the prostate.

Less commonly, another imaging study called an intravenous pyelogram may be performed. It involves taking x-rays of the urinary tract after a dye is injected into the body. The dye makes urine visible on the x-rays and shows any obstructions of the urinary tract and any urinary tract stones.

Filling cystometry. This test involves filling the bladder with fluid and measuring how much pressure builds up in the bladder and how full it is when the urge to urinate occurs. Filling cystometry is recommended only for evaluating bladder function in men who have hematuria, urinary tract infection, renal insufficiency, or a history of urolithiasis (calcium deposits in the urinary tract) or urinary tract surgery.

Cystoscopy. In this procedure, a cystoscope (a type of telescope) is passed through the urethra into the bladder to directly visualize the urethra and bladder. Cystoscopy is usually performed just before prostate surgery to guide the procedure or to look for abnormalities of the urethra or bladder.

WHEN IS BPH TREATMENT NECESSARY?

The progression of BPH cannot be predicted for any individual. Symptoms and objective measurements of urethral obstruction can remain stable for many years and may even improve over time in as many as a third of men. In one study from the Mayo Clinic, urinary symptoms did not worsen over a 3½-year period in 73% of men with mild BPH.

Men who eventually need treatment for BPH usually experience a progressive decrease in the size and force of their urinary stream or a sensation of incomplete emptying of their bladder. Although nocturia (frequent nighttime urination) is one of the most annoying symptoms of BPH, it does not predict the need for future treatment.

If worsening urethral obstruction is left untreated, complications can occur. Some examples are a thickened bladder with a reduced capacity to store urine, infected residual urine, bladder stones, and a backup of pressure that damages the kidneys.

Decisions regarding treatment are based on the severity of symptoms (as assessed by the International Prostate Symptom Score questionnaire), the extent of urinary tract damage, and the man's age and overall health. In general, no treatment (called watchful waiting) is needed in those who have only a few symptoms and are not bothered by them. Treatment—usually surgical—is required in the following situations: kidney damage due to inadequate bladder emptying; complete inability to urinate after treatment of acute urinary retention; incontinence due to overfilling or increased sensitivity of the bladder; bladder stones; infected residual urine; recurrent blood in the urine despite treatment with medication; and symptoms that do not respond to treatment and are troublesome enough to diminish quality of life.

Treatment decisions are most difficult for men with moderate symptoms (International Prostate Symptom Score of 8 to 19). Each of these men must determine whether the symptoms bother him enough, or interfere with his life enough, to merit treatment. When selecting a treatment, both patient and doctor must weigh the effectiveness of various therapies against their side effects and costs.

TREATMENT OPTIONS FOR BPH

The main treatment options for BPH are watchful waiting, phytotherapy, medication, surgery, and minimally invasive therapy. If medications do not relieve symptoms in a man who is not a candidate for surgery (for example, because he is unable to withstand the rigors of surgery), urethral obstruction and incontinence may be managed with intermittent catheterization or with an indwelling Foley catheter (a catheter with an inflated balloon at its end to hold it in place in the bladder). The Foley catheter is usually changed monthly.

Watchful Waiting

Because the progression of and complications from BPH are unpredictable, watchful waiting—meaning that the patient is closely monitored but no immediate treatment is attempted—is best for those with minimal symptoms that are not especially bothersome. With this treatment option, physician visits are needed about once a year to review the progress of symptoms, carry out a physical examination, and perform a few simple laboratory tests.

During watchful waiting, men should adopt certain lifestyle measures to help relieve symptoms and prevent them from worsening. For example, they should not take over-the-counter antihistamines and decongestants and should avoid delaying urination. They also need to be careful about their fluid intake by avoiding beverages that contain caffeine, limiting alcohol intake and the amount of fluid consumed at any one time, and avoiding beverages after 7 P.M. Limiting spicy or salty foods, engaging in regular physical activity, doing Kegel exercises (see page 57), and keeping warm can be helpful as well.

Phytotherapy

Some people elect to use saw palmetto and other phytotherapeutic agents (plant-derived substances), including African plum, trinovin, South African star grass, flower pollen extract, soy, stinging nettle, zinc, rye pollen, selenium, purple cone flower, and pumpkin seeds, to manage their BPH symptoms. Except for saw palmetto, no solid evidence exists that any of these substances are effective in the management of BPH.

A 2002 meta-analysis of saw palmetto that included data from 21 randomized studies and more than 3,000 men with BPH revealed that men taking saw palmetto were 76% more likely to have improved urinary symptoms than men taking a placebo. In addition, saw palmetto produced improvements similar to those seen with finasteride (Proscar; a drug commonly prescribed for BPH) in terms of urinary symptoms and peak urine flow.

Hematuria: Blood in the Urine

This alarming symptom has a variety of possible causes, some not serious.

Hematuria is the presence of red blood cells in the urine. In gross hematuria, these cells are visible to the naked eye, appearing as spots of blood or blood clots in the toilet water or turning the water pink, bright red, reddish-brown, or cola-colored. In microscopic hematuria, the red blood cells can be seen only upon examination of the urine under a microscope. Because hematuria may be caused by a serious condition, all people with gross hematuria and those over age 40 with microscopic hematuria should receive a prompt and thorough medical evaluation.

Causes of the Bleeding

Hematuria is the result of bleeding in the urinary tract—which includes a man's kidneys, bladder, prostate, and urethra. The bleeding can stem from many causes: infection, inflammation, trauma, cancer, or kidney or bladder stones. It also can be a symptom of benign prostatic hyperplasia or prostatitis. Bleeding disorders and anticoagulant medications such as warfarin (Coumadin) may also cause or contribute to hematuria.

However, hematuria is not always indicative of a serious condition. Vigorous exercise can cause blood to be excreted in the urine, but this usually lasts no more than two days. Urethral catheterization can also cause temporary hematuria. Also, pigmenturia—a condition that mimics blood

in the urine—results from eating foods or taking medications that discolor the urine but involves no bleeding. (These foods include beets, blackberries, blueberries, fava beans, rhubarb, paprika, and foods and medications containing red or dark food coloring.) Finally, what may appear to be blood in the urine may actually stem from blood in the semen, which is usually not a serious condition.

Doctors can find no cause for hematuria in up to 10% of cases, and some 9% to 18% of healthy people have microscopic hematuria.

Diagnosing the Bleeding

Both gross hematuria and microscopic hematuria can be evaluated in a doctor's office, although some patients with gross hematuria may seek an emergency room evaluation.

Either way, an assessment includes taking a medical history and asking about recent food and drug intake, exercise, and urological procedures. The doctor will ask about specific features of the blood in the urine, including if there is any associated pain or irritation, whether blood appears at the beginning or end of the urine stream, how much blood is in the urine, and if any blood clots are present.

The doctor will then try to determine the cause of the bleeding by performing a number of tests. These

can include urinalysis (to look for red and white blood cells, protein, or chemicals), urine culture, blood tests, genital and rectal exams (to look for prostate disease), and a study to image the upper part of the urinary tract (kidney and ureters), which might include an intravenous pyelogram (an x-ray of the urinary tract) or computed tomography (CT). In addition, cytoscopy (inserting a flexible tube through the urethra to view the bladder) is performed to directly visualize the lower part or the urinary tract (urethra and bladder).

Microscopic hematuria usually indicates a kidney problem is present, and gross hematuria and blood clots typically result from a problem in the bladder, prostate, or urethra. In addition, doctors assume that painless, gross hematuria is the result of cancer until malignancy is ruled out.

Stopping the Bleeding

Therapy depends on the exact cause, and treating the underlying cause should stop the bleeding. If the cause involves the bladder, prostate, or urethra, the patient should seek treatment from a urologist. If the bleeding originates from kidney disease for which surgery would not be corrective (medical renal disease), follow-up with a nephrologist is necessary. Some patients may require catheter irrigation of the bladder to remove any clots that might be blocking urine flow.

In the meta-analysis, side effects of saw palmetto were mild and infrequent. Erectile dysfunction occurred in 1% of men taking saw palmetto and 5% of men taking finasteride. Other side effects of saw palmetto include headache, dizziness, nausea, and mild abdominal pain.

If saw palmetto is going to work, it usually does so within the first month of treatment. Therefore, saw palmetto should be stopped if no improvement in symptoms occurs after a month of use. If saw palmetto relieves symptoms, continue taking it, but be sure to inform your doctor. The typical dose of saw palmetto is 160 mg taken twice daily. Supplements that contain 85% to 95% free fatty acids and sterols are the most likely to be effective.

Medication

Medication is a relatively new development in the treatment of BPH; data are still being gathered on the benefits and possible side effects of long-term drug therapy. Currently, two types of drugs—5-alpha-reductase inhibitors and alpha-1-adrenergic blockers—are used to treat BPH. Preliminary research suggests that these drugs improve symptoms in 30% to 60% of men, but it is not yet possible to predict who will respond to medication or which drug will work best for which patient.

5-alpha-reductase inhibitors. Two 5-alpha-reductase inhibitors are used to treat BPH: finasteride (Propecia, Proscar) and dutasteride (Avodart). These drugs inhibit the enzyme 5-alpha-reductase, which converts testosterone to dihydrotestosterone, the major male sex hormone within the cells of the prostate. These drugs work best in men with larger prostates (40 g or more), whose symptoms are likely the result of physical obstruction of the urethra.

The two 5-alpha-reductase inhibitors are equally effective. Both can reduce the size of the prostate by 20% to 30%, relieve BPH symptoms, and reduce the risk of acute urinary retention and the need for BPH surgery. However, these drugs must be continued indefinitely to prevent symptom recurrence. Moreover, it may take as long as a year to achieve the maximum benefits from these drugs.

Finasteride and dutasteride cause relatively few side effects. Erectile dysfunction (the inability to achieve a full erection) occurs in 5% to 8% of men, decreased libido (sex drive) in 3% to 6%, reduced ejaculate in 1%, and breast enlargement or tenderness in 0.5%. Sexual side effects tend to decrease with time, and they disappear when the drug is stopped. Breast-related side effects do not diminish with time but often improve once the drug is no longer taken.

Another side effect of 5-alpha-reductase inhibitors is a lowering of PSA levels by about 50%, which may interfere with the results of PSA tests to detect prostate cancer (if not taken into account). To prevent this problem, men should have a PSA test before starting treatment with a 5-alpha-reductase inhibitor so that subsequent PSA values can be interpreted in light of this baseline value. If a man is already taking a 5-alpha-reductase inhibitor and no baseline PSA level was obtained, the results of a current PSA test should be multiplied by two to estimate the true PSA level. A PSA level that falls less than 50% after a year of treatment with a 5-alpha-reductase inhibitor suggests either that the drug is not being taken as directed or that prostate cancer might be present. Any increase in PSA levels while taking a 5-alpha-reductase inhibitor also raises the possibility of prostate cancer. The fall in PSA levels disappears when the 5-alpha-reductase inhibitor is stopped.

Alpha-1-adrenergic blockers (alpha-blockers). These drugs relax smooth muscle tissue within the prostate by blocking the effect of nerve impulses that signal the muscles to contract. As a result, daily use of an alpha-blocker may increase urinary flow and relieve symptoms of urinary frequency, urinary urgency, and nocturia. Several alpha-blockers—alfuzosin (UroXatral), doxazosin (Cardura), tamsulosin (Flomax), and terazosin (Hytrin)—have been approved by the U.S. Food and Drug Administration (FDA) for the treatment of BPH.

An advantage of alpha-blockers over 5-alpha-reductase inhibitors is that they work almost immediately. Another advantage is that they can treat high blood pressure (hypertension) when it is present. However, whether alpha-blockers are superior to 5-alpha-reductase inhibitors may depend more on the size of the prostate. For example, when terazosin and finasteride were compared in a study published in *The New England Journal of Medicine*, terazosin appeared to produce greater improvement in BPH symptoms and urinary flow rate than finasteride. But this difference may have been due to the larger number of men in the study with small prostates, who would be more likely to have BPH symptoms from smooth muscle constriction than from physical obstruction by excess glandular tissue.

A 2004 review article in *The Journal of Urology* found that all four alpha-blockers were effective at relieving BPH symptoms. Men taking alfuzosin had a 19% to 40% improvement in their symptom scores; those taking doxazosin had a 14% to 39% improvement; men taking tamsulosin had a 24% to 50% improvement; and those taking terazosin had a 38% to 64% improvement.

Alpha-blockers can cause such side effects as orthostatic hypotension (dizziness upon standing due to a drop in blood pressure), fatigue, insomnia, and headache. These side effects are less common with tamsulosin, because it does not lower blood pressure as much as the other alpha-blockers. Orthostatic hypotension can be

NEW RESEARCH

Study Finds Long-Term Benefits With Finasteride Treatment

Men with BPH who take finasteride (Proscar) are at reduced risk for acute urinary retention (AUR) and are less likely to require surgery to treat the condition, according to six-year results from the Proscar Long-Term Efficacy and Safety Study (PLESS).

The current study is an extension of a four-year trial of more than 3,000 BPH patients who were randomly assigned to 5 mg of finasteride daily or a placebo. In the four-year trial, patients on the drug had a 57% lower risk of developing AUR compared with men taking a placebo, and were 55% less likely to require surgery to treat BPH symptoms.

After the four years, participants on the placebo were given the option of switching to finasteride. Two years later, results with more than 2,400 men found that those who had taken finasteride for six years continued to have lower rates of AUR and BPH surgery than those taking a placebo. Those who switched to finasteride had reductions in AUR and BPH surgery that approached levels found in the men who had taken the drug long term.

The researchers concluded that "finasteride treatment led to a sustained decrease in the incidence of AUR and/or BPH–related surgery."

THE JOURNAL OF UROLOGY
Volume 171, page 1194
March 2004

Medications Used in the Treatment of Benign Prostatic Hyperplasia 2005

Drug Type	Generic Name	Brand Name	Average Daily Dosage*	Average Retail Cost[†]
Alpha-1-adrenergic blockers (alpha-blockers)	alfuzosin	UroXatral	1 to 10 mg	10 mg: $53
	doxazosin	Cardura	1 to 8 mg	2 mg: $39 ($14)
	tamsulosin	Flomax	0.4 to 0.8 mg	0.4 mg: $56
	terazosin	Hytrin	1 to 10 mg	2 mg: $62 ($25)
5-alpha-reductase inhibitors	dutasteride	Avodart	0.5 mg	0.5 mg: $81
	finasteride	Proscar	5 mg	5 mg: $81

* These dosages represent an average range for the treatment of benign prostatic hyperplasia. The precise effective dosage varies from patient to patient and depends on many factors. Do not make any changes in your medication without consulting your doctor.
[†] Average price for 30 tablets or capsules (unless otherwise indicated) of the dosage strength listed. Actual price may vary. If a generic version is available, the cost is listed in parentheses. Sources: drugstore.com, eckerd.com, and walgreens.com.

minimized by taking the drug in the evening. Men on alpha-blockers should not take the erectile dysfunction medications sildenafil (Viagra) or vardenafil (Levitra), because the combination can produce dangerously low blood pressure levels.

In men taking medication for the treatment of high blood pressure, dosages may need to be adjusted to account for the blood pressure-lowering effects of the alpha-blocker. Alpha-blockers may also induce angina (chest pain resulting from an inadequate supply of oxygen to the heart) in men with coronary heart disease. A doctor will be able to determine which individuals are good candidates for alpha-blockers.

In addition, a 2003 study suggested that men with BPH and overactive bladder may benefit from treatment with an alpha-blocker and a drug used to treat incontinence. After three months, men taking tamsulosin and tolterodine (Detrol) had greater improvements

How They Work	Special Instructions	Possible Side Effects
By blocking alpha-1-adrenergic receptors, these drugs cause relaxation of muscle tissue in the prostate, bladder neck, and prostate capsule. The result is increased urinary flow and fewer urinary symptoms.	For doxazosin and terazosin, the initial dosage is usually 1 mg to avoid low blood pressure and subsequent light-headedness or dizziness. Patients requiring higher doses receive them in incremental increases. Take tamsulosin 30 minutes after the same meal each day.	Consult your doctor if you persistently experience headache, unusual tiredness or sleepiness, irritability or restlessness, nausea, abnormal ejaculation, decreased sex drive, diarrhea, back pain, drowsiness, trouble sleeping, chest pain, or runny or stuffy nose. Seek medical attention as soon as possible if you experience light-headedness or dizziness; a fast, pounding, or irregular heartbeat; chest pain or shortness of breath; dizziness or light-headedness upon rising from a sitting or lying position; a persistent erection; or swelling in the feet or lower legs.
By blocking the enzyme 5-alpha-reductase, which converts testosterone into dihydrotestosterone (a hormone responsible for prostate growth), these drugs cause the prostate to shrink. The drugs are most effective when the prostate is enlarged.	The full effect usually takes about a year to occur. Most men need to take the drug indefinitely to keep symptoms under control. Women who are or may become pregnant should not handle crushed tablets because of the potential risk of birth defects in a male fetus.	Side effects are relatively infrequent but can include erectile dysfunction, decreased libido, and decreased ejaculate volume. Consult your doctor as soon as possible if you notice breast tenderness and enlargement, skin rash, or swelling of the lips.

in quality of life than men taking tamsulosin alone.

Combination therapy. For men with lower urinary tract symptoms due to an enlarged prostate who opt for medication, taking a 5-alpha-reductase inhibitor in combination with an alpha-blocker may be the treatment of choice. And in 2004, the FDA approved the use of finasteride together with doxazosin for treating BPH symptoms due to an enlarged prostate.

Recently, the National Institutes of Health sponsored a trial called Medical Therapy of Prostate Symptoms (MTOPS) that is the largest trial ever to compare various types of medication for BPH. The 4½-year trial involved more than 3,000 men with BPH symptoms. The men were treated with finasteride, doxazosin, a combination of finasteride and doxazosin, or a placebo.

The results, which were published in 2003 in *The New England Journal of Medicine*, revealed that not only is combination therapy safe, it appears to be more effective than monotherapy (either finasteride or doxazosin alone) for men with enlarged prostates. For example, men on combination therapy were 67% less likely to have their BPH progress than men who took the placebo. Men who took either finasteride or doxazosin alone also had a reduced risk of progression (34% and 39%, respectively). Also, the combination therapy reduced the risk of acute urinary retention by 79% compared with the placebo. Finasteride reduced this risk by 67%, but doxazosin did not significantly affect rates of urinary retention.

Combination therapy works best in men with larger prostates because finasteride works by reducing prostate size. Older men, those with higher PSA levels, and men with low urinary flow rates are more likely than others to have prostate enlargement.

Surgery

Surgery for BPH, known as simple prostatectomy, typically involves removing only the inner portion of the prostate and is performed either transurethrally (through the urethra) or by making an incision in the lower abdomen. Simple prostatectomy for BPH differs from radical prostatectomy for prostate cancer, in which the entire prostate and the seminal vesicles are removed (see pages 40–44).

Surgery offers the fastest, most certain way to improve BPH symptoms, and less than 10% of patients will require retreatment 5 to 10 years later. But surgery is associated with a greater risk of long-term complications, such as erectile dysfunction, incontinence, and retrograde ejaculation, compared with other treatment options for BPH. (Retrograde ejaculation—ejaculation of semen into the bladder rather than through the penis—is not dangerous but may cause infertility and anxiety.) The frequency of these complications varies with the type of surgical procedure. Now that medications are available to treat BPH, fewer patients are opting for surgical procedures.

Surgery is not performed until any urinary tract infection or kidney damage from urinary retention is successfully treated. Because blood loss is a common complication during and immediately following most types of BPH surgery, men taking aspirin should stop taking it 7 to 10 days prior to surgery. Aspirin interferes with blood clot formation.

Transurethral prostatectomy (TURP). Transurethral prostatectomy, also called transurethral resection of the prostate (TURP), is considered the gold standard for BPH treatment—the one against which other therapies are compared. More than 90% of simple prostatectomies for BPH are performed transurethrally by TURP.

The procedure is typically done in the hospital under general or spinal anesthesia. In patients with smaller prostates and no other medical problems, TURP may be done as an outpatient procedure.

The procedure involves removal of tissue from the inner portion of the prostate with a long, thin instrument called a resectoscope, which is passed through the urethra into the bladder. A wire loop attached to the end of the resectoscope cuts away prostate tissue and seals blood vessels with an electric current or laser energy. When laser energy is used (usually a holmium laser), the procedure is called laser prostatectomy. The resulting, loose bits of tissue collect in the bladder and are flushed out of the body through the resectoscope; a sample of the tissue is examined in the laboratory for the presence of prostate cancer.

Once the surgery is complete, a catheter is inserted through the urethra into the bladder to prevent blood clot formation; the catheter remains in place for one to three days. After the catheter is removed, most men experience a greater urgency to urinate for 12 to 24 hours. A hospital stay of one to two days is common. Most men experience little or no pain after the procedure, and a full recovery can be expected within three weeks.

Improvement in symptoms is noticeable almost immediately after surgery and is greatest in those who have the worst symptoms before the surgery. Marked improvement occurs in about 90% to 95% of men with severe symptoms and in about 80% of those with moderate symptoms—a rate of improvement that is significantly better than that achieved with medication or watchful waiting. In addition, more than 95% of men who undergo TURP require no further treatment over the next five years.

The most common complications immediately following TURP are bleeding, urinary tract infection, and urinary retention. Longer-term complications can include erectile dysfunction, retrograde ejaculation, and incontinence. However, evidence is growing that TURP may cause no more sexual function problems than other treatments for BPH and, in some cases, may even bring about improvements. (Erectile dysfunction and incontinence can be treated, as discussed on pages 56–62.) Risk of death from TURP is very low (0.1%).

Open prostatectomy. An open prostatectomy is the operation of choice when the prostate is so large (larger than 80 to 100 g) that TURP cannot be performed safely. There are two types of open prostatectomy for BPH: suprapubic and retropubic. Both require an incision extending from below the navel to the pubic bone. A supra-

NEW RESEARCH

Urinary Problems Tied to Sexual Dysfunction in Older Men

Middle-aged and older men with urinary tract problems may be at increased risk for sexual dysfunction, suggesting the two may share underlying causes, according to researchers.

Their study of more than 2,100 men age 40 to 79 showed that as lower urinary tract symptoms grew in severity, sexual function tended to decline, mainly in men younger than 70. The authors say the findings suggest that doctors should consider a man's sexual function when treating urinary tract problems, and that research should look into whether common mechanisms underlie both types of problems.

Both urinary symptoms (such as weak urine flow, straining, and a feeling of urgency) and sexual dysfunction (such as impotence and ejaculation problems) grow more common as men age. But whether these conditions have anything in common beyond older age has been unclear.

In this study, the link between urinary symptoms and sexual dysfunction was strongest among younger men, suggesting, the researchers state, that the association is not simply an "age-related phenomenon."

MAYO CLINIC PROCEEDINGS
Volume 79, page 745
June 2004

pubic prostatectomy involves opening the bladder and removing the inner portion of the prostate through the bladder. In a retropubic prostatectomy, the bladder is moved aside and the inner prostate tissue is removed without entering the bladder. Both procedures are performed in a hospital under general or spinal anesthesia. As in TURP, removed tissue is checked for prostate cancer.

After a suprapubic prostatectomy, two catheters are placed in the bladder, one through the urethra and the other through an opening made in the lower abdominal wall. The catheters remain in place for three to seven days after surgery. Following a retropubic prostatectomy, a catheter is placed in the bladder through the urethra and remains in place for a week. The hospital stay (five to seven days) and the recovery period (four to six weeks) are longer for open prostatectomy than for TURP.

Like TURP, an open prostatectomy is an effective way to relieve symptoms of BPH. But because complications are more common with open prostatectomy than with TURP—and, in some cases, the complications can be life-threatening—open prostatectomy is reserved for otherwise healthy men with the largest prostates. The most common complications immediately after open prostatectomy are excessive bleeding, which may require a transfusion, and wound infection. Because an open prostatectomy is elective surgery, men can donate their own blood in advance, in case they need a transfusion during or after the procedure. More serious complications of an open prostatectomy, though rare, include heart attack, pneumonia, and pulmonary embolism (a blood clot that moves to the lungs). Breathing exercises, leg movements in bed, and walking soon after the surgery can reduce the risk of these complications. Long-term complications, including erectile dysfunction, incontinence, and retrograde ejaculation, are slightly more frequent with open prostatectomy than with TURP.

Transurethral electrovaporization. One of the most promising advances in the surgical treatment of BPH is transurethral electrovaporization, a modification of TURP. As in TURP, the procedure involves inserting a resectoscope through the urethra. But instead of cutting away tissue with a wire loop, a powerful electrical current, delivered by a grooved roller at the end of the resectoscope, vaporizes prostate tissue with minimal bleeding. A catheter is placed in the urethra after the procedure. Preliminary experience suggests that the procedure can be performed on an outpatient basis, with removal of the catheter within 24 hours.

Transurethral electrovaporization appears to be as effective as

TURP. It also offers a reduced risk of bleeding, no need to stay overnight in the hospital, and lower cost. Compared with TURP, however, men undergoing transurethral electrovaporization may have higher rates of symptoms such as postoperative irritative voiding, dysuria, urinary retention, and unplanned secondary catheterization. Other disadvantages of transurethral electrovaporization include less certainty about the long-term effectiveness of the procedure and the lack of a tissue sample to check for prostate cancer.

Transurethral incision of the prostate (TUIP). First used in the United States in the early 1970s, TUIP also employs an instrument inserted through the urethra. But instead of cutting away prostate tissue, one or two small incisions are made in the prostate with an electrical knife or laser. These incisions alleviate the symptoms of BPH by decreasing the pressure exerted by prostate tissue on the urethra. A sample of tissue is often taken during the procedure to check for prostate cancer. TUIP takes less time to perform than TURP and can be done, in most cases, on an outpatient basis under local anesthesia.

TUIP is effective only in men with prostates smaller than 30 g. The degree of symptom improvement in these men is similar to that achieved with TURP, but patients may be more likely to need a second procedure. Since the incidence of retrograde ejaculation is lower than with TURP, TUIP is an option for men concerned about their fertility.

Minimally Invasive Therapy

A variety of minimally invasive procedures have been introduced over the past decade as alternatives to TURP. The goal of these procedures is to alleviate lower urinary tract symptoms while reducing the risk of complications associated with surgery.

Minimally invasive therapy for BPH uses heat to vaporize tissue in the prostate, a procedure known as thermoablation. Researchers are unclear exactly how thermoablation works—it may improve symptoms by reducing smooth muscle tone within the prostate, or simply by destroying prostate tissue.

The advantages of minimally invasive therapy over TURP are that it is performed on an outpatient basis and that there are fewer adverse events such as bleeding, incontinence, and retrograde ejaculation. But minimally invasive therapy has a number of disadvantages relative to TURP. First, it takes more time after the procedure for symptoms to improve. Second, the risk of urinary retention is as high as 40%. Third, more than 50% of men need further treatments.

Comparing Treatments for BPH

The table below can help you compare the benefits and risks of various treatment options for benign prostatic hyperplasia (BPH). Factors specific to your condition may make a particular treatment more or less beneficial than indicated in the table. When considering treatment options for BPH, discuss all the benefits and risks with your doctor.

Treatment	Usual Effect on Symptoms (Points on BPH Symptom Score)	Most Common Adverse Events
Watchful waiting	Symptoms will come and go	Small risk of worsening symptoms; acute urinary retention
Alpha-blockers	Moderate (6 to 8)	Stomach/intestinal discomfort (11%); stuffy nose (11%); headache (12%); dizziness (15%)
5-alpha-reductase inhibitors	Modest (3 to 4)	Erection problems (8%); decreased sexual desire (5%); reduced amount of semen (4%)
Combination drug therapy	Moderate (6 to 7)*	Combination of above
Transurethral microwave thermotherapy (TUMT)	Moderate to large (9 to 11)	Urgency/frequency (28% to 74%); infection (9%); second procedure needed (10% to 16%)
Transurethral needle ablation (TUNA)	Moderate (9)	Urgency/frequency (31%); infection (17%); second procedure needed (23%)
Transurethral prostatectomy (TURP), laser, and similar surgeries	Large (14 to 20)	Urgency/frequency (6% to 99%); urinary retention (1% to 21%); erection difficulty (3% to 13%); second procedure needed (1% to 14%)
Open surgery for large prostate glands	Large	Incontinence (6%)

Source: The American Urological Association.
* Combination therapy has been shown to reduce the risk of adverse outcomes (such as progression of symptoms, urinary retention, incontinence, renal insufficiency, or urinary tract infection) to a greater extent than either treatment alone.

Fourth, no tissue sample is available to test for prostate cancer. And fifth, the long-term effectiveness of these treatments has not been established.

The most commonly used minimally invasive therapies for BPH are transurethral microwave thermotherapy (TUMT), transurethral needle ablation (TUNA), interstitial laser coagulation (ILC), and water-induced thermotherapy (WIT).

ime Lost From Work	Hospitalization	Anesthesia	Pain and Discomfort
day each year for office follow-up	None	None	None
irst year, 1 day every 3 to 4 months or office follow-up; after 1 year, 1 day ach year for office follow-up	None	None	None
irst year, 1 day every 3 to 4 months or office follow-up; after 1 year, 1 day ach year for office follow-up	None	None	None
irst year, 1 day every 3 to 4 months or office follow-up; after 1 year, 1 day ach year for office follow-up	None	None	None
day for treatment; up to 1 week for ecovery; first year, 1 day every 6 onths for office follow-up	None (outpatient procedure)	Oral or injected sedatives or pain killers	During procedure, mild to moderate with use of anesthesia; after treatment, mild (urinary symptoms)
day for treatment; up to 1 week for ecovery; first year, 1 day every 6 onths for office follow-up	None (outpatient procedure)	Oral or injected sedatives and pain killers; spinal or general anesthesia	During procedure, mild to moderate with use of anesthesia; after treatment, mild (urinary symptoms)
to 4 weeks	1 to 2 days	Spinal or general	Moderate
to 6 weeks	3 to 7 days	General	Moderate

Transurethral microwave thermotherapy (TUMT). In TUMT, a catheter is inserted through the urethra and microwave energy is sent through the catheter to heat the prostate to temperatures above 113° F. At the same time, a cooling system prevents damage to the surrounding tissues, particularly the urethra. TUMT requires a local anesthetic, which is placed within the urethra. A new microwave thermotherapy device approved in February 2004 (called the Prolieve system) uses warm instead of cool water and appears to have similar results.

TUMT is most appropriate for men with moderately sized prostates (30 to 100 g) and moderate to severe symptoms (International Prostate Symptom Score of 12 or more). Research shows that TUMT typically produces a 40% to 70% reduction in symptom scores, but the improvements tend not to last as long as those with TURP. For example, about 20% of men need retreatment (either with TUMT or TURP) after two years; this rate increases to about 33% after five years.

Side effects from TUMT are usually minor and generally pass with time. TUMT is less likely to cause bleeding and sexual function problems than TURP, but it is associated with a higher risk of urinary tract infection. These infections usually result from catheterization, and the longer the catheter is in place, the higher the risk of infection. Men undergoing TUMT usually have a catheter in place for 2 to 14 days. To reduce the risk of infection, antibiotics are often prescribed either after the procedure or after catheter removal. Other side effects of TUMT include short-term incontinence and urinary retention.

Transurethral needle ablation (TUNA) and interstitial laser coagulation (ILC). With TUNA and ILC, a needle is placed through the urethra to delivery radiofrequency energy (TUNA) or laser energy (ILC) into the prostate tissue. Men with larger prostates may require several needle punctures.

One advantage of these approaches is that the surgeon can target specific areas of the prostate; other minimally invasive therapies deliver heat to the entire prostate. However, TUNA and ILC usually require intravenous sedation in addition to local anesthesia.

In a randomized study that compared TUNA and TURP, improvements in symptom scores were similar to those of TUMT. But in a multicenter study in the United States, TUNA did not improve symptoms adequately in 27% of men, who then underwent TURP. Like TUMT, the benefits of TUNA are not always long lasting. After two years, about 20% of men need retreatment (either with TUNA or TURP), and this rate increases to about 33% after five years. The American Urological Association recommends that TUNA be limited to men with obstructive BPH, prostates of 60 g or less, and enlargement predominantly in the lateral lobe.

A multicenter trial of ILC demonstrated a 60% improvement in symptom scores with a major complication rate lower than 2%. Catheterization was required for an average of five days after the procedure. In a 2003 study, men who underwent ILC had reductions in symptoms and improvements in quality of life that were similar to those in men who underwent TURP, but the ILC group had shorter hospitals stays and less serious complications. In addition, 16% of the men who received ILC required treatment with TURP in the following year. However, the American Urological Association recommends that more research be conducted before ILC is routinely offered to patients.

Water-induced thermotherapy (WIT). WIT involves the insertion of a balloon-containing catheter through the urethra and into the bladder. Once in place, the balloon is inflated inside the prostatic urethra (the portion of the urethra that is located within the prostate) and is filled with water heated to 140° F. The catheter is insulated to prevent damage to tissues other than the prostate. The procedure can be performed using local anesthesia. The duration of catheterization (one to five weeks) may be longer than for other minimally invasive therapies.

A study of 125 men treated with WIT found that the improvement in symptom scores was significant and that treatment results tended to last. Side effects were infrequent and manageable, and no sexual function problems were reported. Ongoing randomized studies will help determine the value of WIT compared with other minimally invasive therapies.

Stents

Stents are plastic or metal devices that are placed in the urethra via a catheter to keep the urethra open. Currently, only a metal stent is available in the United States. This option is used most often in elderly men who have acute urinary retention and whose ill health makes them unable to withstand more aggressive treatments such as TURP. The primary advantages of stents are that they can be placed quickly (in about 15 minutes) under spinal anesthesia, men can leave the hospital the same day or the next morning, long-term catheterization is not required, and the recovery time is short. However, patients may experience bothersome urinary symptoms (urgency, frequency, or painful urination) for days to weeks after the procedure. Other concerns include the need for precise positioning of the stent within the urethra and the possibility of deposits forming around the stent. Additionally, little is known about the long-term effects of stents. If necessary, a stent can be removed, in most cases without damaging the urethra.

NEW RESEARCH

Needle Procedure Helps Ease BPH Symptoms Over Long Term

A procedure known as transurethral needle ablation of the prostate (TUNA) is sometimes used instead of transurethral resection of the prostate (TURP) to treat urinary symptoms caused by BPH, but the long-term results were unclear. Now a study reveals that TUNA continues to have advantages over TURP after five years of follow-up.

The researchers compared TUNA and TURP in 121 men ages 50 and older who had experienced lower urinary tract symptoms from BPH for at least three months. Five years later, urinary symptoms and quality-of-life measures showed improvement in both groups, but improvement was greater among men who had TURP.

Impotence and incontinence were less common among the men who had TUNA, with erectile dysfunction occurring in 3% of TUNA patients and 21% of men in the TURP group. Retrograde ejaculation occurred in 41% of patients in the TURP group and none of those in the TUNA group. Overall, there were fewer adverse events in the men who had TUNA compared with TURP.

"In appropriately selected patients who have bothersome voiding symptoms due to BPH," the researchers conclude, "TUNA is an attractive treatment option."

THE JOURNAL OF UROLOGY
Volume 171, page 2336
June 2004

Prostate Cancer

Some experts theorize that every man will develop some degree of prostate cancer if he lives long enough. Autopsy studies have shown microscopic evidence of prostate cancer in 15% to 30% of men over the age of 50 and in 60% to 70% of men who reach age 80.

The number of men diagnosed with prostate cancer is on the rise, but the death rate from the disease is on the decline. Widespread use of the prostate specific antigen (PSA) test to screen for prostate cancer and the aging of the population is likely responsible for the increase in prostate cancer cases. Whether the PSA test is also responsible for the declining death rate is a matter of great debate.

A male born today has a 16% chance of being diagnosed with prostate cancer at some time in his life and a 3% chance of dying of the disease.

CAUSES OF PROSTATE CANCER

The underlying cause of prostate cancer is unknown. Like other cancers, however, multiple sequential events over a period of many years are probably necessary to produce a cancerous change in a prostate cell. The first step in the cancer process is the action of an initiator that produces a mutation (alteration) in the genetic make-up of a cell. But the subsequent action of a cancer promoter, which stimulates growth of the abnormal cell, is necessary for cancer to progress.

Age, race, and family history are important risk factors for prostate cancer. Environmental factors such as diet may also play a role. No clear association has been found between the development of prostate cancer and alcohol intake (although binge drinking may have an effect; see the sidebar on the opposite page), physical activity, smoking, vasectomy, or the presence of benign prostatic hyperplasia (BPH).

Age

As a man ages, his risk of having prostate cancer increases dramatically. This age-related increase is greater for prostate cancer than for any other type of cancer. The average age at the time of diagnosis is between 65 and 70, and the average age of death is between 77 and 80.

NEW RESEARCH

Benefits of Testosterone Replacement Outweigh Risks

Researchers have concluded that testosterone replacement therapy does not increase the risk of heart disease, prostate cancer, or elevated cholesterol levels in men.

Testosterone replacement therapy is used to counteract the effects of hypogonadism, a condition characterized by low testosterone levels. The condition affects 2 to 4 million older American men, causing decreased sex drive, erectile dysfunction, reduced muscle mass and bone density, anemia, and depression.

The researchers combined and analyzed the results of 72 studies that evaluated testosterone replacement therapy. They found no evidence suggesting any relationship between testosterone and increased risk of heart attack, stroke, angina, or other problems related to heart disease. In fact, some studies indicated that testosterone may even decrease the risk of heart disease.

The researchers also found no link between testosterone and an increased risk of prostate cancer, although the authors emphasized the need to monitor patients closely who take testosterone for early signs of the disease.

In addition, an Institute of Medicine committee has stressed that future research should establish a clear benefit of testosterone therapy for hypogonadal men as well as assess any long-term risks.

THE NEW ENGLAND JOURNAL OF MEDICINE
Volume 350, page 482
January 29, 2004

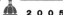

Race

The incidence of prostate cancer in the United States varies by race. The rate for white men is 101 per 100,000 each year. Black men are at higher risk (137 per 100,000), and Asian-Americans are at the lowest risk (20 to 47 per 100,000).

Family History

Studies of identical and fraternal twins show that prostate cancer has a stronger hereditary component than any other type of cancer. Having a first-degree relative (a brother or father) with prostate cancer doubles the risk of prostate cancer; having a second-degree relative (an uncle or grandfather) with the disease confers only a small risk.

A number of genetic alterations are linked with prostate cancer. The most studied of these is known as HPC1. Although some analyses have confirmed that mutations in HPC1 (a region of chromosome 1 that may be involved in protecting against prostate inflammation) increase the risk of prostate cancer, other studies have failed to find an association. Other genes involved in the binding or metabolism of androgens and the body's reaction to inflammation or infection may be important.

Although genes can affect the risk of prostate cancer, other factors are also at work. The likelihood that identical twins (who share all genetic information) will both develop prostate cancer is 19% to 27%, emphasizing the importance of lifestyle and environmental factors in the risk of prostate cancer.

Environmental Factors

Much effort has been devoted to a search for environmental factors that might serve as promoters for prostate cancer. The incidence of microscopic prostate cancer is similar among men in the United States and in all the other countries that have been examined. But the mortality rates from prostate cancer differ from one country to another and even within different regions of the United States. These differences suggest that some environmental factor or factors influence the progression of prostate cancer from microscopic tumors to clinically significant ones. Two possible factors are diet and sunlight exposure.

Diet. The majority of studies on the relationship between dietary fat and prostate cancer have found that a higher fat intake is associated with an increased risk of prostate cancer. Fat makes up 30% to 40% of the calories in the American diet, compared with 15% in Japan. These differences in fat intake may help explain the much

Binge Drinking Increases Prostate Cancer Risk

Men who binge drink increase their risk of getting prostate cancer, while men who regularly drink moderate or even heavy amounts of alcohol don't expose themselves to the same danger, according to new research. Several previous studies have noted an increased risk of prostate cancer among men who consume a lot of alcohol or who have been long-time drinkers, but none examined drinking patterns.

Researchers evaluated the association between drinking habits and the risk of prostate cancer among nearly 48,000 men over a 12-year period. Men who regularly drank large quantities of alcohol and men who were former drinkers were at no greater risk for prostate cancer than nondrinkers or men who drank less than one day a week. But for men who went on drinking binges—consuming at least the equivalent of at least eight cans of beer in just a day or two—increased their risk by 64% over nondrinkers. The association between alcohol intake and prostate cancer was strongest among men with type 2 diabetes.

Overall, the authors concluded, alcohol doesn't appear to contribute to prostate cancer risk, except for men who infrequently drink large amounts. The results warrant further evaluation.

AMERICAN JOURNAL OF EPIDEMIOLOGY
Volume 159, page 444
March 1, 2004

lower death rate from prostate cancer in Japan, as well as the great variability in mortality rates around the world. Another possibility is that people who eat a high-fat diet are less likely to eat healthful foods such as vegetables.

A high intake of vegetables may lower the risk of prostate cancer. According to a study of 628 men with prostate cancer published in the *Journal of the National Cancer Institute* in 2000, men who ate 28 or more servings of vegetables a week had a 35% lower risk of prostate cancer than those who ate 14 or fewer servings per week.

Cruciferous vegetables, such as cabbage and broccoli, appeared to provide a further protective effect: Men who ate three or more servings of cruciferous vegetables a week (in addition to other vegetables) had a 41% lower risk of prostate cancer than those who ate less than one serving a week. Cruciferous vegetables are rich in substances that induce enzymes to detoxify environmental carcinogens, including the free radicals found in the human diet.

Moderate evidence suggests that other dietary components also may help prevent prostate cancer. High intakes of lycopene (an antioxidant found in tomatoes and tomato-based products) are associated with a 16% to 21% reduced risk of prostate cancer. Taking supplements of selenium (a trace element) reduced the risk of prostate cancer by 66% in one study, and another study found that the incidence of prostate cancer was reduced by 34% in men taking vitamin E supplements.

Calorie intake may also affect prostate cancer risk. A 2003 study found that men who ate the most calories (around 2,600 per day) were nearly four times as likely to have prostate cancer as men who ate the least calories (1,100 per day). However, previous studies on the link between prostate cancer and high-calorie diets have produced inconsistent results, so more research on this topic is needed before recommendations on calorie intake can be made.

Weight. Obesity (having a body mass index [BMI]—an expression of weight and height—of 30 or more) is known to increase the risk of cancer as well as its severity. A 2003 study found that men who were obese were 20% more likely to die of prostate cancer than normal-weight men. Obesity may contribute to cancer by increasing blood levels of sex hormones or insulin.

Sunlight exposure. According to one study, sunlight may protect against prostate cancer by promoting the body's production of vitamin D. Vitamin D is synthesized in the skin during exposure to the ultraviolet (UV) radiation in sunlight. When the incidence of prostate cancer mortality was examined in white men in 3,073 counties

---

NEW RESEARCH

More Evidence Selenium Fights Prostate Cancer

Adding to evidence that the mineral selenium may be helpful in men with prostate cancer, new research suggests that high selenium levels in the blood may help slow prostate tumor growth.

The study of nearly 1,200 men followed for 13 years found that those with the highest blood levels of selenium at the outset were half as likely as men with the lowest levels to develop advanced prostate cancer. Higher selenium levels showed no clear effect on earlier prostate cancer, suggesting that the mineral may slow a tumor's progression rather than prevent its initial development.

Selenium has many jobs in the body, including protecting cells from DNA damage that can spark cancer, and pushing abnormal cells to commit suicide. There is evidence that selenium accumulates in the prostate, and some studies have suggested it helps ward off prostate cancer. The new findings, according to an accompanying editorial, underscore selenium's "tremendous potential" as a weapon against prostate cancer.

However, it's still unknown whether taking supplements that contain selenium cuts the risk of prostate cancer or slows its growth. Only large clinical trials, such as the ongoing Selenium and Vitamin E Cancer Prevention Trial (SELECT), can answer this question, the study authors note.

JOURNAL OF THE NATIONAL CANCER INSTITUTE
Volume 96, page 696
May 5, 2004

DRE: Don't Skip It

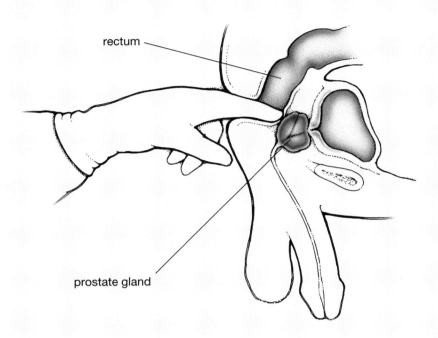

rectum

prostate gland

Because the prostate cannot be seen or felt externally, doctors perform a digital rectal examination (DRE) to assess its size, shape, and consistency. Along with prostate specific antigen (PSA) testing, a DRE is an essential screening tool for prostate cancer.

The American Cancer Society and American Urology Association recommend that all men over age 50 have a DRE and a PSA test at least once a year. Men at high risk for prostate cancer—black men and any man with two or more first-degree relatives (father or brothers) with the disease—should begin annual DRE and PSA screening at age 40 or 45.

Despite this recommendation, a study published in the *Archives of Internal Medicine* in 2004 found that only 47% of 588 men who underwent PSA testing had a DRE performed along with it. Skipping this exam means that many men with prostate cancer and a normal PSA result will go undiagnosed.

Some men avoid getting a DRE because they feel uncomfortable about the procedure, but it is not painful and lasts less than a minute. During a DRE, the patient either bends forward over the examination table, lies on his side, or kneels on the table. As shown in the illustration above, the doctor then inserts a gloved, lubricated finger a few inches into the rectum and gently palpates the prostate gland to feel for a nodule or lump, change in size, hard tissue, or any other abnormality that might indicate a tumor is present.

in the United States, areas with the lowest amounts of UV radiation had the highest mortality rates. Overall, deaths from prostate cancer were highest in the Northeast and lowest in the Southwest.

In addition, a laboratory study found that physiological concentrations of the active form of vitamin D change the makeup of prostate cancer cells so that they are less likely to spread. Further studies are needed to determine whether vitamin D supplements can prevent or treat prostate cancer. Spending at least half an hour in the sunlight each day and drinking fortified milk are the best ways to get vitamin D; megadose supplements can be toxic. For those who take supplements, the recommended dosage of vitamin D is 400 to 800 IU daily.

PREVENTION OF PROSTATE CANCER

Finasteride (Proscar), which is used to treat benign prostatic hyperplasia (BPH), has been hypothesized to decrease the risk of prostate cancer. However, a 2003 study found that although finasteride does appear to reduce the overall risk of prostate cancer, but it seems to increase the risk of high-grade prostate cancer. After seven years, 18.4% of the men taking finasteride developed prostate cancer, compared with 24.4% of men taking a placebo. However, more serious tumors (Gleason score of 7 to 10) occurred in 6.4% of the finasteride group, compared with 5.1% of the placebo group. Based on these findings, men should not take finasteride solely to prevent prostate cancer, and men taking finasteride for BPH should undergo careful monitoring for cancer.

SYMPTOMS OF PROSTATE CANCER

In its early stages, prostate cancer usually causes no symptoms. As the prostate enlarges, however, a man may experience difficulty in beginning to urinate, nocturia, and urinary urgency and frequency—symptoms indistinguishable from those of BPH, except that they may appear more abruptly when due to cancer. The onset of erectile dysfunction or a decrease in the firmness of erections may occur when the cancer invades the nerves that control erections. In some men, the first symptoms of prostate cancer result from its spread to distant sites—for example, severe back pain from cancer that has spread to the spine.

DIAGNOSIS OF PROSTATE CANCER

Abnormalities in either a digital rectal exam or PSA test raise the suspicion of cancer in most cases, and further tests such as transrectal ultrasound and prostate biopsy are then required. Diagnosing prostate cancer at an early stage can be difficult with a digital rectal exam alone, because the cancer cells tend to spread diffusely through the prostate and into surrounding tissues, rather than forming a solid mass as do most other forms of cancer.

NEW RESEARCH

Study Quantifies Time Advantage Of Prostate Cancer Screening

Prostate cancer is detected more than 10 years earlier in men who undergo early screening for the disease than in those who aren't screened, a new study suggests.

Researchers in Sweden screened 946 randomly selected men for prostate cancer with prostate-specific antigen (PSA) testing, digital rectal exam, and ultrasound, with prostate biopsies for suspicious findings (the screening group). The reference group consisted of 657 men who had their PSA measured using blood that had been collected and frozen at the same time that screening took place for the screening group.

Among men with a PSA level of 3 ng/mL or greater, it took 10.6 years for the incidence of cancer in the reference to catch up to that of the screening group. Men with a PSA level of 3 ng/mL or greater had an average time between screening and cancer diagnosis of 4.5 years in the screening group and 7.8 years in the reference group.

The authors concluded that PSA screening did not result in overdetection of the disease. However, others have found that overdiagnosis rates with prostate cancer screening are as high as 50% in men at age 65.

INTERNATIONAL JOURNAL OF CANCER
Volume 108, page 122
January 1, 2004

Digital Rectal Examination

The frequent absence of a solid, palpable mass makes it difficult to detect early prostate cancer with a digital rectal exam. Used alone, a digital rectal exam misses 30% to 40% of prostate cancers, and most cancers found with the exam are detected when it is too late for treatment to be effective. The most reliable way to detect prostate cancer in its early stages is to combine digital rectal exams with measurements of PSA levels in the blood. (For more information on the digital rectal examination, see the feature on page 27.)

Prostate Specific Antigen (PSA) Test

The PSA test was first approved by the FDA in 1986 as a way to determine whether prostate cancer had been treated successfully and to monitor for its recurrence. However, PSA tests are now FDA approved for detection and are widely used to screen for the presence of prostate cancer.

Clinical studies have demonstrated the following benefits of PSA testing: 1) An elevated PSA is the single best predictor of the presence of prostate cancer; 2) PSA testing detects prostate cancer about 5 to 10 years earlier than digital rectal exams; 3) Most cancers detected with PSA testing are curable; and 4) Serial PSA testing of a population leads to virtual elimination of advanced prostate cancer at the time of diagnosis.

However, it is not clear whether using the PSA test to screen for prostate cancer actually reduces the risk of death from the disease. In addition, some men with an elevated PSA do not have prostate cancer, and some of the cancers detected by the PSA test are too small or too slow growing to be life-threatening. These men may undergo unnecessary diagnostic tests and treatments and may experience undue anxiety. Consequently, men should discuss the benefits and drawbacks of PSA testing with their physician before having their PSA levels measured.

PSA is an enzyme produced almost exclusively by the glandular cells of the prostate. It is secreted during ejaculation into the prostatic ducts that empty into the urethra. PSA liquefies semen after ejaculation so that sperm are released. Normally, only very small amounts of PSA are present in the blood. But an abnormality of the prostate can disrupt the normal architecture of the gland and create an opening for PSA to pass into the bloodstream. Thus, high blood levels of PSA can indicate the presence of cancer. The percentage risks of cancer based on PSA levels are as follows:

NEW RESEARCH

Many Men With Prostate Cancer May Get 'Normal' Test Result

A study is calling into question the definition of "normal" on the PSA test used to screen for prostate cancer, adding to the controversy over when a man's PSA levels should prompt action.

The study of nearly 3,000 men ages 62 to 91 found that 15% of those who over a 7-year period maintained PSA results in what's considered the normal range (below 4 ng/mL) and had no abnormality on digital rectal examination were found to have cancer when their prostate tissue was biopsied. Of the total cohort (3,000 men) about 2% were found to have aggressive, "high-grade" tumors.

The findings, the authors report, show that prostate cancer—even more-serious forms—is "not rare" among men with normal PSA results. However, they and other experts say, the question of what to do with the findings is complicated. Lowering the PSA threshold for "normal" would boost the odds of overtreatment, but keeping it at 4 ng/mL means that some tumors will go undetected longer—a "dilemma," the authors conclude, that "must be resolved."

An accompanying editorial cautions against lowering the PSA threshold for now, citing, among other reasons, the lack of proof that screening at the current threshold saves men's lives.

THE NEW ENGLAND JOURNAL OF MEDICINE
Volume 350, pages 2239 and 2292
May 27, 2004

- PSA levels under 4 nanograms per milliliter (ng/mL) are "normal" at age 50 and older; levels below 2.5 ng/mL are "normal" at age 40 to 49. These levels are associated with less than a 15% to 19% risk of cancer;
- 4 to 10 ng/mL, 20% to 30% risk;
- 10 to 20 ng/mL, 50% to 75% risk; and
- above 20 ng/mL, 90% risk.

The American Cancer Society and the American Urological Association recommend an annual PSA test beginning at age 50. Men at increased risk for prostate cancer—black men and men with a family history of the disease—should begin annual screening at age 40 or 45. A recent study by H. Ballentine Carter, M.D., author of this White Paper, found that testing all men at age 40, age 45, and then every other year after age 50 may be a better strategy—it saved more lives and was less expensive. Another recent study suggests that men age 50 and older who have PSA levels below 2 ng/mL do not need annual testing.

A number of factors may affect the results of a PSA test. For example, some studies show that ejaculation one or two days before a PSA test may increase PSA levels in the blood. Consequently, men should abstain from sex for two days prior to a PSA test. Digital rectal exams and biopsies of the prostate may also affect PSA levels, though the increase in PSA caused by a digital rectal exam is not thought to be significant enough to result in a false-positive test result. A biopsy, however, may elevate PSA levels for as long as four weeks. In addition, other prostate problems (such as BPH or prostatitis) can inflate PSA levels, and BPH medications (such as finasteride and dutasteride) can lower PSA levels by about 50%.

Researchers have developed several ways to improve the ability of PSA to detect prostate cancer. These improvements include assessing PSA in relation to prostate size (PSA density); monitoring annual changes in PSA (PSA velocity); measuring the ratio of free to total PSA (percent free PSA); and adjusting PSA for a patient's age (age-specific PSA).

PSA density. PSA density takes into account the size of a man's prostate when evaluating his PSA level. It is calculated by dividing the PSA value by the size of the prostate (as determined by transrectal ultrasound; see page 32). This measurement helps doctors distinguish between BPH and cancer: The higher the PSA density, the greater the chance of cancer, because elevated PSA is less likely the result of prostate enlargement. According to several studies, a PSA density greater than 0.15 indicates a higher risk of cancer. PSA den-

NEW RESEARCH

Rate of PSA Rise May Predict Men's Death Risk

Men whose PSA levels rapidly rise in the year before prostate cancer diagnosis may face a relatively high risk of death despite surgery, study findings suggest.

The results imply that for these men, "watchful waiting" may not be the best option, according to researchers. They found that among nearly 1,100 men with cancer confined to the prostate, those whose PSA levels rose more than 2 ng/mL in the year prior to diagnosis were more likely than other men to die over the seven years following surgery.

Although the large majority of men with a quickly rising PSA at diagnosis were still alive at the end of the study, they had a nearly 10-times greater risk of dying from prostate cancer as other men did. Given this, watchful waiting—the practice of delaying treatment to see if a prostate tumor progresses—may not be the best choice for men with a high PSA velocity, the study authors conclude.

However, they stress, it's unclear whether such patients' death rates would in fact be higher if they were treated with watchful waiting rather than surgery. Clinical trials, the authors conclude, are needed to figure out the best treatment approach for these men.

THE NEW ENGLAND JOURNAL OF MEDICINE
Volume 351, page 125
July 8, 2004

A Precursor to Prostate Cancer

Men who develop a particular type of prostatic lesion may require close follow-up.

A prostate biopsy that reveals prostatic intraepithelial neoplasia (PIN) may leave men unsure of how to react. Although PIN is thought to be a pre-malignant lesion that has the potential to evolve into cancer, it is not cancer itself. But certain men with this finding require careful follow-up, because sometimes a second biopsy will reveal a previously undetected tumor.

Diagnosing PIN

PIN used to go by several different names (such as dysplasia, intraductal dysplasia, or atypical hyperplasia), and doctors may still use some of these terms. In addition, PIN used to be classified as grade I, II, or III (with I being the least serious and III being the most). Now, pathologists classify PIN as high-grade only, which encompasses grades II and III. Grade I—or low-grade PIN—cannot be reliably diagnosed.

Approximately 9% of men who have a prostate biopsy in the United States will be diagnosed with high-grade PIN, which translates to approximately 115,000 men every year. Similar to the rates for prostate cancer, the rates for PIN are higher among blacks than among whites, who have a higher rate than Asian men.

The Implications of PIN

There is controversy among experts as to the appropriate follow-up of men with high-grade PIN. Some studies have shown that men with high-grade PIN are at higher risk of having prostate cancer and should undergo a repeat biopsy. However, several well-designed studies suggest that men with a diagnosis of high-grade PIN have the same risk of prostate cancer as men who have no abnormal findings on a biopsy. If a man with high-grade PIN had a well-performed, extended biopsy that included sampling of the entire peripheral zone of the prostate, then a repeat biopsy is not mandatory. A reasonable follow-up plan would be a digital rectal examination and yearly or biennial testing of PSA levels. Most experts agree that PIN does not have an effect on PSA levels.

Some evidence suggests that PIN lesions may be part of a multi-step process that leads to invasive prostate cancer since PIN shares many of the genetic hallmarks of "true" prostate cancer.

How To Proceed

Like some prostate cancers, premalignant lesions don't require treatment—especially since they may never develop into cancer. However, researchers are exploring the possibility of preventing the progression of PIN to prostate cancer with supplements or drugs that may decrease inflammation within the prostate, reduce oxidative damage that can affect genes, and reduce the effects of testosterone within the prostate.

In the meantime, men with high-grade PIN should continue to have their PSA levels checked and undergo periodic prostate exams. They should also keep their weight under control, exercise regularly, and eat a low-fat diet rich in fruits, vegetables, and fiber.

sity appears most useful for diagnosing prostate cancer in men with PSA levels between 4 and 10 ng/mL.

PSA velocity. This measurement takes into account annual changes in PSA values, which rise more rapidly in men with prostate cancer than in men without the disease. A study from Johns Hopkins and the National Institute of Aging found that an increase in PSA levels of greater than 0.75 ng/mL per year was an early predictor of prostate cancer in men with PSA levels between 4 and 10 ng/mL. PSA velocity is especially helpful in detecting early cancer in men with mildly elevated PSA levels and a normal digital rectal exam; it is not useful in predicting the presence of cancer unless changes in PSA are evaluated over at least 1½ to 2 years.

Percent free PSA. PSA in the blood is either bound (attached to proteins) or unbound (free). Men with prostate cancer have a higher percentage of bound PSA and a lower percentage of free PSA than men with BPH. Research suggests that determining the ratio of free to total PSA in the blood helps distinguish between PSA elevations due to cancer and those caused by BPH. In men with PSA levels between 4 and 10 ng/mL, performing a prostate biopsy only when the percent free PSA is 24% or below would result in the detection of more than 90% of prostate cancers and reduce by 20% the number of unnecessary biopsies. Percent free PSA, as well as PSA density and PSA velocity, can also be used to determine the need for a repeat biopsy when the initial biopsy shows no evidence of cancer but cancer is still suspected.

Age-specific PSA. PSA increases with age because the prostate gradually enlarges as men grow older. Some years ago, researchers suggested adjusting PSA levels for the age of the patient: Higher levels would be considered normal in older men and lower levels considered normal in younger men. However, research has not shown that using lower levels to prompt biopsy in younger men increases the likelihood of finding curable cancers, nor that using higher levels in older men interferes with the chance of detecting curable cancer. For now, a level of 4 ng/mL is considered the upper limit of normal in men age 50 and older. For men younger than age 50, the upper limit of normal is 2.5 ng/mL.

Transrectal Ultrasound

If the results of a digital rectal exam, a PSA test, or both are suspicious for cancer, transrectal ultrasound is used to determine the size of the prostate, identify areas of possible cancer, and direct the needles used for prostate biopsy. The procedure takes 15 to 20 minutes and is performed on an outpatient basis. Some physicians use a local anesthetic such as lidocaine (Xylocaine) to reduce discomfort during the procedure. While the patient is lying on his side, an ultrasound probe (about the size of a finger) is gently inserted three to four inches into the rectum. The probe emits sound waves that are converted into video images. The images are generated with the probe in several positions as it is gradually withdrawn from the rectum.

Prostate Biopsy

When prostate cancer is suspected, either from the results of a digital rectal exam, a PSA test, or both, a prostate biopsy is performed. The procedure involves taking samples of prostate tissue and examining them under a microscope for the presence of cancer. Each year, about 800,000 men undergo prostate biopsy.

The most common biopsy method is transrectal ultrasound-guided biopsy, also known as TRUS. The procedure is usually done in a urologist's office and takes about 20 minutes to perform. While the patient is lying on his side, an ultrasound probe is inserted into the rectum to visualize the prostate. Fitted to the probe is a biopsy gun that drives small needles through the wall of the rectum and into the prostate. In less than a second, the needle removes a small tissue sample. Usually, 8 to 12 tissue samples are taken throughout the prostate.

After the procedure, the tissue samples are sent to the laboratory to be examined under a microscope by a pathologist. The results are usually ready in three to five days. Nearly 75% of the time, no prostate cancer is detected in the samples, usually because the elevated PSA levels that prompted the biopsy were due to another prostate condition (such as BPH or prostatitis) or a nonmedical reason (such as recent sexual activity). A second biopsy is required when the pathologist finds atypical cells (cells suspicious but not diagnostic of cancer) or when the biopsy does not indicate cancer but the results of the digital rectal exam or PSA test were highly suggestive of cancer.

Many men worry that prostate biopsy will be painful, but it usually causes only minor discomfort. Common side effects include minor rectal bleeding; blood in the stool, urine, or semen; and soreness in the biopsied area. All of these side effects disappear with time.

Other Diagnostic Tests

Other routine tests include urinalysis and blood tests for anemia. If surgery is contemplated, general health status—particularly cardiovascular and pulmonary function—is assessed to decide whether the man is a suitable candidate for surgery.

Determining the Extent of Cancer

Determining the extent of prostate cancer is important in predicting the course of the disease and choosing the best treatment. The results from the digital rectal exam, PSA tests, and prostate biopsy give the urologist a good idea of whether the cancer is confined to the prostate or has spread outside the gland.

In some cases, patients may undergo a bone scan to determine whether prostate cancer has spread to the bones. The bone scan involves an intravenous injection of a radioactive material, which settles in damaged bone. (Bone can be damaged by cancer as well as by arthritis and other bone diseases.) A special scanner is then

---

NEW RESEARCH

Study IDs Possible Marker Of Early Prostate Cancer

Testing biopsy samples for a protein present throughout cancerous prostates may help men avoid unnecessary repeat biopsies and help catch early tumors that would have been missed on biopsy, preliminary research suggests.

The study looked at prostate tissue samples from men without prostate cancer and from men who had initially negative biopsies but were diagnosed with the disease after subsequent biopsies. The researchers found that a protein known as EPCA was present throughout the prostates of men with cancer but not in those without the disease. What's more, for 21 of the 25 cancer patients, EPCA was detectable in the tissue samples that initial biopsies had deemed negative.

Though much more work is needed, the authors conclude, the findings suggest that EPCA tests could be used with biopsies to catch cancer earlier, and to help confirm that cancer is not present. Men with negative EPCA results could be followed less aggressively, while those with positive findings could be followed closely and get repeat biopsies.

Work is under way, the researchers note, to develop a blood test for EPCA. Two authors on the study are with Tessera Diagnostics Inc., which is developing the EPCA technology.

THE JOURNAL OF UROLOGY
Volume 171, page 1419
April 2004

Understanding the Grade and Stage of Your Cancer

Obtaining and reading a copy of your pathology report can prove helpful in understanding your cancer and deciding on the best treatment.

A pathology report outlines the diagnostic results of the prostate needle biopsy (or the biopsy specimen taken during prostatectomy). The pathologist who examined the biopsy specimen prepares the report.

Although you may not be offered a copy of your pathology report, your doctor will provide one if asked. Alternatively, you can obtain your report from the pathology laboratory where the biopsy specimen was sent. The report will have your name, patient number, and case number (which usually appears as S-year-number).

Noncancerous Findings

While benign (noncancerous) findings on the biopsied tissue cannot completely rule out cancer—it's always possible that the cancer lurks in other, unbiopsied prostate tissue—such findings indicate that an elevated PSA is likely due to other causes. These causes include chronic or acute inflammation and benign prostatic hyperplasia (BPH).

A prostate biopsy that indicates prostatic intraepithelial neoplasia (PIN; see the feature on page 31) could mean that prostate cancer has been missed. But recent studies show that men with PIN on biopsy have a similar chance of cancer on repeat biopsy, compared with those with benign findings on biopsy.

Cancer Grade

Described most often as adenocarcinoma, a malignant (cancerous) tissue specimen is assigned a Gleason score—the most important factor in predicting the state of the disease and the probable outcome. The Gleason score is the sum of the grades of the two most prevalent malignancy patterns in the specimen. Assigned by the pathologist, these grades characterize the tumor and describe how closely the malignant cells resemble normal ones. Grades range from 1 to 5, with 1 being the closest to normal and having the least potential to spread. A Gleason score of 7 results from a grade of 3 for the predominant pattern of cancer cells and a grade of 4 for the secondary one. You may also find the percentage of each grade in your pathology report, but the Gleason score is most commonly reported.

Cancer Stage

Two systems—the Whitmore-Jewett and the TNM (tumor, node, metastasis) systems (see the inset box, opposite)—are used by physicians to describe how far the prostate cancer has spread. The Whitmore-Jewett system uses stages A, B, C, and D—with A indicating the earliest cancer and D the most advanced—to describe the extent of the tumor. The stage is further subdivided with numbers, for example, stage A1 or A2, for a more specific indication of the percentage of cancerous tissue.

The TNM system assigns a T number (T1 to T4) to a tumor according to its extent on a digital rectal examination; an N number (N0 to N3) indicating lymph node involvement; and an M number (M0 to M1) to indicate the presence of distant metastases.

used to detect the radioactivity. Areas of the body with increased radioactivity have bone damage, possibly because cancer has spread to the bone.

Some physicians do not order a bone scan when PSA levels are less than 10 ng/mL, because the chance of a positive scan is very low. Other physicians prefer to have the scan done even if the risk of spread is low, so that a baseline measurement is available for comparison if a bone scan is needed at a later date. People with PSA levels of 20 ng/mL and higher, Gleason scores of 8 to 10 (see page 36), or palpable disease on both sides of the prostate or beyond the prostate should have a bone scan.

A test called the ProstaScint scan is also available to detect prostate cancer cells that have spread, in this case to the lymph nodes or soft organs. ProstaScint uses antibodies that attach to a protein,

Cancer Staging System

TNM	Whitmore-Jewett	Description
T1	A	Cancer nonpalpable by DRE
T1a	A1	Less than 5% of sample from TURP malignant and low-grade
T1b	A2	More than 5% of sample from TURP malignant and/or not low-grade
T1c	(BO)	PSA elevated, nonpalpable by DRE
T2	B	Tumor digitally palpable by DRE and thought to be confined
T2a	B1	Confined to one lobe of gland <1.5 cm
T2b	B2	Confined to one lobe of gland >1.5 cm
T2c		Palpable in both lobes by DRE
T3	C	Locally extensive beyond capsule
T4		Tumor extension to adjacent organs
Tx, N1, or M1	D	Distant metastases
Tx, N1, or M0	D1	Pelvic lymph node involvement
Tx, Nx, M1	D2	Metastasis to distant sites other than lymph nodes (bone)

These stages are further subdivided into a, b, and c to describe how the cancer was diagnosed and the extent of cancerous tissue. The most commonly diagnosed stage of cancer today is T1c, indicating that the cancer was not found during a digital rectal exam (DRE), but was identified by needle biopsy performed after finding an elevated PSA.

Other Information
Your pathology report will also include the name of the pathologist and address of the laboratory where the specimen was analyzed. If the report indicates "outside consultation," the pathologist determined the case to be difficult and therefore sent it to another laboratory for a second opinion. Patients, and increasingly urologists, are rarely able to choose which pathologist reviews the biopsy specimen.

called prostate specific membrane antigen, on prostate cancer cells. These antibodies mark cancer cells with a radioactive isotope that is then picked up by a special scanner. The ProstaScint scan is not considered to be very accurate. It is usually used when PSA levels start to rise again after surgery or radiation therapy.

Computed tomography (CT) or magnetic resonance imaging (MRI) may be done to look for enlarged lymph nodes if the spread of cancer is suspected. In some cases, the urologist may recommend a laparoscopic biopsy, in which a surgeon uses a laparoscope (an instrument with a light and camera) to view the lymph nodes near the prostate.

After determining the extent of the cancer, doctors use one of two methods to describe the cancer's clinical stage. These are the Whitmore-Jewett and TNM (tumor, node, metastasis) systems. For more information about these methods, see the feature on pages 34–35.

CHOOSING A PROSTATE CANCER TREATMENT

The choice of treatment for prostate cancer—watchful waiting, surgery, radiation therapy, or hormone therapy—depends on the clinical stage of the cancer (extent of disease) and the age and general health of the individual. Investigators have found that, in healthy men who have more than a 10-year life expectancy, about 80% of prostate cancers detected by PSA testing have the potential to progress and thus warrant treatment. Still, with increased use of PSA testing, some men will be diagnosed with small prostate cancers (which cannot be felt during a digital rectal exam but are suspected from PSA tests and confirmed by biopsy) that pose no immediate threat and, indeed, may never need treatment. Two recent studies suggest that 30% to 50% of cancers detected by PSA screening would never have become apparent otherwise.

Possible complications also must be considered when deciding on a treatment option. If a man opts for surgery or radiation therapy, he risks the possibility of bowel, urinary, or sexual problems. If he chooses watchful waiting (no treatment is provided, but the patient is closely monitored for cancer growth), he may be anxious about the progress of the disease and urinary or sexual symptoms may arise if the disease progresses.

Doctors use several methods to help predict the seriousness of the cancer, which is factored into the treatment decision. One method is the Gleason score, which ranges from 2 to 10. A score of 2 to 4 indicates a greater probability of an insignificant cancer—a cancer that is unlikely to grow rapidly and spread. Higher scores suggest a greater likelihood of a significant, life-threatening cancer. Men with "high-grade" disease (defined as a Gleason score of 7 to 10) are considered poor candidates for watchful waiting, since the high score indicates an aggressive cancer. (For more information about cancer grade, see the feature on pages 34–35.)

Another method helpful in determining the best treatment option is the Partin tables (named after the Johns Hopkins physician who developed them). The tables help doctors predict whether cancer is confined to the prostate or has spread to adjacent tissue, seminal vesicles, or lymph nodes. The prediction is based on the patient's PSA levels, biopsy Gleason score, and TNM cancer stage. If cancer has spread outside the prostate, surgery may not be the best treatment option.

Johns Hopkins researchers have also developed a way of determining which men are good candidates for watchful waiting. They have found that the best candidates have prostate cancers that cannot be felt on a digital rectal exam; PSA density of less than 0.15; signs of cancer in no more than two biopsy samples; cancer cells in less than 50% of any single biopsy sample; and a Gleason score of less than 7.

Age also plays an important part in deciding whether to choose watchful waiting or to treat prostate cancer more aggressively. Because prostate cancer generally progresses slowly, older men with small tumors can choose watchful waiting more safely than younger men. Men in their 50s and early 60s with prostate cancer are more likely to live long enough for their disease to become life-threatening; men in their late 70s and 80s are more likely to die of another cause.

For example, in the study described in the sidebar at right, most of the prostate cancers grew slowly for up to 15 years after the initial diagnosis.

TREATMENT OPTIONS FOR PROSTATE CANCER

The standard treatment options for prostate cancer include watchful waiting, radical prostatectomy, radiation therapy, and hormone treatment. Radiation therapy can be delivered from an external source (external beam radiation therapy) or by implantation of radioactive seeds (brachytherapy). Cryotherapy (freezing the prostate) is also used to treat prostate cancer.

Radical prostatectomy and radiation therapy can potentially cure prostate cancer when the disease is detected in its early stages. Hormone therapy is not curative and is generally used to slow the progression of the disease once it has spread to other sites. Though chemotherapy is effective in treating some types of cancer, it has been less successful for prostate cancer. (Men with prostate cancer who wish to discuss specific treatments with other men who have already undergone them should contact the support groups listed on page 68.)

Because prostate cancer progresses more slowly than other types of cancer, men can take some time to carefully consider the various treatment options. They should talk to their doctor about the relative risks and benefits of each treatment and consider consulting physicians from different fields (urologists, radiation oncologists,

NEW RESEARCH

Study Supports Early Prostate Cancer Therapy for Younger Men

Opting for aggressive treatment over "watchful waiting" may be the better choice for younger men with prostate cancer, according to researchers.

Their study of 223 Swedish men with early-stage, initially untreated prostate cancer found that while most tumors lay dormant for 10 to 15 years after diagnosis, there was a surprising acceleration in the rates of tumor progression and death beyond the 15-year mark. The findings, the authors say, support aggressive treatment for otherwise healthy men diagnosed in their 60s or younger, who are likely to live for at least another 15 years.

The new study is the first to have followed prostate cancer patients for such a long time after diagnosis—an average of 21 years. While the cancer did not progress during the first 15 years in most cases, the rates of progression and death from prostate cancer tripled after the 15-year point among the 49 patients who were still alive. The findings "argue for" early surgery in men with long life expectancies, the authors conclude.

However, an editorial published with the findings points out that while surgery appears to boost men's survival in the five years after the procedure, the long-term benefits are unknown.

JOURNAL OF THE AMERICAN MEDICAL ASSOCIATION
Volume 291, pages 2713 and 2757
June 9, 2004

Seeking a Second (or Third or Fourth) Opinion

Getting a balanced view of all your options for prostate cancer may involve consulting with several specialists.

Determining a course of treatment for prostate cancer is one of the most harrowing decisions in modern medicine. Not only do treatments such as surgery and radiation therapy have troubling side effects, doctors can't agree on which treatments work best—and are more likely to recommend the option that they specialize in. Hence, to be in the best position for making decisions about your own treatment, it's vital to get more than one opinion.

Three Types of Specialists
In an often-cited study published in the *Journal of the American Medical Association* in 2000, researchers asked more than 1,000 specialists what treatment they would recommend for a man with early-stage prostate cancer who was expected to live at least 10 more years. Nearly all the urologists (93%)—who perform surgery—chose surgery as the preferred treatment, while most of the radiation oncologists (72%) responded that radiation therapy and surgery were equally effective treatments. The study authors' conclusion? Patients should schedule a consultation with a member of each specialty

before making a decision.

If these specialists don't agree, one option is to schedule a consultation with a medical oncologist, a specialist in cancer treatment who does not perform radiation or surgery. Another option is to see a second urologist or radiation oncologist. Doctors of the same specialty often have different approaches to treatment: For example, some radiation oncologists will recommend external beam radiation therapy; others, brachytherapy; and still others, a combination.

The Importance of the Pathologist
A final but not-to-be-overlooked reason to seek a second opinion is that if done at a center that specializes in prostate cancer treatments, it involves having another pathologist review the slides from your biopsy specimen. An accurate pathology reading is essential because it forms the basis for treatment decisions.

Unfortunately, spotting cancerous cells and determining how abnormal they appear are difficult, and pathologists sometimes make errors. In one study, pathologists at Johns Hopkins

reviewed biopsy samples of 535 men who had been referred for radical prostatectomy and reclassified 7 (1.3%) as benign. Upon subsequent clinical workup, 6 of 7 men were considered not to have prostate cancer, and their surgery was canceled. Getting an incorrect reading can limit your treatment options—or lead to having treatments that you don't need.

How To Get a Second Opinion
Some patients are reluctant to bring up the matter of second opinions, thinking that their doctor may not be receptive to involving another physician. Today, however, doctors in step with current medical standards welcome such discussions and support their patients' desire for additional information whenever appropriate. Health insurers generally pay for second opinions, and some even require them before certain procedures.

Your primary care doctor and the urologist who performed the biopsy are the best sources for referrals. Request that, if possible, they suggest a colleague affiliated with a different hospital. Although this is not absolutely necessary, the practice is

and medical oncologists) to get a broader spectrum of opinions. Making a treatment decision is most difficult for men with early-stage prostate cancer, since more treatment options are available.

Watchful Waiting
Watchful waiting involves no immediate treatment but does involve close monitoring for cancer progression. This treatment approach is most often recommended for men who are unlikely to live long enough to benefit from treatment and for those who have disease that is too far advanced to cure. In addition, some men who are thought to have small prostate cancers that are likely to grow very

prudent, because doctors who work at the same institution often share similar views and may be reluctant to contradict one another. Also check to be certain the consultant is board certified in the appropriate specialty. The American Medical Association (www.ama-assn.org) and the American Urological Association (www.urologyhealth.org) offer referral services. Hospitals, local health departments, family, and friends are other possible resources.

If your referring doctor is unwilling to discuss the possibility of a second opinion or makes you feel uncomfortable about the matter, strongly consider changing doctors.

Before meeting with you, the consultant will require all relevant medical records. The first doctor's office can send written reports and test results directly to the consultant. Be sure to call before your appointment to confirm their arrival, as it will be impossible to proceed without proper documentation; you can also choose to collect the records and deliver them personally.

During the consultation, the doctor will review the information and may perform a physical examination or order more tests. Recommendations made in a written report will be sent to the referring physician—and also to you if you request them.

Making an Appointment at Hopkins

Many people facing a serious health crisis wish to get a second opinion from a leading academic medical center such as Johns Hopkins. There are several ways to make appointments at Hopkins. The most direct way is for your physician to call the Hopkins Access Line (410-955-9444 in Baltimore and internationally or 800-765-5447 in the rest of the United States).

If you prefer to make an appointment yourself, you may call the appointment service line (410-955-5464 in Baltimore, or 410-955-8032 outside Baltimore, including international calls).

Finally, Johns Hopkins USA provides one point of contact for out-of-town patients. A representative can help you identify an appropriate physician or specialist, coordinate multiple medical appointments, arrange second opinions, and obtain general information about Johns Hopkins's many services. To talk with a representative, call 443-287-0528 weekdays, 8:30 A.M. to 5 P.M. Eastern Time.

Be sure that the specialists address all treatment options—surgery, radiation therapy, and watchful waiting—and discuss the advantages and disadvantages of each. If your doctors don't agree and you don't know what to do, one or more of the following approaches can help you reach a decision:

- Have the specialists explain to you why they came to their respective conclusions.
- Suggest that the specialists discuss the matter with each other; sometimes such conversations produce an acceptable consensus.
- Ask your general practitioner—or, if you wish, another specialist—to help you sort through the options.
- Consider seeking an opinion at a nationally recognized cancer center, such as one affiliated with the National Comprehensive Cancer Network (www.nccn.org).
- Try talking to men who have been treated for prostate cancer.

Don't panic if you're having trouble making a decision. Prostate cancer is generally a slow-growing malignancy, which means that most people can safely spend up to three months learning about the disease and consulting with the appropriate specialists.

---

slowly may opt for this approach.

Men who choose watchful waiting must see their doctor regularly to determine whether the cancer is progressing. If the cancer progresses, treatment options such as radical prostatectomy or radiation therapy may be considered, particularly in younger men. Recommendations on the frequency of visits and the tests conducted at each visit vary from doctor to doctor. H. Ballentine Carter, M.D., author of this White Paper, uses the following guidelines for men age 75 and younger who are in otherwise good health: PSA testing and a digital rectal exam twice a year, in addition to transrectal ultrasound and prostate biopsy once a year. The recommendations for PSA testing and digital rectal exams remain the same after age 75, but yearly ultrasound and biopsy are no longer performed routinely. Between appointments, men of any age should call their doctor if they experience blood in the urine, difficulty urinating, or new onset of pain.

Radical Prostatectomy

Radical prostatectomy offers the possibility of a cure only if the cancer has not spread to the lymph nodes in the pelvis or to other parts of the body. Therefore, when the risk of spread is judged to be high, some surgeons perform a laparoscopic biopsy to obtain samples of the lymph nodes before the planned prostatectomy; others sample the lymph nodes at the time of the scheduled prostatectomy and discontinue the operation if the cancer has spread. However, it is uncommon today (because of PSA testing) to find disease that has spread to lymph nodes at the time of surgery. If enlarged lymph nodes are discovered on a CT scan or MRI, a fine needle biopsy to remove some cells from the lymph nodes may be performed to determine whether the cancer has spread.

Radical prostatectomy is the only treatment for localized prostate cancer (cancer confined to the prostate) that has been proven to reduce deaths from the disease. A study published in 2002 found that Swedish men randomized to radical prostatectomy had a 50% reduction in their risk of dying of prostate cancer eight years after diagnosis, compared with men randomized to watchful waiting.

Radical prostatectomy was developed at Johns Hopkins at the beginning of the 20th century. The operation was not popular at first because of the high frequency of erectile dysfunction and urinary incontinence. But in the early 1980s, Patrick Walsh, M.D., a urologist at Johns Hopkins, developed a new approach to the operation. He devised a "road map" that allows surgeons to remove the prostate with a lower chance of damaging the structures important for erections and urinary control.

This anatomical, or "nerve-sparing," technique has reduced the risk of severe incontinence to 1% to 3% and the chance of mild incontinence to around 10%. The risk of erectile dysfunction varies with the age of man and the skill of the surgeon. One group of researchers reported successful recovery of erections in 68% of men treated with nerve-sparing surgery. Dr. Walsh has performed the procedure on more than 2,000 men with early prostate cancer, preserving erectile function in 90% of men in their 40s, 75% of those in their 50s, and 60% of those in their 60s. Full recovery of erectile

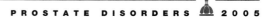

function can take more than a year in some cases, however. When erectile dysfunction does occur after surgery, it usually can be treated successfully (see pages 58–62).

Nerve-sparing radical retropubic prostatectomy begins with a vertical incision in the abdomen—from the pubic area to the navel. (Some surgeons make the incision in the perineum, which is located between the scrotum and rectum; in this case the procedure is called a perineal prostatectomy.) If appropriate, samples of tissue from the pelvic lymph nodes may be removed and tested for signs of cancer. To minimize bleeding, which can obscure the surgeon's view and increase the risk of complications, the surgeon then cuts and ties off the group of veins (the dorsal vein complex) that lie atop the prostate and urethra. Next, the surgeon severs the urethra, taking care to avoid the urethral sphincter muscles in order to preserve urinary continence.

At this point, the "nerve-sparing" aspect of the procedure comes into play: The tiny nerve bundles that sit on either side of the prostate and that are required for an erection are carefully dissected away from the prostate but are otherwise left intact. (If the cancer is suspected to have spread to these nerves, however, they will be removed.) The surgeon then cuts through the bladder neck (the junction between the bladder and the prostate) to completely separate the prostate and removes some of the surrounding tissues, including the seminal vesicles and vas deferens (the main duct that carries semen). Finally, the bladder neck is narrowed with stitches and reconnected to the urethra. A Foley catheter (inserted through the urethra to drain urine from the bladder) is left in place for two to three weeks to allow the rebuilt urinary tract to heal. Rare complications of radical prostatectomy include narrowing of the urethra (urethral stricture), damage to the rectum, and the surgical and anesthetic risks (including death) that accompany any operation.

Some surgeons are using laparoscopy to perform radical prostatectomy. The laparoscopic procedure is less invasive than traditional prostatectomy; it requires five tiny incisions in the abdomen rather than one long one. A 2003 study found that men who had the laparoscopic prostatectomy had less blood loss, required fewer pain pills after hospital discharge, had a shorter time to recovery, and had their catheters removed sooner than men who had a traditional prostatectomy. But the laparoscopic procedure takes two to three times as long to perform, so it is 15% to 30% more expensive than a traditional prostatectomy. Also, it is unclear how rates of cancer recurrence and erectile dysfunction compare with those of the

Advancements in Radiation Therapy

Newer techniques may make this prostate cancer treatment even more effective.

Radiation therapy is the second most common treatment for early-stage prostate cancer (radical prostatectomy is the first). Like radical prostatectomy, radiation therapy has the potential to cure prostate cancer when the disease is detected in its early stages.

Radiation can be delivered to the prostate either externally or internally. The standard external delivery method is called external beam radiation therapy (EBRT), in which beams of radiation are aimed at the tumor from outside the body. Because radiation to the prostate can damage the nearby rectum, bowel, and bladder, researchers have refined and developed alternatives to standard EBRT. Three-dimensional conformal radiation therapy (3DCRT) is the most popular refinement; intensity-modulated radiation therapy (IMRT) is a further refinement. The newest technique is proton-beam radiation.

Brachytherapy, also known as seed therapy, is a common method of internal radiation and is considered an option for men who choose radiation therapy. The two main refinements of brachytherapy are MRI-guided brachytherapy and high-dose-rate brachytherapy.

Talk to your doctor about which of these treatments, if any, may be appropriate for you.

3DCRT

In 3DCRT, the radiation oncologist (also known as the radiologist) uses dozens of computed tomography (CT) scans to "conform" the radiation beams to the precise shape of the tumor. Custom shaping of the beams permits higher dosing of radiation to the tumor while avoiding healthy tissue and nearby organs.

3DCRT has distinct advantages over standard EBRT. Studies have shown that 3DCRT markedly reduces the acute side effects that occur during traditional radiation treatment. For example, in one study, symptoms of bowel and bladder irritation requiring medication were reduced from 57% with conventional EBRT to 36% with 3DCRT.

Because the radiation doses used with 3DCRT are significantly higher than those delivered with conventional EBRT, 3DCRT may increase the chance of a cure. In a 2003 review article in *The Lancet Oncology*, the authors cited several published studies showing better disease-free survival rates with 3DCRT than with standard EBRT. In addition, they found that for men with clinical stage T1c or T2 and a Gleason score of less than 8, the five-year biochemical disease-free survival rates for 3DCRT were similar to those for radical

prostatectomy, standard brachytherapy, and IMRT. Until longer follow-up is done, however, the effectiveness of 3DCRT remains uncertain.

IMRT

A further refinement of 3DCRT is intensity-modulated radiation therapy (IMRT), in which the intensity of each beam is raised or lowered to meet the needs of the patient. Unlike 3DCRT, in which the radiation oncologist must arrange the beams by hand and determine the total dose of radiation to give, IMRT software determines the number, orientation, and intensity of beams. More research is needed, but several studies suggest that IMRT may allow for higher (and more effective) doses of radiation with fewer side effects than 3DCRT.

One concern with IMRT is that it's so precise, tissue adjacent to tumors may receive inadequate irradiation. But so far, short-term data indicate that disease-free survival at three years is 92% for low-risk tumors, 86% for intermediate-risk tumors, and 81% for high-risk tumors. The usefulness of IMRT will become apparent with longer follow-up.

Proton Beam Radiation Therapy

Proton beam radiation therapy employs the specialized targeting of

standard approach. Laparoscopic prostatectomy is being performed at Johns Hopkins in some patients, but it is still considered an evolving procedure. The surgeons at Johns Hopkins recommend that it be done only in otherwise healthy men with smaller tumors (PSA levels of less than 10 mg/dL, a Gleason score of 7 or less, and a normal digital rectal exam) who are not overly concerned about the possibility of loss of erectile function (as a nerve-sparing procedure is more difficult using the laparoscopic technique).

After radical prostatectomy, PSA tests are used to evaluate the

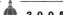

3DCRT, but it uses proton beams instead of x-rays. Protons, which are positively charged subatomic particles, are effective at killing cells at the end of their path while causing minimal damage to the tissues they pass through. The theory is that these particles can allow for higher radiation doses with fewer side effects.

Researchers from Loma Linda University recently published their results on 1,255 men with T1 or T2 prostate cancer treated with either proton beam radiation therapy or a combination of proton beam radiation therapy and x-rays. They found that 10 years after treatment, overall disease-free survival was 73%—similar to results with other forms of therapy—but with a low rate of side effects. A further refinement of this technique called proton beam IMRT is currently being investigated in an attempt to improve upon these excellent results.

Only a few centers currently offer proton beam radiation therapy, but that may change if studies continue to produce good results.

Brachytherapy

In standard brachytherapy, 80 to 120 radioactive "seeds" (tiny metal pellets) are implanted directly into the tumor under ultrasound guidance. The radiation works in the immediate area of the tumor and delivers a highly concentrated, yet confined, dose of radiation over a continuous period—24 hours a day for several months. The pellets remain in the body after they lose their radioactive energy. The seeds can migrate to other parts of the body, such as the lungs, but so far this migration does not appear to cause any complications.

Brachytherapy is an increasingly popular treatment option. In 1994, less than 4% of men who opted for radiation therapy for their cancer chose brachytherapy. By 1999, that figure had climbed to 36%. Some radiation experts believe that in the near future, the procedure will surpass radical prostatectomy as the treatment of choice for less aggressive forms of prostate cancer.

MRI-Guided Brachytherapy

In a further refinement of this process, Anthony D'Amico, M.D., Ph.D., of Harvard Medical School, has pioneered the technique of using magnetic resonance imaging (MRI) to guide seed implantation. An MRI allows for a much more precise placement of the seeds than ultrasound, according to Dr. D'Amico.

MRI-guided brachytherapy is not widely available because few oncologists have access to the necessary equipment, and only a few centers of excellence in the United States offer it at this time. However, Dr. D'Amico predicts that more treatment centers will begin using it in the near future.

High-Dose-Rate Brachytherapy

Another refinement to the brachytherapy procedure is high-dose-rate brachytherapy, in which the seeds are inserted into the prostate temporarily, rather than permanently.

Ultrasound is used to guide the placement of approximately 25 tiny hollow plastic needles into the prostate. While the patient remains in the hospital, a single radioactive pellet is delivered through each needle several times over a 24- to 48-hour period. After each treatment, the pellet is removed. After the final treatment, the needles are removed as well, and the patient is discharged.

High-dose-rate brachytherapy is thought to be superior to standard brachytherapy because a targeted level of radiation can be delivered through each needle, and because the radioactive seeds do not remain in the body. This level of control may mean the tumor is targeted more precisely and surrounding tissues are spared as much as possible.

A short-term study of 149 men published in *The Journal of Urology* in 2004 found that those who received high-dose-rate brachytherapy had similar disease-free rates after three years compared with the standard brachytherapy group. However, the high-dose group had reduced rates of several side effects, including urinary frequency, rectal pain, incontinence, and hematuria (blood in the urine).

success of the surgery and to monitor for disease recurrence. An undetectable PSA level (usually less than 0.2 ng/mL) after radical prostatectomy indicates that all the prostate tissue (both benign and malignant) has been removed. A detectable PSA immediately after surgery means that the tumor had already spread to other tissues before the surgery and thus could not be totally removed. A subsequent rise in PSA levels indicates the cancer has recurred in the area of the prostate or in another place in the body.

For men with cancer confined to the prostate (stage T1 or T2) before treatment, the chance of a cancer recurrence—indicated by detectable PSA levels—10 years after treatment is around 30%. A detectable PSA indicates a cancer recurrence months to years before the cancer is visible by a CT or bone scan. When evidence indicates that residual cancer is limited to the pelvis, radiation therapy is a treatment option. A detectable PSA in the first year after surgery indicates a high probability that the disease has spread beyond the pelvis and that radiation will not successfully eradicate the cancer. In this case, hormone therapy is considered, particularly if the cancer has spread to the bones.

Researchers at Johns Hopkins have studied the outcome for men with a detectable PSA after surgery. They followed nearly 2,000 patients who had cancer confined to the prostate and underwent radical prostatectomy by the same surgeon. Of the 304 men (15%) who had detectable PSA levels in the years following surgery, their five-year disease-free survival rate was 63% following the first detectable PSA, and metastatic cancer (cancer that has spread to other parts of the body) was not apparent for an average of eight years. These results should reassure men who experience rising PSA levels following surgery. At the same time, these findings serve as a reminder that continued regular monitoring is essential after surgery.

External Beam Radiation Therapy

External beam radiation therapy involves aiming beams of radiation at the tumor from outside of the body. It is a treatment option for men with localized prostate cancer (stage T2) or locally advanced disease (stage T3). Although no randomized trial has directly compared radical prostatectomy with radiation, available evidence suggests that, for patients with cancer confined to the prostate, either approach is associated with a good chance of being cancer free 5 to 10 years after treatment.

External beam radiation therapy is also used as a palliative treatment (a treatment aimed at relieving pain and limiting disease complications, rather than curing a disease). For a patient with prostate cancer that has spread to the bones, radiation therapy can reduce pain and lessen the likelihood of bone fractures. It can also be used to treat neurological symptoms resulting from compression of the spinal cord if cancer has spread to the spine.

Radiation oncologists are making improvements in external beam radiation therapy in an attempt to increase cure rates and reduce the risk of complications. These improvements include three-dimensional conformal radiation therapy (3DCRT), intensity-modulated radiation therapy, and proton-beam radiation. For more information on these advances, see the feature on pages 42–43.

Complications of radiation therapy mostly involve adverse effects on the urinary tract and bowel, and usually disappear days to weeks after completing treatment. The risk of long-term urinary complications, such as blood in the urine, bladder problems, or narrowing of the urethra, is about 8%. The risk of long-term rectal complications, such as bleeding, ulceration, rectal inflammation, narrowing of the rectum, or chronic diarrhea, is about 3%.

The risk of erectile dysfunction becomes more likely with time. In one recent study of 434 men, 86% were potent 15 months after treatment but only 50% were potent 6 years later. Younger men and those with normal sexual function before radiation therapy are the most likely to maintain potency.

PSA levels greater than 0.5 to 1 ng/mL indicate a high likelihood of residual cancer after radiation therapy; rising PSA tests after radiation therapy are evidence of disease progression. If cancer recurs after radiation therapy—and there is no evidence of distant disease—some patients can benefit from removal of the prostate or cryotherapy in an attempt to eradicate remaining disease within the prostate. Hormone therapy is used to treat recurrent disease at distant sites.

Brachytherapy

Another method of treating prostate cancer with radiation is brachytherapy, in which radioactive seeds (tiny metal pellets) are implanted directly into the tumor in the prostate. (For more information on brachytherapy and other internal radiation therapy techniques, see the feature on pages 42–43.)

Brachytherapy is appropriate for men with early-stage prostate cancer (stage T1) who have a Gleason score of 6 or less and a PSA level less than 10 ng/mL. But the procedure does not appear to be as effective as radical prostatectomy or external beam radiation therapy for men with higher stages or grades of disease. Consequently, an expert panel recently recommended against using brachytherapy in men with cancer graded T2 or higher, Gleason scores of 7 or more, or PSA levels above 10 mg/mL. The same panel also recommended against combining brachytherapy with external beam radiation therapy because of a high risk of side effects.

The side effects of brachytherapy are similar to those of external beam radiation therapy—urinary and bowel problems. But these complications may occur more often with brachytherapy than with

Radiation May Help Treat Recurrent Prostate Cancer

Timely radiation therapy for recurrent prostate cancer may offer hope for some men whose outlook traditionally has been regarded as grim, a study suggests.

Reviewing the cases of 501 men who received external beam radiation for cancer that had returned after radical prostatectomy, researchers found that the therapy offered men a 45% chance of remaining progression-free for four years. Moreover, the treatment, known as salvage radiotherapy, even helped some men with aggressive tumors who have previously been seen as "destined" to develop widespread cancer.

After cancerous prostate tissue is removed, a man's PSA levels should be undetectable. In cases where PSA levels quickly shoot up after surgery, the odds are high that the cancer has spread to distant sites. But in this study, even some men with rapidly rising PSA readings and aggressive, "high-grade" tumors did well after salvage radiotherapy.

An accompanying editorial notes that salvage radiation is typically used "too infrequently and too late," and should be offered early on to men at high risk for developing widespread cancer. However, the four-year follow-up does not answer the question whether salvage radiotherapy improves the survival of men with recurrent disease after surgery.

JOURNAL OF THE AMERICAN MEDICAL ASSOCIATION
Volume 291, pages 1325 and 1380
March 17, 2004

external beam radiation. In addition, the radioactive seeds can migrate to other parts of the body, such as the lungs, although research suggests that seed migration has no negative consequences.

Because brachytherapy is associated with a lower chance of a cure and a somewhat higher rate of complications than external beam radiation therapy, the latter is still considered the gold standard of radiation treatment for prostate cancer.

Two refinements of brachytherapy are MRI-guided brachytherapy and high dose rate brachytherapy; these are discussed in the features on pages 42–43.

Cryotherapy

Cryotherapy is accomplished by placing a probe through the perineum and into the prostate. The probe is attached to a source of nitrogen or argon, which cools the tip of the probe to extremely low temperatures. The low temperature freezes and destroys the prostate cancer cells. Although cryotherapy is a minimally invasive procedure, the long-term effectiveness of this technique is not well known and the risk of side effects such as erectile dysfunction is high. As a result, enthusiasm for cryotherapy as an initial treatment for prostate cancer has diminished. Men in whom radiation fails to eradicate disease locally are sometimes treated with cryotherapy.

Hormone Therapy

The discovery that male sex hormones (androgens), testosterone in particular, are required to maintain the size and function of the prostate led to the development of treatments designed to interfere with these effects of testosterone. Preventing testosterone from acting on prostate cancer cells can temporarily cause the cancer to regress, or at least to grow more slowly. However, because some prostate cancer cells are able to grow without testosterone (they are called androgen-independent or androgen-insensitive cells), the tumor will continue to grow despite the withdrawal of this hormone. Thus, hormone therapy is useful for the treatment of prostate cancer, but it does not offer a cure.

Hormone therapy used to be reserved for men whose prostate cancer has spread to other tissues (such as the lymph nodes or the bones) and cannot be completely eradicated by surgery or radiation. Now, hormone therapy also can be used to treat men whose disease has not spread but is expected to. According to a study published in the *Journal of the National Cancer Society* in 2003, hormone therapy should be considered for men whose PSA values double

A Common Complication After Radiation Therapy

Bowel disorders can develop months or years after treatment.

Because of the prostate's close proximity to the rectum, radiation therapy to treat prostate cancer can cause rectal inflammation (proctitis). Symptoms include diarrhea, straining when emptying the bowel, urgency, pain, and, sometimes, bleeding.

Although contemporary radiation techniques have made proctitis less common, it still affects many men undergoing radiation therapy. Some studies estimate that 10% to 20% of men experience bowel problems such as pain, burning, and/or diarrhea after radiation therapy. Men with circulation problems, such as peripheral arterial disease, heart disease, or high blood pressure, may be at increased risk because good blood flow is needed to heal rectal injury.

Symptoms may not appear until months or even years after therapy is completed, as radiation doses are cumulative and the effects take time to manifest in the body. When they do occur, however, symptoms can be severe—as many as 85% of affected men require treatment. Some cases of acute proctitis resolve within a few months, but a 2003 study found that 47% of radiation patients were still experiencing rectal bleeding two years after treatment had ended, as were 33% after three years. More severe complications, such as new blood vessel growth in the damaged rectum or fecal incontinence, are rare.

For most men, warm baths and over-the-counter pain relievers can help ease discomfort. There are, however, no proven standard treatments. Anti-inflammatory drugs, such as sulfasalazine (Azulfidine) or corticosteroids, taken orally or in an enema, may help. One study showed good results using oral metronidazole (Flagyl), an antibiotic, with a combination of anti-inflammatory medications. Another study found sucralfate (Carafate), a prescription medication used orally to treat and prevent ulcers, provided some relief when administered rectally.

If bleeding is a problem, endoscopic laser surgery or heated probes can be used to seal off the leaky vessels. More invasive surgical techniques are available but rarely required.

within the first three months of treatment with radical prostatectomy or radiation therapy.

The goals of hormone therapy for men with advanced prostate cancer are to prolong life and relieve symptoms, such as bone pain and urinary problems. Most men with M+ stage cancer live for six months to ten years; on average, about half survive for three years or less, and about a quarter live for five years. The survival rate for a man who chooses hormone therapy depends on the type of cells that make up his prostate cancer—that is, the ratio of androgen-dependent cells to androgen-independent cells. The greater the number of androgen-dependent cells within the tumor, the more likely the cancer will respond to hormone therapy. A PSA level of less than 4 ng/mL within three to six months of initiating hormone therapy predicts a good response to the treatment. A rising PSA level while on hormone therapy means that the disease is progressing.

There is no consensus as to when to begin hormone treatment. Whether hormone treatment is started before or after a bone scan detects the spread of prostate cancer may or may not make a difference in the survival rate. Because all effective forms of hormone therapy produce erectile dysfunction and loss of libido (sex drive)—and none is curative regardless of when treatment begins—

an earlier start may not be worth the risks of these and other side effects (such as hot flashes or loss of energy) or the costs of hormone therapy. However, the short-term use of hormone therapy in men with early-stage prostate cancer—particularly in combination with surgery or radiation therapy—has grown in popularity.

There is general consensus that hormone therapy prior to radical prostatectomy provides no benefit in terms of cancer cure. Hormone therapy is sometimes given to men with larger prostates (greater than 40 g) who are undergoing brachytherapy because hormone therapy helps to shrink the prostate before implanting the radioactive seeds. However, no well-designed randomized clinical trial has yet shown a survival benefit for men who receive hormone therapy prior to brachytherapy compared with men who do not.

There is general consensus that men with higher-grade cancer (grade D2 or greater, a Gleason score of 7 or more, or a PSA level of 10 or more) have better disease-free outcomes when hormone therapy is used in combination with radiation therapy as compared to radiation therapy alone.

There are two approaches to hormone therapy, also called testosterone withdrawal, androgen blockade, or castration. The first is surgical removal of the testicles, which produce about 95% of the body's testosterone (surgical castration). The second is the use of medications that interfere with the manufacture or actions of testosterone (medical castration). These medications include estrogens, luteinizing hormone-releasing hormone (LH-RH) analogs, gonadotropin-releasing hormone antagonists, and antiandrogens.

The signal to synthesize testosterone originates in an area of the brain called the hypothalamus. At regular intervals, the hypothalamus secretes luteinizing hormone-releasing hormone (LH-RH), which stimulates the pituitary gland to produce luteinizing hormone and follicle-stimulating hormone. Luteinizing hormone signals Leydig cells in the testicles to secrete testosterone into the bloodstream; follicle-stimulating hormone stimulates sperm production. When testosterone reaches the prostate, it is converted to dihydrotestosterone—a more potent form of testosterone—by the enzyme 5-alpha-reductase. The medications used for medical castration inhibit this sequence of events at various stages.

The most significant side effects of hormone therapy are erectile dysfunction in about 90% of patients and loss of libido. Other side effects include breast enlargement, weight gain, loss of muscle mass, osteoporosis (decreased bone mass), and fatigue. About two thirds of men have hot flashes—like those experienced by women during menopause. Hot flashes are not harmful and are probably caused by the effects of low androgen levels on the hypothalamus, which regulates body temperature. Hot flashes often can be managed with low doses of oral estrogen or with formulations of the hormone progesterone, such as medroxyprogesterone (Provera) or megestrol acetate (Megace). Hormone therapy does not cause the voice to change in pitch, as some men fear.

Surgical castration. Surgical removal of the testicles, known as bilateral orchiectomy, is the easiest and oldest way to interrupt the effect of testosterone on prostate cancer cells. The operation can be performed in about 20 minutes under spinal or local anesthesia, and the patient can usually go home the same day. People on anticoagulant therapy may not be candidates for surgical castration, since they are at risk for uncontrolled bleeding.

Surgical castration involves making a small incision in the scrotum and removing each testicle. Neither the operation nor the recovery is painful. In a variation of this procedure, called a subcapsular orchiectomy, only the contents of the testicles are removed. The empty shell of each testicle is left in place, resulting in a more satisfactory outward appearance. However, some surgeons do not use this technique because there is a risk that some testosterone-producing cells may be left behind.

The effect of orchiectomy is almost immediate. Within 12 hours of the procedure, testosterone levels fall to what is known as the castrate range. Because it is so effective, orchiectomy is the standard to which all other hormone therapies are compared.

Even though it is the most effective and least expensive form of hormone therapy, only about a quarter of men choose surgical castration. Obviously, psychological issues influence the decision to have this operation, which cannot be reversed. Men who are psychologically troubled by orchiectomy may prefer medical castration. Medical treatments can be as effective as orchiectomy, and the side effects are similar. Despite these side effects, hormone therapy—whether surgical or medical—prolongs the life of most men.

Estrogen preparations. A synthetic form of the female hormone estrogen can lower testosterone levels to the castrate range by blocking the release of luteinizing hormone from the pituitary gland, thereby shutting down the production of testosterone. Daily doses of synthetic estrogen (Premarin) are as effective as surgical castration, though the hormone takes longer to work; testosterone levels fall over a two-week period.

The most significant side effect of synthetic estrogen is an

Medications Used in Hormone Treatment of Prostate Cancer 2005

Drug Type	Generic Name	Brand Name	Average Dosage*	Average Retail Cost[†]
Estrogens	estrogen, conjugated	Premarin	3.75 mg daily	1.25 mg: $38
Gonadotropin-releasing hormone antagonist	abarelix	Plenaxis	100 mg injected monthly	100 mg: [price n/a]
Luteinizing hormone-releasing hormone (LH-RH) analogs	goserelin	Zoladex 3.6 Zoladex 10.8	3.6 mg injected monthly 10.8 mg injected every 3 months	3.6 mg: $514 10.8 mg: [price n/a]
	leuprolide	Eligard Lupron	7.5 mg injected monthly 7.5 mg injected monthly	7.5 mg/mL, 1 mL vial: [price n/a] 5 mg/mL, 2.8 mL vial: $421 ($335)
	leuprolide implant	Viadur	65 mg released annually 3.75 mg injected monthly	65 mg: [price n/a] 3.75 mg: [price n/a]
	triptorelin	Trelstar Depot Trelstar LA	11.25 mg injected every 3 months	11.25 mg: [price n/a]
Antiandrogens	bicalutamide flutamide nilutamide	Casodex Eulexin Nilandron	50 mg daily 750 mg daily 300 mg daily	50 mg: $410 125 mg: $73 ($46) 150 mg: $307

* These dosages represent an average range for the treatment of prostate cancer. The precise effective dosage varies from patient to patient and depends on many factors. Do not make any changes in your medication without consulting your doctor.

† Average price for 30 tablets or capsules (unless otherwise indicated) of the dosage strength listed. Actual price may vary. If a generic version is available, the cost is listed in parentheses. Sources: drugstore.com, eckerd.com, and walgreens.com.

increased risk of cardiovascular complications. These include heart attack, stroke, blood clots in the lungs or legs, phlebitis (inflammation of the veins), and edema (swelling of the legs). Because of these risks, people with a history of heart disease or thrombophlebitis (vein inflammation due to a blood clot) should not use estrogen therapy. In other people, these side effects can be minimized by using low doses of estrogen. In addition, taking an aspirin every other day helps to lower the risk of heart attack and blood clots; edema can be treated with diuretics (drugs that promote water loss through the urine). Estrogen can also cause nausea and vomiting. And like surgical castration, estrogen can cause breast enlargement and erectile dysfunction.

With the approval of LH-RH analogs, estrogens are no longer

How They Work	Comments
Estrogen targets the hypothalamus to block the release of luteinizing hormone-releasing hormone (LH-RH). In the absence of LH-RH, the pituitary gland does not release luteinizing hormone (LH), which is required to stimulate the production of testosterone by the testicles. Estrogen also acts directly on the pituitary.	Estrogen tablets lower testosterone to the castrate range over a two-week period. If estrogen is discontinued, testosterone levels return to normal. Side effects include possible cardiovascular problems (such as heart attack or blood clots), enlargement of the breasts, nausea, vomiting, fluid retention, erectile dysfunction, and loss of libido.
Inhibits gonadotropin and related androgen production by directly blocking gonadotropin-releasing hormone (GnRH) receptors in the pituitary. Also suppresses luteinizing hormone (LH) and follicle stimulating hormone (FSH) secretion, reducing the secretion of testosterone by the testes.	Used for men who are not candidates for treatment with LH-RH analogs. Equivalent to treatment by surgical castration in delaying progression of cancer initially, but effectiveness decreases over time. Side effects include hot flashes, sleep disturbance, breast enlargement, and dizziness.
Initially, these drugs stimulate the release of LH by the pituitary gland, prompting a jump in testosterone production. After several weeks, however, they block LH formation by the pituitary, and testosterone levels fall to the castrate range.	These drugs are equivalent to treatment by surgical castration in delaying progression of cancer. LH-RH analogs pose less cardiovascular risk than estrogen. Their side effects include erectile dysfunction, loss of libido, hot flashes, weight gain, fatigue, and loss of bone and muscle mass. Viadur is an implant that must be replaced annually.
To stimulate prostate cells, testosterone must first bind to specific androgen receptors within the cells. Antiandrogens bind to these androgen receptors, thus preventing androgens (including testosterone) from stimulating the cell.	Since antiandrogens do not block testosterone production, erectile function is preserved in some men. These drugs are used in combination with surgical castration or LH-RH analogs, since they are not as effective when used alone. Side effects are breast enlargement, diarrhea, and possible liver damage. Men taking flutamide should have their liver function checked after the first few months of treatment.

widely used. However, there is renewed interest in diethylstilbestrol (DES), a form of estrogen used in the 1960s for advanced prostate cancer. In addition, researchers are investigating the potential of an estrogen patch to lower testosterone levels without the side effects associated with other types of hormone therapy.

LH-RH analogs. These are synthetic products with chemical structures almost identical to natural LH-RH. Initially, they behave like LH-RH and stimulate the release of luteinizing hormone from the pituitary gland, causing an increase in testosterone production. But after a short period, they block the release of luteinizing hormone and reduce testosterone secretion from the testicles. The result is testosterone levels similar to those that occur after surgical castration or with estrogen. LH-RH analogs are equivalent to surgical castration and estrogen in their ability to delay progression of cancer and prolong survival.

Commonly used LH-RH analogs are goserelin (Zoladex), leuprolide (Eligard, Lupron), and triptorelin (Trelstar). LH-RH analogs are traditionally given as injections every month or every three months. Another option is an implanted drug delivery system (Viadur) that releases leuprolide continuously for one year.

The initial increase in testosterone with LH-RH analogs may be severe enough to exacerbate bone pain in men with prostate cancer that has spread to the bones and can be prevented with an antiandrogen (see below) until testosterone levels fall to the castrate range about two to three weeks later.

Other side effects of the LH-RH analogs include erectile dysfunction, loss of libido, hot flashes, weight gain, fatigue, and decreased bone and muscle mass. (The bisphosphonates pamidronate [Aredia] and zoledronic acid [Zometa] have been shown to prevent bone loss associated with LH-RH analogs, and zoledronic acid may actually boost bone density.) In addition, some men experience irritation at the injection sites. LH-RH analogs are less likely than estrogen to cause breast enlargement, nausea, vomiting, and cardiovascular problems.

Gonadotropin-releasing hormone antagonist. In 2003, the FDA approved abarelix (Plenaxis) for the treatment of advanced prostate cancer that does not respond to other hormone therapies. Abarelix works by lowering levels of testosterone in the blood. It is equivalent to treatment by surgical castration in delaying progression of cancer initially, but effectiveness decreases over time. The drug is given by injection every two weeks for the first month, then every four weeks. Because it can cause life-threatening allergic reactions in some men, the drug is available only through doctors participating in a risk management program. Side effects include hot flashes, sleep disturbance, breast enlargement, and dizziness.

Antiandrogens. To stimulate prostate cells (both cancerous and noncancerous), testosterone must first bind to specific androgen receptors within the cells. Drugs called antiandrogens can bind to these receptors and prevent testosterone from stimulating the cells. Since antiandrogens do not block testosterone production—which sets them apart from the other types of hormone therapy—their use may preserve erectile function in some patients. Three antiandrogens are approved by the FDA for the treatment of advanced prostate cancer: bicalutamide (Casodex), flutamide (Eulexin), and nilutamide (Nilandron).

When used alone, antiandrogens may not be as effective as other forms of castration. In addition, antiandrogens can cause hot flashes, breast enlargement, diarrhea, and, in rare instances, liver damage. To monitor for liver damage, men taking an antiandrogen must have their liver function tested a few months after starting treatment. Signs of liver problems include nausea, vomiting, fatigue, and jaundice. Nilutamide may slow the ability of the eyes to adapt to darkness. This side effect lasts for about four to six weeks.

In 40% to 75% of men taking an antiandrogen, an increase in PSA levels occurs, indicating disease progression. But if the medication is discontinued, PSA levels will fall. Why this occurs is not clear. It is possible that a mutation in the cancer cells results in their response to stimulation by antiandrogens.

Total androgen blockade. Since the adrenal glands also produce small amounts of androgens, including testosterone, some doctors use antiandrogens in combination with surgical or medical castration to block the possible effect of adrenal androgens on prostate cells. The combination of an antiandrogen (to block the effect of adrenal androgens) and surgical castration, an LH-RH analog, or a gonadotropin-releasing hormone antagonist (to halt production of testicular androgens) is referred to as total androgen blockade or total androgen suppression. Despite promising preliminary findings, numerous studies have failed to demonstrate that total androgen blockade prolongs life more than simply halting the production of testicular androgens alone. For example, a recent analysis of numerous studies found no difference in survival between men treated with total androgen blockade and those who underwent surgical castration or took LH-RH analogs alone. In addition, the results of the largest clinical trial to date, which compared total androgen blockade (orchiectomy plus flutamide) to orchiectomy alone, demonstrated no survival advantage with total androgen blockade.

Intermittent androgen suppression. In this approach, androgen blockade is achieved chemically (using an LH-RH analog or gonadotropin-releasing hormone antagonist alone or in combination with an antiandrogen) until PSA levels fall to the castrate range. Treatment is then discontinued until PSA begins to climb again. The rationale for this approach is the belief that hormone therapy encourages the growth of androgen-insensitive cancer cells (the cells that cause the tumor to continue to grow despite hormone therapy). Some doctors believe that cycling therapy on and off may delay the emergence of these deadly cells. In addition,

NEW RESEARCH

Ethnicity Influences Treatment Of Prostate Cancer

Black and Hispanic men receive definitive treatment for prostate cancer less often than white men, according to researchers. Previous studies have reported that care for black men with prostate cancer differs from that offered to their white counterparts, but few studies have examined care given to Hispanic men.

In this study, researchers analyzed data on more than 142,000 men with prostate cancer from a large national database to determine if the rates of definitive treatment (which includes surgery and various types of radiation therapy) differed among white, black, and Hispanic patients.

It turned out that black men with moderate-grade prostate cancer were 36% less likely than white men to receive definitive therapy, while Hispanic men were 16% less likely. The disparities were even more pronounced for men with more aggressive cancers. The study also showed that treatment differences narrowed over time for Hispanic men but far less for black men. Overall, black men are at greater risk for dying of prostate cancer than men of other races, though the reasons are unclear.

The authors concluded that further studies are necessary to determine the impact this phenomenon has on prostate cancer mortality in Hispanic and black American men.

THE JOURNAL OF UROLOGY
Volume 171, page 1504
April 2004

intermittent androgen suppression is associated with fewer side effects, since men discontinue therapy for periods of time.

More studies are needed to determine whether intermittent androgen suppression is as effective at slowing disease progression as continuous androgen support. But many oncologists use this approach routinely.

PC-SPES. PC-SPES was an over-the-counter product marketed as an herbal remedy for prostate cancer in the United States. It was removed from the market in 2002 after the discovery that the product contained several prescription drugs: the synthetic estrogen DES, the potent anti-inflammatory drug indomethacin (Indocin), and the blood thinner warfarin (Coumadin). Men who had good results with PC-SPES should ask their doctor about taking DES.

Other options. Testosterone levels can be reduced within 24 hours with ketoconazole (Nizoral)—a drug approved by the FDA to treat fungal infections that also inhibits the synthesis of adrenal and testicular androgens. Ketoconazole is used only when lowering androgens rapidly might be beneficial (for example, to alleviate pain). It is used only in the short term, because it raises luteinizing hormone levels, which can cause testosterone levels to rise and disease progression to occur. Ketoconazole can also cause liver problems.

Flutamide in combination with finasteride has been studied as a treatment option for advanced prostate cancer. Researchers hoped this combination would be effective, since finasteride lowers levels of dihydrotestosterone and could potentially enhance the ability of flutamide to block androgen action. But this approach is less effective than standard hormone therapy using an LH-RH analog or surgical castration.

Once hormone therapy is no longer effective, other treatment options are available to relieve cancer pain and improve quality of life. Effective pain relief is always possible with large enough doses of the proper medications. A wide range of medications—nonsteroidal anti-inflammatory drugs and corticosteroids, as well as morphine and other narcotics—may be used to stop pain. Mitoxantrone (Novantrone)—a chemotherapy drug used to treat a form of leukemia—is also approved for reducing pain from metastatic prostate cancer. It is used in combination with the steroid prednisone (Deltasone and other brands). Also, in 2004 the FDA approved docetaxel (Taxotere), a drug already used to treat advanced breast and lung cancer. Docetaxel, which is given as an injection with prednisone, may help prolong survival in men who do not respond to hormone therapy.

Dealing With the Side Effects of Hormone Therapy

While hormone therapy can be effective, it is often approached with trepidation because of its side effects.

Hormone therapy is used to slow the spread of incurable prostate cancer and to palliate symptoms. More recently, it has also been used as an adjunct to either radiation or surgery for locally advanced disease that is potentially curable.

But hormone therapy is associated with a number of undesirable side effects. For example, surgical castration by removal of the testicles or medical castration by using luteinizing hormone-releasing hormone (LH-RH) analogs such as goserelin (Zoladex) and leuprolide (Lupron) can cause both erectile dysfunction (ED) and loss of libido (sexual drive) because of reduced testosterone levels. Other side effects range from the annoying—like hot flashes—to the dangerous—for example, osteoporosis (bone loss).

Fortunately, many of these symptoms can be managed, if not eliminated. Discussed below are some of the more common symptoms of hormone therapy and the strategies for treating them.

Loss of Libido

Decreased testosterone levels result in a loss of libido. But one type of hormone therapy—antiandrogen therapy (see pages 52–53)—does not disrupt the production of testosterone by the testicles in the same way as castration. Rather, because antiandrogens block the action of testosterone by selectively binding to testosterone receptors, testosterone is rendered ineffective, but remains in the bloodstream. This may spare libido.

Antiandrogens are currently under investigation as a method of preserving libido during hormone treatment. Unfortunately, antiandrogens are not as effective for treating prostate can-

cer as castration and cannot be used as a solo therapy.

Erectile Dysfunction

Lowering testosterone levels by castration may cause ED. As with libido, antiandrogens appear to have less impact on potency since testosterone is not eliminated. Therefore, oral ED drugs like sildenafil (Viagra) may work in men taking antiandrogens alone. But because antiandrogens are not as effective when used alone, they are most often combined with surgical castration or LH-RH analogs.

Researchers have explored the possibility of using antiandrogens in combination with finasteride (Proscar), which blocks the conversion of testosterone to a more active androgen within prostate cells. This approach may result in a lower rate of ED, but it is not as effective against cancer as surgical castration or LH-RH analogs.

Hot Flashes

Similar to those experienced by women during menopause, hot flashes are sudden, brief periods of warmth and flushing followed by perspiration. The majority of patients who receive hormone therapy experience hot flashes and approximately 10% of men continue to have them after hormone therapy is terminated. They are probably due to the effects of low levels of androgens on the hypothalamus, which regulates body temperature.

Some men can successfully ignore or tolerate hot flashes, or manage them by wearing layers of clothing or opening windows. But if hot flashes continue to be bothersome, low doses of oral estrogen (1 mg per day), medroxyproges-

terone (Provera), or megestrol acetate (Megace) may be prescribed to alleviate them.

Osteoporosis

Osteoporosis is a decrease in bone mass that causes bones to become weak, brittle, and prone to fracture. Testosterone deficiency increases the risk of osteoporosis in men, and a recent study demonstrated that castration results in a reduction of bone mass to 70% of normal after 10 years of treatment.

For this reason, calcium supplements are recommended for men undergoing hormone therapy. The National Institutes of Health (NIH) recommends that men over age 65 take 1,500 mg of calcium a day, and men receiving hormone therapy should be sure to get at least that much. Also, they should take daily vitamin D supplements (400 IU for men age 51 to 70 and 600 IU for those over age 70) to promote the absorption of calcium from the intestine.

Exercise is another important way to prevent osteoporosis. Weight-bearing exercise, such as walking and lifting weights, helps to increase muscle mass, which stimulates bone growth. Finally, a number of medications, such as pamidronate (Aredia) and zoledronic acid (Zometa), are used to prevent and treat osteoporosis in men with prostate cancer.

Liver Damage

Liver damage is a rare but serious side effect of the antiandrogen flutamide (Eulexin). Patients receiving flutamide should be monitored regularly and carefully for liver problems with blood tests and examinations. Signs of liver problems include nausea, vomiting, fatigue, and jaundice.

Bone pain can be treated with bisphosphonate drugs such as zo-ledronic acid (Zometa), radiation therapy, or injections of a radio-active substance called strontium-89. Surgery, such as transurethral prostatectomy (also called transurethral resection of the prostate, or TURP), can be performed to treat urinary symptoms caused by locally advanced disease (see pages 16–17).

MANAGING SIDE EFFECTS OF TREATMENT

The two side effects of prostate cancer treatment that concern men the most are urinary incontinence and erectile dysfunction. As treatments for prostate cancer improve, these complications will become less common. When they do occur, however, there are effective ways to alleviate them.

Urinary Incontinence

Because surgery or radiation therapy may irritate the urethra or bladder or damage the urinary sphincter muscles that contract to prevent urine from flowing out of the bladder, some degree of incontinence is common immediately after treatment.

For example, urge incontinence (the strong, sudden need to urinate that is followed by a bladder contraction and results in invol-untary loss of urine) is common for a few days after catheter removal in men who have undergone TURP for the treatment of BPH. In the initial period after radical prostatectomy for prostate cancer, men typically experience stress incontinence, in which leak-age of urine occurs during moments of physical strain (such as sneezing, coughing, or lifting heavy objects). Recovering bladder control can be a slow process after treatment for BPH or prostate cancer and may take up to six months. Fortunately, severe inconti-nence occurs in less than 1% of men after surgery for BPH and in less than 10% of men after radical prostatectomy or radiation thera-py for prostate cancer.

A number of methods can be used to reduce incontinence. These include lifestyle measures, Kegel exercises, collagen injec-tions, and artificial sphincter implantation. In addition, absorbent products, penile clamps, external collection devices, catheters, and medications can help men cope with incontinence.

Lifestyle measures. Simple changes in behavior can be helpful. A high-calorie diet and lack of exercise can lead to obesity, which increases pressure on the bladder and exacerbates incontinence. Because constipation can also worsen symptoms, it is important to eat high-fiber foods, such as leafy green vegetables, fruits, whole grains, and legumes. Caffeine and alcohol consumption should be limited since they increase frequency of urination. If nighttime urination is a problem, avoid consuming liquids several hours before bedtime.

Kegel exercises. Kegel exercises are performed by squeezing and relaxing the pelvic floor muscles that support the bladder and surround the urethra. By strengthening these muscles, bladder control may improve. In a 2003 study, 68% of men who did Kegel exercises after radical prostatectomy for prostate cancer regained urinary continence within three months, compared with 37% of men who did not do these exercises.

To locate the pelvic floor muscles, try slowing or stopping the flow of urine midstream. Although there is no standard routine for performing Kegel exercises, a good starting point is 45 repetitions a day. Each repetition involves contracting the pelvic floor muscles for three seconds, then releasing them for another three seconds. Divide the 45 repetitions into three sets of 15. Do each set in a different position: sitting, standing, and lying down, respectively.

Collagen injections. Collagen can be injected around the bladder neck to add bulk and provide increased resistance to urine flow during times of physical strain. However, repeat injections often are needed because collagen is a naturally occurring protein and is broken down by the body.

Artificial sphincter implantation. In this procedure, a doughnut-shaped rubber cuff is implanted around the urethra. The cuff is filled with fluid and is connected by a thin tube to a bulb implanted in the scrotum. In turn, the bulb is connected to a reservoir within the abdomen. The fluid in the cuff creates pressure around the urethra to hold urine inside the bladder. When the urge to urinate is felt, squeezing the bulb transfers fluid from the cuff to the reservoir and deflates the cuff for three minutes so urine can drain through the urethra. Afterward, the cuff automatically refills with fluid and urine flow is again impeded.

Absorbent products. Wearing absorbent pads or undergarments is the most common way to manage incontinence. Typically used right after surgery, these products are effective for minor to severe incontinence.

Penile clamps. These devices, which compress the penis to prevent urine from leaking, are an option for severe incontinence. Penile clamps are not recommended immediately after treatment because they prevent the development of muscle control that is

NEW RESEARCH

Frequent Ejaculation Linked to Lower Prostate Cancer Risk

Frequent ejaculation does not appear to raise a man's odds of prostate cancer—and may help lower the risk for some, new research suggests. Previous studies that were not as well designed had found a link between frequent ejaculation and an increased risk of prostate cancer.

Investigators found that for most of the 29,000-plus men they followed, self-reported ejaculation frequency did not sway the risk of developing prostate cancer. However, the most active group—the 2,000 who ejaculated at least 21 times per month—did show a lower risk of the disease.

The new study asked male health professionals ages 46 to 81 to estimate how many times per month they ejaculated during the past year and throughout their 40s and 20s. Those who fell into the 21-plus category at any age—but particularly in the last year—were less likely to develop prostate cancer over the next eight years than men who ejaculated four to seven times per month.

Since the study factored in diet and other lifestyle habits, it seems unlikely that generally better health explains the finding, the authors say. Some hypothesize that ejaculation helps "flush out" potentially cancer-promoting compounds from the prostate. However, more research is needed to understand the relationship.

JOURNAL OF THE AMERICAN MEDICAL ASSOCIATION
Volume 291, page 1578
April 7, 2004

needed to regain urinary continence.

External collection devices. These condom-like devices can be pulled over the penis and held in place with adhesive, Velcro straps, or elastic bands. A tube drains fluid from the device to a bag secured on the leg. Often used with a penile clamp, these devices should not be used immediately after surgery, because muscle control needed for bladder control will not develop.

Catheters. A Foley catheter is a small tube that is inserted through the urethra and allows urine to flow continuously from the bladder into a bag after prostate treatment. This option is not recommended for long-term use because it can cause irritation, infection, and, possibly, loss of muscle control.

Medications. Medication can be used to control mild to moderate incontinence but is not effective for severe cases. Medications such as oxybutynin (Ditropan), tolterodine (Detrol), and propantheline (Pro-Banthine) may reduce urge incontinence by decreasing involuntary bladder contractions. Nasal decongestants, like pseudoephedrine, or the antidepressant imipramine (Tofranil) can reduce stress incontinence by increasing smooth muscle tone in the bladder neck. Because pseudoephedrine is a stimulant that can increase heart rate and blood pressure, it should be used only under a doctor's supervision. The drug also may cause nervousness, restlessness, and insomnia and may have adverse effects in people with asthma or cardiovascular disease.

Erectile Dysfunction

Men who must undergo radical prostatectomy or radiation therapy for prostate cancer often fear they will be unable to resume sexual activity after treatment. While these procedures may result in erectile dysfunction, they do not directly affect libido or the ability to achieve orgasm. This is in contrast to hormone therapy, which lowers testosterone levels and decreases libido.

The penis is made up of nerves, smooth muscle, and blood vessels. Within the penis are two cylindrical chambers—the corpora cavernosa, or corporal bodies—that extend from the base to the tip. When a man has an erection, smooth muscle tissue within the penis relaxes, causing these spongy chambers to dilate and fill with blood. The swollen corporal bodies press against and close the veins that normally allow blood to flow away from the penis; as a result, the penis remains engorged with blood. After orgasm, the smooth muscle tissue contracts and blood once again flows out of the penis.

This process is initiated by signals passing through nerve bundles that run toward the penis along both sides of the prostate. Radical prostatectomy can cause erectile dysfunction when one or both of these nerve bundles is damaged during surgery. Nerve damage does not affect sensation in the penis, but it does impair the ability to achieve a normal erection. Radiation treatment can also result in erectile dysfunction by damaging these nerve bundles or the arteries that carry blood to the penis.

The first treatment used in erectile dysfunction is either a vacuum pump or an oral medication. If these are ineffective or inappropriate, another option is vasodilators, which are injected or inserted into the penis. Surgical implantation of a prosthesis is an option for men who do not respond to less invasive forms of treatment.

Vacuum pumps. A simple, noninvasive treatment for erectile dysfunction is the vacuum pump—an airtight tube that is placed around the penis before intercourse. The tube is attached to a pump, which withdraws air from the tube and creates a partial vacuum that causes the penis to become engorged with blood. A constricting ring is then placed at the base of the penis to prevent blood from flowing out. Erections last about half an hour; leaving the constricting ring on for a longer period may be harmful. Vacuum pumps are highly effective devices, but many men find them cumbersome to use.

Oral medications. Oral drugs are the newest advance in the treatment of erectile dysfunction. Three oral drugs are currently available: sildenafil (Viagra), vardenafil (Levitra), and the newly approved tadalafil (Cialis). All three belong to a class of drugs known as phosphodiesterase type 5 inhibitors. Unlike other therapies for erectile dysfunction, these drugs do not produce erections in the absence of sexual stimulation.

Normally, sexual arousal increases levels of a substance called cyclic guanosine monophosphate (cGMP) in the penis. Higher levels of cGMP relax smooth muscles in the penis and allow blood to flow into its two inner chambers. Sildenafil, vardenafil, and tadalafil work by blocking the actions of an enzyme called phosphodiesterase type 5, which is found primarily in the penis. This enzyme causes erections to subside by breaking down cGMP. By maintaining increased cGMP levels, the drugs enhance both relaxation of smooth muscles in the corpora cavernosa and engorgement of these chambers with blood. As a result, men with erectile dysfunction can respond naturally to sexual arousal.

Oral drugs have been tested in a wide range of men with erectile dysfunction. For a discussion of their effectiveness and side effects, see the feature on the opposite page.

Vasodilators. Erections can be produced with vasodilators, drugs that widen the blood vessels and allow the penis to become engorged with blood. The most commonly used vasodilator for erectile dysfunction is alprostadil. Other vasodilators include papaverine and phentolamine.

Alprostadil can be injected directly into the base of the penis with a needle or inserted into the urethra in pellet form through a delivery system called MUSE. Both approaches have drawbacks. Injections can cause pain, scarring, and priapism—a painful, prolonged erection that must be treated medically. MUSE can cause urethral burning. Using low doses can minimize the risk of such side effects.

Since vasodilators cause erections by dilating blood vessels—an event that occurs after the nerve signal travels along the nerve bundles to the penis—they may work when sildenafil does not (such as when the nerve bundles are no longer intact). Moreover, researchers recently theorized that regular injections of vasodilators (regardless of whether the injections were followed by sexual activity) might help bring about the return of normal erections—presumably by re-establishing blood flow to the penis.

In a small 12-week study, 67% of radical prostatectomy patients who received alprostadil injections eventually achieved normal erections, compared with just 20% of those who did not receive injections. In addition, an Israeli study found that vasodilator injections were more effective than vacuum pumps or sildenafil for regaining erectile function.

A study of 270 radical prostatectomy patients who used MUSE suggested that this approach may be successful in stimulating erections in 40% of cases. MUSE is not effective in men with incontinence, because urine leakage washes the pellet out of the urethra before it can be absorbed.

Surgery. Several types of surgically implanted devices can provide erections sufficient for sexual intercourse. In one approach, a semi-rigid device—a rod-shaped piece of silicone inserted into the penis—is bent downward into the erect position before intercourse; afterward, it is folded upward close to the body. A more commonly used device consists of two hydraulic chambers implanted into the penis and connected to a fluid-filled pump placed in the scrotum. An erection is created by pumping fluid into the chambers.

Future treatments. Erectile dysfunction is an expanding field of

Choosing a Drug for Erectile Dysfunction

Men who have difficulty achieving or maintaining an erection now have three medications available. How do they compare?

Erectile dysfunction (ED) is an important concern for men with prostate disorders because it is a potential complication of treatment. Sildenafil (Viagra), the first oral medication for this condition, became available in 1998. Since then, two additional ED drugs have become available: vardenafil (Levitra) and tadalafil (Cialis). All three of these drugs are phosphodiesterase type 5 (PDE5) inhibitors, and they work in the same way: by permitting more blood to flow into the penis during sexual stimulation.

How They Compare

There are no studies that directly compare one PDE5 inhibitor with another, but some differences exist. For example, although data suggest that all three drugs become effective in about 20 minutes, some research suggests that higher doses of Levitra may "peak" faster. Levitra's faster peaking time means a faster effect. In addition, Viagra and Levitra typically improve erections for about four hours, and they cannot be taken more than once daily. By contrast, Cialis is effective for 24 to 36 hours, meaning you can take your pill Friday night, for example, and have it last for much of the weekend.

Side effects are also slightly different for the three drugs. Viagra and Levitra may cause facial flushing, nasal congestion, or nausea. At high doses, Viagra may make objects appear tinged with blue. Cialis can cause muscle aches, and Levitra can prompt a drop in blood pressure (hypotension), which can result in fainting. However, not all men experience these problems, and side effects often lessen with repeated use.

Special Considerations

Men with or at risk for cardiovascular disease should receive a thorough medical workup before initiating sexual activity regardless of which medication is chosen. PDE5 inhibitors are not recommended for men who use nitroglycerin tablets or patches, which are prescribed for heart-related chest pain, or for those who've had a heart attack, stroke, or life-threatening arrhythmia during the last six months. Deaths associated with PDE5 inhibitors have been related to severe hypotension caused by taking nitroglycerin with a PDE5 inhibitor or heart attacks triggered by strenuous physical activity (including sex).

Liver or kidney impairment may preclude taking a PDE5 inhibitor or affect the dosage you can take. Simultaneous administration of Viagra to patients taking alpha-blocker therapy may lead to symptomatic hypotension in some patients. Therefore, Viagra doses above 25 mg should not be taken within four hours of taking an alpha-blocker. Cialis can be taken with 0.4 mg of the alpha-blocker tamsulosin (Flomax), but not with other alpha-blockers. Because the coadministration of alpha-blockers and Levitra can produce hypotension, Levitra is contraindicated in patients taking alpha-blockers. (The bottom line is that none of the PDE5 inhibitors should be taken with alpha-blockers with the exception of Cialis and 0.4-mg of Flomax or Tamsulosin.) Other medications that may require special consideration include erythromycin (an antibiotic), ketoconazole (an antifungal drug), and ritonavir (Norvir), a protease inhibitor used to treat HIV infection.

Keeping Expectations Realistic

Although PDE5 inhibitors can restore the ability to achieve a healthy erection, they will not increase libido (the desire for sex), improve a flawed relationship, or create intimacy where little exists. In fact, introducing an ED medication into a formerly sexless partnership could be a destabilizing force, particularly if other aspects of the relationship are troubled. In such cases, counseling may be recommended in addition to drug therapy.

research, with new treatments on the horizon. One experimental drug called apomorphine (Uprima) targets mechanisms in the brain to stimulate an erection. It may be available within the next year or two. Although apomorphine may not be as effective as sildenafil, vardenafil, or tadalafil, it may provide another option for men who cannot take these oral medications.

A topical preparation of alprostadil (Topiglan) has shown some promise for men with erectile dysfunction. This preparation is applied to the head of the penis. Further research is necessary, but absorption will likely be a problem with this approach. An ointment is easier to use than alprostadil injections or the MUSE delivery system, and it would be associated with fewer side effects, but it is more difficult to achieve efficient absorption of the drug through the skin.

Prostatitis

Prostatitis is a common condition in which the prostate becomes infected or inflamed. The disorder usually causes severe pain in the perineum—the area between the rectum and scrotum. Men may also feel pain in their groin, genitals, and lower back. Another possible symptom is an urgent or frequent need to urinate, which can be mistaken for benign prostatic hyperplasia (BPH). Some men complain of painful ejaculation, while others say that ejaculation provides pain relief. According to one study, men with prostatitis have a diminished quality of life that is on par with those who have recently suffered a heart attack.

Prostatitis is often difficult to treat, and part of the problem is that the disease comes in several forms. Some patients experience acute flare-ups, with sudden and continuous pain that lasts for several days. More common, however, is chronic prostatitis, which may last for several weeks, only to disappear and then start up again. It usually affects men in their early 40s, and it is one of the leading reasons why men visit a urologist.

Prostatitis is further differentiated by bacterial and nonbacterial causes. Nearly 95% of patients are thought to develop prostatitis from nonbacterial causes, which have yet to be identified. In addition, some men have signs of inflammation, such as white blood cells in their semen, but none of the painful symptoms of prostatitis. A related condition, called prostatodynia, causes the same symptoms as prostatitis, but with no signs of infection or inflammation on laboratory tests.

CAUSES OF PROSTATITIS

While the causes of bacterial prostatitis are obvious and easy to detect, researchers are unsure why men develop the more prevalent, nonbacterial form. Some men find that stress, emotional problems, or even coffee may trigger flare-ups. Other possible culprits include

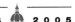

zinc deficiency, tight urinary sphincter muscles, infrequent ejaculation, and dehydration. Researchers have yet to confirm whether these are possible causes of nonbacterial prostatitis.

Some experts suggest that nonbacterial prostatitis is not really a prostate problem at all. Rather, flare-ups could be the result of a pelvic muscle spasm or some other cause that mimics symptoms originating in the prostate. Another theory under investigation is that prostatitis is caused by an autoimmune disorder, in which the immune system mistakenly attacks healthy prostate tissue and promotes inflammation—not unlike the way rheumatoid arthritis targets the joints. Indeed, researchers recently found that men with chronic prostatitis had increased levels of the same pro-inflammatory molecules that are elevated in the joint tissue of people with rheumatoid arthritis.

DIAGNOSIS OF PROSTATITIS

As part of the initial evaluation, the patient's urine is examined to determine if the disease stems from a bacterial cause. In the past, cultures were taken from normal urine flow (both urethral and bladder specimens) and from urine voided after a prostate massage—a process in which the doctor methodically strokes the prostate until fluid is pushed out into the urethra. But these cultures have not been found helpful in distinguishing between the types of prostatitis.

A prostate massage is not performed if a bout of acute prostatitis is accompanied by fever and chills. Acute flare-ups may also cause a steep rise in prostate specific antigen (PSA) levels, so PSA testing for prostate cancer should be avoided during these episodes.

A symptom questionnaire recently developed by the National Institutes of Health (NIH) may also help in assessing the disease. The questionnaire asks about three aspects of prostatitis: pain, urinary symptoms, and quality of life. After scoring the answers, a physician can determine the impact of a patient's symptoms and the degree to which treatments are working.

TREATMENT OF PROSTATITIS

Treatment is fairly straightforward for bacterial prostatitis. A patient is given antibiotics for a period of 4 to 16 weeks. Appropriate antibiotics include carbenicillin (Geocillin, Geopen), trimethoprim/sulfamethoxazole (Bactrim, Cotrim), doxycycline (Apo-Doxy, Doryx),

NEW RESEARCH

Painful Ejaculation Signals More Severe Prostatitis

Men with chronic prostatitis who experience painful ejaculation have worse symptoms and poorer outcomes than those who never have pain after ejaculation, according to a new study.

Researchers surveyed 486 men with chronic prostatitis from the NIH Chronic Prostatitis Cohort study over a three-month period. Of these, 24% reported frequent pain after ejaculation and 26% never had pain after ejaculation. The other 50% reported intermittent pain after ejaculation.

The more often a man reported painful ejaculation, the researchers found, the worse his symptoms of chronic prostatitis were and the less likely he was to experience improvement. People with pain after ejaculation were also more likely to be younger, have a worse quality of life, live alone, and have a lower income.

People with pain after ejaculation may have a specific form of prostatitis, which would explain why the disease affects them differently. Alternately, postejaculatory pain may be a marker for increased disease severity, or increased sensitivity to pain.

THE JOURNAL OF UROLOGY
Volume 172, pages 432 and 542
August 2004

and fluoroquinolones like ciprofloxacin (Cipro). Bacterial prostatitis is the most curable form of the disease, although some patients may not respond to treatment, or symptoms may reappear once the antibiotics are stopped.

Treatment of nonbacterial prostatitis is more difficult, and no one treatment has been proven to improve symptoms for most men. Several possible treatments are available, and some can be used separately or in combination It may take some trial and error to find a combination of therapies and self-care techniques to obtain symptom relief.

While antibiotics typically are reserved only for bacterial diseases, many patients with nonbacterial prostatitis receive antibiotics and a prostate massage, followed by high doses of alpha-blocker drugs (typically used for BPH). Prostatodynia (painful prostate) may improve when treated with muscle relaxants and alpha-blockers. Men who experience pain are usually helped by anti-inflammatory medications. A warm bath may also work for some men, while ice packs are more effective for others.

If ejaculation is not painful, sex or masturbation may improve symptoms. Still, many men are frustrated because no therapy exists that provides consistent relief from nonbacterial prostatitis. Fortunately, major research efforts are currently under way, such as the NIH-funded Chronic Prostatitis Cohort Study. Experts are optimistic that this study and other research will provide important new insights on improving the management of chronic prostatitis. ■

GLOSSARY

5-alpha-reductase inhibitors—A class of drugs used to treat benign prostatic hyperplasia (BPH). They block the conversion of testosterone into dihydrotestosterone, the major male sex hormone within the cells of the prostate.

acute urinary retention—A complete inability to urinate that requires immediate medical attention.

age-specific PSA—An adjustment of the PSA value that accounts for the natural, gradual increase in PSA that occurs with age as the prostate enlarges.

alpha-1-adrenergic blockers—A class of drugs used to treat benign prostatic hyperplasia (BPH) that work by relaxing smooth muscle tissue within the prostate. Also called alpha-blockers.

androgens—Sex hormones, such as testosterone, found in higher levels in males than in females.

antiandrogens—Drugs that bind to androgen receptors in cells, preventing androgens from stimulating the cells.

benign prostatic hyperplasia (BPH)—Noncancerous enlargement of the prostate gland due to an increase in the number of prostate cells.

bladder neck—The junction between the bladder and the prostate.

brachytherapy—A treatment for prostate cancer that involves the implantation of radioactive seeds into the prostate.

catheterization—A procedure in which a tube is inserted into the urethra to drain urine from the bladder. Used after prostate surgery and in the treatment of acute urinary retention.

cryotherapy—The use of extreme cold to treat a disease, such as prostate cancer.

cystoscopy—Passage of a cystoscope (a type of telescope) through the urethra into the bladder to directly view the urethra and bladder.

digital rectal exam—An examination in which a doctor inserts a lubricated, gloved finger into the rectum to feel for abnormalities of the prostate and rectum.

dihydrotestosterone—The most potent androgen inside prostate cells; formed from testosterone by the enzyme 5-alpha-reductase.

external beam radiation therapy—A therapy for prostate cancer that uses an x-ray machine to aim high-energy radiation at the prostate.

filling cystometry—A test that involves filling the bladder with fluid, measuring how much pressure builds up in the bladder, and how full it is when the urge to urinate occurs.

Foley catheter—A small tube inserted through the ure-thra that allows urine to drain from the bladder into a bag. Has a balloon at its tip so that it remains in place when filled with water.

follicle-stimulating hormone—A pituitary hormone that stimulates sperm production by the testicles.

glandular cells—Cells in the prostate that produce part of the fluid portion of semen. Also called epithelial cells.

Gleason score—A classification system for prostate cancer, based on the microscopic appearance of cancer cells; it is used to predict the seriousness of the cancer and the need for treatment. Scores range from 2 to 10 and are derived by adding the two most prevalent cancer grades, which range from 1 to 5. A lower score indicates that the cancer is less aggressive.

hematuria—Blood in the urine.

hormone therapy—Usually a treatment for prostate cancer that has spread beyond the prostate. Slows the progression of cancer by preventing testosterone from acting on cancer cells but does not cure the cancer.

imaging studies—Tests that produce an image of the inside of the body. Some examples of these tests are ultrasound, computed tomography (CT), magnetic resonance imaging (MRI), and x-rays.

incontinence—An inability to control bladder function.

intermittent androgen suppression—A technique in which androgen blockade with medications is discontinued once PSA levels fall and restarted when PSA levels begin to rise again.

interstitial laser coagulation—A minimally invasive therapy for BPH, in which a needle is placed through the urethra to deliver laser energy to the prostate.

Kegel exercises—Exercises to strengthen the pelvic floor muscles. May help men recover bladder function more quickly after prostate surgery.

laparoscopy—A technique in which a tiny instrument containing a light and camera at one end is inserted into the body through a small incision. Used for a variety of surgical and diagnostic procedures, including radical prostatectomy.

laser prostatectomy—A treatment for BPH in which laser energy is used to destroy excess prostate tissue.

libido—Sex drive.

luteinizing hormone—A pituitary hormone that stimulates the release of testosterone from the testicles.

luteinizing hormone-releasing hormone (LH-RH)—A hormone released by the hypothalamus that stimulates the pituitary gland to produce luteinizing hormone and follicle-stimulating hormone.

GLOSSARY—continued

luteinizing hormone-releasing hormone (LH-RH) analogs—Medications with chemical structures almost identical to natural LH-RH. They block the release of luteinizing hormone from the pituitary gland, thus reducing testosterone secretion from the testicles.

medical castration—The use of medication to interfere with the manufacture or actions of testosterone.

metastatic prostate cancer—Prostate cancer that has spread from the prostate to other parts of the body.

nerve-sparing radical prostatectomy—A type of surgery for prostate cancer in which structures important for erectile and bladder function are left intact. Associated with a lower risk of erectile dysfunction and severe incontinence than traditional radical prostatectomy.

neurogenic bladder—A dysfunction of the bladder due to a malfunction of the nerves that control the bladder.

nocturia—Frequent nighttime urination; a symptom of benign prostatic hyperplasia (BPH) and other diseases.

orchiectomy—See **surgical castration**.

penile clamp—A device that compresses the penis to prevent urine from leaking.

percent free PSA—The amount of PSA not attached to blood proteins divided by the total amount of PSA. Men with prostate cancer have a lower percentage of free PSA than men with benign prostatic hyperplasia (BPH).

perineal prostatectomy—A type of radical prostatectomy in which the incision is made into the perineum instead of into the abdomen.

perineum—The area between the scrotum and rectum.

phytotherapy—The use of plant-derived substances to treat a medical condition such as benign prostatic hyperplasia (BPH).

pressure-flow urodynamic studies—Tests that measure bladder pressure during urination by placing a recording device into the bladder and often into the rectum as well.

ProstaScint—A test for detecting prostate cancer that has spread to other parts of the body (except the bones).

prostate—A gland the size and shape of a crab apple that surrounds the upper portion of the male urethra. Its main function is to produce part of the fluid that makes up semen.

prostate specific antigen (PSA)—An enzyme produced by the glandular cells of the prostate and secreted into the seminal fluid that is released during ejaculation. High blood levels may indicate the presence of prostate cancer but can also be caused by benign prostatic hyperplasia (BPH) and infection.

prostatitis—An inflammation of the prostate that may cause pain in the lower back and in the area between the scrotum and rectum.

prostatodynia—A condition that causes the same symptoms as prostatitis but is not associated with infection or inflammation.

PSA density—The PSA level divided by the size of the prostate. Allows the doctor to better distinguish between benign prostatic hyperplasia (BPH) and prostate cancer by taking prostate size into account when assessing the PSA level.

PSA velocity—A measurement of the changes in PSA values over time. PSA velocity is greater in men with prostate cancer than in those without the disease.

radical prostatectomy—A type of surgery for prostate cancer that removes the entire prostate and the seminal vesicles.

residual urine—Urine retained in the bladder after voiding. It can become infected or lead to the formation of bladder stones.

retrograde ejaculation—Ejaculation of semen into the bladder rather than through the penis. Can lead to infertility.

retropubic open prostatectomy—An operation for benign prostatic hyperplasia (BPH). Used when the prostate is too large for the surgeon to perform transurethral prostatectomy (TURP). It involves moving aside the bladder so that the inner prostate tissue can be removed without entering the bladder.

seminal vesicles—Glands located on each side of the male bladder that secrete seminal fluid.

simple prostatectomy—A type of surgery for benign prostatic hyperplasia (BPH) that typically involves removing only the inner portion of the prostate. It is performed either through the urethra (TURP) or by making an incision in the lower abdomen (retropubic or suprapubic prostatectomy).

smooth muscle cells—Muscle cells in the prostate that contract to push prostatic fluid into the urethra during ejaculation.

stent—A plastic or metal device placed in the urethra to keep it open.

suprapubic open prostatectomy—An operation for benign prostatic hyperplasia (BPH) performed when the prostate is too large to allow for TURP. Involves opening the bladder and removing the inner portion of the prostate through the bladder.

surgical castration—Surgical removal of either the testicles (bilateral orchiectomy) or the contents of the testicles (subcapsular orchiectomy).

thermotherapy—A treatment for benign prostatic hyperplasia (BPH) that involves heating the prostate to more than 110° F. Resulting tissue and nerve damage alleviates symptoms.

thromboembolism—Vein inflammation due to a blood clot.

TNM system—A system for describing the clinical stage of a cancerous tumor using T numbers (T1 to T4) to indicate whether the tumor can be felt or not and if it can be felt, the extent of the tumor. In addition, an N+ is used to indicate cancer that has spread to the lymph nodes and an M+ for cancer that has spread to other parts of the body.

total androgen blockade—A treatment for prostate cancer that interferes with the production and action of both testicular and adrenal androgens by combining an antiandrogen with a luteinizing hormone-releasing hormone analog or surgical castration.

transrectal ultrasound—A procedure that uses an ultrasound probe inserted into the rectum to create images of the prostate. Used during prostate biopsy to diagnose prostate cancer.

transurethral incision of the prostate (TUIP)—A benign prostatic hyperplasia (BPH) treatment in which one or two small incisions are made in the prostate with an electrical knife or laser. Symptoms of BPH are alleviated by decreasing the pressure the prostate exerts on the urethra.

transurethral microwave therapy (TUMT)—A benign prostatic hyperplasia (BPH) treatment that uses microwave energy to heat and destroy prostate tissue. The microwave energy is emitted from a catheter inserted in the urethra.

transurethral needle ablation (TUNA)—A benign prostatic hyperplasia (BPH) treatment in which prostate tissue is destroyed with heat delivered by low-energy radio waves through tiny needles at the tip of a catheter inserted into the prostate through the urethra.

transurethral prostatectomy (TURP)—The "gold standard" treatment for benign prostatic hyperplasia (BPH). A long, thin instrument called a resectoscope is passed through the urethra into the bladder and used to cut away prostate tissue and seal blood vessels with an electric current. Also called transurethral resection of the prostate.

transurethral vaporization of the prostate (TVP)—A procedure for benign prostatic hyperplasia (BPH) that uses a powerful electrical current to vaporize the prostate tissue with minimal bleeding.

urethra—The canal through which urine is carried from the bladder and out of the body. In men, the urethra also carries semen that is released during ejaculation.

urethral stricture—Narrowing of the urethra.

uroflowmetry—A noninvasive test for benign prostatic hyperplasia (BPH) that measures the speed of urine flow.

vasodilator—A drug that allows the penis to become engorged with blood by widening the blood vessels. Used as a treatment for erectile dysfunction. Examples are alprostadil, papaverine, and phentolamine.

watchful waiting—An approach to the management of benign prostatic hyperplasia (BPH) or prostate cancer in which no treatment is immediately attempted, but the patient is carefully monitored. Also known as expectant management.

water-induced thermotherapy—In this minimally invasive therapy for BPH, a water-filled balloon inflated in the urethra heats the prostate to temperatures that destroy prostate tissue.

Whitmore-Jewett system—A system for describing the clinical stage of a cancerous tumor using the letters A, B, C, and D, with D denoting the most advanced stage.

HEALTH INFORMATION ORGANIZATIONS AND SUPPORT GROUPS

American Cancer Society
1599 Clifton Rd. NE
Atlanta, GA 30329
☎ 800-ACS-2345
www.cancer.org
National, community-based organization that answers questions about cancer, provides information on specific cancer topics, and makes referrals to treatment centers or self-help organizations. Free publications on prostate cancer. Sponsors a support group called Man to Man.

American Foundation for Urologic Disease
1128 North Charles St.
Baltimore, MD 21201
☎ 800-242-2383
   800-808-7866 (US TOO)
www.afud.org
Supports research and seeks to educate the public with brochures and educational packets on urological diseases. Call for information about US TOO, a support group for prostate cancer survivors and their families.

Cancer Care
275 7th Ave.
New York, NY 10001
☎ 800-813-HOPE/212-712-8080
www.cancercare.org
Provides support for patients and families through financial assistance, educational materials, referrals to local community resources, and one-on-one counseling (at the 800 number).

Cancer Information Service
National Cancer Institute
Public Inquiries Office
31 Center Dr., MSC 2580
Building 31, Room 10A03
Bethesda, MD 20892-2580
☎ 800-4CANCER
cis.nci.nih.gov
Nationwide network with 19 regional offices. Provides information about early detection, risk, and prevention of cancer; local services; and details of ongoing clinical trials. Publishes free literature.

The National Kidney and Urologic Diseases Information Clearinghouse
3 Information Way
Bethesda, MD 20892-3580
☎ 800-891-5390/301-654-4415
www.kidney.niddk.nih.gov/
   index.htm
National clearinghouse that provides access to a health information database. Also publishes a newsletter and provides educational material. Write, call, or visit the Web site for information.

Prostate Cancer Education Council
1800 Jackson St.
Golden, CO 80401
☎ 303-316-4685
www.pcaw.com
The Council is a group of doctors and health professionals who produce educational materials on prostate cancer and are working on a long-term study on prostate screening.

LEADING HOSPITALS FOR UROLOGY

U.S. News & World Report and the National Opinion Research Center, a social-science research group at the University of Chicago, recently conducted their 15th annual nationwide survey of 8,160 board-certified physicians in 17 medical specialties. The doctors nominated the hospitals that they considered to be the best from among 6,012 U.S. medical centers. This is the current list of the best hospitals for urology, as determined by a combination of factors: doctors' recommendations from 2002, 2003, and 2004; federal death rates; and factual data regarding quality indicators, such as the ratio of registered nurses to patients and use of advanced technology. However, because the results reflect the doctors' opinions to some extent, they are partly subjective. Any institution listed is considered a leading center, and the rankings do not imply that other hospitals cannot or do not deliver excellent care.

1. **Johns Hopkins Hospital**
   Baltimore, MD
   ☎ 410-955-5000
   www.hopkinsmedicine.org

2. **Cleveland Clinic**
   Cleveland, OH
   ☎ 800-223-2273/216-444-2200
   www.clevelandclinic.org

3. **Mayo Clinic**
   Rochester, MN
   ☎ 507-284-2511
   www.mayoclinic.org

4. **University of California, Los Angeles, Medical Center**
   Los Angeles, CA
   ☎ 800-825-2631/310-825-9111
   www.healthcare.ucla.edu

5. **Barnes-Jewish Hospital**
   St. Louis, MO
   ☎ 314-747-3000
   www.barnesjewish.org

6. **New York-Presbyterian Hospital**
   New York, NY
   ☎ 212-305-2500
   www.nyp.org

7. **Duke University Medical Center**
   Durham, NC
   ☎ 919-684-8111
   www.mc.duke.edu

8. **Massachusetts General Hospital**
   Boston, MA
   ☎ 617-726-2000
   www.mgh.harvard.edu

9. **Memorial Sloan-Kettering Cancer Center**
   New York, NY
   ☎ 800-525-2225
   www.mskcc.org

10. **University of Texas, M.D. Anderson Cancer Center**
    Houston, TX
    ☎ 713-792-2121
    www.mdanderson.org

Source: *U.S. News & World Report,* July 12, 2004.

THE JOHNS HOPKINS WHITE PAPERS

Selected Medical Journal Article

OSTEOPOROSIS AND PROSTATE CANCER

Men with advanced prostate cancer face an elevated risk of developing the bone-thin-ning disease osteoporosis. This can lead to fractures, which are painful, lessen quality of life, and may decrease life span. For these reasons, men with prostate cancer who face the greatest fracture risk should be screened for weak bones and receive protective treatment if necessary, Michael G. Oefelein, M.D., and Martin I. Resnick, M.D., recommend in the article reprinted here from the *Urologic Clinics of North America.*

Advanced prostate cancer tends to spread, or metastasize, to the skeleton, weakening bone structure and making fractures more likely. Late-stage disease is often treated with androgen-deprivation therapy, which inhibits the growth and spread of prostate tumors in some patients. But because androgens also help maintain bone mineral density, androgen-deprivation treatment can increase osteoporosis risk. Some studies have also shown that prostate cancer patients with no bone metastases who have not yet received androgen-deprivation treatment have reduced bone mineral density, Drs. Oefelein and Resnick note, suggesting there may be other bone-weakening mechanisms at work in prostate cancer patients.

Risk factors for developing osteoporosis include white race, sedentary lifestyle, smoking cigarettes, and drinking alcohol. Thin men also are at higher risk. Being African-American, getting regular weight-bearing exercise, and having a high body mass index are protective against loss of bone mineral density, and men who don't drink or smoke also are at lower risk for weakened bones. Specific osteoporosis risk factors among prostate cancer patients include having disease that does not respond to hormone treatment or disease that has spread to the bones.

The most accurate screening test for osteoporosis and a less-severe condition known as osteopenia is dual-energy x-ray absorptiometry (DEXA), which usually measures bone density at the lumbar spine, hip, and forearm. Blood and urine tests also can measure the rate of bone formation and breakdown, the authors note.

To maintain bone strength prostate cancer patients can take vitamin D and calcium and engage in weight-bearing exercise. Other options include estrogen and bone-building drugs known as bisphosphonates. Several studies have shown that zoledronic acid (Zometa), a member of this class of drugs, can help prevent bone loss, pain, and fractures in men with prostate cancer.

Drs. Oefelein and Resnick conclude by recommending that slender white men with prostate cancer, as well as those with disease that does not respond to hormone treatment or has metastasized to the bone, receive osteoporosis screening and preventive treatment if necessary.

REPRINT

ELSEVIER
SAUNDERS

Urol Clin N Am 31 (2004)

UROLOGIC
CLINICS
of North America

The impact of osteoporosis in men treated for prostate cancer

Michael G. Oefelein, MD*, Martin I. Resnick, MD

*Department of Urology, Case Western Reserve University School of Medicine,
University Hospitals of Cleveland, 11100 Euclid Avenue, Cleveland, OH 44106, USA*

A unique interaction exists between the skeletal organ system and prostate cancer. Over a century ago, Paget described the predilection of cancer for a specific organ system according to the seed and soil analogy. Metastatic prostate cancer specifically targets bone, and metastatic disease to bone initiates the pathophysiologic cascade culminating in the cachexia of bone. Specifically, osteoblastic bone metastases result in excess and disorganized bone formation with decreased bone strength. Weak, disorganized bone becomes clinically apparent through an increase in skeletal-related events (SREs), and the patient experiences skeletal fracture after trivial injury, intractable pain, and a progressive decline in quality of life. In addition to these disease-related effects on the skeletal organ system, treatment-induced effects include cancer treatment–related osteoporosis, particularly androgen deprivation–associated bone mineral density (BMD) loss. This article focuses on prostate cancer treatment androgen deprivation–induced osteoporosis, but does not neglect non–treatment-related mechanisms.

Definition and diagnosis of osteoporosis

The definition of *male osteoporosis* is derived from the World Health Organization definition of osteoporosis in white women [1]. *Osteoporosis* is defined as a BMD of less than or equal to −2.5 standard deviations below the young adult mean

BMD. *Osteopenia* is defined as a BMD between −1 and −2.5 standard deviations below this mean [1].

Biochemical and radiologic testing can evaluate BMD. Of the numerous radiologic techniques, dual-energy x-ray absorptiometry (DEXA) is considered the most accurate, and exposes the patient to less radiation than quantitative CT (QCT) scan [2]. Determining bone site–specific BMD seems to allow greater precision in predicting fractures at that site [3]. Unlike QCT, which is excellent for determining spine BMD, DEXA scanning has a site-specific capability. The lumbar spine, hip, and forearm are the sites most frequently assessed.

Laboratory tests are also useful in assessing bone formation and resorption, and include serum and urine studies. The heat-labile fraction of alkaline phosphatase is the most widely used marker of bone formation. Urinary levels of collagen cross-links, such as N-telopeptide, pyridinoline, and deoxypyridinoline, are the most commonly used markers for bone resorption [4].

Etiology and epidemiology of prostate cancer–associated osteoporosis

Prostate cancer–related osteoporosis

Several investigators have identified osteopenia and osteoporosis in men with prostate cancer before initiating androgen-deprivation therapy (ADT) [5,6]. Wei and colleagues [5] identified five of eight (63%) hormonally naïve prostate cancer patients with osteopenia or osteoporosis, and Smith and colleagues [6] identified 14 of 41 (34%) hormonally naïve, bone-scan negative

---

* Corresponding author.

patients with carcinoma of the prostate as fulfilling the DEXA-scan criteria for osteopenia or osteoporosis. QCT methods also were used, and identified 39 of these 41 (95%) patients as having osteopenia or osteoporosis. Hypogonadism, hypovitaminosis D, and dietary calcium levels below the recommended daily allowance were observed in 20%, 17%, and 59% of these study participants, respectively. These observations indicate that a significant proportion of hormonally naïve patients with carcinoma of the prostate but without clinical evidence of skeletal metastatses manifest evidence of reduced BMD. Whether these observations differ significantly from those of age-matched control subjects without carcinoma of the prostate is unknown, but it seems that BMD may decline in prostate cancer patients by mechanisms other than those of treatment-related osteoporosis [7].

Mechanisms independent of androgen-deprived BMD loss have been reviewed recently [7]. Metastatic prostate cancer cells in bone lead to a disruption of physiologic bone remodeling by abnormally stimulating osteoclasts and osteoblasts through the local release of paracrine substances (eg, transforming growth factor [TGF] and parathyroid hormone–related protein) (Fig. 1) [8,9]. Although bone formation (osteoblastic) predominates, bone resorption (osteolysis) also is increased, as demonstrated by several biochemical and histomorphometric studies [8–10]. Most sclerotic lesions are of a mixed type, in which excessive new bone is deposited away from sites of bone resorption and does not contribute to bone strength. Increased bone resorption also may be caused by calcium entrapment in bone as a consequence of excessive bone formation. An increased serum parathyroid hormone level results from calcium demand and parathyroid hormone–mediated stimulation of osteoclast activity at sites distant from those involved by the tumor [8–10]. The results of this complicated cascade are diminished bone strength and an increased risk for skeletal complications. Therefore, bone is not an inanimate, fixed substance—it is a continuously changing organ system. As the body wastes from cancer, so does bone.

These treatment-independent mechanisms of osteoporosis are potentially significant. Evidence of skeletal fractures after the diagnosis of prostate cancer and before initiating ADT combined with fractures after initiating ADT significantly correlate with overall survival [11]. Whether earlier intervention or treatment to prevent bone cachexia

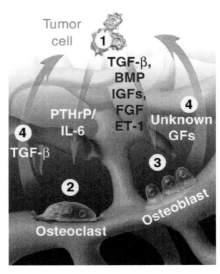

Fig. 1. Pathogenesis of osteoblastic bone metastases. Factors are released by tumor cells (*1*) that stimulate osteoclast (*2*) and osteoblast (*3*) activity. Excessive abnormal bone formation around tumor cell deposits results in low bone strength. Osteoclastic and osteoblastic activity releases growth factors (*4*) that stimulate tumor cell growth, perpetuating the cycle. BMP, bone morphogenetic protein; IGF, insulin growth factor; FGF, fibroblast growth factor; ET-1, endothelin-1. (Courtesy of Novartis Oncology, Inc., East Hanover, NJ.)

will improve health-related quality of life (HRQOL) and overall survival remains unknown.

Prostate cancer treatment–related osteoporosis

Androgen-deprivation cancer treatment–associated osteoporosis is observed frequently, but its effects on men, and prostate cancer patients in particular, has been appreciated only recently. Although men experience a gradual, age-related BMD loss of 7% to 12% per decade beginning at 30 years of age, osteoporosis in males is rare, probably because they have a greater peak bone mass and no menopause equivalent [12,13]. Most men with osteoporosis have secondary causes, which include hypogonadism, glucocorticoid excess, alcoholism, thyroid and parathyroid disorders, osteomalacia, and cancer [13]. Tobacco and alcohol consumption are independent risk factors for osteoporosis in men, whereas obesity has been reported to be protective [14].

Prostate cancer treatment–related androgen suppression reduces BMD 3% to 7% per year

(Table 1) [15–22]. The pathophysiologic mechanism by which testosterone deprivation reduces BMD has not been characterized completely. Androgens mediate osteoblast development and growth and augment bone-matrix production and osteocalcin secretion [23]. Growth factors important in osteoblast proliferation (eg, TGF-β and insulin growth factors) potentially are mediated by testosterone [23]. Aromatase, which converts androgens to estrogens, is active in bone. The protective effects of androgens on bone may be mediated by the local production of estrogens [23]. Scherr and colleagues [24] proposed that the estrogen-deficient hypogonadal state reduces BMD by a similar mechanism [25].

Prostate cancer patients' risk for cancer treatment–related osteoporosis varies. African-American race, higher body mass index (BMI), participation in weight-bearing exercise, and abstinence from tobacco and alcohol protect against BMD loss, and reduce risk for treatment-associated skeletal fractures [26]. Conversely, thin, sedentary white men who drink alcohol and smoke tobacco are at greatest risk [26].

Therapies to achieve androgen deprivation are known and used widely (eg, orchiectomy, estrogen administration, and gonadotrophin-releasing hormone agonist and antagonist administration) and remain the initial treatment of choice for patients with metastatic prostate adenocarcinoma. Not all methods to achieve androgen suppression have the same impact on bone health, however. Methods that provide androgen deprivation without estrogen ablation (eg, nonsteroidal anti-androgens and estrogens) may provide a relative degree of protection [24,25].

Estrogen therapy has been revived recently as a method to suppress androgens because of the BMD-sparing side effect [15,24,25,27,28]. The thromboembolic risks historically associated with oral estrogen therapy may be minimized through use of lower oral dosages and parenteral administration [27,28]. Using parenteral estrogen (polyestradiol phosphate [PEP], 240 mg, every 2 weeks for five doses followed by a maintenance dose of 240 mg every month), Hedlund and Henriksson [27] reported comparable efficacy in overall survival and cardiovascular safety compared with a cohort of men randomized to combined androgen blockade (CAB). Cardiovascular mortality was 3.5% in the PEP group and 3.1% in the CAB group. Additional advantages of PEP

Table 1
Available therapeutic modalities to achieve androgen-suppression treatment and the effect on bone mineral density and fracture risk

Androgen-suppression treatment	BMD effect at femoral neck (12 mo)	Osteoporotic fracture risk	References	Comments
Estrogens	Increased BMD, N-telopeptide reduced	Not reported	[15,24,25,27]	BMD-protective; parenteral administration has no higher CV toxicity [27,28]
Orchiectomy	2.4%–7.6% reduction	12%–40%; 3.9 fold increase	[15–17]	BMD-adverse with a 3.9 fold higher risk for fracture than age-matched control subjects
GnRH Agonists	3.3%–9.6% reduction	4%–50%; fivefold increase	[11,18–20]	BMD-adverse with a fivefold higher risk for fracture than age-matched control subjects
NSAA-monotherapy	Urinary N-telopeptide levels reduced; increases serum testosterone and estradiol levels	Not reported	[21]	May maintain BMD and prevent fractures
Combined androgen blockade	6.5%	Not reported	[22]	BMD-adverse

Abbreviations: CV, cardiovascular; GnRH, gonadotrophin-releasing hormone; NSAA, nonsteroidal antiandrogens.

treatment include a significantly lower cost of care than CAB [27].

These observations, and the realization that prolonged nonestrogen ADT has a detrimental effect on BMD, have increased interest in estrogen-mediated or -augmented ADT [27]. Scherr and colleagues [24] reported that diesthylstilbesterol (DES), 1 mg/d, significantly reduced urinary N-telopeptides levels compared with patients on ADT without estrogens. These authors concluded that rapid bone turnover and resorption can be prevented with DES, 1 mg, alone or in combination with other modes of androgen deprivation. Whether DES, 1 mg, effectively suppresses testosterone in all patients requires individual patient monitoring [29]. DES is inexpensive ($0.75 per day), effective, and potentially useful in reducing an individual's risk for osteoporosis [24,25].

Ockrim and colleagues [28], using transdermal estradiol therapy in 20 prostate cancer patients, reported effective testosterone suppression and tumor response without significant cardiovascular toxicity. These authors also reported diminished andropause symptoms, improved quality of life, and increased BMD. The authors emphasized the cost savings of transdermal estradiol over conventional hormone therapies.

The BMD-preserving effects of estrogen-mediated ADT mirror those reported for bisphosphonates [30]. The average daily costs of bisphosphonate therapy, however, are considerable compared to other treatments (alendronate, 10 mg/d for 30 days, $61.50; zoledronic acid, 4 mg/mo intravenously, $850 plus infusion costs) [31], and do not include the cost of ADT. Proponents of bisphosphonate therapy emphasize the reduction of SREs with the newer, more potent, intravenous bisphosphonates, which potentially balances the added cost of bisphosphonate therapy [32,33].

The clinical impact of skeletal-related events

Prostate cancer patients, especially those undergoing ADT, are at risk for SREs, and this risk increases with the duration of therapy. Daniell [34] first reported an association between androgen deprivation and SREs. In a group of 49 surgically castrated prostate cancer patients, eight fractures were identified at variable time intervals after bilateral orchiectomy [34]. Townsend and colleagues [35] reported 20 of 224 patients (9%) treated with luteinizing hormone–releasing hormone (LHRH) agonists for prostate cancer

developed skeletal fractures; 11 of these patients (4.9%) had fractures attributed to androgen deprivation–associated osteoporosis. The median follow-up of this population was not reported, but the mean number of 1-month LHRH injections was 20.

Oefelein and colleagues [26] reported on prostate cancer– and prostate cancer treatment–related skeletal fractures in nearly 200 men with a median follow-up of 47 months. Prostate cancer patients undergoing ADT were at a fivefold increased risk for androgen suppression–associated skeletal fractures compared to reported rates in age-matched control subjects. The 5- and 10-year fracture rates after the diagnosis of prostate cancer were 13% and 33%, respectively. The duration of androgen suppression, race, and BMI less than 25 kg/m^2 were associated significantly with the risk for skeletal fracture. Slender, white prostate cancer patients seem to be at greatest risk for androgen suppression–associated fractures. Conversely, African-American men and men with BMIs greater than normal (25 kg/m^2) are at minimal risk despite prolonged durations (more than 10 years) of androgen suppression.

These observations illustrate the cumulative long-term risk to prostate cancer patients on ADT, and support the finding that the duration of androgen suppression is associated significantly with skeletal fractures in these patients. A relatively high percentage (9%) of prostate cancer patients develop skeletal fractures before starting androgen suppression. Thus, it is possible that mechanisms in addition to that of androgen deprivation may be important in the pathogenesis of BMD loss and its association with skeletal fractures in prostate cancer patients [7].

Berruti and colleagues [36] reported the incidence of skeletal complications in prostate cancer patients with bone metastasis and hormone refractory disease. In the 112 patients, 27 had a vertebral body collapse or compression, and 10 had a pathologic fracture, for an overall incidence of 30%. A significant proportion of these patients received corticosteroid therapy (49 of 112), chemotherapy (68 of 112), and palliative radiotherapy (52 of 112). Clinical variables associated with increased skeletal events included increasing bone pain, tumor burden, reduced performance status, increased total alkaline phosphatase, and urinary deoxypyridinoline.

Saad and colleagues [37] reported SREs in androgen-insensitive prostate cancer patients randomized to treatment with zoledronic acid or placebo. SREs were defined prospectively as pathologic bone fractures, spinal cord compression, surgery to bone, radiation therapy to bone, or a change in antineoplastic therapy to treat bone pain. The 24-month incidence of SREs in the placebo arm was 49%. Zoledronic acid reduced SREs by 36% by multiple event analysis, and delayed the time to the first SRE by 5 months ($P = 0.009$). All SREs and pathologic fractures were reduced significantly in the zoladronic acid treatment arm, but overall survival and HRQOL as assessed by the Functional Assessment of Cancer Therapy-General (FACT-G) were not impacted significantly. Regarding the natural history of SREs in men with hormone refractory prostate cancer, the major observation is the high (49%) rate of SREs in the control group.

Recent evidence presented in abstract form supports the concept that each SRE has a significant economic as well as quality-of-life impact. SREs may increase morbidity and medical care costs. In the Netherlands, the estimated average cost attributable to SREs in prostate cancer patients in 1998 was 6973 euros (2002 US $7300) [32]. Clinically significant decrements in multiple domains of HRQOL were observed in prostate cancer patients who experienced SREs [33].

Despite these consistent reports identifying men with prostate cancer to be at increased risk for skeletal complications, limited information exists regarding the influence skeletal fractures may have on prostate cancer patient survival. Atraumatic hip fractures in men are associated with a 32% excess mortality in the year following the fracture [38]. Oefelein and colleagues [11] identified a significant negative association between skeletal fracture and overall survival in a cohort of 192 prostate cancer patients on ADT (Fig. 2). This observation remained significant in a multivariate analysis of 11 input variables, as did the presence of skeletal metastases and the pretreatment prostate-specific antigen (PSA) level. In the subset analysis, the location of fracture (eg, hip, spine, or extremity) was not associated significantly with overall survival.

In sum, prostate cancer and prostate cancer treatment result in a specific targeting and cachexia of bone, reduce BMD, cause osteoporosis, and predispose these men to SREs. Slender white men are at greatest risk for cancer treatment–related SREs. Skeletal fractures independently predict overall survival; hence, preventing skeletal fracture is paramount.

Treatment options

Therapeutic options for maintaining bone health in prostate cancer patients include vitamin

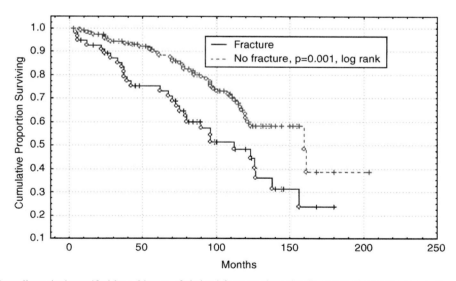

Fig. 2. Overall survival stratified by a history of skeletal fracture since the diagnosis of prostate cancer (log rank test, $P = 0.001$). Circles indicate complete responses. Ticks indicate censored responses.

D (800 IU/d), calcium supplementation (1200 mg/d), weight-bearing exercise, parenteral estrogen therapy, and the use of bisphosphonate therapy. Recently, Orwoll and colleagues [39] reported a significant reduction in vertebral fractures in osteoporotic men without prostate cancer on the oral bisphosphonate alendronate. No reduction in the rate of hip or extremity fractures was observed in these men.

Zolendronic acid, a third-generation bisphosphonate, is approved for use in patients with androgen-insensitive prostate cancer with skeletal metastases. The approval of this agent was based on the results of a randomized, prospective, phase-III trial comparing zoledronic acid, 4 mg, with placebo [37]. The primary endpoint was SREs. Secondary endpoints included overall survival, HRQOL, pain scores, and PSA level. The treatment arm had significantly fewer SREs, with significantly fewer recurrent events in patients who had an SRE. Pain scores also were significantly less at 3 months and 6 months. Overall survival rate, PSA level, and HRQOL as assessed by the FACT-G were no different from placebo.

Smith and colleagues [30] recently reported on the results of a multicenter, double-blind, randomized, placebo-controlled clinical trial designed to assess the effect of zoledronic acid on BMD during ADT for nonmetastatic prostate cancer. A total of 106 men were enrolled. Mean BMD of the lumbar spine increased by 5.6% in men receiving zoledronic acid and decreased by 2.2% in men given placebo ($P < 0.001$). Mean BMD of the femoral neck, trochanter, and total hip also increased in the zoledronic acid group and decreased in the placebo group. These authors concluded that zoledronic acid increased BMD in the hip and spine during ADT for patients with nonmetastatic prostate cancer.

Summary

Prostate cancer patients are at significant risk for SREs, with up to 50% of androgen-insensitive patients experiencing an SRE at 24 months. The risk increases with the duration and type of cancer treatment. SREs decrease HRQOL, increase the cost of care, and are associated negatively with overall survival. Screening men at greatest risk (slender white men and men with hormone refractory disease or metastatic disease) with BMD measurements, and initiating empiric therapy (vitamin D_3, calcium, parenteral estrogens, bisphosphates) may be warranted.

References

[1] WHO Study Group on Assessment of Fracture Risk and its Application to Screening for Postmenopausal Osteoporosis. Assessment of fracture risk and its application to screening for postmenopausal osteoporosis. Geneva (Switzerland): World Health Organization; 1994.

[2] Raisz LG, Kream BE, Lorenzo JA. Metabolic bone disease. In: Wilson JD, editor. William's textbook of endocrinology. 9th edition. Philadelphia: W.B. Saunders; 1998. p. 1211–28.

[3] Marshall D, Johnell O, Wedel H. Meta-analysis of how well measures of bone mineral density predict occurrence of osteoporotic fractures. BMJ 1996; 312:1254–61.

[4] Ross RW, Small EJ. Osteoporosis in men treated with androgen deprivation therapy for prostate cancer. J Urol 2002;167:1952–6.

[5] Wei JT, Gross M, Jaffe CA, Gravlin K, Lahaie M, Faerber GJ, et al. Androgen deprivation therapy for prostate cancer results in significant loss of bone density. Urology 1999;54:607–11.

[6] Smith MR, McGovern FJ, Fallon MA, Schoenfeld D, Kantoff PW, Finkelstein JS. Low bone mineral density in hormone-naive men with prostate carcinoma. Cancer 2001;91:2238–45.

[7] Berruti A, Dogliotti L, Tucci M, Tarabuzzi D, Fontana D, Angeli A. Metabolic bone disease induced by prostate cancer: rationale for the use of bisphosphonates. J Urol 2001;166:2023–31.

[8] Dowell DJ. Malignant bone resorption: cellular and biochemical mechanisms. Ann Oncol 1992;3:257.

[9] Guise TA, Mundy GR. Cancer and bone. Endocr Rev 1998;19:18.

[10] Urwin GH, Percival RC, Harris S. Generalised increase in bone resorption in carcinoma of the prostate. Br J Urol 1985;57:721.

[11] Oefelein MG, Ricchiuti V, Conrad W, Resnick MI. Skeletal fractures negatively correlate with overall survival in men with prostate cancer. J Urol 2002; 168:1005–7.

[12] Jackson JA, Kleerekoper M. Osteoporosis in men: diagnosis, pathophysiology and prevention. Medicine 1990;69:137.

[13] Kelepouris N, Harper KD, Gannon FM. Severe osteoporosis in men. Ann Intern Med 1995;123:452.

[14] Seeman E, Melton LK. Risk factors for spinal osteoporosis in men. Am J Med 1983;75:977–83.

[15] Eriksson S, Eriksson A, Stege R, Carlstrom K. Bone mineral density in patients with prostatic cancer treated with orchidectomy and with estrogens. Calcif Tissue Int 1995;57:97–9.

[16] Daniell HW, Dunn SR, Ferguson DW, Lomas G, Niazi Z, Stratte T. Progressive osteoporosis during

androgen depravation therapy for prostate cancer. J Urol 2000;163:181–6.

[17] Melton LJ III, Alothman KI, Khosla S, Achenbach SJ, Oberg AL, Zincke H. Fracture risk following bilateral orchiectomy. J Urol 2003;169(5):1747–50.

[18] Maillefert JF, Sibilia J, Michel F, Saussine C, Javier RM, Tavernier C. Bone-mineral density in men treated with synthetic gonadotrophin-releasing hormone agonists for prostatic carcinoma. J Urol 1999; 161:1219.

[19] Stoch SA, Parker RA, Chen L, Bubley G, Ko YJ, Vincelette A, et al. Bone loss in men with prostate cancer treated with gonadotropin-releasing hormone agonists. J Clin Endocrinol 2001;86:2787–91.

[20] Mittan D, Lee S, Miller E, Perez RC, Basler JW, Bruder JM. Bone loss following hypogonadism in men with prostate cancer treated with GnRH analogs. J Clin Endocrinol Metab 2002;87:3656–61.

[21] Smith MR, Fallon MA, Goode MJ. Cross-sectional study of bone turnover during bicalutamide monotherapy for prostate cancer. Urology 2003;61: 127–31.

[22] Diamond T, Campbell J, Bryant C, et al. The effect of combined androgen blockade on bone turnover and bone mineral densities in men treated for prostate carcinoma. Cancer 1998;83:1561.

[23] Wiren K, Orwoll E. Androgens and bone: basic aspects. In: Orwoll E, editor. Osteoporosis in men. San Diego (CA): Academic Press; 1999. p. 211–74.

[24] Scherr D, Pitts WR, Vaughan ED. Diethylstilbesterol revisited: androgen deprivation, osteoporosis and prostate cancer. J Urol 2002;167:535–8.

[25] Pitts WR Jr. Diethylstilbesterol revised: androgen deprivation, osteoporosis and prostate cancer. J Urol 2002;168:2131–2.

[26] Oefelein MG, Ricchuiti V, Conrad W, Seftel A, Bodner D, Goldman H, et al. Skeletal fracture associated with androgen suppression induced osteoporosis: the clinical incidence and risk factors for patients with prostate cancer. J Urol 2001; 166(5):1724–8.

[27] Hedlund PO, Henriksson P. Parenteral estrogen versus total androgen ablation in the treatment of advanced prostate carcinoma: effects on overall survival and cardiovascular mortality. The Scandinavian Prostate Cancer Group (SPCG)-5 Trial Study. Urology 2000;55:328–33.

[28] Ockrim JL, Lalani EN, Laniado ME, Carter SC, Abel PD. Transdermal estradiol therapy for ad- vanced prostate cancer—forward to the past?. J Urol 2003;169:1735–7.

[29] Kent JR, Bischoff AJ, Arduino LJ. Estrogen dosage and suppression of testosterone levels in patients with prostatic carcinoma. J Urol 1973;109: 858–60.

[30] Smith MR, Eastham J, Gleason DM, Shasha D, Tchekmedyian S, Zinner N. Randomized controlled trial of zoledronic acid to prevent bone loss in men receiving androgen deprivation therapy for non-metastatic prostate cancer. J Urology 2003;169: 2008–12.

[31] Drugstore.com. Available at http://www.drugstore. com. Accessed June 2003.

[32] Groot MT, Boeken Kruger CGG, Pelger RCM, Uyl-de Groot CA. Costs of prostate cancer, metastatic to the bone, in The Netherlands. Eur Urol 2003;43:226–32.

[33] Wiefurt KP, Yun L, Castel LD, Timbie JW, Glendenning A, Schulman KA. The impact of skeletal-related events on health-related quality of life of patients with metastatic prostate cancer. Ann Oncol 2002;13(Suppl 5):180.

[34] Daniell HW. Osteoporosis after orchiectomy for prostate cancer. J Urol 1997;157:439–44.

[35] Townsend MF, Sanders WH, Northway RO, Graham SD. Bone fractures associated with luteinizing hormone-releasing hormone agonists used in the treatment of prostate cancer. Cancer 1997;79: 545–50.

[36] Berruti A, Dogliotti L, Bitossi R, et al. Incidence of skeletal complications in patients with bone metastatic cancer and hormone refractory disease: predictive role of bone resorption and formation markers evaluated at baseline. J Urol 2000;164: 1248–53.

[37] Saad F, Gleason DM, Murray R, Tchekmedyian S, Venner P, Lacombe L, et al. A randomized, placebo-controlled trial of zoledronic acid in patients with hormone-refractory metastatic prostate carcinoma. J Natl Cancer Inst 2002;94: 1458–68.

[38] Kiebzak GM, Beinart GA, Perser K, Ambrose CG, Siff SJ, Heggeness MH. Under treatment of osteoporosis in men with hip fracture. Arch Intern Med 2002;162:2217–22.

[39] Orwoll E, Ettinger M, Weiss S, Miller P, et al. Alendronate for the treatment of osteoporosis in men. N Engl J Med 2000;343:604–10.

ISBN 1-933087-12-9
ISSN 1542-1716
Twelfth Printing
Printed in the United States of America

Oefelein, M.G. and Resnick, M.I. "The impact of osteoporosis in men treated for prostate cancer." Reprinted with permission from *Urologic Clinics of North America* Vol. 31, No. 2 (May 2004): 313–319. Copyright © 2004, Elsevier Ltd.

The Johns Hopkins White Papers are published yearly by Medletter Associates, Inc.

Visit our Web site for information on Johns Hopkins Health After 50 publications, which include White Papers on specific disorders, home medical encyclopedias, consumer reference guides to drugs and medical tests, and our monthly newsletter
The Johns Hopkins Medical Letter: Health After 50.
www.HopkinsAfter50.com

VISION

Andrew P. Schachat, M.D.,

Harry A. Quigley, M.D.,

and

Oliver D. Schein, M.D., M.P.H.

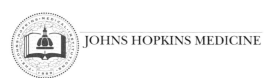 JOHNS HOPKINS MEDICINE

Dear Readers:

Do you have trouble reading, recognizing the faces of friends or relatives, or seeing street signs—even when you're wearing your glasses or contact lenses? If so, you may have low vision. The most common causes of low vision are cataracts, glaucoma, age-related macular degeneration (AMD), and diabetic retinopathy. Fortunately, medical treatments are available for all of these conditions. And even when vision remains poor, low-vision resources and strategies can minimize the impact of low vision on one's life.

This White Paper reviews the most up-to-date information on the causes, prevention, symptoms, diagnosis, and treatment of vision disorders that are likely to affect older adults.

Here are some of this year's highlights:

• When **floaters and flashes** are a sign of something serious. (page 11)
• The benefits of **cataract surgery** for people with usable vision in just one eye. (page 13)
• Could cholesterol-lowering **statin drugs** protect against glaucoma? (page 19)
• **Medications** that have the potential to cause vision problems. (page 25)
• What you can do to **reduce the risk of AMD**. (pages 35 and 36)
• Selecting the best treatment for **AMD**. (page 39)
• An **experimental treatment** for people with diabetic retinopathy. (page 45)
• High-tech and low-tech relief for **dry, itchy eyes**. (page 46)

I hope that this knowledge will greatly improve the treatment and quality of life of people experiencing vision problems.

Sincerely,

Andrew P. Schachat, M.D.
Professor
Department of Ophthalmology
Johns Hopkins University School of Medicine

P. S. Don't forget to visit HopkinsWhitePapers.com for the latest news on vision disorders and other information that will complement your Johns Hopkins White Paper.

THE AUTHORS

Andrew P. Schachat, M.D., graduated from Princeton University and the Johns Hopkins University School of Medicine. He did his ophthalmology residency at the Wilmer Eye Institute at Johns Hopkins Hospital and a vitreoretinal and oncology fellowship at the Wills Eye Hospital in Philadelphia. Currently, he is the Karl Hagen Professor of Ophthalmology and director of the Retinal Vascular Center and the Ocular Oncology Service at the Wilmer Eye Institute. In addition, he is the editor of *Ophthalmology* and is on the editorial board of *The Johns Hopkins Medical Letter: Health After 50*. Dr. Schachat is also the editor of the first two volumes of Steven Ryan's *Retina,* a three-volume textbook of retinal disease for ophthalmologists. He was a principal investigator on the Macular Photocoagulation Study, which proved the benefit of laser treatment for some patients with age-related macular degeneration, and, more recently, on the trials showing the safety and efficacy of photodynamic therapy with verteporfin.

■ ■ ■

Harry A. Quigley, M.D., is the A. Edward Maumenee Professor of Ophthalmology and the director of both the Glaucoma Service and the Dana Center for Preventive Ophthalmology at the Wilmer Eye Institute at Johns Hopkins Hospital. He was a founding member of the American Glaucoma Society and served as its secretary for eight years. He was elected chief executive officer of the Association for Research in Vision and Ophthalmology and editor-in-chief of *Investigative Ophthalmology and Visual Science.*

■ ■ ■

Oliver D. Schein, M.D., M.P.H., is the Burton E. Grossman Professor of Ophthalmology at the Wilmer Eye Institute and carries a joint appointment in the department of epidemiology at the Johns Hopkins University School of Hygiene and Public Health. Dr. Schein's clinical expertise is in medical and surgical conditions of the anterior segment of the eye involving cataracts and complications of cataract surgery, corneal scarring, and corneal surgery. He is an author of the American Academy of Ophthalmology's "Preferred Practice Pattern" on Cataract.

CONTENTS

Anatomy of the Eye . . . . .p. 1
Refractive Errors . . . . .p. 2

Cataracts
Types of Cataracts . . . . .p. 4
Causes of Cataracts . . . . .p. 5
Symptoms of Cataracts . . . . .p. 8
Prevention of Cataracts . . . . .p. 9
Treatment of Cataracts . . . . .p. 10

Glaucoma
Causes of Glaucoma . . . . .p. 19
Symptoms of Glaucoma . . . . .p. 22
Prevention of Glaucoma . . . . .p. 22
Diagnosis of Glaucoma . . . . .p. 22
Treatment of Glaucoma . . . . .p. 24

Age-related Macular Degeneration
Anatomy of the Retina . . . . .p. 32
Types of Age-related Macular Degeneration . . . . .p. 32
Causes of Age-related Macular Degeneration . . . . .p. 34
Symptoms of Age-related Macular Degeneration . . . . .p. 34
Prevention of Age-related Macular Degeneration . . . . .p. 35
Diagnosis of Age-related Macular Degeneration . . . . .p. 36
Treatment of Age-related Macular Degeneration . . . . .p. 37

Diabetic Retinopathy
Causes of Diabetic Retinopathy . . . . .p. 42
Symptoms of Diabetic Retinopathy . . . . .p. 44
Prevention of Diabetic Retinopathy . . . . .p. 44
Diagnosis of Diabetic Retinopathy . . . . .p. 45
Treatment of Diabetic Retinopathy . . . . .p. 45

Chart: Glaucoma Drugs . . . . .p. 28

Glossary . . . . .p. 48
Health Information Organizations and Support Groups . . . . .p. 51
Leading Hospitals for Ophthalmology . . . . .p. 52
Selected Medical Journal Article . . . . .p. 53

VISION

The most common eye diseases in people over age 50 are cataracts, glaucoma, age-related macular degeneration, and diabetic retinopathy. Fortunately, if treated early enough, progression of these eye disorders can often be slowed or halted with medication, surgery, or a combination of both. Moreover, treatment of vision problems may allow a person to return to such daily activities as driving, grocery shopping, reading, and performing household tasks, thus improving their quality of life. Besides medication and surgery, people can take steps on their own to make it easier to live with an eye disorder, and low vision aids are available to enhance visual acuity for those whose disorder cannot be treated.

Because most eye disorders are symptomless in their early stages, many people are unaware that they have one. Surveys by researchers at Johns Hopkins have found that about one third of people with eye disease were unaware of it and that more than one third of those age 65 to 84 had not visited an ophthalmologist (eye doctor) in the last year. Periodic visits to an eye care specialist are needed to detect conditions early enough to allow effective treatment. Regular check-ups are particularly important for people over age 65, those with risk factors for serious eye disease, those in fair or poor general health, and those with diabetes.

ANATOMY OF THE EYE

The eye is a complex structure that sends nerve impulses to the brain when stimulated by light rays reflected from an object. The brain then processes these impulses to create the perception of vision.

The *iris,* the colored circle in the middle of the eye, is the eye's most prominent structure. Also visible from the front of the eye are the *pupil,* the opening in the center of the iris that resembles a large black dot, and the *sclera,* which makes up part of the outer layer of the eye. The iris is composed of smooth muscles that contract and expand to alter the size of the pupil and control the amount of light that enters the eye. The sclera is the tough, white connective tissue that covers and protects the majority of the eye.

Also at the front of the eye are the *cornea, lens,* and *conjunctiva.* The cornea is a transparent, dome-shaped disk that covers the iris and pupil. Beneath the cornea is a transparent, elastic structure called the lens. The cornea does about three quarters of the work of focusing light on the retina; the lens does the rest. The conjunctiva is a thin, lubricating mucous membrane that covers the sclera and lines the inside of the eyelids.

Inside the sclera lie two more layers. The middle layer, the *choroid*, contains a dark pigment that minimizes scattering of light inside the eye. It is rich in blood vessels that supply nutrients to the *retina*, the innermost layer of the eye that consists of light-sensitive nerve tissue. The retina functions like film in a camera, receiving an imprint of an image and sending it via the *optic nerve* to the brain to be "developed." At the center of the retina is a small area called the *macula*; it is responsible for central vision and for seeing detail and color.

The *vitreous humor* is a thick, gel-like substance that fills the back of the eyeball behind the lens. A watery fluid called the *aqueous humor* is located in front of the lens. These two humors help to maintain intraocular pressure (the internal pressure of the eye), which is needed to prevent the eyeball from collapsing. Intraocular pressure is controlled by specialized cells that produce aqueous humor and by ducts and canals that drain this fluid from the eye.

REFRACTIVE ERRORS

The major role of the lens is to refract and focus light from both distant and near objects. This process is achieved by changes in the shape of the lens (accommodation). To see at a distance, muscle fibers attached to the lens tighten to flatten the shape of the lens and focus light coming from a distance onto the retina. For close vision, these muscle fibers relax, and the lens reverts to its naturally rounder shape, which focuses light from close objects onto the retina.

Refractive errors are caused by a deviation in the way light focuses on the retina. The four types of refractive errors are nearsightedness (myopia), farsightedness (hyperopia), astigmatism, and presbyopia. All four conditions can be corrected with eyeglasses or contact lenses. An increasingly popular alternative to glasses and contacts, especially for nearsightedness, is laser vision correction (see the reprint on page 53).

In nearsighted people, the eyeball is too long or the cornea has too much curvature. Light focuses on a point in front of the retina; as a result, near objects can be seen clearly, but distant ones do not come into proper focus. More than 30 million Americans age 40 and older are nearsighted.

If the eyeball is too short or the cornea is too flat, light focuses

NEW DEVICE APPROVAL

Permanent Implanted Contact Lens Corrects Nearsightedness

The U.S. Food and Drug Administration (FDA) recently approved a new type of permanent contact lens called the Artisan that is surgically inserted into the eye. The device sits in front of the pupil, where it is held in place with two tiny clips.

To investigate the benefits of the Artisan, its manufacturer, Ophtec USA Inc., studied the use of the device in 662 people with moderate to severe nearsightedness. Three years after the procedure, 92% of the participants had vision of at least 20/40 and 44% had vision of at least 20/20.

However, over time, Artisan recipients began slowly and steadily to lose endothelial cells, which line the cornea and keep it clear. For that reason, the FDA requires that only patients with corneal endothelial cells dense enough to withstand some loss receive the device.

Other side effects included retinal detachment, cataracts, and corneal swelling.

Even after surgery, people may need glasses in situations of low light, such as night driving, and for reading.

Although the Artisan is intended to be permanent, it can be replaced or removed if needed.

APPROVED BY THE FDA
September 13, 2004

Low Vision: Breaking Down the Statistics

Just how common are low vision and blindness? According to a new study in the *Archives of Ophthalmology*, some 2.4 million Americans over age 40 have low vision (a corrected visual acuity of 20/40 or worse in the better eye) and a further 937,000 are blind (a corrected visual acuity of 20/200 or worse in the better eye). These numbers are expected to rise as the population ages.

The most common causes of low vision and blindness vary according to race and ethnicity. These variations, according to the authors, may be the result of differences in access to and use of eye and overall health care, the prevalence of other health factors such as high blood pressure and high blood glucose (particularly for diabetic retinopathy), and access to and awareness of health-related information. The bar graph below breaks down the causes of low vision by race and ethnicity.

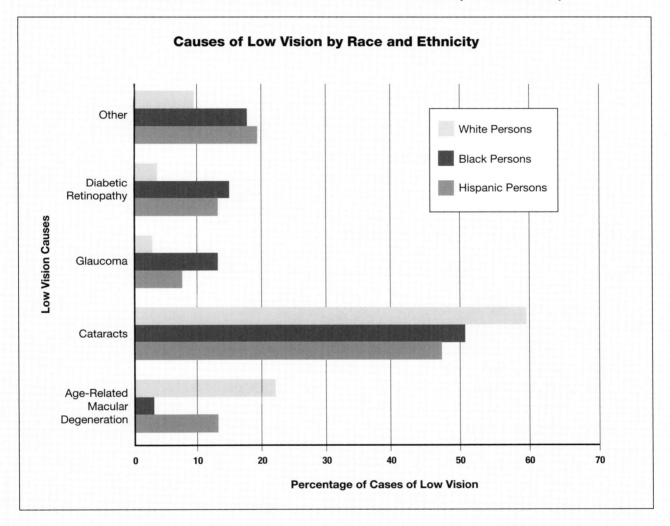

on a point behind the retina. In this condition, called farsighted-ness, distant objects can be seen clearly, but close ones do not come into proper focus. About 12 million people age 40 and older in the United States are farsighted.

Astigmatism occurs when the cornea or lens is slightly irregular in shape. This causes light to focus at different points in the eye. The result is blurred or distorted vision. Astigmatism is common in people with nearsightedness.

Presbyopia occurs when the lens begins to lose its ability to accommodate. As we age, the lens gradually becomes thicker and more rigid and is less able to change its shape to bring close objects into focus. Presbyopia affects almost all people over age 45. The primary treatment is reading glasses. Some surgical treatments are available now, and others are being investigated. If the person is also nearsighted or has astigmatism, prescription bifocals, trifocals, or contact lenses are required.

Cataracts

A cloudiness or opacification of the lens is called a cataract. Derived from the Latin word meaning "waterfall," the term *cataract* arose from the ancient misconception that cataract symptoms were caused by evil liquids that mysteriously flowed into the eye.

Cataracts can occur at any age—in fact, babies can be born with them—but they are most common later in life. About 50% of people age 65 to 74 and 70% of those age 75 and older have cataracts. In 2004, an estimated 20.5 million Americans over 40 (approximately 17%) had a cataract; that number is expected to reach 30.1 million by 2020. However, not all cataracts affect vision significantly or require treatment.

Ordinarily, light rays reflected from an object enter the eye through the cornea and lens, which together focus the light onto the retina to produce a sharp image. When a cataract develops, however, light rays are no longer precisely focused. Instead, the rays are scattered before reaching the retina.

TYPES OF CATARACTS

The lens is made of protein fibers arranged in a specialized way so that the lens is transparent. The lens is composed of four distinct structures: At the center is the *nucleus,* which is surrounded by the *cortex,* then the lens *epithelium,* and finally the lens *capsule.* Protein fibers are secreted by the lens epithelium throughout life.

The three common types of cataracts are defined by where they occur in the lens: nuclear, cortical, and posterior subcapsular (in the rear of the lens capsule). Nuclear cataracts are the most common, and their incidence increases with age. Cortical cataracts also become more common with age and are related to lifetime exposure to ultraviolet light. Posterior subcapsular cataracts are most likely to occur in younger people and are often the result of prolonged use of corticosteroids (such as prednisone), inflammation, trauma, or diabetes. People often have more than one type of cataract in the same eye.

The extent of vision damage and how quickly vision becomes impaired depend not only on the size and density of the cataract, but also its location in the lens. For example, a cataract on the outside edge of the cortex has little effect on vision because it does not interfere with the passage of light through the center of the lens, while a dense nuclear cataract causes severe blurring of vision.

CAUSES OF CATARACTS

The cause of most cataracts is unknown, but at least two factors associated with aging contribute to cataract development. One, clumping (aggregation) of lens proteins leads to scattering of light and a decrease in the transparency of the lens. Two, the breakdown of lens proteins leads to the accumulation of a yellow-brown pigment that clouds the lens.

Certain chemical changes have been noted in the eyes of people with cataracts. These changes include a reduced uptake of oxygen by the lens and a rise in the water content of the lens, which is later followed by dehydration. Amounts of calcium and sodium in the lens increase, while levels of potassium, vitamin C, and protein decrease during cataract formation. In addition, glutathione (an antioxidant) appears to be deficient in lenses with cataracts. Studies on the use of medications or vitamins to alter the levels of these substances in the lens have not produced promising results, however.

Currently, there is no effective drug therapy to prevent cataract formation. But cigarette smoking, medications such as corticosteroids, eye injuries, sunlight, diabetes, and even obesity can increase the risk of cataracts.

Cigarette Smoking

Cigarette smoking is associated with an increased risk of cataracts. Studies of male physicians and female nurses found an increased incidence of nuclear and posterior subcapsular cataracts in those who smoked the most. Smoking at least 20 cigarettes a day more than doubled the risk of these types of cataracts in men; in women,

NEW RESEARCH

Eye Disorders Tied To Mortality, Though Reasons Remain Unclear

Scientists have observed that some eye disorders are significant predictors of decreased life span, though the relationship between the two is not clear. In a new study, researchers have once again described an association between eye disease and mortality, but they also found a possible life-prolonging effect for people with eye disease who took zinc supplements.

The investigators randomly assigned more than 4,700 individuals with either cataracts or age-related macular degeneration (AMD), age 55 to 81, to receive oral supplements of zinc, antioxidants, antioxidants plus zinc, or a placebo. Half the participants were followed for 6½ years or longer. By the end of the study, 534 subjects had died.

Patients with advanced AMD were 41% more likely to die than those without AMD or with a mild case of the disease. Participants with severe visual impairment in one eye or who had cataract surgery also were at increased risk for dying. Surprisingly, subjects who took zinc supplements had a 27% lower risk of death than those who did not take zinc.

The authors concluded that the strong link between eye disorders and life expectancy suggests that cataracts and AMD reflect systemic rather than local disease processes.

ARCHIVES OF OPHTHALMOLOGY
Volume 122, page 716
May 2004

smoking at least 35 cigarettes a day raised the risk by about half. It is not clear why cigarette smoking has an adverse effect on the lens. One possibility is that smoking might reduce blood levels of nutrients required for lens maintenance.

Corticosteroids

Long-term use of corticosteroids, especially at high doses, is the most common drug-related cause of cataracts. In one study of individuals taking oral prednisone for prolonged periods, cataracts developed in 11% of those taking less than 10 mg a day, in 30% of those taking 10 to 15 mg a day, and in 80% of those taking more than 15 mg a day. Short-term use of oral corticosteroids is unlikely to lead to cataracts.

Inhaled corticosteroids also can raise the risk of cataracts. In one study, people who had used inhaled corticosteroids had a 50% greater prevalence of nuclear cataracts and a 90% greater prevalence of posterior subcapsular cataracts than those who had not used inhaled corticosteroids. In another study, people using inhaled corticosteroids for more than three years were three times more likely to need cataract surgery than those who did not use these medications. In addition, the likelihood of cataract surgery increased with higher doses of inhaled corticosteroids. These results may cause concern for people with asthma, who often rely on inhaled corticosteroids to treat their condition. However, the benefits of inhaled corticosteroids for asthma outweigh the long-term risk of cataracts, which are treatable.

Cataracts can also develop from applying topical corticosteroids to the eyelids or using corticosteroid-containing eyedrops (though the more common side effect is elevated intraocular pressure, which may lead to glaucoma). To reduce the chance of these adverse effects, topical corticosteroids applied to the eye and corticosteroid-containing eyedrops should be used only under the supervision of an ophthalmologist.

Eye Injuries

Blunt trauma to the eye or damage to the eye from alkaline chemicals can cause opacification of the lens, either immediately or later on. Rapid cataract formation commonly occurs after a penetrating eye injury.

Sunlight and Ionizing Radiation

Population studies have shown that prolonged exposure to the ultraviolet (UV) radiation in sunlight more than doubles the risk of

How Cataracts Affect Vision

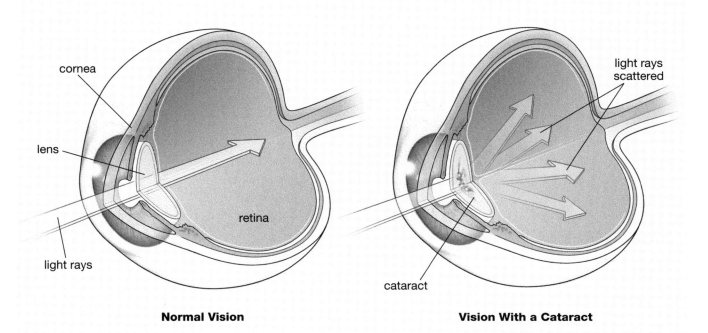

Normal Vision   **Vision With a Cataract**

Although the eye is an extremely complex organ, the principles of vision are actually quite simple: The eye allows us to see by processing the light that reflects off objects in the world around us.

As light rays enter the eye, they pass through the cornea and lens, which focus the light to produce a sharp image on the retina—much like the lens of a camera focuses light onto film. When energy from the light rays hits the retina, it is transformed into electrical signals that travel through the optic nerve to the brain, which interprets these signals as a visual image.

A cataract is a clouding of the lens of the eye that interferes with clear vision. A healthy lens, which consists primarily of water and protein, is normally transparent. Light passing through the lens is refracted and focused onto the retina—which (sometimes with the help of glasses or contact lenses) sends a crisp visual image to the brain. With age, however, changes occur in the lens—including the clumping together of proteins and other chemical transformations—that can lead to the development of a cataract. The resulting opacity blocks light entering the eye, so that the rays reaching the retina are scattered and diffuse rather than focused and precise.

The extent of a cataract's effect on vision depends largely on its location. Cataracts covering the entire lens or those in the center of the lens (nuclear cataracts) result in such symptoms as blurred vision, double vision, and sensitivity to light and glare; cataracts located on the outer edge of the lens may cause only slight visual disturbances that may not be noticed.

cortical cataracts. In one study, the risk of developing cortical cataracts was two times greater in people with the highest levels of sunlight exposure than in those with the lowest exposure levels. In addition, the more sunlight exposure, the higher the risk of cortical cataracts. However, the study found that nuclear cataracts were not linked to sunlight exposure. Ionizing radiation (from x-rays, for example) also can cause cataracts.

Diabetes

People with diabetes are at increased risk for cataracts, particularly the posterior subcapsular type, and these cataracts tend to occur at an earlier age in people with diabetes than in the general population. Some evidence indicates that the accumulation of sorbitol (a sugar formed from glucose) in the lens promotes cataract formation in people with diabetes.

Obesity

Excess weight also may increase the odds of developing cataracts. Proper weight is often determined using body mass index (BMI), a measure of weight in relation to height. To calculate BMI, weight in pounds is multiplied by 704 and divided by the square of height in inches. Overweight is defined as a BMI of 25 to 29.9 and obesity as a BMI of 30 or greater.

In one study of men between the ages of 40 and 84, those whose BMI was between 22 and 28 had roughly a 50% increase in cataract risk compared with those whose BMI was less than 22. A BMI higher than 28 more than doubled cataract risk. Posterior subcapsular cataracts were most often associated with a high BMI. Other studies have found similar results in women.

Although the reason for the link between obesity and cataracts is unclear, it is thought that a low-calorie intake may reduce cataract formation by decreasing blood glucose levels or improving the antioxidant properties of the blood.

SYMPTOMS OF CATARACTS

The most common symptom of cataracts is a painless blurring of vision. Everything becomes dimmer, as if seen through glasses that need cleaning. Most often, both eyes are affected, though vision is usually more compromised in one eye than the other. Changes in vision can occur rapidly—in a matter of months—or almost imperceptibly over many years. In some cases, double vision occurs. This is caused by the passage of light through a lens that has irregular areas of opacity, which can split the rays of light from a single object and focus them on different parts of the retina. Other possible symptoms of cataracts include increasingly frequent changes in eyeglass and contact lens prescriptions and a yellowish tinge to objects.

In the early stages of a nuclear cataract, some people who previously needed reading glasses for presbyopia are able to read without them, a change referred to as second sight. This improvement occurs because the cataract alters the shape of the lens, making it better able to focus on nearby objects. Over time, however, progression of the cataract generally impairs vision.

Individuals with cortical or posterior subcapsular cataracts often have worse vision in bright light; for example, they may have problems with night driving because of the brightness of oncoming headlights. Bright light causes the pupils to contract and restricts the passage of light to the center of the lens—the part that may be most severely affected by the cataract.

PREVENTION OF CATARACTS

Since smoking contributes to the risk of developing cataracts, smoking cessation is a vital step in cataract prevention. Studies show that former smokers have a lower risk of cataracts than current smokers, although their risk is not as low as that of someone who has never smoked. Other benefits of quitting smoking include a reduced risk of cancer, lung disease, and coronary heart disease.

Wearing UV-light-blocking sunglasses and a hat with a wide brim will help reduce eye exposure to UV radiation and may reduce the risk of cataracts. Virtually all sunglasses with tinted plastic lenses provide protection against UV radiation; there is no relationship between the cost of a pair of sunglasses and its UV-blocking ability. The American Academy of Ophthalmology recommends wearing sunglasses when in the sun for extended periods.

Whether certain medications can reduce the risk of cataracts is controversial. The results of trials of medications, such as aspirin or hormone replacement therapy, have been contradictory.

Some researchers have proposed that antioxidant vitamins from foods or vitamin supplements might help prevent cataracts by protecting against free radicals—unstable oxygen molecules that over time can damage various components of the lens. Abundant in fruits and vegetables, antioxidants include beta-carotene, vitamin C, vitamin E, and selenium. Population studies have found a link between high intakes of antioxidants and a reduced incidence of cataracts, but results from the Age-Related Eye Disease Study, a large, randomized, placebo-controlled trial, found no such benefit from antioxidant supplements.

NEW RESEARCH

Cataracts Leading Cause of Vision Loss in Nursing Home Patients

More than one third of nursing home residents in a recent study had poor vision, with vision loss due to cataracts more common among blacks than whites.

The findings underscore the need for better vision screening and care in nursing home patients, the researchers say, noting that the longer a person was in the nursing home, the more likely he or she was to have vision loss.

The researchers surveyed residents of 28 nursing homes and were able to complete vision screening of 1,307 individuals. Thirty-seven percent had vision worse than 20/40 in their best-seeing eye, when corrected with glasses. Although the rate of vision loss and blindness was not significantly different in whites and blacks, the researchers found that cataracts accounted for more cases of vision loss in blacks than in whites (54% vs. 37%). Cataracts were the most common cause of vision loss in both groups, the researchers note, and can easily be treated with surgery.

Although blindness due to macular degeneration was more common among whites, glaucoma was more common among blacks. Both findings have been seen in past studies.

ARCHIVES OF OPHTHALMOLOGY
Volume 122, page 1019
July 2004

TREATMENT OF CATARACTS

About 1.5 million cataract surgeries are performed each year in the United States. Surgery is the only way to cure cataracts, but not everyone with cataracts requires surgery. Some people can improve their vision with lifestyle measures.

Lifestyle Measures

Lifestyle measures can help improve vision in some people with cataracts. These measures include reducing glare by wearing sunglasses and a wide-brimmed hat when outdoors; choosing the appropriate type and amount of indoor lighting; using a magnifying glass; and buying large-print reading materials. Getting a stronger prescription for eyeglasses or contact lenses sometimes can be helpful as well.

Cataract Surgery

Surgery for cataracts involves removing all or part of the lens and replacing it with an intraocular lens implant. Cataract removal is the most frequently performed surgery in people over age 65 and is considered by many doctors to be the most effective surgical procedure in all of medicine.

If the eye is normal except for the cataract, surgery will improve vision in more than 95% of cases. Because the intraocular lens implant is designed to correct nearsightedness or farsightedness, 85% of people undergoing cataract surgery achieve at least 20/40 vision—good enough to drive a car—one year after the operation. (People with 20/40 vision are able to see at 20 feet what a person with normal vision can see at 40 feet.) After cataract surgery, however, most people will still need to wear glasses to read small print or do close handwork.

Significant postsurgical complications occur in only 1% to 2% of operations (see page 17) and include inflammation, infection, bleeding, swelling, retinal detachment, and glaucoma. People with other eye diseases and serious medical problems are most at risk for complications.

Deciding Whether To Have Cataract Surgery

Immediate removal of a cataract is rarely necessary. Instead, the decision of when to have the surgery almost always rests with the patient. The decision is based on the cataract's interference with day-to-day activities like reading and driving, the balance between

Dealing With a Detached Retina

Floaters and flashes that appear suddenly may signal a serious eye problem.

Nearly everyone experiences floaters—small dots, lines, clouds, or "cobwebs" across the visual field—from time to time. This phenomenon is caused by shadows cast on the retina by microscopic structures within the vitreous humor (a thick, gel-like substance that fills the back of the eyeball behind the lens). Seeing flashes of light, which occurs when this fluid shifts, is another common ocular phenomenon.

In most cases, flashes and floaters are harmless and temporary, though they can be frequent and annoying. Sometimes, though, they indicate that the retina (the innermost layer of the eye that consists of light-sensitive nerve tissue) is tearing or in danger of detaching from the underlying layers of the eyeball. Retinal detachment may be a medical emergency that can result in blindness, but prompt treatment generally preserves vision.

How the Retina Detaches

Vitreous humor is a gelatinous fluid that adheres to the retina and fills most of the space inside the eye. As we age, the fluid gradually liquifies and becomes more mobile. Eventually, the vitreous humor begins to shift within the eye. Sometimes, this movement prompts the posterior surface of the vitreous to slide or pull away from the retina, a condition called posterior vitreous detachment (PVD).

PVD develops in 10% of adults by age 50 and in two thirds of those age 70 and older. In most instances it causes no problems. But sometimes the vitreous humor remains adherent to the retina in some areas; as it pulls away, it can tear the retina. Tears are not necessarily harmful, but they may permit fluid to collect underneath the retina. If the fluid spreads, the retina may peel away and detach from the

back of the eye—a so-called retinal detachment.

Who's At Risk

Retinal detachment is a serious complication associated with cataract surgery. The problem develops in up to 1% to 2% of those who have a cataract removed, about half the time within a year of surgery. People who are severely nearsighted are also at increased risk, possibly because the elongated eyeball characteristic of the condition stretches and weakens the retina.

Additional risk factors include a personal or family history of retinal detachment, other eye problems (such as lattice degeneration, which causes retinal thinning), and eye trauma. People with diabetes are vulnerable to another, less common mechanism of retinal detachment related to the formation of scar tissue within the eye.

When To Worry

Retinal tears are not painful, and symptoms may vary. Symptoms that do occur often appear in only one eye at a time and may develop either gradually or suddenly. The most distinctive clue is a shower of hundreds or thousands of little black dots across the field of vision, which may signal a hemorrhage caused by tearing across a blood vessel. Floaters or sudden flashes of white light also are characteristic. If the retina detaches, it may seem that a dark curtain or shade is spreading across the visual field.

Prompt evaluation by an ophthalmologist is necessary if you experience a shower of dots or a curtain spreading across the visual field; new unexplained blurred vision; or an unusually high number of floaters or intensity of light flashes. Call your eye

doctor and do as he or she advises. If you don't have an eye doctor and can't locate one, you can go to an emergency room. Not all hospitals provide emergency eye care on site, however, so calling the hospital first may help you locate an appropriate facility.

Treating a Tear or Retinal Detachment

Numerous procedures may be used to treat retinal tearing and detachment, depending on their extent and location. In certain cases, small holes in the retina require no treatment. In others, combinations of more than one surgical approach may be required. Many are performed on an outpatient basis. The amount of vision restored and preserved with all procedures is greater if the macula is still attached—but even if the prognosis is poor, treatment usually is still advisable.

After treatment, medication can be prescribed to ease any pain. For the first few days following surgery, physical activity is usually restricted, although reading, writing, and watching television are generally possible soon after surgery. Improvement of vision in the affected eye may take weeks or months.

The chances of reattaching the retina are high for all types of retinal detachment surgery for uncomplicated cases, as more than 90% of retinal detachments can be repaired. The actual amount of vision restored, however, can vary greatly. A great advantage of the available techniques—laser therapy, cryotherapy, scleral buckling, vitrectomy, and pneumatic retinopexy—is that if one fails, another can be undertaken immediately or in a matter of days.

the operation's benefits and risks, and the presence of other health conditions that might affect the outcome. In some cases, people with another major vision disorder, such as advanced glaucoma or age-related macular degeneration, may be discouraged from having cataract surgery because it may not improve their vision. On the other hand, cataract removal might benefit people with certain types of retinal damage.

Below are some questions to consider before deciding on cataract surgery. Answering yes to several of the questions suggests that a cataract is interfering with daily life and that surgery might be beneficial.

- Am I having trouble performing my job duties because I cannot see clearly? Do I have to strain to read computer screens?
- Am I constantly squinting?
- Am I inhibited when participating in activities I enjoy—such as reading, watching television, or going out with friends—because of vision limitations?
- Do I stay in at night because of vision problems?
- Does glare from the sun or car headlights interfere with or prevent me from driving?
- Am I fearful of bumping into something or falling because of my eyesight?
- Do I need help performing daily activities—such as preparing food or doing laundry—because of my vision? Could I be more independent if my vision were improved?
- Am I becoming increasingly nearsighted? Despite frequent prescription changes, do I still have trouble seeing with my glasses or contacts?
- Does my eyesight bother me all the time?

Presurgical Tests

Before cataract surgery, the ophthalmologist will obtain a medical history, which includes past and current medical conditions, current medications, and allergies. A-scan ultrasonography, a test that uses sound waves or a laser to measure the length of the eyeball, is routinely performed. The eyeball length is used to determine the appropriate focusing power of the intraocular lens implant. If the surgeon cannot see the retina in the back of the eye because the cataract is too opaque, another test called B-scan ultrasonography is used. This test uses reflected sound waves to look at structures in the back of the eye.

Types of Cataract Surgery

Before the 1970s, most surgeons performed cataract surgery with the naked eye or with the aid of loupes—specialized glasses that provide a small amount of magnification. Today, microsurgery is the rule: An operating microscope is placed over the eye undergoing surgery. The microscope magnifies the eye four to six times its normal size.

If both eyes have cataracts that require surgery, they are most often operated on one at a time, with at least several weeks—and more often months—between the two operations. There are several reasons for the delay. First, it gives the first eye time to recover. Second, should any complications arise, the surgeon might perform the second operation differently. Third, if the results with the first eye are good enough, a second operation may not be needed.

Cataract surgery usually takes less than an hour to perform. About 90% of the surgeries are done on an outpatient basis with a local anesthetic, given either by injection or eyedrops. (General anesthesia is used only in people who are extremely anxious or allergic to local anesthetics.) Patients often are given a sedative before the surgery to make them drowsy.

The two main types of cataract surgery are intracapsular and extracapsular.

Intracapsular surgery. Intracapsular cataract surgery removes the entire lens—the capsule, cortex, and nucleus. The procedure is rarely performed today but still is used in some situations, such as when the lens is partially or completely dislocated.

An incision is made at the side of the cornea, and the surgeon inserts a cryoprobe (a rod with an extremely cold tip) through the incision. When the lens is touched by the tip of the probe, it adheres—as a tongue might stick to a cold metal object in the winter—and the surgeon guides the lens out of the eye as the probe is withdrawn. The incision is closed with fine sutures.

Extracapsular surgery. Extracapsular surgery is by far the most common type of cataract surgery because it minimizes trauma to the eye and is associated with fewer postoperative complications than intracapsular surgery. In extracapsular surgery, the surgeon makes an incision at the side of the cornea and removes the front of the lens capsule, followed by the nucleus and cortex. The back of the lens capsule remains intact. This back portion of the capsule provides support for the intraocular lens implant. Most extracapsular surgery is performed using phacoemulsification.

Phacoemulsification. As with the traditional extracapsular pro-

NEW RESEARCH

Cataract Surgery Benefits People Who Are Blind in One Eye

People who can see with only one eye (monocular) experience twice as much improvement in visual function after cataract surgery as those who can see with both eyes (binocular), a new study shows.

The findings are not surprising, the researchers note, because monocular individuals have worse vision than binocular ones before surgery. However, they add, some ophthalmologists are reluctant to remove cataracts from individuals with only one seeing eye owing to the risk of damaging that eye.

The researchers compared outcomes of cataract surgery in 100 monocular patients (meaning their best-corrected vision was 20/200 or better in one eye and below 20/200 in the other eye) with 100 binocular patients (meaning their best-corrected vision was better than 20/200 in both eyes).

Monocular and binocular patients showed equal improvement in visual acuity after cataract removal, but monocular patients improved twice as much as binocular individuals in a test of visual function.

Six to eight months after surgery, 10 patients in the monocular group showed a decline in visual acuity. It remains unclear whether they would have been better off without having the surgery; the researchers conclude that a clinical trial would be necessary to answer this question.

AMERICAN JOURNAL OF OPHTHALMOLOGY
Volume 138, page 125
July 2004

cedure, the surgeon makes an incision at the outer edge of the cornea and inserts a needle to cut away the front of the lens capsule. Rather than using standard surgical tools to remove the cataract, the surgeon then inserts a thin probe. Once activated, the probe emits ultrasonic vibrations that break the cortex and nucleus of the lens into tiny fragments, which are then vacuumed away through a thin tube. At this point, an intraocular lens implant can be inserted to replace the missing lens.

The major advantage of phacoemulsification is that its smaller surgical incision may hasten postoperative healing. Recovery time can be further reduced when phacoemulsification is used in conjunction with a foldable intraocular lens implant, which is unfurled inside the eye. When these techniques are combined, the incision can be up to 70% smaller than that with standard extracapsular surgery—so small that it heals without stitches.

Lens Replacement

Once a lens has been removed, the patient is referred to as *aphakic,* which is Greek for "without lens." To see clearly, the refractive power of the lens must be replaced so that light can focus onto the retina. The three most common replacement options are intraocular lens implants, glasses, and contact lenses.

Intraocular lens implants. By far the most frequent type of lens replacement is an intraocular lens implant, which is placed at the time of cataract surgery. The quarter-inch plastic lens implant is inserted either just in front of the iris (anterior implant) or just behind it (posterior implant). More than a hundred brands of implants are available; most of them are posterior implants. Posterior implants rest against the back wall of the lens capsule and have plastic loops that jut out to hold the implant in position behind the iris. In general, posterior implants can be used only in conjunction with extracapsular surgery. Intraocular lens implants have been in wide use since 1977, and most ophthalmologists believe they are very safe.

Not all people who undergo cataract surgery are able to receive an intraocular lens implant, however. For example, lens implantation may not be possible in people with certain eye diseases including severe, recurrent uveitis (inflammation of the iris, ciliary body, or choroid), some cases of proliferative diabetic retinopathy (new blood vessel growth onto the back surface of the vitreous humor), and rubeosis iridis (new blood vessel growth on the iris, which usually occurs in people with diabetes).

The most common type of lens implant is the single-focus lens.

Remedies for Red Eye

Allergic conjunctivitis is a common cause of red, itchy eyes. It is also highly treatable.

Although allergies are best known for causing nasal symptoms, they also can be irritating to the eyes. The affected part of the eye is the conjunctiva, the thin, elastic tissue that covers the white of the eye and lines the inside of the eyelid. Fortunately, doctors and patients have an array of therapies at their disposal to prevent or treat allergic conjunctivitis.

Symptoms and Causes

Conjunctivitis can be caused by either allergies or infection. In allergic conjunctivitis, the eyes become red and itchy, with a watery, stringy, or rope-like discharge. Both eyes are usually affected. In addition, people with allergic conjunctivitis often have a history of allergic rhinitis, asthma, or eczema.

Infectious conjunctivitis also leads to eye redness but is more likely to produce tearing and discharge in one or both eyes. People with these symptoms may need antibiotics and should see a doctor.

Allergic conjunctivitis can be seasonal (occurring only at specific times of the year) or perennial (occurring year-round). Seasonal allergic conjunctivitis is typically caused by outdoor allergens, such as pollen, and the perennial form is usually caused by indoor allergens, such as cockroaches, dust mites, or pet dander. Skin or blood testing by an allergist can pinpoint a patient's specific triggers.

Treatment

To prevent symptoms, patients should learn to avoid or limit their exposure to triggering substances. When symptoms do erupt, cold compresses on the eyes may help relieve symptoms in the short term.

Drug Class	Medication
Mast-cell stabilizers	• cromolyn (Crolom, Opticrom) • ketotifen (Zaditor) • lodoxamide (Alomide) • olopatadine (Patanol)
Antihistamines	• azelastine (Astelin, Optivar) • emedastine (Emadine) • epinastine (Elestat) • levocabastine (Livostin) • nedocromil (Alocril) • pemirolast (Alamast)
Nonsteroidal anti-inflammatory drugs	• diclofenac (Voltaren) • ketorolac (Acular)
Corticosteroid	• loteprednol (Alrex, Lotemax)
Vasoconstrictors	• naphazoline (Albalon and other brands)* • oxymetazoline (OcuClear, Visine L.R.)† • tetrahydrozoline (Tyzine)

* Some versions of naphazoline are available over the counter.
† Oxymetazoline is available over the counter.
The rest of the medications in the chart are prescriptions.

Medications are a mainstay of treatment for allergic conjunctivitis. Some doctors recommend using artificial tears, which provide a barrier between allergens and the eye; they also help dilute and flush out the allergens that contact the eye. Antihistamine eyedrops are often effective for acute treatment of redness and itching. Sometimes doctors will prescribe oral antihistamine medication to reduce itching.

Vasoconstrictors may be good for short-term treatment of redness and swelling that can occur. Nonsteroidal anti-inflammatory eyedrops may also be good for reducing symptoms in some patients. Mast-cell inhibitors help treat a range of symptoms, including itching, swelling, and watery eyes.

Doctors usually prescribe corticosteroid eyedrops only for severe cases and only for short periods because of the risk of side effects, including cataract and elevated eye pressure, which may lead to glaucoma. The chart above lists some medicated eyedrops commonly used for allergic conjunctivitis.

For some patients, immunotherapy (allergy shots) may be a useful way to prevent allergies from recurring.

Unlike the natural lens of the eye, a single-focus lens cannot alter its shape to bring objects at different distances into focus. As a result, the surgeon generally selects a lens that will provide good distance vision, and the person wears reading glasses for near vision. Alternately, the surgeon can correct one eye for distance and the other for near vision; this is called monovision. In general, new eyeglasses cannot be prescribed until about three weeks after cataract surgery because the prescription changes as the eye heals. Still, if the eye is otherwise normal, people with lens implants often have functional vision as early as the first day after surgery.

The first multifocal lens implant, which provides both distance and near vision, was approved by the U.S. Food and Drug Administration (FDA) several years ago. Multifocal lenses contain several concentric rings, each of which permits the user to see at a different distance. Although these lenses reduce the need for eyeglasses, many people still have to wear glasses for certain tasks. In addition, multifocal lenses can cause visual side effects such as glare and halos. Newer multifocal implants are currently in development.

The newest type of lens implant, called an accommodating lens, contains a hinge that allows for both distance and near vision. The FDA approved the first of these devices, the CrystaLens, in 2003. Although most people do achieve 20/40 vision or better with the implant, the range of vision varies, and improvements in near vision may decrease over time.

Many of the single-focus and all of the multifocal lens implants available today are foldable. Foldable implants, which have been available since the early 1990s, are made from silicone, acrylic, or hydrogel, and can be inserted into a smaller surgical opening than that required for other types of implants. The smaller opening may cause less trauma to the eye and lead to quicker recovery.

Once inserted, lens implants require no care of any kind. Like any device, however, complications can occur. The most common complication is glare or reduced vision when the intraocular lens is not aligned with the pupil.

Glasses. Another option for lens replacement is cataract glasses. Although effective, these glasses are rarely used after routine cataract surgery because they are heavy and awkward. The glasses magnify objects by about 25%, causing them to appear closer than they actually are—a somewhat disorienting sensation. Because of the thickness and curvature of the lenses, cataract glasses magnify objects unequally and so have a distorting effect as well. In addition, they tend to limit peripheral vision. When used, cataract glasses are prescribed four to eight weeks after surgery.

Contact lenses. Like cataract glasses, contact lenses are not routinely used after cataract surgery. The lenses provide almost normal vision, but their major drawback is that people often have difficulty handling, removing, and cleaning them. The frequent handling of contact lenses may also increase the risk of eye infection. Because the patient must be able to see when the contacts are not in place, a pair of cataract glasses is also necessary. Both the contacts and glasses can be prescribed four to eight weeks after surgery.

After Surgery

Most people experience minimal discomfort after cataract surgery; a mild painkiller (such as Tylenol) can be taken if needed. Some redness, scratchiness, or morning discharge may be present during the first few days after surgery. In addition, it is common to see a few black spots or shapes (called floaters) drifting through the field of vision. A protective patch is generally worn over the eye for 24 hours. Glasses must be worn during the day to avoid trauma to the eye, and an eye shield is used at night for several days to a few weeks to prevent accidentally rubbing or poking the eye while asleep.

Vision varies widely when the patch is first removed. In most people, vision remains blurred for several days to weeks, then gradually improves as the eye heals. In some cases, the sutures in the eye alter the shape of the cornea and result in temporary blurring or astigmatism. This problem generally goes away on its own, though it may require removal of the sutures—a simple and painless procedure. In general, vision improves faster in those who receive intraocular lens implants than in those with cataract glasses or contact lenses. However, surgery usually changes the corrective prescription for the eye (even in those with lens implants), and new eyeglasses will be needed to correct any remaining near- or farsightedness. The patient is considered fully recovered when the eye is completely healed and vision has stabilized so that a final corrective prescription can be obtained.

Possible Complications of Surgery

Though cataract surgery is associated with a low rate of complications, problems may arise, especially in older adults or those with general health problems such as diabetes. Patients should contact their doctor if any of the following symptoms develop during

NEW RESEARCH

Multifocal Lenses Don't Boost Satisfaction With Cataract Surgery

People who have multifocal lenses implanted after cataract surgery are less likely to need reading glasses afterwards than those who receive monofocal lenses, but they aren't any happier about their quality of vision. The reason is that people who get multifocal lenses appear to have unrealistic expectations about the device, according to a new study.

Dutch researchers randomized 75 people who needed cataract surgery to receive either monofocal or multifocal lenses. Patients were counseled about what to expect from each of the implants.

Three months after both eyes had been operated on, about 90% of the patients in both groups were satisfied with their quality of near and far vision when using glasses. Although more people in the multifocal group were able to see well without reading glasses most of the time (43% vs. 22%), they were no more likely than those in the monofocal group to state that their expectations of surgery were met (62% vs. 63%).

The researchers conclude that although multifocal lenses can reduce people's dependence on reading glasses, more than half of people who receive them still need glasses—and that patients should be aware of this before surgery.

OPHTHALMOLOGY
Volume 111, page 1832
October 2004

recovery from surgery: unusual pain or aching; persistent redness; bleeding; excessive tearing or discharge; any sudden vision changes; or seeing many bright flashes of light.

About 1% of people, particularly those who are very nearsighted, may develop retinal detachment after cataract surgery. Retinal detachment is a vision-threatening condition in which the retina becomes separated from the underlying layers of the eye. Disruption of the back of the lens capsule during or after surgery (such as during follow-up laser treatment for postsurgical clouding of the capsule) can increase the risk. Cystoid macular edema (a specific pattern of swelling of the central retina) is another common eye-related complication of cataract surgery. The swelling can result in visual impairment that is usually temporary. If the swelling does not go down on its own, eyedrops may be prescribed.

About 1 in 1,000 people develop an infection of the vitreous humor, called endophthalmitis, after cataract surgery. Patients who experience an increasingly red eye, blurred vision, and pain should see their ophthalmologist promptly. Typically, this condition can be treated with antibiotics and removal of some of the vitreous humor. Other complications of cataract surgery, such as significant bleeding inside the eye or large pieces of the cataract falling into the back of the eye (dropped nucleus), are rare.

In up to 20% of extracapsular surgeries, the back of the lens capsule subsequently becomes cloudy and causes vision difficulties similar to those of the original cataract. Fortunately, recent advances in lens material and design have substantially reduced the risk of this complication. When cloudiness occurs, laser treatment (see below) is an effective remedy.

Laser Treatment Following Extracapsular Surgery

A YAG (yttrium, aluminum, and garnet) laser is used if vision is blurred by clouding of the back of the lens capsule that remains in the eye following extracapsular surgery. The YAG laser produces a hole in the back of the lens capsule by focusing a burst of energy on it. The procedure, called a YAG capsulotomy, leads to prompt clearing of vision.

The risk of retinal detachment with YAG capsulotomy is small, affecting approximately 1 in 300 people within three to four years of surgery. This risk is increased in younger people and those who are extremely nearsighted. Therefore, just as the initial decision to have cataract surgery is based in part on balancing possible risks and benefits, similar issues are weighed prior to YAG treatment.

Glaucoma

Glaucoma, the second leading cause of adult blindness in the United States after age-related macular degeneration, often results from an intraocular pressure (IOP) that is too high for the optic nerve to tolerate. About 2.2 million Americans age 40 and over have glaucoma and, because the condition does not cause symptoms in its early stages, half of them do not know it. Another 5 to 10 million people are at increased risk for the disorder.

The risk of glaucoma varies with race and age. The condition is more common in blacks and Hispanics than in whites, and it occurs more frequently with increasing age. In one study, the prevalence of glaucoma was about 1% in people age 40 to 49; in those over age 70, it reached 10% in whites and 20% in blacks.

The two main forms of glaucoma are open-angle and closed-angle. Open-angle glaucoma, which accounts for 90% of all glaucoma cases in the United States, progresses slowly and produces no obvious symptoms until its late stages. It is equally common in men and women. Closed-angle glaucoma accounts for the remaining 10% of glaucoma cases and occurs most often in people of Chinese descent and some other Asian groups. Women are at greater risk than men.

Both types of glaucoma can lead to blindness by damaging the optic nerve. Even people with normal IOP can suffer damage to the optic nerve—in fact, 25% to 30% of people with glaucoma do not have elevated IOP levels. Susceptibility to IOP varies from person to person, and risk factors other than IOP play a role in the development of glaucoma. Early detection and treatment of elevated IOP levels can help prevent optic nerve damage.

CAUSES OF GLAUCOMA

Each day, the eye produces about 1 teaspoon of aqueous humor—a clear fluid that provides nutrients to, and carries waste products away from, the lens and cornea. (In other parts of the body, these functions are carried out by the blood, but the lens and cornea have no blood supply.) The aqueous humor is produced by the ciliary body (which surrounds the lens). Aqueous humor flows from behind the iris through the pupil and into the front chamber of the eye; it then drains from the eye through a spongy network of connective tissue called the trabecular meshwork, where it ultimately enters the bloodstream. An alternate drainage system, the

NEW RESEARCH

Anticholesterol Drugs Protect Against Glaucoma

Long-term use of cholesterol-lowering drugs called statins appears to reduce the risk of glaucoma among men, particularly those with cardiovascular disease and high cholesterol, according to new research. Statins have previously been linked to possible decreased risk of age-related macular degeneration, and there are sound scientific reasons why these drugs may also protect against glaucoma.

Researchers evaluated the medical records of 667 men age 50 or older who had recently developed glaucoma, then determined their statin use. For comparison, statin use was also recorded for 6,667 control subjects without glaucoma.

Patients who had used statins for two years or longer were 40% less likely to develop glaucoma than those who had used the drugs for less time. The benefits were most pronounced for men with cardiovascular disease and high cholesterol. A protective effect against glaucoma was also observed for nonstatin anticholesterol drugs.

The researchers hypothesize that statins might reduce the risk of glaucoma directly, by reducing atherosclerosis in the optic nerve, or indirectly, by improving blood flow in the eye. Statins might also enhance the ability of cells in the trabecular meshwork to drain excess fluid.

ARCHIVES OF OPHTHALMOLOGY
Volume 122, page 822
June 2004

uveoscleral pathway, is located behind the trabecular meshwork. Ordinarily, fluid production and drainage are in balance, and IOP is between 12 and 22 mm Hg (millimeters of mercury, the same units of measurement used for blood pressure).

In people with open-angle glaucoma who have higher-than-normal IOP levels, ophthalmologists suspect that a partial blockage of the trabecular meshwork traps the aqueous humor. Exactly how this happens is unclear. As more aqueous humor is produced than is removed, the blockage causes an increase in IOP. Initially, IOP does not rise high enough to cause discomfort or any easily perceived changes in vision. But when IOP remains elevated or continues to rise, fibers in the optic nerve are compressed and eventually die, leading to a gradual loss of vision over a period of several years.

In some people, even a normal level of IOP is sufficient to contribute to optic nerve damage. These individuals may have thinner-than-normal corneas that make IOP measurements appear to be lower than they actually are. Therefore, thin corneas may be a risk factor for glaucoma, and the American Academy of Ophthalmology now recommends that people with other risk factors for glaucoma (for example, advanced age, elevated IOP, and black ancestry) have their corneal thickness measured.

Heredity may also play a role in glaucoma risk. Mutations causing glaucoma have been identified in the chromosome 1 open-angle glaucoma gene (GLC1A), which directs the production of myocilin. Myocilin is a protein expressed by trabecular meshwork cells, and mutated forms of myocilin are thought to obstruct the outflow of aqueous humor. Mutations in the gene that directs the production of optineurin have also been associated with glaucoma. Optineurin is another protein found in the trabecular meshwork and retina of the eye, but its role is not yet clear.

Inhaled corticosteroids—commonly used to treat asthma—and nasal sprays containing corticosteroids appear to raise the risk of elevated IOP and open-angle glaucoma, possibly by inhibiting the drainage of aqueous humor. Oral corticosteroids may have the same effect. People who must use corticosteroids (for conditions such as asthma, arthritis, sinusitis, or chronic bronchitis) should have their IOP and vision monitored regularly.

Closed-angle glaucoma is caused by a blockage of aqueous humor at the pupil, leading to a bowing forward of the iris that prevents aqueous humor from reaching the trabecular meshwork. The blockage of the outflow of aqueous humor results in a sudden

NEW RESEARCH

Corneal Thickness Related To Glaucoma Severity

The thickness of the cornea is strongly correlated with the severity of glaucoma, a new study finds. This information may aid ophthalmologists in identifying which patients are at the greatest risk for progression of the disease.

Researcher examined medical records that contained information on 190 patients and 350 eyes afflicted by glaucoma. They found that patients with thinner corneas consistently had worse cases of glaucoma and greater eye damage than those with thicker corneas. Corneal thickness was not, however, associated with the number of glaucoma medications taken by patients. This study was the first to demonstrate that thinner corneas are predictive of more severe glaucoma.

The study also confirmed previous findings that average corneal thickness among black patients is lower than for white patients, which may explain why blacks are four to five times more likely than whites to develop glaucoma. In addition, family history of glaucoma was associated with worse disease.

The authors concluded that measuring corneal thickness may help ophthalmologists identify patients who are at higher risk for developing severe glaucoma-related problems and prompt them to treat their disease more aggressively.

ARCHIVES OF OPHTHALMOLOGY
Volume 122, page 17
January 2004

How Glaucoma Affects Vision

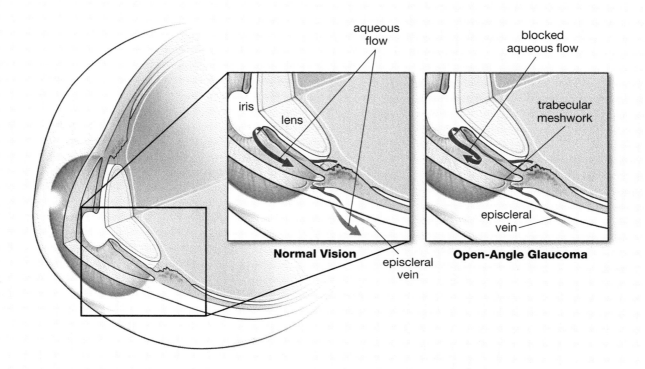

aqueous
flow

blocked
aqueous flow

iris

lens

trabecular
meshwork

Normal Vision

episcleral
vein

Open-Angle Glaucoma

episcleral
vein

Glaucoma occurs when the clear liquid in the front of the eye, called the aqueous humor, places enough pressure on the optic nerve to damage it. Often this damage is caused by elevated pressure within the eye, but in some cases normal pressure damages the nerve.

Internal pressure in the eye, or intraocular pressure (IOP), is primarily regulated by the aqueous humor. Continually manufactured by the ciliary body (a ring of tissue that is located behind the iris), aqueous humor flows through the pupil into the anterior chamber. After delivering nutrients to the lens and cornea, the fluid drains from the eye through a spongy network of connective tissue known as the trabecular meshwork. From these tiny channels, the fluid passes into a larger opening—the canal of Schlemm—and eventually drains into the veins of the sclera (episcleral veins) for disposal. Normally, the steady production and drainage of aqueous humor

maintain a stable balance of fluid in the eye and keep IOP within a safe range.

Open-angle glaucoma caused by high IOP may develop when, for unknown reasons, the trabecular meshwork becomes partially blocked, hindering the outflow of aqueous humor and throwing off the eye's fluid balance. The buildup of aqueous humor causes IOP to rise gradually. Over time, the constant elevation of pressure may damage the optic nerve and impair vision. Treatment with medication or surgery reduces the chance of progressive vision loss. Closed-angle glaucoma, on the other hand, is much more rare and occurs suddenly when IOP rises rapidly. Signs of an attack—including severe pain in the eye, nausea and vomiting, blurred vision, and rainbow-colored halos around lights—should prompt an immediate call to the ophthalmologist.

increase in IOP that can lead to severe, permanent vision damage within one or two days if not treated.

SYMPTOMS OF GLAUCOMA

Open-angle glaucoma generally affects both eyes, although IOP levels and the extent of damage to the optic nerve often differ. Because of the way the optic nerve is structured, the first nerve fibers damaged are those necessary for peripheral vision. People with advanced open-angle glaucoma can have 20/20 vision when looking straight ahead but may have blind spots (scotomas) for images located outside the center of the visual field. The damage often is not detectable by visual field tests (perimetry; see page 24) until as much as 40% of the optic nerve fibers are destroyed. Eventually, the fibers needed for central vision may be lost as well.

Unlike the open-angle form, closed-angle glaucoma sometimes occurs as acute attacks, as IOP rises rapidly to a dangerous level. Signs of an attack include severe pain in the eye, nausea and vomiting, blurred vision, and rainbow-colored halos around lights. Attacks typically do not occur in both eyes at once, but after an initial attack there is a 40% to 80% chance of a similar attack occurring in the other eye within the next 5 to 10 years if no treatment is provided.

PREVENTION OF GLAUCOMA

Until recently, glaucoma was not considered preventable. But a 2002 study of more than 1,600 people with elevated IOP and no signs of glaucoma suggested that IOP-lowering eyedrops may help delay or even prevent the onset of glaucoma. In the study, 4% of those who took IOP-lowering medication developed glaucoma over a five-year period, compared with 10% of those who did not take these medications. If glaucoma does develop, regular eye examinations can help detect the disease in its early stages and reduce the likelihood of damage to the optic nerve.

DIAGNOSIS OF GLAUCOMA

An eye examination for glaucoma involves measuring IOP, viewing the optic nerve, and testing the visual fields. In general, whites should be examined for glaucoma every two years after age 50 and blacks every two years after age 40; optic nerve damage is uncommon before age 50 in whites but can occur up to 10 years earlier in blacks. People with cardiovascular disease or high degrees of near-sightedness may need to begin examinations at a younger age and undergo them more often because of their increased risk of nerve damage from glaucoma.

IOP measurements alone are no longer used to diagnose glaucoma, because some people with elevated IOP do not develop optic nerve damage, while others develop glaucoma despite normal IOP. A high IOP raises the suspicion of glaucoma, but other tests are required to make a diagnosis.

Tests for Glaucoma

Ophthalmologists use three types of tests to screen for glaucoma in people at risk, make the diagnosis, and follow people during treatment. The three tests are tonometry to measure IOP, ophthalmoscopy to inspect the optic nerve, and perimetry to test the visual fields. A high IOP warrants further testing, and the final diagnosis is made by also finding evidence of optic nerve damage typical of glaucoma or by identifying defects in the visual fields characteristic of glaucoma. The distinction between open-angle and closed-angle glaucoma is made by examining the front part of the eye to check the angle where the iris meets the cornea. This is done using a special technique known as gonioscopy.

Tonometry. Tonometry measures IOP by assessing the amount of force necessary to make a slight indentation in a small area of the cornea. The most effective way to do this is with applanation tonometry. In this test, anesthetic eyedrops are administered to numb the eye. Then, slight pressure is applied to the cornea with a small instrument while the doctor looks through a table-mounted microscope (called a slit lamp). A handheld tonometry device (Tono-Pen) also is sometimes used and is relatively accurate. Tonometry is painless and poses virtually no risk to the cornea.

Air-puff tonometry, in which IOP is measured with a quick puff of warm air, is being reevaluated as a diagnostic tool. Anesthetic eyedrops are not needed for this procedure because the air-puff tonometer does not touch the eye.

Ophthalmoscopy. Examination of the optic nerve is required for the diagnosis of glaucoma, and periodic examinations of the nerve are valuable to follow the progress of the disorder during treatment. To perform ophthalmoscopy, the doctor dilates the patient's pupils with eyedrops and then uses an ophthalmoscope—a special instrument with a small light on the end—to magnify and examine the optic nerve. Another type of ophthalmoscopy, called a slit lamp, uses

NEW RESEARCH

LASIK Eye Surgery May Affect Glaucoma Care

Reductions in corneal thickness after laser in situ keratomileusis (LASIK) eye surgery may affect the detection and treatment of glaucoma, ophthalmologist experts report.

Since its introduction, millions of patients worldwide have undergone LASIK vision-correction surgery, which involves the removal of a layer of corneal tissue—resulting in a thinner cornea. Although changes in corneal thickness can affect measurements of intraocular pressure (IOP), ophthalmologists have only recently begun to take corneal thickness into account when measuring IOP.

To determine how LASIK–linked reductions in corneal thickness might affect IOP measurements, researchers measured corneal thickness in 188 patients at a glaucoma clinic. When corneal thickness was factored into IOP readings, approximately half of patients required an adjustment in their IOP readings, the researchers report.

These alterations in IOP readings led to a change in recommendations concerning medication therapy for 8.5% of the patients, a change regarding laser therapy decisions in 2.1%, and a change in the decision regarding glaucoma surgery in 3.2%.

Based on these findings, the researchers urge further study to determine whether measurements of corneal thickness should become standard in glaucoma diagnosis and treatment.

ARCHIVES OF OPHTHALMOLOGY
Volume 122, page 1270
September 2004

a specialized microscope that allows three-dimensional visualization of the optic nerve. Signs of a damaged optic nerve include "cupping" in its center and a loss of its normal pink color. A number of other imaging systems are used to supplement ophthalmoscopy, including laser-based image formation and special polarized light reflection measurement.

Perimetry. This test is used to help diagnose glaucoma and monitor progression of the disease during treatment. The patient wears a patch over one eye and looks straight ahead at a bowl-shaped white area, while a computer presents lights in fixed locations around the bowl. The patient indicates each time he or she sees a light. Perimetry provides a "map" of the visual fields. The type of vision loss associated with glaucoma is relatively specific, and perimetry can detect the typical visual-field defects of glaucoma. The test takes about four minutes to perform in each eye.

Quicker methods of perimetry that take only two minutes per eye are now being used for screening purposes. Among the most promising is Frequency Doubling Technology. This test measures damage to the larger ganglion cells in the retina, which may be more likely damaged by glaucoma than the optic nerve.

TREATMENT OF GLAUCOMA

Glaucoma is a chronic disorder that cannot be cured. Open-angle glaucoma often can be treated safely and effectively with medication or surgery, though lifelong therapy is almost always necessary. Decisions on when to start treatment are based on evidence of optic nerve damage, visual field loss, and risk factors (such as elevated IOP, increasing age, and black or Hispanic background). Acute closed-angle glaucoma is a medical emergency. People with symptoms of closed-angle glaucoma (see page 22) should contact their ophthalmologist immediately.

The overall aim in the treatment of glaucoma—either open-angle or closed-angle—is to prevent damage to the optic nerve by lowering IOP and maintaining it at a level that is unlikely to cause further nerve damage. The appropriate target for IOP is generally 25% below the IOP level at the time of diagnosis. In a small number of people with extremely high IOP levels (above 35 mm Hg), the percent decrease to reach the target IOP is substantially more. Once the target IOP is achieved, patients are monitored to confirm that damage to the optic nerve is not progressing. If progressive damage is detected at the target IOP, a lower target is selected.

Medications That May Cause Vision Problems

Vision problems can be an unwanted side effect of many different medications. Most of these drugs will cause only temporary visual disturbances—such as blurred or double vision, dry eyes, excessive tearing, puffy eyelids, sensitivity to light, seeing a yellow or blue tinge, or a change in eye color—that disappear with time or once the medication is discontinued. However, long-term use of some medications may result in more serious vision disorders.

Always consider drug side effects when visual symptoms develop, and be sure to tell your ophthalmologist about all medications you are taking. Regular use of any drug associated with serious vision disorders merits periodic monitoring of the eyes. Listed below are some of the most common drugs associated with vision problems.

- Antiarrhythmia drugs, such as amiodarone (Cordarone) and digoxin (Lanoxin), are used to treat abnormal heart rhythms and may cause visual disturbances such as blurred vision, yellow vision, or blue-green halos around objects.

- Antimalarial drugs, such as chloroquine (Aralen) and hydroxychloroquine (Plaquenil), are used not only for malaria, but also for rheumatoid arthritis and lupus. They may cause visual disturbances such as blurred vision, and prolonged therapy may lead to irreversible retinopathy.

- Corticosteroids such as prednisone (Deltasone and other brands) may lead to glaucoma or cataracts. Oral treatments (commonly used for arthritis) are linked to cataracts, while the inhaled versions used to treat asthma are associated with both cataracts and glaucoma.

- Erectile dysfunction drugs, like sildenafil (Viagra), tadalafil (Cialis), and vardenafil (Levitra), can temporarily cause objects to have a blue tinge to them, blurred vision, and sensitivity to light.

- Phenothiazines, like chlorpromazine (Thorazine) and thioridazine (Mellaril), are used to treat schizophrenia. These drugs may lead to blurred vision, changes in color vision, and difficulty seeing at night.

- Tamoxifen (Nolvadex), which is used to reduce the risk of breast cancer recurrences, may lead to blurred vision, changes to the retina and cornea, and cataracts.

Unfortunately, treatment cannot reverse optic nerve damage or improve vision.

Choosing a treatment for glaucoma is based on achieving the greatest benefits at the lowest risk and minimizing cost and inconvenience. Medication and surgery are both first-line treatments for glaucoma; each has its own complications and possible side effects. In some cases, medication does not stop the progression of optic nerve damage or visual field loss, possibly because the doctor has selected a target IOP that is not low enough or because the target IOP is not reached (often because the patient does not take the medication as prescribed). Surgical complications such as the development of cataracts occur in only a small number of people, and the risk is lower with laser trabecular surgery than with traditional filtration surgery.

Medication

In people with glaucoma, periodic visits to the ophthalmologist to monitor IOP, visual fields, treatment side effects, and the appearance of the optic nerve are essential. Visits may be as frequent as daily or weekly when treatment is being initiated or adjusted in people with severe optic nerve damage or extremely high IOP levels, or only every three to six months in people with stable IOP levels and minimal optic nerve damage.

Some people do not closely follow their glaucoma treatment regimen. Two main factors contribute to this problem: taking a large number of other prescription medications and having to take glaucoma medication more than twice a day. In addition, the cost or side effects of glaucoma medication may be to blame. If any of these factors are affecting your ability to follow your treatment regimen, ask your doctor if any changes can be made to the regimen.

Two forms of medication are used to treat glaucoma: eyedrops and oral drugs.

Eyedrops. Eyedrops are the most common medication for glaucoma. In general, eyedrops are applied one to four times a day on a regular schedule. Drops can cause local side effects such as burning, stinging, tearing, itching, or redness in the eye. Because some of the drug is absorbed into the body, systemic side effects may occur but are less common than with oral medications. One example of a common side effect is that beta-blocker eyedrops can lower blood pressure at the same time as they lower IOP.

Systemic side effects can be minimized by carefully following instructions for using eyedrops, including placing a finger on the inside corner of the eye for two to three minutes to prevent the eyedrops from entering the nasal ducts.

Five types of eyedrops are currently used: beta-blockers, topical prostaglandins, carbonic anhydrase inhibitors, adrenergic agonists, and miotics (see the text below and the chart on pages 28–29).

Beta-blockers. These drugs lower IOP by reducing the production of aqueous humor. The most commonly used beta-blocker is timolol (Timoptic). Newer beta-blockers such as betaxolol (Betoptic), carteolol (Ocupress), levobunolol (Betagan), and metipranolol (OptiPranolol) are just as effective. Systemic side effects of beta-blockers include slower heart rate, reduced blood pressure, reduced libido, anxiety, nausea and vomiting, and breathing difficulties.

Topical prostaglandins. The topical prostaglandins bimatoprost (Lumigan), latanoprost (Xalatan), and travoprost (Travatan) reduce IOP by increasing drainage of aqueous humor through the uveoscleral pathway. These medications appear to be at least as effective as the beta-blocker timolol and are associated with fewer side effects. Consequently, topical prostaglandins are now the most frequently used drugs for glaucoma. Topical prostaglandins also are sometimes used in combination with another glaucoma medication to produce greater reductions in IOP. About 3% of people taking topical prostaglandins for six months or more experience gradual changes in eye color—from blue or green to brown. Other possible side effects include burning, stinging, and increased eyelash growth.

Carbonic anhydrase inhibitors. Two carbonic anhydrase inhibitors are available as eyedrops: brinzolamide (Azopt) and dorzolamide (Trusopt). These eyedrops lower IOP by decreasing production of aqueous humor. They are used when other glaucoma medications are ineffective. Common side effects include fatigue, stinging in the eyes, and loss of appetite.

Adrenergic agonists. Adrenergic agonists, such as dipivefrin (Propine) and epinephrine (Epifrin), can increase the drainage of aqueous humor but work primarily by decreasing its production. Possible side effects include burning in the eyes, enlarged pupils, and allergic reactions. Brimonidine (Alphagan) and apraclonidine (Iopidine) also are adrenergic agonists. They reduce IOP by decreasing production of aqueous humor and increasing its drainage through the uveoscleral pathway. Their most common side effects are dry mouth and altered taste. Allergic reactions also are a possibility.

Miotics. Miotics, such as pilocarpine (Isopto Carpine and other brands) and carbachol (Isopto Carbachol), increase the drainage of aqueous humor by improving its flow through the trabecular meshwork. Side effects of these drugs include nearsightedness and reduced night vision. Excessive tearing, eye pain, and allergic reactions may also occur.

Combination agent. A medication containing both dorzolamide and timolol is available (Cosopt). This drug reduces the production of aqueous humor and has shown to be more effective in lowering IOP than either agent alone. However, a 2003 study found that dorzolamide-timolol did not lower IOP as effectively as bimatoprost. The drug is often used together with a topical prostaglandin to reduce IOP in patients in whom single-drug therapy has not been successful.

Oral medications. Acetazolamide (Diamox) and methazolamide, both carbonic anhydrase inhibitors, are the only glaucoma medications that are taken orally. Because of their side effects, they are generally used only when optic nerve damage continues despite the use of eyedrops at the highest tolerable dose. The drugs initially lower IOP by 20% to 30% but are associated with significant systemic side effects (such as numbness or tingling in the hands and feet, malaise, and loss of appetite) and occasional serious complications (such as depression, kidney stones, diarrhea, and damage to blood cells).

NEW RESEARCH

Health Information on the Internet Often Commercial

Consumers who scour the Internet for health-related information can expect very different results depending on which search engine they use, according to a new study. While some searches turn up predominantly noncommercial sources, others are heavily weighted toward Web sites peddling products such as vitamin supplements or unconventional and unproven treatments.

Investigators used seven search engines to look for information on macular degeneration and categorized the top 10 results as either strictly commercial, primarily or exclusively informational or governmental, or strictly educational. Each search result was also weighted by its position on the results list.

Overall, commercial sites accounted for 25% of all results, and most appeared relatively high up on the results list. Large variabilities were found among the search engines: While one listed 80% commercial sites, another listed only 30%. Also, some search engines receive a fee from companies in exchange for greater search visibility.

A good way to locate authoritative Web sites and screen out commercial ones is to use www.medlineplus.gov when searching for health information. Patients can use information from such Web sites to help them formulate questions for their health care provider.

ARCHIVES OF OPHTHALMOLOGY
Volume 122, page 380
March 2004

Glaucoma Drugs 2005

Drug Type	Generic Name	Brand Name	Average Retail Price per 5-mL Bottle *
Beta-blockers	betaxolol	Betoptic S	0.25%: $44 (0.5%: $22)
	carteolol	Ocupress	1%: $37 ($16)
	levobunolol	Betagan	0.25%: $28 ($9)
	metipranolol	OptiPranolol	0.3%: $29 ($11)
	timolol	Timoptic Ocumeter	0.25%: $20 ($13)
		Timoptic-XE Ocumeter	0.25%: $29 ($21)
Adrenergic agonists	apraclonidine	Iopidine	0.5%: $74
	brimonidine	Alphagan	0.15%: $39
	dipivefrin	Propine	0.1%: $25 ($10)
	epinephrine	Epifrin	0.5%: $50
Miotics	carbachol	Isopto Carbachol	1.5%: $40
	echothiophate	Phospholine Iodide	0.125%: $43
	pilocarpine	Isopto Carpine	2% (15-mL bottle): $29 ($9)
		Pilocar	2% (15-mL bottle): $17
		Pilopine HS	4 g of gel: $49
Carbonic anhydrase inhibitors	acetazolamide	Diamox	500 mg (30 tablets): $140 (9) 1%: $36
	brinzolamide	Azopt	2%: $30
	dorzolamide	Trusopt Ocumeter	50 mg (30 tablets): ($12)
	methazolamide	—	
Topical prostaglandins	bimatoprost	Lumigan	0.03%: $109
	latanoprost	Xalatan	0.005% (2.5-mL bottle): $51
	travoprost	Travatan	0.004% (2.5-mL bottle): $62
Combination product	dorzolamine-timolol	Cosopt	2-0.5% (10-mL bottle): $94

* Average price per 5-mL bottle (unless otherwise indicated) of the dosage strength listed. Actual price may vary. If a generic version is available, the cost is listed in parentheses. Sources: drugstore.com, eckerd.com, walgreens.com.

Surgery

About 10% of people with open-angle glaucoma undergo surgery. They choose surgery because they prefer it or because they experience serious side effects from medications, do not respond adequately to drug treatment, are unable to take their medications properly, or have medical conditions or allergies that do not permit optimal drug therapy. The two most common surgical procedures for open-angle glaucoma are laser trabecular surgery and filtration surgery. While surgery cannot restore lost vision, it can reduce IOP by improving the drainage of aqueous humor. As a result, surgery can halt the progression of optic nerve damage and vision loss.

Laser trabecular surgery. In this procedure, 80 to 100 tiny laser burns are made in the area of the trabecular meshwork. The proce-

How They Work	Comments
These eyedrops decrease the production of aqueous humor.	Lowered pulse rate, low blood pressure, asthma, fainting, drowsiness, confusion, depression, and dry eyes may occur in some people. Beta-blockers usually should not be used by people who have severe lung or heart ailments.
These eyedrops decrease aqueous humor production and increase its drainage.	Associated with the highest rate of allergic reactions. People may also experience red eyes, pain, headaches, eye irritation, high blood pressure, or rapid heart rate. The drops may stain contact lenses (except dipivefrin). Use with caution in people with heart ailments or high blood pressure.
These eyedrops or ointment increase drainage of aqueous humor through the trabecular meshwork by constricting the pupil.	People may experience dim vision (especially at night) or increased nearsightedness. Echothiophate may cause cataracts; in general, it is used only when cataracts have been removed.
These oral drugs (acetazolamide and methazolamide) and eyedrops (brinzolamide and dorzolamide) decrease the production of aqueous humor.	Up to 50% of people taking oral carbonic anhydrase inhibitors have side effects, including tingling of hands and feet, stomach upset, depression, kidney stones, and, more rarely, anemia; thus, these drugs are used only when absolutely necessary to avoid surgery and preserve eyesight. Brinzolamide and dorzolamide eyedrops do not have such side effects.
These eyedrops increase the drainage of aqueous humor from the eye.	A change in eye color is the most noticeable side effect, with about 3% of people experiencing an increase in brown pigmentation. Other side effects include stinging, burning, redness, and foreign body sensation.
See **Carbonic anhydrase inhibitors** and **Beta-blockers**, above	See **Carbonic anhydrase inhibitors** and **Beta-blockers**, above

dure increases the drainage of aqueous humor, most likely by stimulating the metabolic activity of trabecular cells. The procedure takes about 15 minutes and is performed on an outpatient basis using eyedrops for anesthesia. IOP must be measured one hour after surgery because it may rise as a result of the treatment. Postoperative complications are minimal and include eye inflammation, blurred vision, and minimal discomfort, which usually last for about 24 hours.

It takes up to six weeks to determine whether the procedure has been effective. IOP-lowering medication is still required after surgery, but if the procedure reduces IOP considerably, medication sometimes can be taken at a lower dose. As with many treatments, however, the effect of surgery diminishes with time in some people. About 40% of people need additional medication or some other form of surgery within five years.

Filtration surgery. Filtration surgery (trabeculectomy) uses conventional surgical instruments to open a passage through the trabecular meshwork so that aqueous humor can drain into surrounding tissues. The operation takes about 20 minutes, is performed on an outpatient basis under local anesthesia, and is relatively safe and long lasting. In general, a protective eye patch must be worn for one day after the procedure, and patients are advised to avoid driving, bending over, and performing strenuous activity for at least a week. If necessary, the drainage flap created during the surgery can be loosened or tightened later on with a new laser procedure called suture lysis or with the use of special adjustable sutures.

About half of patients are able to discontinue their glaucoma medication after filtration surgery; 35% to 40% still need some medication; and 10% to 15% need additional surgery, such as shunts or cyclodestructive surgery (see below). Filtration surgery is associated with a risk of infection and bleeding in the eye and requires a longer recovery period than laser trabecular surgery. About one third of people develop cataracts within five years of filtration surgery. It is not clear whether the surgery itself causes the cataracts or whether they would have occurred anyway, but the cataracts can be surgically removed when necessary.

Researchers are working to improve the effectiveness of filtration surgery. One of the most promising approaches is the use of antimetabolites (substances that block biological processes) such as mitomycin (Mutamycin) or 5-fluorouracil (Efudex). Both mitomycin and 5-fluorouracil can be applied as a liquid during surgery; 5-fluorouracil can also be injected under the surface of the eye after surgery. These drugs interfere with normal wound healing so that the openings created by the procedure do not close. Currently, these antimetabolites are used in people who have had unsuccessful filtration surgery and in younger individuals who normally have strong wound-healing abilities.

Shunts. If filtration surgery is unsuccessful, one alternative is to drain excess aqueous humor using a shunt made of plastic tubing. The shunt is implanted into the front chamber of the eye, and the aqueous humor drains onto a plate sewn onto the side of the eye. Fluid on the plate is then absorbed by the tissues surrounding the eye. In one study, a shunt called the Baerveldt implant lowered IOP in 72% of people with previously uncontrolled glaucoma.

Cyclodestructive surgery. This form of glaucoma surgery uses a laser to destroy the ciliary body, which produces aqueous humor.

Recovery time depends on the type and extent of surgery. The procedure does not require an incision, so normal activity can be resumed earlier than after filtration surgery. Cyclodestructive surgery is usually used only when other measures have failed.

Treatment of Closed-angle Glaucoma

During an acute attack of closed-angle glaucoma, IOP may be high enough to damage the optic nerve or obstruct one of the blood vessels carrying blood and oxygen to the retina. Unless IOP is lowered promptly, blindness can occur within one or two days. The goals of treatment are to protect the optic nerve and prevent a future attack in the other eye. IOP in the affected eye is lowered with medication followed by surgery, either laser (iridotomy) or conventional (iridectomy). In both cases, surgery involves making a tiny hole in the iris to allow a path for the flow of aqueous humor. Surgery is almost always successful, and repeat treatment is rarely necessary. A preventive iridotomy or iridectomy in the other eye is usually performed because of the high likelihood of a future acute attack in that eye. In some people, a chronic form of closed-angle glaucoma may require filtration surgery or long-term use of eyedrops.

Age-related Macular Degeneration

Age-related macular degeneration (AMD) affects the macula, the central, most sensitive part of the retina. In the United States, AMD is the leading cause of severe and irreversible loss of central vision in people over age 40, affecting 1.7 million Americans, or 1.47% of people in this age group. This number is expected to reach 2.95 million people by 2020. Severe vision loss is commonly defined as a decline in visual acuity to 20/200 or less. People with corrected vision of 20/200 or less in both eyes are considered to be legally blind. (Visual acuity of 20/200 corresponds to seeing only the big "E" on an eye chart.)

The prevalence of severe vision loss from AMD increases with age, and most people with impaired vision from AMD are age 60 or older. Evidence of AMD can be detected in up to one fourth of people over age 65 and one third of those over age 80. About 2% of people age 65 or older are legally blind because of AMD. Fortunately, most cases of AMD do not result in severe vision loss.

NEW RESEARCH

Poor Vision Leads to More Tumbles

Older women with deteriorating vision are more likely to fall and hurt themselves than their peers whose visual acuity remains stable or improves, according to new research. Falls are a common cause of injury and even death among the elderly. Approximately one third of older individuals fall each year, and 7% of those older than 75 years go to the emergency room each year as the result of a fall.

Researchers tested visual acuity in more than 2,000 women, once at the beginning of the study and again an average of 5½ years later. For one year following the second exam, study participants were asked to send in postcards every four months to report any falls.

Overall, 16% of the women reported one fall, and 11% reported two or more. Women with declining vision were more than twice as likely to fall frequently as those whose vision was unchanged or improved. The effect of a decline in visual acuity was most pronounced among women whose vision was relatively poor to begin with.

The findings suggest that elderly people with impaired or declining vision should seek treatment in an effort to reduce the risk of falling.

OPHTHALMOLOGY
Volume 111, page 857
May 2004

ANATOMY OF THE RETINA

The retina is the light-sensitive layer of nerve tissue that lines the inner eye. It is made up of millions of tiny nerve receptor cells called cones and rods. Light rays reflected from an object are focused by the cornea and lens onto the retina; the cones and rods send impulses through the optic nerve to the brain in response to light.

The most sensitive portion of the retina is a small area at its center, called the macula. The macula is about one fiftieth of an inch across and is responsible for central and fine-detail vision. In the middle of the macula is a small indentation, the fovea. It contains the highest concentration of cones (the most sensitive receptors of light) and provides the sharpest vision. When you look directly at an object, the light rays focus onto the fovea.

Central and detailed vision require an intact macula. If function of the macula is lost, the eye must rely on peripheral vision, which is less sensitive than central vision. As a result, activities such as reading normal-sized print are impossible without the use of low-vision aids.

TYPES OF AGE-RELATED
MACULAR DEGENERATION

The two forms of AMD are non-neovascular (also known as nonexudative, atrophic, or dry) AMD and neovascular (also called exudative or wet) AMD.

Non-neovascular AMD. About 90% of people with AMD have the non-neovascular form. Non-neovascular AMD usually is characterized by shrinkage of tissues in the retina and formation of drusen, which are small accumulations of debris underneath the retina. Although this form of AMD cannot be prevented or reversed, the disease progresses slowly and may stabilize for periods of time. In fact, vision is not seriously impaired in many people with non-neovascular AMD.

Neovascular AMD. This is the more serious form of the disorder and is the primary cause of AMD-related vision loss. Loss of vision from neovascular AMD results from either the growth of new blood vessels (neovascularization) in the choroid layer of the eye (the layer between the retina and sclera) or the subsequent detachment of the layer of pigment epithelial cells just beneath the retina. The new blood vessels tend to leak fluid (including lipids, or

How Age-related Macular Degeneration Affects Vision

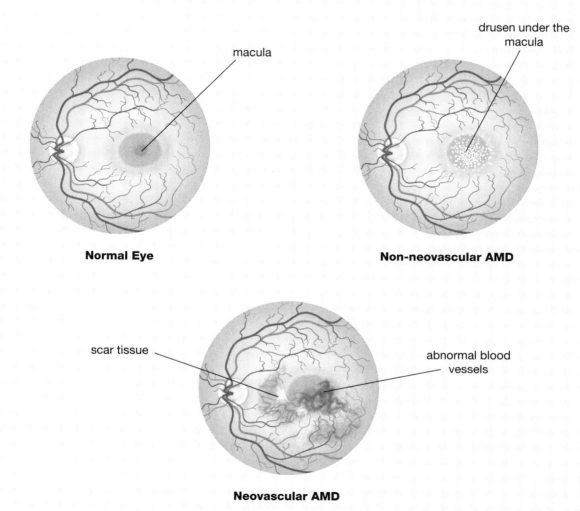

macula

Normal Eye

drusen under the macula

Non-neovascular AMD

scar tissue

abnormal blood vessels

Neovascular AMD

Illustrations: Jacqueline Schaffer

Age-related macular degeneration (AMD) affects the macula, which is the central, most sensitive part of the retina. The macula is responsible for central vision and for seeing details and colors. As the condition progresses, the eye must rely on peripheral vision because central vision is compromised.

There are two types of AMD: dry (non-neovascular) and wet (neovascular). In the non-neovascular form, which makes up about 90% of cases, degeneration of the layer of pigment epithelial cells causes the retina to become thinner, and small yellow deposits (drusen) develop beneath the surface of the retina. Patients with the non-neovascular type usually do not lose vision unless they develop advanced non-neovascular AMD or the neovascular form. In neovascular AMD, abnormal blood vessels develop and may begin bleeding. The body heals these blood vessels, but the remaining scar tissue prevents the macula from functioning properly.

There is no cure for AMD, though only 1% to 2% of people who have it will lose vision from it. The progression of the condition can be arrested in some patients with vitamin and mineral supplements to reduce the risk of neovascularization. If the neovascular form develops, laser surgery may be helpful.

fats) under the retina.

Neovascular AMD may develop at any time in people with non-neovascular AMD. Those with more or larger drusen and more changes in the pigment epithelial layer in the macula have a greater chance of developing the neovascular form. People with neovascular AMD in one eye have up to a 60% chance that the other eye will become similarly affected within five years.

Neovascular AMD is further classified by the location of the new blood vessels and the pattern of fluid leakage. The location of the neovascularization is described in terms of its proximity to the fovea. New vessels most distant from the fovea are termed extrafoveal; those at the fovea itself are called subfoveal; and those in between are named juxtafoveal. The pattern of fluid leakage is described as classic or occult. When examined by fluorescein angiography (see page 36), classic new blood vessels tend to leak more than occult new blood vessels in the early frames of the angiogram, and the extent of the leakage tends to be better delineated with classic than with occult new vessels.

CAUSES OF AGE-RELATED MACULAR DEGENERATION

The causes of both non-neovascular and neovascular AMD are unknown. But increasing age, farsightedness, cigarette smoking, a light-colored iris, and a family history of the disorder are known to increase the risk of both forms. In addition, high blood pressure appears to be associated with a higher risk of neovascular AMD.

A defect in a gene called ABCR may also play a role in AMD. A study found that 16% of people with AMD had a mutation in this gene, compared with only 0.5% of people in the general population without AMD. ABCR directs the production of a protein found in the rods of the retina.

SYMPTOMS OF AGE-RELATED MACULAR DEGENERATION

In most cases, AMD produces no symptoms. When symptoms occur in people with non-neovascular AMD, they develop gradually. In contrast, symptoms can be severe and occur in a matter of days or weeks in people with neovascular AMD. Symptoms of AMD include a grayness, haziness, or blank spot in the area of central vision; words on a page may be blurred; straight lines may appear to have a kink in them; and objects may seem smaller than they are. Alternatively, color vision may become dimmer, since the receptors involved in color discrimination (cones) are most dense in the fovea.

People can monitor themselves for AMD-related vision changes using an Amsler grid, a diagram of a box subdivided into smaller boxes by a series of cross-connecting perpendicular lines. Patients hold the grid at reading distance, fix one eye on its center, and cover the other eye. Minor blurring or wavy or distorted lines may indicate early AMD. More advanced cases of AMD are indicated by gray areas or blind spots around the center of the grid.

The Amsler grid alone, however, is not a reliable indicator of AMD. People are advised to monitor their vision in several ways, such as during reading, while watching television, and by noting the appearance of various objects.

PREVENTION OF AGE-RELATED MACULAR DEGENERATION

Some studies indicate that people can take steps to prevent AMD or slow its progression. These steps include dietary supplements, diet, and, possibly, reduced exposure to sunlight.

The effect of dietary supplements on the risk and progression of AMD was investigated in the Age-Related Eye Disease Study, which included more than 3,500 people (age 55 to 80). For an average of six years, participants took dietary supplements (containing antioxidants, zinc, or antioxidants plus zinc) or a placebo. None of the dietary supplements reduced the risk of developing AMD. But in those with intermediate or advanced AMD, the supplement containing antioxidants plus zinc reduced the risk of more advanced AMD by 25%.

The antioxidant plus zinc supplement used in the study contained 500 mg of vitamin C, 400 IU of vitamin E, 15 mg of beta-carotene, 80 mg of zinc oxide, and 2 mg of cupric oxide. It is is sold under the brand name Ocuvite PreserVision and is available without a prescription. Smokers and people who have recently quit smoking should not use this supplement, because the beta-carotene in it has been found to increase the risk of lung cancer in smokers.

Other studies have suggested that eating fruits and vegetables high in carotenoids, especially those high in beta-carotene (carrots,

NEW RESEARCH

Few Ways To Reduce Risk Of Macular Degeneration

The strongest risk factors for age-related macular degeneration (AMD) are impossible to change: getting older and having a family history of the disease. So what can people do to reduce their risk?

According to a recent review article, although some research indicates that high blood pressure, smoking, and previous cataract surgery all raise the risk of advanced AMD, not all studies have found these links—and it's unclear whether quitting smoking or getting blood pressure under control can prevent AMD. Other suspected risk factors, such as high cholesterol, obesity, and artery disease, have been only weakly associated with the eye disease, the review authors note.

One study, they point out, has demonstrated that supplements containing antioxidants and zinc may cut the risk of blindness for people with intermediate or advanced AMD. Still, with the lack of modifiable risk factors solidly linked to AMD, there remains a large number of people with early AMD for whom "no preventive approaches, as yet, can be recommended."

AMERICAN JOURNAL OF OPHTHALMOLOGY
Volume 137, page 486
March 2004

spinach, and cantaloupes, for example), might help prevent AMD. In addition, avoiding excessive exposure to sunlight has been found to be protective in some studies. In the Beaver Dam Eye Study, people who spent at least five hours a day in the summer engaged in leisure activities outdoors in their teens and 30s had twice the rate of AMD as those who spent fewer than two hours outside each day. In addition, people who wore hats and sunglasses tended to have a lower rate of AMD (see the sidebar on the opposite page).

Based on these findings, it is probably worthwhile to protect the eyes from UV rays (for example, by wearing sunglasses and a wide-brimmed hat when outdoors) and to eat plenty of fruits and vegetables rich in carotenoids. Taking vitamin and mineral supplements will not help prevent AMD in healthy people or protect against the progression of AMD in people with early AMD. But people with intermediate or advanced AMD may benefit from these supplements and should ask their doctor about them.

In addition, some current trials are testing whether low-powered laser treatment can help prevent AMD, while other studies are investigating injections of drugs that prevent new blood vessel growth before it begins.

Other suspected risk factors are high blood pressure, smoking, high cholesterol, obesity, and artery disease, but any association with AMD is likely to be weak.

DIAGNOSIS OF AGE-RELATED MACULAR DEGENERATION

Ophthalmoscopy is used to diagnose non-neovascular AMD. To perform ophthalmoscopy, the doctor dilates the patient's pupils with eyedrops and uses an ophthalmoscope—a special instrument with a light at the end—to magnify and examine the back of the eye. Non-neovascular AMD is diagnosed when the doctor sees drusen or other pigment changes in the macula.

A diagnosis of neovascular AMD is suspected when a person experiences new symptoms and ophthalmoscopy shows leakage of fluid or blood in the area of the macula. The diagnosis is then confirmed by fluorescein angiography. This test must be performed and interpreted promptly because neovascular AMD can progress within days.

Using fluorescein angiography, the doctor examines the blood vessels in the eye. A dye called fluorescein is injected into a vein in the arm. Photographs of the retina are taken with a special camera as the dye circulates through the blood vessels of the eye. The light

NEW RESEARCH

Fruit-Rich Diet May Protect Against Developing AMD

A diet rich in fruits may protect against the development of age-related macular degeneration (AMD), researchers report. This finding adds to previous research suggesting that fruit might reduce the risk of AMD.

The researchers followed more than 77,000 women for up to 18 years, and nearly 41,000 men for up to 12 years, none of whom had signs of AMD. All the participants submitted periodic food consumption questionnaires. By the end of follow-up, a total of 464 cases of early-stage AMD and 316 cases of neovascular AMD (a more severe type of the disease) had been diagnosed.

Fruit intake was inversely proportional to the risk of AMD, particularly neovascular AMD: Participants who consumed three or more servings per day of fruit had a 36% lower risk than those who ate fewer than 1½ servings daily. The results were similar for men and women. No substantial associations were observed between vegetable intake and AMD.

The authors concluded that further studies are needed to confirm their findings and to identify the compounds in fruits that might protect against AMD.

ARCHIVES OF OPHTHALMOLOGY
Volume 122, page 883
June 2004

from the camera flash passes through a blue filter, and the resulting blue light stimulates the fluorescein to emit a yellow-green light. This allows the doctor to view the fluorescein in the blood vessels of the retina and choroid and to see if any fluorescein has leaked from damaged vessels. The procedure is associated with serious risks— death in about 1 in 225,000 people and major complications in 1 in 2,000 people—as well as a small chance of nausea or vomiting. But the test is essential to diagnose neovascular AMD and to identify the sites of neovascularization.

A newer test called indocyanine green angiography, which uses a similar procedure but a different dye, may be employed if fluorescein angiography does not adequately delineate the abnormal vessels. The green dye can sometimes provide a clear image despite such barriers as bleeding or changes in pigmentation.

Some people with cataracts may need to have them removed, since the cataracts can obstruct the view of the back of the eye and interfere with diagnosis or treatment. In some cases, removal of cataracts improves vision in people with AMD.

TREATMENT OF AGE-RELATED MACULAR DEGENERATION

Non-neovascular AMD usually is not treated. Instead, people are monitored for the possible development of neovascular AMD. Based on results from the Age-Related Eye Disease Study, people with intermediate non-neovascular AMD in one or both eyes or advanced non-neovascular AMD in one eye should consider taking supplemental antioxidants and zinc to slow the progression of the disease. These supplements are available commercially in a product called Ocuvite PreserVision.

Neovascular AMD can be treated about 20% of the time with photocoagulation or photodynamic therapy. When these therapies are ineffective or cannot be performed, low-vision aids can help people go about their daily activities despite vision loss in both eyes. Researchers also are working on a number of new drugs and surgical procedures that may one day prove beneficial for people with neovascular AMD.

Photocoagulation

The standard treatment for neovascular AMD in which new blood vessel growth is not located directly under the fovea is coagulation of the blood vessels with a laser, a procedure called photocoagula-

NEW RESEARCH

Too Much Sun May Lead To Macular Degeneration

Extended exposure to strong sunlight may increase the risk of age-related macular degeneration (AMD), according to 10-year results from the Beaver Dam Eye Study.

For a decade, researchers followed nearly 2,800 individuals who lived in a small Wisconsin town. All participants responded to questionnaires designed to gauge sunlight exposure and had their eyes examined.

Those exposed to summer sun for more than five hours a day during their teens, in their 30s, and at the time of the study had double the risk of developing early AMD compared with those exposed for fewer than two hours a day during the same periods.

Wearing hats and sunglasses at least half the time was associated with a decreased risk of developing macular abnormalities (soft indistinct drusen and retinal pigment epithelium depigmentation), but only among people reporting the highest levels of exposure to summer sun. Hat and sunglass use had no effect on the risk of AMD.

The study authors hypothesize that AMD risk may be related to visible light, not ultraviolet light, which would help explain the lack of effect from wearing sunglasses. But UV–blocking sunglasses are still recommended as a possible way to reduce the risk of cataracts.

ARCHIVES OF OPHTHALMOLOGY
Volume 122, page 750
May 2004

tion. The procedure is noninvasive, is performed on an outpatient basis by an ophthalmologist with special training and experience, and takes about 15 to 20 minutes. Before the procedure, the pupil is dilated with eyedrops and anesthetized with drops or an injection. The doctor then aims a high-energy laser beam at the new blood vessels to destroy them.

According to the Macular Photocoagulation Study, photocoagulation decreases the risk of vision loss when well-defined new blood vessels can be identified in extrafoveal, juxtafoveal, or subfoveal sites. For example, in participants with extrafoveal AMD, severe vision loss occurred after 18 months in 60% of untreated eyes but in only 25% of treated eyes. The risk of severe vision loss was also lowered after photocoagulation of juxtafoveal and subfoveal vessels. Although benefits of photocoagulation persisted for five years, they did diminish over time. Recurrence of neovascularization after successful photocoagulation was 10% at one to two months, 24% after six months, and 54% after three years.

Because of this high rate of recurrence of neovascularization after photocoagulation, patients need to be carefully monitored and periodically undergo fluorescein angiography. Immediate reexamination is required if new symptoms of vision loss or distortion are noted. A close watch must be maintained on the other eye as well. Some people use an Amsler grid for self-monitoring, but this method is not particularly reliable.

The major potential complication of photocoagulation is damage to the macula, which can result in a permanent blind spot in the center of the visual field. This complication is most likely in people with neovascularization close to or at the center of the macula.

Photodynamic Therapy

A newer option for treating neovascular AMD is photodynamic therapy, which was approved by the FDA in 2000. The procedure is particularly helpful for people with neovascularization directly under the fovea who cannot undergo photocoagulation because of a high risk of vision loss.

Photodynamic therapy is a two-step procedure performed in a doctor's office. It involves injection of a light-sensitive drug called verteporfin (Visudyne) into the patient's arm. The drug preferentially binds to cells in the new blood vessels. A low-powered laser is then beamed into the eye to activate the drug and produce a toxic, reactive form of oxygen that destroys abnormal tissue, while leaving normal tissue intact. As a result, growth of abnormal vessels is halted

Which AMD Treatment Is Best for You?

Several treatments are available for age-related macular degeneration (AMD). The type of AMD you have (non-neovascular or neovascular)—as well as the location of any leaking blood vessels—will determine which treatment, if any, is most appropriate. The following chart presents the 2004 recommenda- tions from the American Academy of Ophthalmology regarding the most appropriate candidates for vari- ous AMD treatments. Bear in mind that these recom- mendations are only guidelines, and your doctor may make a different treatment decision based on your specific condition.

Treatment Type	Most Appropriate for People With...	Follow-up Care
Observation (no medica- tion or surgery)	• No clinical signs of AMD • Early AMD • Advanced AMD with one of the fol- lowing problems in both eyes: thin- ning of the central retina or residual scar tissue from new blood vessels	• A dilated-eye exam at least once a year • Fundus photography or fluorescein angiog- raphy required only if symptomatic
Antioxidant vitamin and mineral supplements (sold under the brand name Ocuvite PreserVision)	• Intermediate AMD • Advanced AMD in one eye only	• Monitoring of near vision with reading test or the Amsler grid • Eye exam within 6 to 24 months if no symptoms • If new symptoms (such as waviness, dis- tortion, or blurred vision) suggest choroidal neovascularization (CNV; growth of new blood vessels in the layer between the reti- na and sclera), call your doctor promptly • Fundus photography as needed • Fluorescein angiography if there is evi- dence of edema (swelling) or other CNV symptoms
Photocoagulation	• New or recurrent extrafoveal classic CNV (fluid leakage from blood vessels distant from the fovea, the indentation in the center of the macula) • Juxtafoveal classic CNV (leakage from blood vessels closer to the fovea) • May be considered for some types of new or recurrent subfoveal CNV (leak- age at the fovea itself), as well as for juxtapapillary CNV (leakage adjacent to the optic nerve)	• Eye exam with fluorescein angiography 2 to 4 weeks after treatment, then 4 to 6 weeks later, then every three months, depending on results of eye exam • Retreatment if new blood vessels develop • Monitoring of near vision with reading test or the Amsler grid
Photodynamic therapy	• Many patients with predominantly classic new or recurrent subfoveal CNV • Some patients with occult CNV (fluid leakage with different characteristics than classic CNV)	• Fluorescein angiography every 3 months until the patient's exam is no longer chang- ing and the leaking has stopped, with retreatment for recurrent leaking or devel- opment of new vessels • Monitoring of near vision with reading test or the Amsler grid

Source: The American Academy of Ophthalmology.

and vision loss is stabilized with minimal damage to the retina.

In two randomized trials led by researchers at Johns Hopkins, 402 patients with neovascularization received photodynamic therapy and 207 patients received placebo therapy. After two years, 53% of the people in the photodynamic group had no further vision loss, compared with 38% of those in the placebo group. In the third year, further vision loss in the photodynamic group was minimal, particularly in people with predominantly classic neovascularization. Adverse side effects of photodynamic therapy included pain, swelling, hemorrhage, and inflammation at the injection site. Photosensitivity reactions were seen in about 1% of the participants.

Experimental Treatments

Researchers are working on a number of new treatments that may one day help prevent vision loss—or even improve vision—in people with AMD. The most promising medications under investigation are vascular endothelial growth factor (VEGF) inhibitors (including rhuFab V2 and pegatanib [Macugen]) and angiostatic corticosteroids (such as anecortave, triamcinolone, and flucinolone). These treatments may help prevent new blood vessel growth as well as leakage from blood vessels in the eye. Other treatments under investigation are radiation therapy, thermotherapy, and surgery.

New surgical techniques are also being developed. In one procedure called subfoveal surgery, which is being investigated at Johns Hopkins and other medical centers, abnormal new blood vessels are surgically removed from behind the retina. The results so far are promising, although the procedure has led to blindness in some people.

Several years ago, researchers at Johns Hopkins began investigating macular translocation, a surgical technique to move the retina. In people with subfoveal neovascularization, the retina is detached, moved, and reattached so that the subfoveal vessels become extrafoveal, where they then can be treated with photocoagulation without harming central vision. Early results showed improvement in up to one third of patients. However, interest in macular translocation has dwindled since the advent of photodynamic therapy.

Low-Vision Aids

In people with AMD, low-vision aids can help optimize remaining vision and improve the ability to perform daily activities. Some

NEW RESEARCH

Common Drugs Don't Increase Risk of Macular Degeneration

Ophthalmologists have suspected that some commonly used drugs might increase the chances of developing age-related macular degeneration (AMD). Now researchers find that no strong relationship exists between medication use and early AMD, although people who use drugs to lower blood pressure are at slightly increased risk.

Researchers pooled the results of three large studies that included more than 4,600 patients at risk for AMD and who were taking one or more commonly used prescription and over-the-counter medications. Using a special camera, they examined patients' eyes at the beginning of the study and then again five to six years later.

Patients who took blood-pressure–lowering drugs—and particularly beta-blockers—were at slightly increased risk for developing early AMD, but the association was weak. By contrast, women on hormone replacement therapy (HRT) and certain antidepressant drugs appeared to be at decreased risk for AMD.

The authors noted that people taking drugs for high blood pressure may be at increased risk for AMD because they have uncontrolled high blood pressure, not because of the medication. Alternately, the finding could have been by chance. Additional research is needed to explore the effects of common drugs on the development of AMD.

OPHTHALMOLOGY
Volume 111, page 1169
June 2004

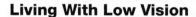

Living With Low Vision

A few small changes can make life easier for someone with vision impairment.

Mild vision impairment has little effect on day-to-day activities, but moderate to severe damage can make it difficult for people to perform common household tasks. Ophthalmologists and low-vision counselors recommend these simple, practical strategies to help visually impaired patients maintain their independence.

Always leave doors completely open or completely closed. This reduces the risk of accidentally walking into the door edge.

Choose a tablecloth that contrasts with the color of your dishes; for example, a dark cloth under white dishes provides enhanced contrast. Similarly, use dark-colored cups or mugs for light liquids and vice versa. This will minimize spilling.

Tack down loose rugs, use nonslip mats beneath them, or use furniture to hold them down to prevent slipping and tripping.

Use a brightly colored sticker or tape a colorful piece of paper to all clear glass doors to help you determine whether the door is open or closed and prevent collisions.

Avoid buying or consider replacing glass-topped coffee or end tables; the edges are extremely difficult to see, making bumping injuries more likely.

Mark the important settings on the dials of the stove, washer, dryer, and other appliances using brightly colored tape.

Mark the outer edge of all indoor and outdoor stairs with a strip of paint or non-skid material in a color that contrasts with the rest of the step. The strip should extend about 2 inches from the edge—both horizontally and vertically—and should go across the full width of the step. This reduces the chances of tripping or falling on the stairs.

When loading knives into the dishwasher or drainboard, be sure to place them sharp-side down.

Examine unidentified objects with the hands before bringing them near the face for a closer view; this will prevent inadvertent poking of the eyes.

Have someone help you arrange clothing if you have color-vision problems. Separate items according to color and then use labeled dividers to identify them.

examples of low-vision aids are telescopes, closed-circuit televisions, magnifying glasses, clocks and phones with large numbers, and large-print reading materials. Telescopes and closed-circuit televisions require an evaluation and prescription from an eye care professional, as well as training in their use. Many low-vision aids are available through low-vision clinics and low vision rehabilitation services. For more tips on living with low vision, see the feature above.

Diabetic Retinopathy

About 18 million Americans have diabetes, a condition characterized by abnormally high levels of glucose (sugar) in the blood. Although no cure exists for diabetes, blood glucose levels can be controlled by carefully following a program of diet, exercise, and (if necessary) medication.

High blood glucose levels can damage small blood vessels in the retina, a condition called diabetic retinopathy. The condition affects more than 4.1 million Americans age 40 and over and is more common in people with poorly controlled diabetes. Nearly 900,000 Americans have diabetic retinopathy severe enough to cause vision loss.

CAUSES OF DIABETIC RETINOPATHY

There are two forms of diabetes: type 1 and type 2. In type 1 diabetes, mild abnormalities in the retina begin to appear an average of seven years after the onset of diabetes; damage that threatens vision usually does not develop until much later, however. In people with type 2 diabetes—the more common type—retinopathy may be present at the time of diagnosis or relatively soon afterward. This is because the onset of type 2 diabetes is gradual, and changes in the retina may have already taken place before diabetes is diagnosed. Almost all people with type 1 diabetes will eventually develop retinopathy, compared with 70% of those with type 2 diabetes. However, people with type 2 diabetes are less likely to develop more advanced retinopathy than people with type 1 diabetes. Currently, an estimated 32% of people age 18 and over diagnosed with type 1 diabetes before the age of 30 have vision-threatening retinopathy.

In the early, or nonproliferative, stages of diabetic retinopathy, blood vessels in the retina develop weak spots that bulge outward (microaneurysms) and may leak fluid and blood into the surrounding retinal tissue. These initial abnormalities usually cause no visual symptoms, and in many people the disease progresses no further.

Macular edema—swelling around the macula caused by the leakage and accumulation of fluid—can occur in people with diabetes. The swelling alters the position of the retina and causes blurred vision. Loss of vision is more pronounced when the center of the macula is affected.

The most dangerous form of diabetic retinopathy is proliferative retinopathy. It is characterized by neovascularization—the growth of small, new blood vessels onto the back surface of the vitreous humor. Acute loss of vision can occur when the new blood vessels rupture and bleed into the vitreous humor or when scar tissue pulls the retina away from the back of the eye (retinal detachment).

Researchers are uncertain exactly how high blood glucose levels lead to diabetic retinopathy, but one possibility is a substance known

How Diabetic Retinopathy Affects Vision

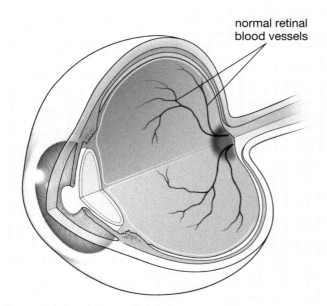

Normal Retina

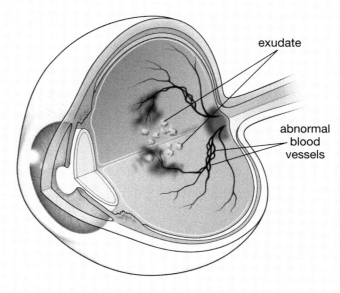

Diabetic Retinopathy

Diabetic retinopathy begins with mild deterioration of the tiny blood vessels that nourish the retina. Portions of the vessels may develop bulges (microaneurysms) that leak blood (hemorrhages) or fluid (exudates) into the surrounding tissue. Generally, vision remains stable during these early, or nonproliferative, changes unless swelling in the macula (the central, most sensitive portion of the retina) develops.

Later on, some individuals may develop the more serious stage, called proliferative retinopathy, in which abnormal blood vessels begin growing on the retina and onto the back surface of the vitreous humor. These fragile vessels are prone to rupture and bleed into the vitreous, causing blurred vision or temporary blindness. Scar tissue may form, pulling the retina away from the back of the eye

(retinal detachment)—a condition that may require treatment to minimize vision loss.

The type of visual damage caused by diabetic retinopathy is highly variable, depending on the location of retinal damage. Possible effects include blurring, distortion, or blind spots. In either stage of the disease, a vision-threatening complication called macular edema—in which fluid accumulates in the macula—may develop.

Because even advanced retinopathy may be asymptomatic, it is essential for people with diabetes to have regular check-ups by an ophthalmologist and to report any vision changes immediately. If detected early enough, the most frequent causes of vision loss—new blood vessel growth, retinal detachment, and macular edema—can be minimized with laser treatment or surgery in many cases.

as vascular endothelial growth factor (VEGF). VEGF promotes the growth of new blood vessels in the eye and is secreted into the eye in response to damage caused by diabetes. Studies also suggest that elevated levels of cholesterol and triglycerides in the blood and high blood pressure can increase the risk of diabetic retinopathy. These conditions are more common in people with diabetes than in the general population.

SYMPTOMS OF DIABETIC RETINOPATHY

The early stages of diabetic retinopathy generally cause no symptoms, so periodic eye exams are necessary to detect the condition. Even proliferative retinopathy does not produce symptoms initially. Symptoms develop only when there is bleeding—the patient sees spots or showers of small spots called floaters, which can be severe enough to block vision entirely. Sudden bleeding into the vitreous humor can also cause rapid vision loss. If blood vessel changes cause macular edema or closure of the small vessels supplying the macula (macular nonperfusion), blurring of vision can occur. In addition, scar tissue on the macula due to proliferative retinopathy can blur vision. Symptoms of retinal detachment include wavy or watery vision, a dark shadow in part of the peripheral field of vision, and sudden blindness in one eye.

PREVENTION OF DIABETIC RETINOPATHY

People with diabetes can take several steps to prevent the development of diabetic retinopathy or slow its progression. These steps include regular eye exams and keeping blood glucose and blood pressure under control.

Two large studies have shown the benefits of controlling blood glucose levels. In the Diabetes Control and Complications Trial, people with type 1 diabetes who gave themselves multiple insulin injections each day reduced their risk of diabetic retinopathy by 76% and their risk of retinopathy progressing by 54%, compared with people who followed a less rigorous treatment regimen. In the United Kingdom Prospective Diabetes Study, people with type 2 diabetes who controlled their blood glucose levels with medication were 30% less likely to have retinopathy that required laser treatment than people who relied on diet and exercise alone. Blood glucose levels are considered well controlled when hemoglobin A1c levels are less than 7%.

Blood pressure reduction also appears to lower the risk and progression of diabetic retinopathy. For example, a recent study found that every 10 mm Hg reduction in systolic blood pressure (the top number) decreased the incidence of retinopathy and other diabetic complications by 12%. Blood pressure reduction may even help people with diabetes who do not have high blood pressure. In a study of people with type 2 diabetes whose blood pressure was below 140/90 mm Hg, lowering blood pressure to about 128/75 mm Hg with medication resulted in less progression of diabetic retinopathy over a five-

NEW RESEARCH

Eye Complication Seen In Many U.S. Diabetics

Researchers estimate that more than 40% of middle-aged and older Americans with diabetes have the potentially vision-threatening eye complication retinopathy.

A review of eight diabetic retinopathy studies, a federal health survey, and Census data suggests that retinopathy affects just over 4 million of the roughly 10 million U.S. adults age 40 and up who have diabetes. Moreover, 1 in every 12 diabetics in this age group may have advanced, vision-threatening retinopathy.

The new findings reveal a high prevalence of diabetic retinopathy in the United States, yet the study authors say the actual number many be higher because it's believed that many people with type 2 diabetes are unaware they have the disease. The researchers estimate that by 2020, as many as 7.2 million Americans age 40 and older will have diabetic retinopathy, and 1.6 million may have a vision-threatening form. Currently, Hispanic and black adults appear to have higher rates than whites of both milder and advanced retinopathy.

Calling diabetic retinopathy a "substantial public health problem," the researchers conclude that more attention needs to be paid to preventing the development and progression of the eye disease.

ARCHIVES OF OPHTHALMOLOGY
Volume 122, page 552
April 2004

year period than that seen in people whose blood pressure was 137/81 mm Hg on average. People with diabetes should keep their blood pressure below 130/80 mm Hg.

Some research also suggests that lowering blood cholesterol levels and quitting smoking may be helpful in preventing the development and progression of diabetic retinopathy.

DIAGNOSIS OF DIABETIC RETINOPATHY

Because diabetic retinopathy often produces no symptoms—even in its advanced stages—and early treatment of advanced retinopathy can usually halt vision loss, people with diabetes need to visit their ophthalmologist regularly. People with type 1 diabetes should begin seeing an ophthalmologist for annual eye exams no later than five years after diabetes is diagnosed. Because significant retinopathy may be present at the time of diagnosis in people with type 2 diabetes, an eye examination by an ophthalmologist is advised at that time and annually thereafter. More frequent exams are needed for people with more advanced retinopathy.

At the exam, the ophthalmologist dilates the pupils with eyedrops and directly views the retina with an ophthalmoscope—a special instrument with a light on the end. The ophthalmologist will look for signs of edema, fluid leakage, new blood vessel growth, bleeding, and other abnormalities. Because the eyedrops cause the eyes to be extremely sensitive to light, people should bring a pair of sunglasses with them and may want to ask someone else to drive them home afterward. Fluorescein angiography (see page 36) is also used to examine the retina for blood vessel changes.

TREATMENT OF DIABETIC RETINOPATHY

Good blood glucose control lessens the risk that retinopathy will progress. Treating other conditions, such as high blood pressure and abnormal cholesterol levels, may also slow progression. In most cases, no treatment is required for nonproliferative retinopathy, though the retina is carefully monitored for the development of macular edema or proliferative retinopathy. These two conditions can be treated with laser photocoagulation or vitrectomy.

Laser photocoagulation. Photocoagulation, which uses lasers to promote closure of new blood vessels, can halt or retard vision loss in most people if performed before too much damage has occurred. In

NEW RESEARCH

Steroid Injections May Aid Diabetic Eye Disease

Laser photocoagulation is the standard treatment for macular edema, but the tactic doesn't work for a significant portion of patients. Now a small study shows that injections of a corticosteroid drug may help treat this condition when standard therapy fails.

The study included 12 patients with macular edema that had failed to improve with laser treatment. A single injection of the drug triamcinolone into the eye reduced thickening in the macula for several months in most patients. There was no significant improvement in their vision, but there was a "trend" toward sharper vision in the treated eyes three months after the injection, according to the authors.

They conclude that triamcinolone injections look like a "promising" treatment for macular edema that fails to respond to standard surgery, although further studies are needed to see whether the therapy actually improves vision and if the rate of side effects is acceptable. Large trials are now under way to see if this is a safe, effective approach.

OPHTHALMOLOGY
Volume 111, page 218
February 2004

Relief for Dry Eye

Dry eye is a common problem in older people, but many treatments are available.

Normally, tears serve to bathe the eye—washing away irritants like dust and keeping the eye lubricated. When the body fails to produce enough tears or produces tears of poor quality, eyes can burn or feel itchy, sticky, irritated, or gritty. This condition is known as dry eye and most commonly occurs in older individuals.

In a study published in the *Archives of Ophthalmology* in 2004, about 13% of the 2,802 participants (age 48 and older) had experienced dry eye over a five-year period. The study also found that dry eye increased with age and was more common in people with diabetes or allergies than in people without these conditions. In addition, the use of diuretics (blood-pressure medications often called water pills) and antihistamines increased the risk of dry eye, while ACE inhibitors (a different type of blood-pressure medication) appeared to decrease the risk.

There is no cure for dry eye, but the symptoms can be relieved effectively in a number of ways.

Low-Tech Relief
Some simple changes in your everyday life may be enough to avoid dry eye.
• Make sure to blink. Blinking helps circulate tears, moisten the eyes, and keep out irritants. Prolonged computer use, in particular, can decrease the number of times an individual blinks.
• Both heat and air conditioning dry the air and irritate the eyes. Try using a humidifier, or even a fish tank, to replace the moisture in the air.
• Wear sunglasses to protect your eyes from the elements, especially when it's windy.
• Avoid direct heat on your eyes; for example, carefully point a hairdryer to avoid the eyes.

Over-the-Counter Products
A number of over-the-counter tear substitutes are available to soothe irritated eyes. Known as artificial tears or rewetting drops, these products lubricate the surface of the eye, essentially functioning as tears. Some directly mimic tears, while others contain less salt than tears. Ask your ophthalmologist which kind is most appropriate. (For example, if burning is your main symptom, those with less salt may provide the most comfort.)

Be aware that drops come with and without preservatives. Those without preservatives are easiest on the eye because they contain fewer chemicals. They may be best if your problem is more severe and you need to use drops several times an hour. However, they are only available in single-use containers and are more expensive than drops with preservatives.

You should not use products advertised to "get the red out" to relieve dry eye. These decongestant drugs constrict blood vessels and can actually worsen the problem. If your eyes are red because of dryness, the redness should clear up with appropriate use of artificial tears. Moreover, decongestant drops should not be used by people with glaucoma unless specifically approved by their ophthalmologist.

Other Options
Most cases of dry eye can be painlessly managed with artificial tears and daily precautions. But when symptoms persist, other options are available. Thicker lubricating ointments that stay in the eyes longer than drops may be applied at night to rewet the eyes. Another approach is to have the doctor close off the tear-drainage system in at least one eye, either temporarily with collagen plugs or more permanently with silicone plugs or surgery. Closing off a tear duct will force what tears are produced to stay longer in the eye. For patients with severe dry eye syndromes, the use of anti-inflammatory drugs administered as eyedrops may be helpful.

people with macular edema, focal laser photocoagulation is performed to target individual blood vessels. Panretinal photocoagulation, which creates a grid-like pattern across a larger area of the retina, is used to treat proliferative retinopathy.

Panretinal photocoagulation causes new blood vessels to regress and reduces by half the risk of blindness in people with proliferative retinopathy. Focal laser photocoagulation improves vision in only about 10% of people with macular edema. But even when vision does not improve, the risk of further deterioration is halved. Although complications are rare, vision loss can result from both types of laser photocoagulation.

Vitrectomy. If the extent or location of the damage makes photocoagulation ineffective, or if the vitreous humor is too clouded with blood, vision may be improved or stabilized with vitrectomy, a surgical procedure that removes the vitreous humor and replaces it with saline solution. Photocoagulation can also be carried out during vitrectomy with a special laser that is inserted into the eye. About 70% of those who undergo vitrectomy notice improvement or stabilization of their vision, and some recover enough vision to resume reading and driving.

Experimental treatments. Several new treatments are being tested for diabetic retinopathy, including VEGF inhibitors and angiostatic corticosteroids. Because VEGF promotes the growth of new blood vessels in the eye, and leakage from these and other vessels can lead to vision loss in people with diabetic retinopathy, researchers have developed agents that inhibit (block) the activity of VEGF. Two VEGF inhibitors—rhuFab V2 and pegaptanib (Macugen)—are currently being studied in people with diabetic retinopathy.

Corticosteroids are generally prescribed to relieve pain and inflammation, but anecortave, triamcinolone, and flucinolone are corticosteroids that can also prevent new blood vessel growth and leakage from blood vessels in the eye. Researchers hypothesize that these drugs block the growth and migration of cells required for the formation of new blood vessels and prevent leakage by maintaining tight spaces between the cells that line blood vessel walls. Like VEGF inhibitors, angiostatic corticosteroids are investigational therapies and are not approved by the FDA. ■

GLOSSARY

A-scan ultrasonography—A test that uses sound waves to measure the length of the eyeball.

adrenergic agonist eyedrops—A treatment for glaucoma. The eyedrops reduce intraocular pressure by decreasing the production of aqueous humor and increasing its drainage through the uveoscleral pathway.

age-related macular degeneration—A loss of central vision caused by changes in the macula. Commonly abbreviated as AMD.

aqueous humor—A watery fluid that is located in front of the lens and provides nutrients to the lens and cornea.

B-scan ultrasonography—A test that uses sound waves to view structures in the back of the eye.

beta-blocker eyedrops—A treatment for glaucoma. The eyedrops reduce intraocular pressure by decreasing the production of aqueous humor.

bifocals—A pair of glasses with lenses that correct both distant and near vision.

carbonic anhydrase inhibitors—Medications used to treat glaucoma that decrease the production of aqueous humor. Available in both oral and eyedrop forms.

cataract—A cloudiness or opacification of the lens that can lead to visual impairment.

central vision—The middle part of the visual field.

choroid—A layer of the eye inside the sclera. Contains a dark pigment that minimizes scattering of light inside the eye.

ciliary body—A part of the eye that surrounds the lens and produces aqueous humor.

classic AMD—One of two types of neovascular AMD, classified based on fluid leakage patterns during an angiogram. Existing therapies are effective only in classic AMD, although it is the less common type.

closed-angle glaucoma—A type of glaucoma caused by a blockage near the iris that prevents aqueous humor from reaching the trabecular meshwork. It results in a rapid buildup of extremely high intraocular pressure that can lead to severe, permanent vision damage within a day or two.

cones—Nerve cells in the retina that are activated only in bright light and by the colors red, blue, or green.

conjunctiva—A thin, lubricating mucous membrane that covers the sclera and lines the inside of the eyelid.

cornea—The transparent, dome-shaped disk covering the iris and pupil.

coronary heart disease—Abnormality of the arteries that supply blood and oxygen to the heart. Can lead to chest pain or a heart attack.

cortical cataract—A cataract affecting the lens cortex.

cyclodestructive surgery—A treatment for glaucoma that destroys the ciliary body with a laser.

cystoid macular edema—A specific pattern of swelling of the central retina.

diabetes—A disease characterized by abnormally high glucose (sugar) levels in the blood.

diabetic retinopathy—Damage to small blood vessels in the retina resulting from chronic high blood glucose levels; more common in people with poorly controlled diabetes.

drusen—Small accumulations of debris underneath the retina.

endophthalmitis—An infection of the vitreous humor that develops in a small number of people after cataract surgery and other kinds of eye surgery.

extracapsular surgery—Cataract surgery that removes the front of the lens capsule along with the cortex and nucleus of the lens, while leaving the back of the lens capsule intact.

filtration surgery—A treatment for glaucoma that uses conventional surgical instruments to open a passage through the clogged trabecular meshwork, so that excess aqueous humor can drain into surrounding tissues.

floaters—Black spots or shapes that drift through the field of vision.

fluorescein angiography—A diagnostic procedure for age-related macular degeneration and other retinal diseases. A special dye, called fluorescein, is injected into a vein in the arm. Photographs of the retina are taken as the dye circulates through the blood vessels of the eye.

fovea—The small indentation at the center of the macula. Contains the highest concentration of cones and provides the sharpest vision.

glare—Light within the field of vision that is brighter than other objects to which the eyes are adapted.

glaucoma—An eye disease that results in damage to the optic nerve. Not always caused by elevated intraocular pressure.

gonioscopy—A technique used to distinguish between open- and closed-angle glaucoma. It involves an examination of the front part of the eye to check the angle where the iris meets the cornea.

hemorrhage—Leakage of blood from blood vessels.

hyperopia—Farsightedness.

intracapsular surgery—Cataract surgery that removes the entire lens (the front and back of the lens capsule, the cortex, and nucleus). The procedure is rarely performed today.

intraocular lens implant—A plastic lens that replaces the lens removed during cataract surgery.

intraocular pressure (IOP)—The pressure exerted by the fluids inside the eyeball.

iridectomy—A treatment for closed-angle glaucoma that involves removal of part of the iris.

iridotomy—A treatment for closed-angle glaucoma that creates a hole in the iris with a laser.

iris—The colored circle in the middle of the eye that controls the amount of light that enters the eye.

laser trabecular surgery—A treatment for glaucoma that involves making 80 to 100 tiny laser burns in the area of the trabecular meshwork. The procedure increases the drainage of aqueous humor.

legal blindness—Vision that is 20/200 or worse in both eyes. (20/200 vision is the ability to see at 20 feet what a normal eye can see at 200 feet.)

lens—A transparent, dome-shaped disk that is responsible (along with the cornea) for the eye's ability to focus light.

lens capsule—The outermost structure of the lens.

lens cortex—The second innermost structure of the lens. It surrounds the nucleus, and its outer edge is lined with a layer of cells called the epithelium.

lens epithelium—Cells that line the outer surface of the lens cortex.

lens nucleus—The center structure of the lens. It is surrounded by the cortex.

macula—A small area at the center of the retina that is responsible for central and fine-detail vision.

macular edema—A swelling of the macula caused by leakage and accumulation of fluid. It is more common in people with diabetes than in the general population.

macular nonperfusion—Closure of small blood vessels supplying the macula.

microaneurysms—Weak spots that bulge outward from blood vessels, including those of the retina.

miotic eyedrops—Used to treat glaucoma. Increase the outflow of aqueous humor through the trabecular meshwork by constricting the pupil.

myopia—Nearsightedness.

neovascular age-related macular degeneration—A form of age-related macular degeneration in which new blood vessels grow in the choroid layer of the eye.

neovascularization—The growth of new blood vessels.

non-neovascular age-related macular degeneration—A form of age-related macular degeneration characterized by the breakdown or thinning of tissues in the macula. It is characterized by the formation of drusen and shrinkage of tissues in the retina and often does not impair vision.

normal tension glaucoma—Damage to the optic nerve despite normal intraocular pressure.

nuclear cataract—A cataract affecting the nucleus of the lens.

occult AMD—One of two types of neovascular AMD, classified based on fluid leakage patterns during an angiogram. Occult AMD is more common and more difficult to treat.

opacification—The process of becoming impenetrable to light.

open-angle glaucoma—The most common form of glaucoma. It usually produces no obvious symptoms until its late stages.

ophthalmologist—Physician who specializes in the diagnosis and treatment of eye diseases.

ophthalmoscopy—Examination of the interior structures of the eye, especially the retina, using a specialized instrument.

optic nerve—A nerve at the back of the eye. It carries visual information from the retina to the brain.

perimetry—A test used to determine a person's visual fields. While the person looks straight ahead at a bowl-shaped white area, a computer presents lights in fixed locations around the bowl. The patient indicates each time he or she sees the light.

peripheral vision—The ability to see objects at the edges of the visual field.

phacoemulsification—A type of extracapsular surgery that is performed with an ultrasonic device, which nearly liquefies the nucleus and cortex so that they can be removed by suction through a tube.

photocoagulation—The standard treatment for neovascular age-related macular degeneration when the new blood vessels are outside the center of the retina. The procedure involves closing the new blood vessels with a laser.

photodynamic therapy—A newer treatment for age-related macular degeneration that involves the intravenous administration of a special drug to sensitize blood vessels in the eye to light. A low-power laser, directed at the new blood vessels, activates the drug and closes the vessels in a way that causes less damage to the retina than standard laser treatment.

GLOSSARY—continued

posterior subcapsular cataract—A cataract in the rear of the lens capsule.

presbyopia—An inability to focus on near objects.

pupil—The opening in the center of the iris that resembles a large black dot.

retina—The innermost layer of the eye that consists of light-sensitive nerve tissue.

retinal detachment—A vision-threatening condition in which the retina becomes separated from the underlying layers of the eye.

rods—Nerve cells in the retina that are sensitive to dim light.

rubeosis iridis—New blood vessel growth on the iris. It usually occurs in people with diabetes.

sclera—The white outer layer that covers and protects most of the eye.

scotoma—A blind spot in the visual field.

shunt—Used in the treatment of glaucoma when filtration surgery is unsuccessful. A shunt creates a new passage to drain excess aqueous humor.

subfoveal surgery—A procedure for age-related macular degeneration in which abnormal blood vessels beneath the retina are surgically removed.

tonometry—A method of measuring intraocular pressure by determining the amount of force needed to make a slight indentation in a small area of the cornea.

topical prostaglandin eyedrops—A treatment for glaucoma. The eyedrops reduce intraocular pressure by increasing the outflow of aqueous humor through the uveoscleral pathway.

trabecular meshwork—A spongy network of connective tissue through which aqueous humor drains from the eye. Blockage of the meshwork causes a buildup of intraocular pressure.

uveitis—Inflammation of the uvea, the part of the eye that contains the iris, ciliary body, and choroid.

uveoscleral pathway—An alternative drainage system for aqueous humor. It is located behind the trabecular meshwork.

vitrectomy—A surgical procedure that removes the vitreous humor and replaces it with saline solution.

vitreous humor—A thick, gel-like substance that fills the back of the eyeball behind the lens.

YAG laser—A type of laser that contains yttrium, aluminum, and garnet. It is used to clear blurred vision that may occur after extracapsular surgery for cataracts.

HEALTH INFORMATION ORGANIZATIONS AND SUPPORT GROUPS

American Academy of Ophthalmology
P.O. Box 7424
San Francisco, CA 94120-7424
☎ 415-561-8500
www.aao.org
Largest association of ophthalmologists in the United States, with more than 27,000 members. For information on a variety of eye-related diseases and their prevention and treatment, describe your ailment(s) and send a self-addressed, stamped business envelope.

American Council of the Blind
1155 15th St. NW, Ste. 1004
Washington, DC 20005
☎ 800-424-8666/202-467-5081
www.acb.org
National information clearinghouse that also offers group insurance plans and other services.

American Optometric Association
243 North Lindbergh Blvd.
St. Louis, MO 63141
☎ 314-991-4100
www.aoanet.org
A professional group of doctors of optometry that lobbies the government and other organizations on behalf of the optometric profession, provides research and education leadership, and sets professional standards, helping its members conduct patient care efficiently and effectively.

Association for Macular Diseases, Inc.
210 East 64th St.
New York, NY 10021
☎ 212-605-3719
www.macula.org/association/about.html
Not-for-profit corporation devoted solely to macular disease. Membership includes a support group and a newsletter devoted to medical advances, new developments in low vision aids, and advice on coping strategies.

The Foundation Fighting Blindness
11435 Cronhill Dr.
Owings Mills, MD 21117-2220
☎ 800-683-5555
   800-683-5551(TDD)
www.blindness.org
Supports research and provides education about retinal degeneration. Publishes a newsletter titled *Fighting Blindness News*.

Glaucoma Research Foundation
490 Post St., Ste. 1427
San Francisco, CA 94102
☎ 800-826-6693/415-986-3162
www.glaucoma.org
National nonprofit organization committed to protecting the sight of people with glaucoma through research and education. Call the toll-free number for free publications.

Lighthouse International
111 E. 59th St.
New York, NY 10022
☎ 800-829-0500/212-821-9200
www.lighthouse.org
National nonprofit vision rehabilitation organization that conducts research and offers educational opportunities and direct services for people with vision loss.

National Association for the Visually Handicapped
22 W. 21st St., 6th Fl.
New York, NY 10010
☎ 212-889-3141
www.navh.org
Volunteer health agency dedicated to serving the partially seeing. Publishes a quarterly large-print newsletter, medical updates, and other publications. Services include sale and/or referral of currently available vision aids and an extensive free-by-mail library of large-print books.

National Eye Institute Information Office
31 Center Dr., 31/6A32
Bethesda, MD 20892-2510
☎ 800-869-2020 (for publications)
   301-496-5248 (public inquiry)
www.nei.nih.gov
Part of the National Institutes of Health. Provides information packets on a variety of eye ailments and answers inquiries over the phone. Supports more than 75% of the vision research conducted in the United States.

Prevent Blindness America
500 E. Remington Rd.
Schaumburg, IL 60173
☎ 800-331-2020
www.preventblindness.org
Provides public and professional education, vision screenings, community programs, toll-free hotline, and research.

Vision Foundation
23A Elm St.
Watertown, MA 02472
☎ 617-926-4232
Provides peer support, information, resources, and specialized rehabilitation instruction for people losing their sight.

Vision World Wide, Inc.
5707 Brockton Dr., Ste. 302
Indianapolis, IN 46220-5481
☎ 800-431-1739/317-254-1332
www.visionww.org
Provides publications in large print, on audiocassette, on computer disk, or in electronic format (PDF or ASCII text). Call the toll-free number for information and referral services.

LEADING HOSPITALS FOR OPHTHALMOLOGY

U.S. News & World Report and the National Opinion Research Center, a social-science research group at the University of Chicago, recently conducted their 15th annual nationwide survey of 8,160 board-certified physicians in 17 medical specialties. The doctors nominated the hospitals that they considered to be the best from among 6,012 U.S. medical centers. This is the current list of the best hospitals for ophthalmology, as determined by doctors' recommendations from 2002, 2003, and 2004. However, because the results reflect the doctors' opinions, they are subjective. Any institution listed is considered a leading center, and the rankings do not imply that other hospitals cannot or do not deliver excellent care.

1. **University of Miami
   (Bascom Palmer Eye Institute)**
   Miami, FL
   ☎ 305-243-2020
   www.bpei.med.miami.edu

2. **Johns Hopkins Hospital
   (Wilmer Eye Institute)**
   Baltimore, MD
   ☎ 410-955-5080
   www.wilmer.jhu.edu

3. **Wills Eye Hospital**
   Philadelphia, PA
   ☎ 215-928-3000
   www.willseye.org

4. **Massachusetts Eye and
   Ear Infirmary**
   Boston, MA
   ☎ 617-573-5520
   www.meei.harvard.edu

5. **University of California, Los
   Angeles, Medical Center
   (Jules Stein Eye Institute)**
   Los Angeles, CA
   ☎ 310-825-5000
   www.jsei.org

6. **University of Iowa
   Hospitals and Clinics**
   Iowa City, IA
   ☎ 800-777-8442/319-384-8442
   www.uihealthcare.com/
   uihospitalsandclinics

7. **University of Southern California
   University Hospital
   (Doheny Eye Institute)**
   Los Angeles, CA
   ☎ 323-442-6335
   www.usc.edu/hsc/doheny

8. **Duke University
   Medical Center**
   Durham, NC
   ☎ 919-684-8111
   www.mc.duke.edu

9. **Barnes-Jewish Hospital**
   St. Louis, MO
   ☎ 314-747-3000
   www.barnesjewish.org

10. **Mayo Clinic**
    Rochester, MN
    ☎ 507-284-2511
    www.mayoclinic.org

Source: *U.S. News & World Report,* July 12, 2004.

LASER SURGERY FOR NEAR- AND FARSIGHTEDNESS

Surgery in which lasers reshape the cornea has become a relatively safe, effective way to improve vision permanently for many people with near- and far-sightedness. In 2003, 1.1 million excimer laser vision surgeries were performed in the United States. In this article reprinted from *The New England Journal of Medicine*, Steven A. Wilson, M.D., of the Cole Eye Institute at the Cleveland Clinic Foundation in Ohio, reviews the risks and benefits of the two main types of laser surgery used in vision correction.

Photorefractive keratectomy (PRK), the first procedure developed, involves removing the outermost layer (or "epithelium") of the cornea. The surface below the epithelium, called the stroma, is then reshaped with an excimer laser. Vision improves as the stroma heals. Laser-assisted in situ keratomileusis (LASIK) surgery, now the most widely used, involves elevating a tiny flap of epithelial stromal tissue. The flap is pulled to the side as the deeper cornea is reshaped with an excimer laser; then the flap is put back in place. LASIK produces less discomfort and faster healing than PRK, but complications related to the flap surgery can occur.

The better a person's vision to begin with, the better chance he or she has of achieving better eyesight after LASIK or PRK, Dr. Wilson notes. For example, a person with 2 diopters of myopia has a 70% to 80% chance of achieving 20/20 vision and a 98% chance of at least 20/40. (A diopter is a measure of the refractive power of a corrective lens. The higher the diopter, the more correction a person needs.) A person with 9 diopters of myopia has a 95% to 98% chance of 20/40 vision after laser surgery, but a 40% to 55% likelihood of 20/20 vision. In the United States, 20/40 vision is the degree of visual acuity most commonly required for driving.

From 5% to 20% of patients will need a second surgery to achieve the best possible results, according to Dr. Wilson. Among people with myopia up to 6 diopters or hyperopia, or farsightedness, up to 2 diopters, the results of PRK and LASIK are virtually identical. For people with worse vision, LASIK tends to have somewhat better results.

Complications, such as seeing haloes around objects and double vision, are more common among people with worse eyesight—in particular, those with myopia above 7 to 8 diopters or hyperopia above 2 to 3 diopters. Some patients with good vision after LASIK as measured with a vision chart may still have troublesome symptoms such as glare, trouble with night driving, or dry eye.

Complications with LASIK are less likely when an experienced surgeon performs the procedure, Dr. Wilson notes. People who should not have laser vision correction include those younger than 21, people with immune-related disorders such as lupus or rheumatoid arthritis that can interfere with healing, and people with moderate to severe dry eye. The surgery also should not be performed during pregnancy or while a woman is lactating.

CLINICAL PRACTICE

Use of Lasers for Vision Correction of Nearsightedness and Farsightedness

Steven E. Wilson, M.D.

This Journal *feature begins with a case vignette highlighting a common clinical problem. Evidence supporting various strategies is then presented, followed by a review of formal guidelines, when they exist. The article ends with the author's clinical recommendations.*

A 32-year-old woman with moderate myopia and mild dry eye has worn soft contact lenses for 12 years. She notes decreased tolerance of the lenses and must remove them after only four to five hours. On examination, her refraction is −4.25 + 1.0 × 90 (−3.75 diopters of spherical equivalent and 1 diopter of astigmatism at 90 degrees) in the right eye and −3.5 + 0.5 × 88 in the left eye, yielding a best corrected visual acuity of 20/20 in each eye. She asks about refractive surgery. What would you advise?

THE CLINICAL PROBLEM

From Cole Eye Institute, the Cleveland Clinic Foundation, Cleveland. Address reprint requests to Dr. Wilson at Cole Eye Institute, the Cleveland Clinic Foundation, 9500 Euclid Ave., Cleveland, OH 44195

N Engl J Med 2004;351:470-5.

Vision correction for myopia (nearsightedness) with the use of an excimer laser was approved by the Food and Drug Administration in 1995. It is estimated that more than 1.1 million such procedures were performed in 2003 in the United States.

The first procedure performed for the correction of myopia was a form of ablation of the stromal surface, termed photorefractive keratectomy (PRK), in which the epithelium is removed from the center of the cornea, and excimer laser correction is applied to the stromal surface (Fig. 1).[1] Visual function improves as the epithelial defect heals. PRK has proven to be very effective, with a good ratio of risk to benefit.[2] Delayed recovery of vision after PRK and transient discomfort in some patients, as well as the development of visually significant opacity of the corneal stroma (referred to as haze) in a small percentage of cases, led to the development of laser-assisted in situ keratomileusis (LASIK) in the mid 1990s.[3]

The LASIK procedure (Fig. 1) is performed with an instrument called a microkeratome or, more recently, with a femtosecond laser and involves forming an epithelial–stromal flap that is attached to the periphery of the cornea by a hinge of uncut tissue. The flap is typically 8 to 10 mm in diameter and 100 to 180 μm in thickness (approximately 15 to 35 percent of the total corneal thickness), but microkeratomes deviate 20 to 30 μm, so flap thickness varies substantially from eye to eye. The flap is lifted, and the high-energy pulses of the excimer laser are applied to the underlying stromal bed so that the ablated cornea overlies the pupil. The flap is then returned to its original position, without the need for sutures. The greater comfort and faster rate of recovery of vision with LASIK than with PRK led to nearly total abandonment of PRK by many refractive surgeons during the late 1990s.

In an attempt to improve on PRK, another method of surface ablation, called laser-assisted subepithelial keratomileusis (LASEK), has been developed.[4] In LASEK, an epithelial flap, attached to the cornea by an uncut hinge at the periphery of the epithelium, is formed with a trephine after brief exposure of the area to 10 to 20 percent ethanol (Fig. 1). The epithelial flap is lifted, and excimer laser ablation is applied to the surface of the stroma (as in PRK). Then the epithelial flap is replaced. Proponents of LASEK have claimed that there may be faster recovery of vision, less pain, and a decreased tendency for haze than with PRK. Since there are no definitive studies of the outcomes of LASEK, this article focuses on LASIK and PRK, with PRK including LASEK.

STRATEGIES AND EVIDENCE

BENEFITS OF PRK AND LASIK

In the hands of an experienced and competent surgeon, the vast majority of patients who undergo PRK or LASIK have an improvement in uncorrected visual acuity.[5-7] The odds of attaining a desired level of uncorrected visual acuity are inversely related to the baseline level of correction. For example, in an eye with 2 diopters of myopia, the likelihood of attaining uncorrected visual acuity of 20/20 is 70 to 80 percent, and the likelihood of achieving 20/40 or better (the visual acuity, with or without corrective lenses, most often required to drive a motor vehicle in the United States and the United Kingdom) is greater than 98 percent. In contrast, in an eye with 9 diopters of myopia, the likelihood of achieving visual acuity of 20/20 is on the order of 40 to 55 percent, and the likelihood of achieving 20/40 is 95 to 98 percent.[5-7] Substantial improvement over preoperative uncorrected vision is achieved in most eyes after PRK or LASIK, even if a visual acuity of 20/40 is not achieved.[6]

Depending on the surgeon and the initial level of attempted correction, approximately 5 to 20 percent of eyes will need a reoperation with additional laser ablation (commonly referred to as an enhancement) to achieve the best possible results.[8] The results for visual acuity are almost identical with PRK and with LASIK for low-to-moderate myopia (up to approximately 6 diopters) and low hyperopia, or farsightedness (less than 2 diopters).[5] Observational studies show that LASIK performed for myopia or hyperopia above these levels is more likely to yield uncorrected visual acuity of 20/20 or 20/40 than is PRK, because the results of PRK have a greater tendency for regression (the loss of the effect of surgery over time).[6]

In most eyes, corrections of visual acuity with PRK or LASIK are relatively stable over time, and few patients return after one year with a drop in uncorrected visual acuity. In my experience, late refractive instability occurs in less than 0.2 percent of patients. Such a decline is usually due to further lengthening of the eye that is independent of refractive surgery. If the healing epithelium becomes thicker than normal (epithelial hyperplasia) in the early postoperative period, then greater correction, or even mild overcorrection, may occur during the months or years after surgery.

RISKS

There are several complications that can occur with PRK and LASIK.[5-7,9] These include visual disturbances (Fig. 2) such as starbursts, halos, distorted images, and multiple images that are most common at night. These aberrations are more likely to occur with excimer laser ablations that are decentered relative to the pupil, and with corrections that are greater than 7 to 8 diopters of myopia or 2 to 3 diopters of hyperopia. In particular, levels of myopia greater than approximately 10 diopters or of hyperopia greater than approximately 4 diopters are associated with a marked increase in visual complications. The occurrence of such complications has been reduced with improvements in laser technology, such as the development of tracking devices that monitor and adjust for eye movements during ablation, and with better screening of patients to rule out corneal topographic abnormalities, corrections that are too high, or other ocular conditions that increase the chances of diminished vision. Although the incidence of these complications has not been well defined prospectively, retrospective studies have suggested an incidence of less than 1 percent among patients who are considered good candidates for surgery. Other complications, such as infection and ectasia (progressive thinning and irregularity of the cornea), occur at rates much lower than 1 percent.

Physicians and patients should consider procedure-specific complications when deciding between approaches. Complications with LASIK that cannot occur after PRK, since there is no flap in the latter,[5-9] include free caps (severed flap hinges), short flaps (incomplete flaps that must be recut later), flap striae (wrinkles that may cause irregular astigmatism), and diffuse lamellar keratitis (inflammation in the stromal interface beneath the flap). The risk of loss of two or more lines of best corrected visual acuity on a Snellen chart is 1 to 2 percent greater with LASIK than with PRK, owing primarily to flap complications. LASIK also may induce transient dry eye, a condition related to the neurotrophic effects of cutting the nerves during flap formation. This condition typically resolves six to nine months after LASIK, when the nerves grow back into the flap.

Haze in the anterior stroma that is related to

REPRINT

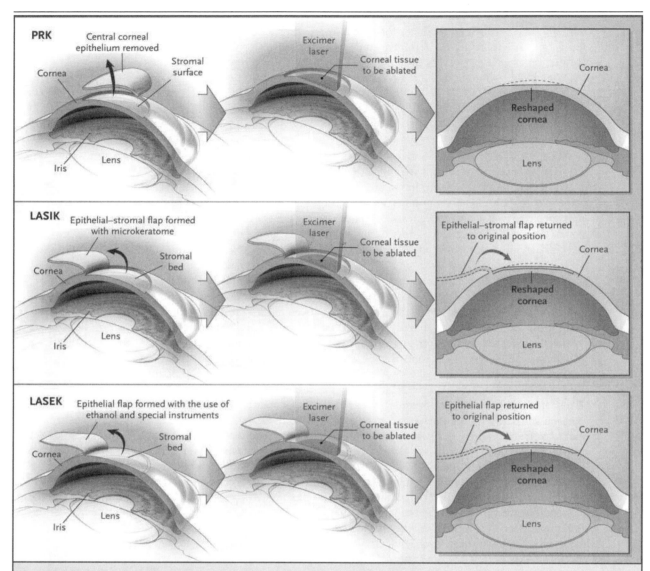

Figure 1. Differences among the PRK, LASIK, and LASEK Procedures.

In PRK (top panel), the central corneal epithelium is removed and stromal tissue is removed from the stromal surface with an excimer laser. The epithelium heals in three to seven days. In LASIK (middle panel), an epithelial–stromal flap is formed with a microkeratome, and a portion of the stromal bed is removed with an excimer laser. In LASEK (bottom panel), an epithelial flap is formed with the use of dilute ethanol and special instruments, and stromal tissue is removed from the stromal bed with an excimer laser. The surgeon hopes to retain the epithelium in LASEK, but in some cases it is lost, and then the procedure is similar to PRK.

wound healing is very rare after LASIK but occurs in 1 to 2 percent of eyes that have been treated with PRK for more than 6 diopters of myopia.[6,7,9] Other advantages of LASIK over PRK include better comfort and vision in the first few days after surgery.

Complications with LASEK tend to be similar to those with PRK, although delayed healing of the epithelium may be more common with LASEK.[4]

Observational data are inconsistent with regard to whether recovery of vision is faster, pain is less, or haze is less with LASEK than with PRK for similar levels of myopia or hyperopia.

The rates of complications with LASIK seem to be lower for more experienced surgeons than for those who are less experienced.[10] Limited training beyond a residency in ophthalmology is required to

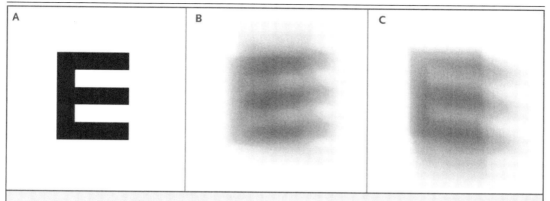

Figure 2. Rare Optical Imperfections after LASIK Procedures.

Panel A shows the letter E as viewed by an eye with few consequential aberrations (optical imperfections) after a LASIK procedure. Panel B shows the letter E as viewed by an eye with severe aberrations after a LASIK procedure. Before the procedure, the eye had serious abnormalities of the corneal topography. This level of distortion is very rare. Panel C shows the letter E as viewed by an eye with a higher order aberration called coma (because items appear to have a tail like that of a comet) after a complicated LASIK procedure. The vision in an eye with this level of coma would probably have substantial starbursts, in which a point of light appears diffuse, with rays extending from the point.

perform LASIK or PRK. An ophthalmologist can perform these procedures after completing approximately two days of training with the specific laser and microkeratome and having a more experienced surgeon serve as proctor during the first few procedures. However, some residents complete one-year or two-year fellowships that focus on refractive surgery.

PREOPERATIVE SCREENING

Preoperative screening is critical to maximize the likelihood of a good outcome of laser surgery for vision correction. A comprehensive eye examination that includes slit-lamp biomicroscopy and a funduscopic examination should be performed in all candidates. In general, patients should have normal, healthy eyes.

Surgery is typically performed only in patients over 21 years of age, owing to concern about ongoing changes in refractive error. Regardless of the patient's age, the refraction should have been relatively stable during the previous one to two years. This may be difficult to verify, and often physicians must rely on the patient's history. There is no upper age limit for the patient who plans to undergo surgery, if the eye is normal aside from refractive error.

Contraindications to laser surgery include systemic diseases such as rheumatoid arthritis, systemic lupus erythematosus, and other active immune-related disorders that may be associated with

healing abnormalities or complications such as corneal melting, which leads to corneal thinning and even perforation. Pregnancy and lactation are contraindications, owing to temporary changes in refraction. Patients with moderate-to-severe dry eye are not considered to be good candidates for LASIK or PRK. Schirmer's test for tear production, in conjunction with slit-lamp biomicroscopy and the history, may be helpful in evaluating patients who have signs or symptoms of dry eye.

Corneal thickness is measured with an ultrasonic pachymeter. The normal thickness of the cornea ranges from 490 to 650 μm.[8] The minimal corneal thickness that is adequate depends on the level of intended correction and the procedure that is planned. The corneal thickness should be considered when deciding whether LASIK, PRK, or no surgery is the best choice in a particular eye. In some cases, LASIK is not a good option, even when the corneal topography is normal, on account of inadequate corneal thickness and an inadequate amount of stromal tissue that will remain untouched posterior to the flap after the laser ablation is completed (residual bed thickness). Many surgeons strive to maintain at least 250 μm of untouched posterior stroma, despite the absence of definitive data suggesting that this is the amount necessary to reduce the risk of corneal ectasia.[8]

The diameter of the pupil in the dark is also relevant. The greater the diameter in the dark, the higher the incidence of glare, halos, and other visual disturbances, especially in eyes with high myopia. The measurements performed during the preoperative eye examination are particularly critical in cases in which high myopia or high hyperopia are present, given the increased associated risk of visual complications.

Topographic maps of the cornea should show no signs of diseases in which progressive thinning of the cornea tends to occur over time. Corneal diseases, such as keratoconus, that are likely to cause progressive corneal thinning and change in the shape of the cornea, are likely to be associated with poor results of PRK or LASIK. Recently, wavefront analysis has been used to identify aberrations affecting the quality of vision throughout the eye, from the tear film to the retina.

AREAS OF UNCERTAINTY

PRK VERSUS LASIK

Data from prospective clinical trials directly comparing LASIK with PRK are lacking. Retrospective studies suggest that these procedures have similar results for patients with low-to-moderate myopia (up to 6 diopters)[6,7] but that for patients with higher levels of myopia, the average uncorrected visual acuity was better after LASIK than after PRK.[6] In eyes with low-to-moderate myopia, the advantages of LASIK over PRK are better comfort and vision during the first few days after surgery. However, the added risk from flap complications with LASIK includes loss of two or more lines of best corrected visual acuity on a Snellen chart.

According to retrospective studies with 6 to 12 months of follow-up, PRK and LASIK have similar results for the correction of low hyperopia (less than 2 diopters).[6,7,9] Most surgeons use LASIK rather than PRK for patients with hyperopia, owing to the faster recovery of vision and the lower likelihood of regression.

Astigmatism is a refractive error in which the correcting lens has greater curvature in one meridian (e.g., vertically) than it does in another (e.g., horizontally); it is measured in magnitude (diopters) and in direction (axes). Astigmatism blurs both distance and near vision. By definition, regular astigmatism can be corrected with lenses in which the maximal and minimal axes of the astigmatism are 90 degrees apart. Irregular astigmatism cannot be corrected with glasses and requires rigid contact lenses or surgery for treatment. Most eyes have at

least a small level of regular astigmatism, along with myopia or hyperopia.[6,7] Regular astigmatism up to approximately 6 diopters can be corrected at the same time as myopia or hyperopia with LASIK or PRK.

PRK is the procedure of choice for the correction of myopia or hyperopia in some eyes.[11,12] These include eyes that have thin but otherwise normal corneas; eyes with anterior basement-membrane dystrophy, in which the microkeratome used to make the LASIK flap commonly produces a large epithelial defect resulting in delayed recovery of vision; and moderately dry eyes.

CUSTOM CORNEAL ABLATION PROCEDURES

Custom corneal ablation procedures involve the use of wavefront analysis to measure the aberrations of the eye and to direct the laser ablation of the cornea. These procedures are an alternative to traditional laser ablation techniques.[13-15] However, there are limited data to compare the custom and the traditional approaches. Studies of one widely used laser system seem to show a modest advantage of custom corneal ablation for lower levels of myopia and hyperopia.[13,14] In general, early results suggest that the benefit of custom corneal ablation may increase as the level of attempted correction increases. Further development and assessment of these techniques are needed to clarify their role.

Data are also lacking to compare various laser systems and other equipment with regard to the outcome of LASIK or PRK. Limited data suggest that microkeratomes now are superior to those that were first developed for LASIK, but rigorous comparisons of equipment have not been performed.

GUIDELINES

General policy statements regarding PRK[16] and LASIK[17] have been published by the American Academy of Ophthalmology (AAO). These statements, based on a review of the literature, indicate that PRK and LASIK are effective and predictable for low-to-moderate myopia (up to 6.0 diopters) with regard to obtaining very good or excellent uncorrected visual acuity and that they are safe in terms of minimal loss of visual acuity in the great majority of eyes. However, the statements also note that the results of PRK and LASIK are more variable in eyes with moderate-to-high myopia (more than 6.0 diopters). Eyes treated with LASIK for low-to-moderate degrees of hyperopia (less than 2.0 diopters) tended to have similar results to eyes treated for low-to-moderate myopia.[17] The AAO summary recommendations for LASIK and PRK can be found at www.aao.org/aao/education/library/recommendations/lasik.cfm and www.aao.org/aao/education/library/recommendations/prk.cfm, respectively. The AAO provides no guidelines for LASEK and no guidance on choosing between LASIK and PRK.

CONCLUSIONS AND RECOMMENDATIONS

PRK, LASIK, and LASEK are relatively effective and predictable surgical procedures for the correction of nearsightedness and farsightedness with or without low-to-moderate astigmatism. LASIK is associated with faster recovery of vision and greater comfort in the early postoperative period but with a somewhat higher risk of complications, such as loss of two or more lines of best corrected visual acuity on a Snellen chart. For levels of myopia from 6 diopters to approximately 10 diopters, LASIK seems to be superior to PRK or LASEK in terms of the predictability of the results and the rate of recovery of vision, although there are no prospective trials directly comparing these procedures. Some patients are not candidates for LASIK owing to inadequate corneal thickness, moderately dry eyes, or other factors.

The patient described in the vignette has relatively low myopia and low astigmatism and should be a reasonable candidate for a laser-ablation procedure. If her corneal thicknesses are in the normal range, LASIK is a good choice, although there is disagreement among surgeons about what constitutes normal corneal thickness. If her corneas are thinner than normal, or if she has mild-to-moderate dry eye, a surface-ablation procedure such as PRK or LASEK is a better choice. I would recommend that the patient consult an experienced surgeon to determine whether either LASIK or PRK is a good choice for her.

I am indebted to Ed Sarver at Sarver and Associates for the images of optical imperfections.

REFERENCES

1. Hersh PS, Stulting RD, Steinert RF, et al. Results of phase III excimer laser photorefractive keratectomy for myopia. Ophthalmology 1997;104:1535-53.
2. Pallikaris IG, Siganos DS. Excimer laser in situ keratomileusis and photorefractive keratectomy for correction of high myopia. J Refract Corneal Surg 1994;10:498-510.
3. Peyman GA. Excimer laser in situ keratomileusis under a corneal flap for myopia of 2 to 20 diopters. Am J Ophthalmol 1996;122:284-5.
4. Vinciguerra P, Camesasca FI. Butterfly laser epithelial keratomileusis for myopia. J Refract Surg 2002;18:Suppl 3:S371-S373.
5. Walker MB, Wilson SE. Recovery of uncorrected visual acuity after laser in situ keratomileusis or photorefractive keratectomy for low myopia. Cornea 2001;20:153-5.
6. Van Gelder RN, Steger-May K, Yang SH, Rattanatam T, Pepose JS. Comparison of photorefractive keratectomy, astigmatic PRK, laser in situ keratomileusis, and astigmatic LASIK in the treatment of myopia. J Cataract Refract Surg 2002;28:462-76.
7. El-Agha MS, Bowman RW, Cavanagh D, McCulley JP. Comparison of photorefractive keratectomy and laser in situ keratomileusis for the treatment of compound hyperopic astigmatism. J Cataract Refract Surg 2003; 29:900-7.
8. Ambrósio R Jr, Wilson SE. Complications of laser in situ keratomileusis: etiology, prevention, and treatment. J Refract Surg 2001;17:350-79.
9. Idem. LASIK vs LASEK vs PRK: advantages and indications. Semin Ophthalmol 2003;18:2-10.
10. Stulting RD, Carr JD, Thompson KP, Waring GO III, Wiley WM, Walker JG. Complications of laser in situ keratomileusis for the correction of myopia. Ophthalmology 1999;106:13-20.
11. Vinciguerra P, Azzolini M, Airaghi P, Radice P, De Molfetta V. Effect of decreasing surface and interface irregularities after photorefractive keratectomy and laser in situ keratomileusis on optical and functional outcomes. J Refract Surg 1998;14:Suppl 2:S199-S203.
12. Autrata R, Rehurek J. Laser-assisted subepithelial keratectomy for myopia: two-year follow-up. J Cataract Refract Surg 2003; 29:661-8.
13. Phusitphoykai N, Tungsiripat T, Siriboonkoom J, Vongthongsri A. Comparison of conventional versus wavefront-guided laser in situ keratomileusis in the same patient. J Refract Surg 2003;19:Suppl 2:S217-S220.
14. Porter J, MacRae S, Yoon G, Roberts C, Cox IG, Williams DR. Separate effects of the microkeratome incision and laser ablation on the eye's wave aberration. Am J Ophthalmol 2003;136:327-37.
15. Vongthongsri A, Phusitphoykai N, Naripthapan P. Comparison of wavefront-guided customized ablation vs. conventional ablation in laser in situ keratomileusis. J Refract Surg 2002;18:Suppl 3:S332-S335.
16. Excimer laser photorefractive keratectomy (PRK) for myopia and astigmatism: American Academy of Ophthalmology. Ophthalmology 1999;106:422-37.
17. Sugar A, Rapuano CJ, Culbertson WW, et al. Laser in situ keratomileusis for myopia and astigmatism: safety and efficacy: a report by the American Academy of Ophthalmology. Ophthalmology 2002;109:175-87.

NOTES

NOTES

NOTES

ISBN 1-933087-13-7
ISSN 1542-1910
Twelfth Printing
Printed in the United States of America

The chart on page 3 is from Congdon, N. et al. "Causes and prevalence of visual impairment among adults in the United States." Adapted with permission from the *Archives of Ophthalmology* Vol. 122, No. 122 (April 2004): 477-485.

The chart on page 39 is from the American Academy of Ophthalmology Retina Panel, Preferred Practice Patterns Committee. "Age-related macular degeneration." San Francisco, CA, 2003. Reprinted with permission from the American Academy of Ophthalmology.

Wilson, S.E. "Clinical practice: Use of lasers for vision correction of nearsightedness and farsightedness." Reprinted with permission from *The New England Journal of Medicine* Vol. 29, No. 5 (July 29, 2004): 470-475. Copyright © 2004, Massachusetts Medical Society.

The Johns Hopkins White Papers are published yearly by Medletter Associates, Inc.

Visit our Web site for information on Johns Hopkins Health After 50 publications, which include White Papers on specific disorders, home medical encyclopedias, consumer reference guides to drugs and medical tests, and our monthly newsletter
The Johns Hopkins Medical Letter: Health After 50.
www.HopkinsAfter50.com

The Johns Hopkins White Papers

Paul Candon
Managing Editor

Catherine Richter
Senior Editor

Devon Schuyler
Consulting Editor

Kimberly Flynn
Writer/Researcher

Leslie Maltese-McGill
Copy Editor

Tim Jeffs
Art Director

Vincent Mejia
Graphic Designer

Betsy Meredith Rigo
Editorial Assistant

Robert Duckwall
Medical Illustrator

Kate Brackney
Intern

Johns Hopkins Health After 50 Publications

Rodney Friedman
Editor and Publisher

Thomas Dickey
Editorial Director

Tom Damrauer, M.L.S.
Chief of Information Resources

Jerry Loo
Product Manager

Darren Leiser
Promotions Coordinator

Joan Mullally
Head of Business Development

Index Abbreviations

HEA=Heart Attack Prevention
HYP=Hypertension and Stroke
LUN=Lung Disorders
MEM=Memory
NUT=Nutrition and Weight Control
PRO=Prostate Disorders
VIS=Vision

A

ACE inhibitors, HEA:42, 44, HYT:24–27, 29–33, 35
Acute bronchitis, LUN:51–52
Adrenal tumors, HYT:6
Adrenergic agonists, VIS:27, 28–29
Age-related macular degeneration (AMD), VIS:31–41
Air pollution, LUN:5, 34–37
Alcohol consumption, HEA:34, 35–36, HYT:19, 23, 54,
    MEM:11–12, NUT:40–42, PRO:25
Aldosterone blockers, HYT:35
Alfuzosin, PRO:5, 13
Allergic rhinitis, LUN:6–7
Alpha-blockers, HYT:33–34, PRO:13–15
5-alpha-reductase inhibitors, PRO:12–13
Alprostadil, PRO:60–62
Alteplase, HYT:38, 69
Alzheimer's disease, MEM:3, 13–19, 22, 23, 26, 27,
    29–52
    causes of, MEM:32
    coping with caregiving, MEM:52–55
    degenerative changes in, MEM:30–32
    diagnosis of, MEM:37
    progression of, MEM:40
    risk factors for, MEM:32–37
    treatment of, MEM:40–52
Alzheimer's vaccine, MEM:45–47
Amnestic syndrome (amnesia), MEM:28–29
Angiography
    cerebral, HYT:66–68
Angioplasty, HYT:62–63
Angiotensin II, HYT:2
Angiotensin II receptor blockers, HEA:44, HYT:33
Antiandrogens, PRO:50–53
Anticoagulant drugs, HYT:52–54, 58–59
Antidepressant medications, HYT:60, 61, NUT:72
Antihypertensive medications, HYT:19–31, 33
Anti-inflammatory drugs, LUN:16–17, MEM:47–48
Antioxidants, HEA:30, MEM:9, NUT:31–36
Antiplatelet drugs, HYT:52–54, 57–58
Aphasia, HYT:47
Apolipoprotein B (apo B), HEA:19
Apolipoprotein E (APOE), MEM:33–34, 37
Aspirin, HEA:44–47, HYT:51–53, 57, 58, LUN:13
Asthma, LUN:1, 3, 11–20, 39
Astigmatism, VIS:2–4
Atherosclerosis, HEA:3, 5, 6, 8, 9, 17, 18, 24, 26, 27, 30,
    37, HYT:12
Atrial fibrillation, HYT:41, LUN:31

B

Bariatric surgery, NUT:73–75
Behavioral modification, NUT:56–58
Benign prostatic hyperplasia (BPH), PRO:1, 2–23
    causes of, PRO:2–4
    diagnosis of, PRO:5–8
    symptoms of, PRO:4–5
    treatment of, PRO:7–23
    medication, PRO:12–16
    minimally invasive therapy, PRO:19–23
    need for, PRO:9
    phytotherapy, PRO:10–12
    stents, PRO:23
    surgery, PRO:16–19
    watchful waiting, PRO:10
Beta$_2$ agonists, LUN:16–18, 24, 67
Beta-blockers, HEA:42, HYT:27–30, 32, VIS:26, 28–29
Beverages, NUT:62, 63
Bile acid sequestrants, HEA:40
Blood clot formation (coronary thrombosis), HEA:6–7
Blood-clotting factors (fibrinogen, factor VII, platelets,
    PAI-1, and PLA-2), HEA:9, 12
Blood gases, LUN:9
Blood pressure, HYT:1–4, MEM:8–9. See also
    Hypertension
    ambulatory monitoring of, HYT:17–18
    classification of, HYT:9–12
    drop during stroke, HYT:63
    evaluating and managing, HYT:9
    home monitoring of, HYT:14, 15–17
    medical evaluation of, HYT:18–19
    systolic vs. diastolic, HYT:10–11
Body mass index (BMI), NUT:53, 54
Brachytherapy, PRO:43, 45–46
Brain, blood supply to, HYT:39
Brain stem, HYT:44
Bronchitis, LUN:3
    acute, LUN:51–52
Bronchodilators, LUN:15–16, 18–20, 24
B vitamins, HYT:49, MEM:14–15, NUT:19–23

C

Calcium, NUT:23, 24, 26–29, 32, 33, 60
Calcium channel blockers, HEA:44, HYT:26–29, 32
Calcium supplements, NUT:28, 29
Calories, NUT:2
Cancer, NUT:10–11, 33–35
    colorectal, NUT:27
    prostate. See Prostate cancer
Carbohydrates, NUT:2, 5
Carbonic anhydrase inhibitors, VIS:27, 28–29
Cardiovascular disease, MEM:35–36, NUT:22
Carotid angioplasty, HYT:62–63
Carotid endarterectomy, HYT:57, 59–62, 65
Carotid stenosis, HYT:51, 54
Castration, surgical, PRO:49
Cataracts, VIS:4–18
    causes of, VIS:5–8
    prevention of, VIS:9
    symptoms of, VIS:8–9
    treatment of, VIS:10–18
    types of, VIS:4–5
Central alpha agonists, HYT:34
Cerebellum, HYT:44, 46
Cerebral angiography, HYT:66–68
Cerebral embolism, HYT:40–42
Cerebral thrombosis, HYT:40
Cerebrovascular disease, HEA:9
Cerebrum, HYT:46
Chemotherapy, LUN:46
Chest imaging, LUN:8
Chest pain, LUN:4
Cholesterol, HEA:5, 14, 26–48, HYT:55–56, NUT:2–3, 5,
    7–8, 10–13, 15, 21, 28, 29, 32, 33, 37, 39–41, 46,
    52, 53, 56, 59, 63, 68, 69, 73

Cholesterol absorption inhibitors, HEA:41
Chronic bronchitis, LUN:20, 22
Chronic kidney disease, HEA:12
Chronic obstructive pulmonary disease (COPD), LUN:1,
    9, 11, 20–28, 55
Cigarette smoking, HEA:12–13, 25, HYT:51, LUN:20, 22,
    39, 40, 43, MEM:11, 12–13, VIS:5–6. See also
    Smoking cessation
Clioquinol, MEM:48
Clopidogrel, HYT:51–53, 57, 58
Coarctation of the aorta, HYT:6
Cognishunt, MEM:44–45
Cognitive rehabilitation therapy, MEM:49
Colorectal cancer, NUT:27
Computed tomography (CT), HYT:65
Contact lenses, VIS:17
Coronary arteries, changes in, HEA:3
Coronary artery spasm, HEA:7–8
Coronary calcium scans, HEA:24–27
Coronary heart disease (CHD), HEA:1–31, 33, 35, 37,
    44–47, HYT:54, NUT:7, 31–33, 39
    screening tests for, HEA:20–25
Coronary thrombosis (blood clot formation), HEA:6–7
Corticosteroids, LUN:16–17, 24, 25, VIS:6, 45
Coughing, LUN:2
C-reactive protein, HEA:6, 18, 20, 21, HYT:56
Creutzfeldt-Jakob disease (CJD), MEM:28
Cryotherapy, PRO:46
CX516 (Ampalex), MEM:44
Cyclodestructive surgery, VIS:30–31
Cystoscopy, PRO:8

D

DASH diet, HYT:22
Delirium, MEM:24–25
Dementia, HYT:66, MEM:18–22, 38
    diagnosis of, MEM:19, 22
    memory and irreversible, MEM:26–52
    memory and reversible, MEM:22
    preventing, MEM:6–16
    tracking, via behavior, MEM:39
Depression, HEA:13, HYT:60–61, LUN:25, 30, MEM:23,
    24–25, 36, 37, 53
Detached retina, VIS:11
Diabetes, HEA:8–9, HYT:25–26, 33, 51, MEM:14,
    NUT:69, VIS:8, 44
Diabetic retinopathy, VIS:41–47
Diet(s), HEA:28, HYT:43, LUN:45, NUT:50–51, 58–66,
    PRO:25–26. See also Nutrition
    fad, NUT:63–66
    very-low-calorie and low-calorie, NUT:68–69
Dietary guidelines, NUT:9
Dietary supplements, NUT:72–73
Digital rectal examination (DRE), PRO:27, 29
Dipyridamole, HYT:58
Direct vasodilators, HYT:34
Diuretics, HEA:42, HYT:24–29
Down syndrome, MEM:36
Driving, MEM:46–47
Drug abuse, HYT:55
Dry eye, VIS:46

E

Echocardiography, HEA:24
Ejaculation, PRO:16, 17, 29, 57, 63
Electrocardiogram (ECG or EKG), HEA:21

Emphysema, LUN:3, 20–22, 25
Enhanced foods, NUT:42–43
EPCA, PRO:33
Erectile dysfunction, PRO:45–48, 50–52, 55, 56, 58–61
Estrogen(s), MEM:48, PRO:49–52
Exercise (physical activity), HEA:32–33, 46, HYT:23, 68, MEM:10–11, NUT:38–39, 51, 55, 58, 66–68
Exercise stress test, HEA:21–22
Exercise testing, LUN:9
Expressive aphasia, HYT:47
External beam radiation therapy, PRO:44–45
Extracapsular surgery, VIS:13–14
Eye, anatomy of the, VIS:1–2
Eye disorders, VIS:1–47
    age-related macular degeneration (AMD), VIS:5, 31–41
    cataracts, VIS:4–18
    diabetic retinopathy, VIS:41–47
    glaucoma, VIS:19–31
    medications that may cause vision problems, VIS:25
    refractive errors, VIS:2–4
Eyedrops, VIS:26–27
Eye injuries, VIS:6
Eyes, HYT:14
Ezetimibe, HEA:38, 39, 41

F

Factor VII, HEA:9
Farsightedness (hyperopia), VIS:2, 3, 10, 17
Fat, body, NUT:56
Fats, dietary, HEA:26–29, MEM:12, NUT:2–14, 59–62
    cancer and, NUT:10–11
    coronary heart disease and, NUT:7
    recommendations for intake of, NUT:11–14
    weight and, NUT:9–10
Fat substitutes, NUT:60, 62
Fatty acids, NUT:5–6
Fiber, dietary, HEA:29, 43, NUT:3, 14–18
Fibrates, HEA:41
Fibrinogen, HEA:9
Filling cystometry, PRO:8
Filtration surgery, VIS:30
Finasteride, PRO:11–13, 15, 16, 28, 54, 55
Fish, NUT:12–14
Flavonoids, NUT:37
Folic acid (folate), NUT:19, 21–23, 32, 33
Food labels, NUT:4–5, 60
Food safety, NUT:45–46
Frontal lobe, HYT:46–47
Frontotemporal dementia, MEM:27
Fruits, NUT:57, VIS:36

G

Gastric bypass, NUT:76–77
Genetically modified food, NUT:43–45
Genetics, HYT:5, MEM:32–33, 35
Ginkgo biloba, MEM:16, 48–49
Glasses, cataract, VIS:16–17
Glaucoma, VIS:19–31
    causes of, VIS:19–20, 22
    diagnosis of, VIS:22–24
    prevention of, VIS:22
    symptoms of, VIS:22
    treatment of, VIS:24–31
Gonadotropin-releasing hormone antagonist, PRO:52, 53

H

Heart attacks, HEA:1–48
    causes of, HEA:5–8
    lifestyle measures to prevent, HEA:25–36
    medications to prevent, HEA:36–48
    prevention of, HEA:1–2
    recognizing, HEA:7
    risk factors for, HEA:8–19
Heart failure, LUN:31
Hematuria, PRO:11
Hemorrhagic stroke, HYT:42–44
Herbal preparations, NUT:72–73
Heredity (genetics), NUT:48–49
High blood pressure. See Hypertension
High-density lipoprotein (HDL) cholesterol, HEA:5, 6, 8–11, 14–17, 19, 20, 28–35, 37, 39–48, MEM:8, NUT:7–8, 10, 12, 15, 21, 32, 39, 41, 46, 52, 56, 63, 68, 73
Homocysteine, HEA:18, HYT:49, NUT:22, 29
Hormonal (endocrine) abnormalities, NUT:51–52
Hormone replacement therapy (HRT), HEA:45, 47–48, HYT:47, 54–55, MEM:16, PRO:46–56
Huntington's disease, MEM:27–28
Hypertension (high blood pressure), HEA:13, 30, 32, 41, HYT:1–38, LUN:31, NUT:26–29
    causes of, HYT:4–8
    complications of, HYT:12–14
    definition of, HYT:10
    diagnosis of, HYT:14–19
    prevalence of, HYT:1
    prevention of, HYT:14
    secondary, HYT:5
    stroke and, HYT:39, 40, 48, 50–51
    symptoms and signs of, HYT:8–9
    treatment of, HYT:19–38
        lifestyle modifications, HYT:20–23
        medical follow-up, HYT:36, 38
        medication, HYT:23–36
        white coat, HYT:11, 13
Hypertensive crisis, HYT:8
Hypertensive emergency, HYT:8
Hypertensive urgency, HYT:8–9

I

IMRT (intensity-modulated radiation therapy), PRO:42
Infections, LUN:1, 51–62
Influenza, LUN:52–55
Inhalers, LUN:10–11
Intermittent androgen suppression, PRO:53–54
Interstitial laser coagulation (ILC), PRO:22–23
Interstitial lung disease, LUN:1, 32–33, 38–39
Intracapsular surgery, VIS:13
Intracerebral hemorrhage, HYT:43
Intraocular lens implants, VIS:14, 16
Iron, NUT:33
Ischemic stroke, HYT:40, 51, 54, 56, 57, 63, 65–66, 68–69

J

J-curve, HYT:36

K

Kegel exercises, PRO:57
Kidneys (kidney damage or disorders), HYT:5–6, 13, 26
    chronic, HEA:12

L

Lacunar strokes, HYT:42
Laparoscopic adjustable gastric banding, NUT:76
Laser photocoagulation, VIS:45–47
Laser trabecular surgery, VIS:28
LASIK eye surgery, VIS:23
Lens replacement, VIS:14, 16
Lewy bodies, dementia with, MEM:27, 29
Light therapy, MEM:51
Limbic system, HYT:46
Lipase inhibitor, NUT:72
Lipid-lowering drugs, HEA:36–39
Lipid profile, HEA:20
Lipoprotein(a) (Lp[a]), HEA:16, MEM:34
Liposuction, NUT:76, 77
Low-density lipoprotein (LDL) cholesterol, HEA:5, 6, 8, 10, 12, 14–17, 19, 20, 27–31, 36, 37, 39–41, 43, 46–48; MEM:8, NUT:7–8, 13, 15, 21, 28, 32, 37, 39, 40, 46
Low vision, VIS:3, 41
Low-vision aids, VIS:40–41
Lung cancer, LUN:1, 39–47
Lung disorders, LUN:1–62
    general approaches to management of, LUN:10–11
    general evaluation of respiratory symptoms, LUN:4–10
    obstructive diseases, LUN:11–28
    symptoms of, LUN:1–4
Lung transplantation, LUN:25–28
Luteinizing hormone-releasing hormone (LH-RH) analogs, PRO:50–55

M

Macular degeneration, age-related, VIS:5, 31–41
Magnetic resonance angiography (MRA), HYT:68
Magnetic resonance imaging (MRI), HYT:65–66
Mediterranean diet, NUT:7
Memory, HYT:47–48, MEM:1–55
    age-associated impairment of, MEM:2–5
    biology of, MEM:1–2
    irreversible dementia and, MEM:26–52
    methods to assist, MEM:5–6
    mild cognitive impairment, MEM:16–18
    reversible dementia and, MEM:22–26
Mental function, medications that may impair, MEM:20–21
Metabolic syndrome, HEA:17–18, 33, HYT:5
Metabolism, NUT:47, 49–50
Mild cognitive impairment, MEM:16–18
Minerals, NUT:3, 18–19, 24, 26–30
Miotics, VIS:27, 28–29
Monoclonal antibody, LUN:17
Monounsaturated fatty acids, HEA:28, NUT:6
Multifocal lenses, VIS:17
Multivitamins, NUT:19, 23

N

Nearsightedness (myopia), VIS:2, 4, 10, 11, 18
Niacin, HEA:40, MEM:15
Niacin (vitamin B$_3$), NUT:21
Nicotine replacement therapy, LUN:43
NMDA receptor antagonist, MEM:42
Noisy breathing, LUN:2, 4
Noradrenergics, NUT:72
NSAIDs, MEM:15–16
Nuclear medicine stress test (nuclear imaging), HEA:23, 24